Cardiovascular/Pulmonary Essentials

Applying the Preferred Physical Therapist Practice Patterns℠

Cardiovascular/Pulmonary Essentials

Applying the Preferred Physical Therapist Practice Patterns℠

Editor
Marilyn Moffat, PT, DPT, PhD, FAPTA, CSCS
Professor, Physical Therapy Department
New York University
New York, New York

Associate Editor
Donna Frownfelter, PT, DPT, MA, CCS, FCCP, RRT
Assistant Professor, Physical Therapy
Program Director, Post-Professional DPT
Rosalind Franklin University of Medicine and Science
College of Health Professions
North Chicago, Illinois

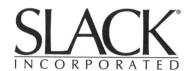

Delivering the best in health care information and education worldwide

www.slackbooks.com

ISBN: 978-1-55642-668-1

Some material contained in this book is reprinted with permission from the American Physical Therapy Association. *Guide to Physical Therapist Practice*. 2nd ed. Alexandria, Va: APTA; 2001 and appears courtesy of the APTA. For more information, please contact the APTA directly at www.apta.org.

Published by: SLACK Incorporated
                 6900 Grove Road
                 Thorofare, NJ 08086 USA
                 Telephone: 856-848-1000
                 Fax: 856-853-5991
                 www.slackbooks.com

Contact SLACK Incorporated for more information about other books in this field or about the availability of our books from distributors outside the United States.

Library of Congress Cataloging-in-Publication Data

Cardiovascular/Pulmonary Essentials : Applying the Preferred Physical Therapist Practice Patterns / editor, Marilyn Moffat ; associate editor, Donna Frownfelter.
        p. ; cm.
    Includes bibliographical references and index.
    ISBN 978-1-55642-668-1 (softcover : alk. paper)
    1. Cardiopulmonary system--Diseases--Physical therapy. I. Moffat, Marilyn. II. Frownfelter, Donna L.
    [DNLM: 1. Respiratory Tract Diseases--therapy. 2. Cardiovascular Diseases--therapy. 3. Physical Therapy Modalities. WF 145 C2667 2007]
RC702.C363 2007
616.1'062--dc22

                                    2007006677

Last digit is print number: 10 9 8 7 6 5 4 3 2 1

Dedication

Undertaking a task of this magnitude is never possible without the utmost support of many individuals to whom I am deeply indebted. Thus this book is dedicated to: all of my Moffat and Salant families; physical therapy collegues; APTA staff; faculty, support staff, and students at New York University; and all of my patients and clients who made this endevour possible.

—*MM*

To our students past, present, and future.

—*DF*

Contents

Dedication .... *v*

Acknowledgments .... *ix*

About the Editors .... *xi*

Contributing Authors .... *xiii*

Preface .... *xv*

Foreword to the Essentials in Physical Therapy *Series by Darcy Umphred, PT, PhD, FAPTA* .... *xvii*

Foreword to Cardiovascular/Pulmonary Essentials *by Cynthia Coffin-Zadai, PT, DPT, CCS, FAPTA* .... *xix*

Introduction .... *xxi*

Chapter One 1
Primary Prevention/Risk Reduction for Cardiovascular/Pulmonary Disorders (Pattern A)
Donna Frownfelter, PT, DPT, MA, CCS, FCCP, RRT
Elizabeth Dean, PT, PhD
Jane L. Wetzel, PT, PhD

Chapter Two 37
Impaired Aerobic Capacity/Endurance Associated With Deconditioning (Pattern B)
Elizabeth Dean, PT, PhD

Chapter Three 83
Impaired Ventilation, Respiration/Gas Exchange and Aerobic Capacity/Endurance
Associated With Airway Clearance Dysfunction (Pattern C)
Dawn M. Stackowicz, PT, MS, CCS
Marilyn Moffat, PT, DPT, PhD, FAPTA, CSCS
Donna Frownfelter, PT, DPT, MA, CCS, FCCP, RRT
Susan M. Butler McNamara, PT, MMSc, CCS

Chapter Four 115
Impaired Aerobic Capacity/Endurance Associated With Cardiovascular Pump Dysfunction
or Failure (Pattern D)
Jane L. Wetzel, PT, PhD

Chapter Five 165
Impaired Ventilation and Respiration/Gas Exchange Associated With Ventilatory Pump Dysfunction
or Failure (Pattern E)
Alexandra Sciaky, PT, MS, CCS

Chapter Six 193
Impaired Ventilation and Respiration/Gas Exchange Associated With Respiratory Failure (Pattern F)
Steven Sadowsky, PT, RRT, MS, CCS
Donna Frownfelter, PT, DPT, MA, CCS, FCCP, RRT
Marilyn Moffat, PT, DPT, PhD, FAPTA, CSCS

Chapter Seven 237
Impaired Ventilation, Respiration/Gas Exchange, and Aerobic Capacity/Endurance Associated
With Respiratory Failure in the Neonate (Pattern G)
Mary Rahlin, PT, MS, PCS

Chapter Eight 267
Impaired Circulation and Anthropometric Dimensions Associated With Lymphatic System
Disorders (Pattern H)
Antoinette P. Sander, PT, DPT, MS, CLT-LANA

Abbreviations 285
Brand Name Drugs and Products 289
Index 291

Acknowledgments

This edited book is one of a series of four books that would not have been possible without the dedication, incredibly hard work, and generosity of so many individuals. I am eternally indebted to each of the following outstanding physical therapists for their willingness to share their expertise, their enthusiasm, and their unbelievable patience in seeing this work come to fruition:

- Associate Editor:
  - Donna Frownfelter, PT, DPT, MA, CCS, FCCP, RRT
- Contributing Authors:
  - Elizabeth Dean, PT, PhD
  - Susan Butler McNamara, PT, MS, CCS
  - Mary Rahlin, PT, MS, PCS
  - Steven Sadowsky, PT, RRT, MS, CCS
  - Antoinette P. Sander, PT, DPT, MS, CLT-LANA
  - Alexandra Sciaky, PT, MS, CCS
  - Dawn M. Stackowitz, PT, MS, CCS
  - Jane L. Wetzel, PT, PhD

The putting together of a book requires the astute skills of both editorial and publishing staff. Working with colleagues and associates at SLACK Incorporated has indeed been a pleasure, and I am indebted to them for their perceptive reviews and their continued encouragement provided along the way. To the following individuals I owe my thanks:

- Carrie Kotlar, who first approached me with the idea of doing this book and stood by throughout the process with unwavering support
- John Bond, who jumped in whenever we needed support from the top
- Jennifer Cahill and Kimberly Shigo, who had the editorial task of making our manuscript into a published book

And last, but not least, are so many who have influenced my life, have challenged me to strive to do the best that I am able, and have supported and encouraged me along the way. My heartfelt thanks are extended to:

- My mother, for her unconditional support
- My father and my husband who were always there for me, were both the epitomy of role models, and were both taken from me too early in life
- My sister and brother-in-law, my stepdaughter, and my grandchildren for always reminding me of what is important in life
- All of my physical therapy colleagues, who have been such an integral part of my life

—MM

I am grateful for Marilyn Moffat's efforts in the development of the *Guide to Physical Therapist Practice* and also for the identification of the need for a book series to demonstrate it's use. Her vision lead to the development of the *Essential Series* and what grew to be a project that went well beyond anything I could have imagined. No matter how hard I felt I worked it seemed Marilyn did a bit more; no sooner would a manuscript be sent than it was being processed again. It made me really understand how the sum of a group working together is always going to be more than the sum of its parts. It was definitely a group dynamic process.

There are so many people to thank, first and foremost the chapter authors who did an incredible job with many revisions and updates as we went through the process. A very special thanks if given to the editors of the *Musculoskeletal Series,* Elaine Rosen and Sandy Rusnak-Smith. Their support with editing and helping to keep the Practice Pattern consistency was so very beneficial. They went above and beyond the call of duty and it was appreciated!

Many thanks go to my family, the faculty of Rosalind Franklin University, the PT Department, and the many friends who supported and encouraged me during this process. Trying to balance teaching, family, and social life is always a challenge during the writing of a book.

My students have been helpful as they reflected on the use of the *Guide to Physical Therapist Practice.* All of our courses at Rosalind Franklin University are team taught and based on case studies and evidence based practice. This rigor has been helpful in identifying students' needs and faculty utilization of the *Guide* in all courses.

The editors and staff at SLACK have been a pleasure to work with and have personified professional support and conduct. All involved have been grateful for their encouragement, deadlines, and facilitation of the completion of this book.

—DF

About the Editors

Marilyn Moffat, PT, DPT, PhD, FAPTA, CSCS, a recognized leader in the United States and internationally, is a practitioner, a teacher, a consultant, a leader, and an author. She received her baccalaureate degree from Queens College and her physical therapy certificate and PhD degrees from New York University. She is a Full Professor of Physical Therapy at New York University, where she directs both the professional doctoral program (DPT) and the post-professional graduate master's degree program in pathokinesiology. She has been in private practice for more than 40 years and currently practices in the New York area.

Dr. Moffat was one of the first individuals to speak and write about the need for a doctoral entry-level degree in physical therapy. Her first presentation on this topic was given to the Section for Education in 1977.

Dr. Moffat completed a 6-year term as the President of the American Physical Therapy Association (APTA) in 1997. Prior to that, she had served on the APTA Board of Directors for 6 years and also as President of the New York Physical Therapy Association for 4 years. During her term as President of the APTA, she played a major role in the development of the Association's *Guide to Physical Therapist Practice* and was project editor of the Second Edition of the *Guide*. Among her many publications is the *American Physical Therapy Association's Book of Body Maintenance and Repair*. As part of her commitment to research, Dr. Moffat is currently a member of the Board of Trustees of the Foundation for Physical Therapy, was a previous member of the Financial Advisory Committee, and has done major fundraising for them over the years.

She is currently on the Executive Committee of the World Confederation for Physical Therapy (WCPT) as the North American/Caribbean Regional Representative, and she was a member of the WCPT Task Force to develop an international definition of physical therapy. She coordinated the efforts to develop international guidelines for physical therapist educational programs around the world. She has given more than 800 professional presentations throughout her practice lifetime, and she has taught and provided consultation services in Taiwan, Thailand, Burma, Vietnam, Panama City, Hong Kong, and Puerto Rico.

Her diversified background is exemplified by the vast number of APTA and New York Physical Therapy Association committees and task forces on which she has served or chaired. She has served as Editor of *Physical Therapy*, the official publication of the Association. She was also instrumental in the early development of the TriAlliance of Rehabilitation Professionals, composed of the APTA, the American Occupational Therapy Association, and the American Speech-Language-Hearing Association. She has been an Associate of the Council of Public Representatives of the National Institutes of Health.

Dr. Moffat is a Catherine Worthingham Fellow of the APTA. She has been the recipient of the APTA's Marilyn Moffat Leadership Award; the WCPT's Mildred Elson Award for International Leadership; the APTA's Lucy Blair Service Award; the Robert G. Dicus Private Practice Section APTA Award for contributions to private practice; Outstanding Service Awards from the New York Physical Therapy Association and from the APTA; the Ambassador Award from the National Strength and Conditioning Association; the Howard A. Rusk Humanitarian Award from the World Rehabilitation Fund; the United Cerebral Palsy Citation for Service; the Sawadi Skulkai Lecture Award from Mahidol University in Bangkok, Thailand; New York University's Founders Day Award; the University of Florida's Barbara C. White Lecture Award; the Massachusetts General's Ionta Lecture Award; the Chartered Society of Physiotherapists' Alan Walker Memorial Lecture Award; the APTA Minority Affairs Diversity 2000 Award; and the Section of Health Policy's R. Charles Harker Policy Maker Award. In addition, the New York Physical Therapy Association also named its leadership award after her. She was the APTA's 2004 Mary McMillan Lecturer, the Association's highest award. Dr. Moffat has been listed in *Who's Who in the East*, *Who's Who in American Women*, *Who's Who in America*, *Who's Who in Education*, *Who's Who in the World*, and *Who's Who in Medicine and Healthcare*.

She is also currently on the Board of Directors of the World Rehabilitation Fund and is a member of the Executive Committee. In addition to her professional associations, she was elected to be a member of Kappa Delta Pi and Pi Lambda Theta.

Donna Frownfelter, PT, DPT, MA, CCS, RRT, FCCP is an internationally known consultant, teacher, clinician, and author. She is coauthor and coeditor of the widely used text, *Cardiovascular and Pulmonary Physical Therapy: Evidence and Practice.* Dr. Frownfelter's varied experiences have included practice in neonate, medical, surgical, and neurological intensive care units, skilled nursing facilities, home care, and pulmonary and cardiac rehabilitation outpatient departments.

Dr. Frownfelter has taught Cardiovascular and Pulmonary Physical Therapy at Northwestern University in the Department of Physical Therapy and Human Movement Science for 30 years. She was honored to receive their first Distinguished Alumni Award for her contributions to Physical Therapy in 2003. She has been elected to serve as Vice President of the NUPT Alumni Association. Currently she is Assistant Professor of Physical Therapy at Rosalind Franklin University of Medicine and Science, where she has received several teaching awards from her students.

She is a frequent speaker in continuing education conferences and has given numerous invited presentations at local, national, and international conferences. Her current clinical research is involved with evaluating the effects of thoracolumbar/sacral othoses on pulmonary function, perceived exertion, and exercise.

She is a past president of the Cardiovascular and Pulmonary Section of the American Physical Therapy Association and also served as their Program Chair and Education Committee Chair. She has been a liaison from the American Physical Therapy Association to the American College of Chest Physicians and the National Emphysema/COPD Association. Dr. Frownfelter initiated the COPD Roundtable at the APTA Annual Conferences. These roundtables bring together persons with COPD and local physical therapists to discuss issues concerning their wants and needs and how physical therapists may facilitate self management of their chronic diseases for optimal function and quality of life.

In 2005 Dr. Frownfelter was elected a Fellow of the American College of Chest Physicians (FCCP) the only physical therapist to receive this honor.

She has been an advocate in the school system for children with asthma and for classroom integration of children who are on ventilatory assist. She is an active member of the Board of Directors of the American Lung Association of Metropolitan Chicago. In this capacity she serves on the COPD Advisory Committee that advocates for and supports people with COPD through educational programs, materials, and social opportunities.

Contributing Authors

Elizabeth Dean, PT, PhD
Professor
School of Rehabilitation Sciences
University of British Columbia
Vancouver, Canada

Donna Frownfelter, DPT, MA, CCS, FCCP, RRT
Assistant Professor, Physical Therapy
Rosalind Franklin University of Medicine and Science
College of Health Professions
North Chicago, Illinois

Susan M. Butler McNamara, PT, MMSc, CCS
Division of Rehabilitation Medicine
Maine Medical Center
Portland, Maine

Marilyn Moffat, PT, DPT, PhD, FAPTA, CSCS
Professor, Physical Therapy Department
New York University
New York, New York

Mary Rahlin, PT, MS, PCS
Rosalind Franklin University of Medicine and Science
North Chicago, Illinois

Steven Sadowsky, PT, RRT, MS, CCS
Assistant Professor and Associate Chair for
Professional Education
Department of Physical Therapy and Human
Movement Sciences
Northwestern University, Feinberg School of
Medicine
Chicago, Illinois

Antoinette P. Sander, PT, DPT, MS, CLT-LANA
Assistant Professor
Department of Physical Therapy and Human
Movement Sciences
Chicago, Illinois

Alexandra Sciaky, PT, MS, CCS
Senior Physical Therapist and Coordinator of Clinical
Education
Ann Arbor Veterans Affairs Healthcare System
Physical Therapy Department
Ann Arbor, Michigan

Dawn M. Stackowitz, PT, MS, CCS
Physical Therapy Supervisor
John H. Stroger, Jr. Hospital of Cook County
Chicago, Illinois

Jane L. Wetzel, PT, PhD
Assistant Professor
Department of Physical Therapy
Duquesne University
Pittsburgh, Pennsylvania

Preface

*Cardiovascular/Pulmonary Essentials: Applying the Preferred Physical Therapist Practice Patterns*SM is part of a series of four books (*Musculosketelal Essentials, Neuromuscular Essentials, Cardiovascular/Pulmonary Essentials,* and *Integumentary Essentials*) aimed at promoting an understanding of physical therapist practice and challenging the clinical thinking and decision making of our practitioners. In this book, 10 distinguished contributors have written chapters to take the *Guide to Physical Therapist Practice* to the next level of practice. Each chapter provides the relevant information for the pattern described by the *Guide* and emphasizes the process through which a physical therapist goes to take the patient from the examination to discharge. The Introduction to this book describes what each chapter contains.

It has been a goal of this entire series, and certainly is a strong hope of each of us involved in editing this series, that these *Essentials* will provide students and practitioners with a valuable reference for physical therapist practice.

As a way of introduction to the *Guide to Physical Therapist Practice,* the information below provides a brief overview of its development. Since I was involved in each step of the entire process, I know the unbelievable amount of work done by so many to see that landmark work reach fruition.

DEVELOPMENT OF THE *GUIDE*

The *Guide to Physical Therapist Practice* was developed based on the needs of membership by the American Physical Therapy Association (APTA) under my leadership as President of the Association. As an integral part of all of the groups responsible for writing the *Guide* and as one of three Project Editors for the latest edition of the *Guide,* I was delighted when SLACK Incorporated approached me to take the *Guide* to the next step for students and clinicians.

HISTORY

In the way of history, the development of the *Guide* began in 1992 with a Board of Directors-appointed task force upon which I served and which culminated in the publication of *A Guide to Physical Therapist Practice, Volume I: A Description of Patient Management* in the August 1995 issue of *Physical Therapy.* The APTA House of Delegates approved the development of Volume II, which was designed to describe the preferred patterns of practice for patient/client groupings commonly referred for physical therapy.

In 1997, Volume I and Volume II became Part One and Part Two of the *Guide,* and the first edition of the *Guide* was published in the November 1997 issue of *Physical Therapy.* In 1998, APTA initiated Parts Three and Four of the *Guide* to catalog the specific tests and measures used by physical therapists in the four system areas and the areas of outcomes, health-related quality of life, and patient/client satisfaction. Additional inclusions in the *Guide* were standardized documentation forms and templates that incorporated the patient/client management process and a patient/client satisfaction instrument.

A CD-ROM version of the *Guide* was developed that included not only Part One and Part Two, but also the varied tests and measures used in practice along with their reliability and validity.

FIVE ELEMENTS OF PATIENT/CLIENT MANAGEMENT

The patient/client management model includes the five essential elements of examination, evaluation, diagnosis, prognosis, and intervention that result in optimal outcomes. The patient/client management process is dynamic and allows the physical therapist to progress the patient/client in the process, return to an earlier element for further analysis, or exit the patient/client from the process when the needs of the patient/client cannot be addressed by the physical therapist. The patient/client management process incorporates the disablement model (pathology/pathophysiology, impairments, functional limitations) throughout the five elements and outcomes, but also includes all aspects of risk reduction/prevention; health, wellness, and fitness; societal resources; and patient/client satisfaction. This is the physical therapist's clinical decision-making model.

APPLICATION OF THE *GUIDE* TO CLINICAL PRACTICE

The *Guide* has its practice patterns grouped according to each of the four systems—musculoskeletal, neuromuscular, cardiovascular/pulmonary, and integumentary. Thus, this *Essentials* series continues where the *Guide* leaves off and brings the *Guide* to meaningful, clinically based examples of each of the patterns. In each chapter in each system area, an overview of the pertinent anatomy, physiology, pathophysiology, imaging, and pharmacology is presented; then three to five cases are presented for each pattern. Each case initially details the physical therapist examination, including the history, systems review, and tests and measures selected for that case. Then the evaluation, diagnosis, and prognosis and plan of care for the case are presented. Prior to the specific interventions for the case is the rationale for the interventions based on the available literature, thus ensuring that, when possible, the interventions are evidence-based. The anticipated goals and expected outcomes for the interventions are put forth as possible in functional and measurable terms. Finally, any special considerations for reexamination, discharge, and psychological aspects are delineated.

Foreword
to the *Essentials in*
Physical Therapy Series

There are many leaders, many educators, and some visionaries, but only a very special few individuals have all three characteristics. The Editor of this series of books, Dr. Marilyn Moffat, certainly has demonstrated these traits and is again helping to guide the profession of physical therapy, as well as all therapists, to a new level of cognitive analysis when implementing and effectively using the *Guide to Physical Therapist Practice*.

Dr. Moffat's dream was for the American Physical Therapy Association to develop the original *Guide*. She nurtured its birth, as well as its development. In 2001, the second edition and evolution of additional practice patterns was introduced to the profession. Although the *Guide* lays the foundation for the entire diagnostic process used by a physical therapist as a movement specialist, many colleagues have difficulty bridging the gap between this model for the entire patient management process and its application to an individual consumer of physical therapy services. Through Dr. Moffat's vision, she recognized this gap and has again tried to link the highest standard of professional process to the patient/client and his or her specific needs.

When you take the leadership of the Editor and combine that with the expertise and clinical mastery of the various chapter authors, the quality of these texts already sets the highest standard of literary reference for an experienced, novel, or student physical therapist.

There are few individuals who could or would take on this dedicated process that will widen the therapist's comprehension of a very difficult and complex process. Dr. Moffat has again contributed, in her typical scholarly fashion, to the world of physical therapy literature and to each practitioner's role as a service provider of health care around the world.

—Darcy Umphred, PT, PhD, FAPTA
University of the Pacific
Stockton, California

Foreword to *Cardiovascular/ Pulmonary Essentials*

The 1995 publication of *The Guide to Physical Therapist Practice* (*The Guide*) provided the internal and external physical therapy (PT) community with a readily accessible document describing the common structure and language for the professional practice of physical therapy. The process for *The Guide*'s development assured that collaborative and representative participation of multiple PT practitioners including: board certified specialists; generalist practitioners from broad and diverse practice settings and geographic regions; and practitioners who managed patients across the lifespan. These individuals collectively created and reviewed all aspects of the document throughout its development. The face validity inherent in such a process could lead to the expectation that *The Guide*'s utility would be readily apparent to each and every PT practitioner.

That unrealistic expectation was not realized for many practical reasons. The simple standardization of language to be consistent with current librarian approved terms allowing *The Guide* to be electronically searched provides an explanation for the obvious change in our description of practice that would make the familiar less recognizable. Similarly, standardization of the practice model and adoption of the World Health Organization approved structures for disablement and enablement provided additional alterations to commonly known and accepted practice. The essential and strategic contemporary updating of PT structure and language within *The Guide* created a disconnect between some practitioners and our current literature.

Dr. Marilyn Moffat and Dr. Donna Frownfelter, along with their colleagues have created a bridge to cross over that gap with the publication of the *Cardiovascular/Pulmonary Essentials*. This text provides a practical case-based approach to managing patients with cardiovascular and pulmonary dysfunction. The brief review of anatomic and physiologic principles in each chapter grounds the reader with the recognizable scientific principles and referenced normative values underlying practice. The standardized Case Format literally brings *The Guide* to life using practical and evidence-based patient examples that all PT's can easily identify. I believe this text will allow either PT students or current PT practitioners with minimal or multiple years of practice to improve their ability to use the Guide as a practical clinical reference, and it will therefore advance PT practice and professionalism.

—*Cynthia Coffin-Zadai, PT, DPT, CCS, FAPTA*
MGH Institute of Health Professions
Boston, Massachusetts

Introduction

The chapters in *Cardiovascular/Pulmonary Essentials* take the *Guide to Physical Therapist Practice*[1] to the next level and parallel the patterns in the *Guide*.

INTRODUCTORY INFORMATION

In each case, where appropriate, a review of the pertinent anatomy, physiology, pathophysiology, imaging, and pharmacology is provided as a means of background material.

PHYSICAL THERAPIST EXAMINATION

Each pattern details three to five case studies appropriate to that pattern in *Guide* format. Thus, the case begins with the physical therapist examination, which is divided into the three parts of the examination—the history, the systems review, and the specific tests and measures selected for that particular case.

HISTORY

The history provides the first information that will be obtained from the patient/client. The history is a crucial first step in the clinical decision-making process as it enables the physical therapist to form an early hypothesis that helps guide the remainder of the clinical examination. The interview with the patient/client and a review of other available information provide the initial facts upon which further testing will be done to determine the concerns, goals, and eventual plan of care.

SYSTEMS REVIEW

After the history has been completed, the next aspect of the examination is the systems review, which is comprised of a quick screen of the four systems areas and a screen of the communication, affect, cognition, language, and learning style. The cardiovascular/pulmonary review includes assessment of blood pressure, edema, heart rate, and respiratory rate. The integumentary review includes assessing for the presence of any scar formation, the skin color, and the skin integrity. The musculoskeletal review includes assessment of gross range of motion, gross strength, gross symmetry, height, and weight. The neuromuscular review consists of an assessment of gross coordinated movements (eg, balance, locomotion, transfers, and transitions). The screen for communication, affect, cognition, language, and learning style includes an assessment of the patient's/client's ability to make needs known, consciousness, expected emotional/behavioral responses, learning preferences, and orientation.

TESTS AND MEASURES

The specific tests and measures to be selected for the patient/client are based upon the results found during the history taking and during the systems review. These latter two portions of the examination identify the clinical indicators for pathology/pathophysiology, impairments, functional limitations, disabilities, risk factors, prevention, and health, wellness, and fitness needs that will enable one to select the most appropriate tests and measures for the patient/client.

EVALUATION, DIAGNOSIS, AND PROGNOSIS AND PLAN OF CARE

The next step in the patient/client management model is evaluation. All of the data obtained from the examination (history, systems review, and tests and measures) are analyzed and synthesized to determine the diagnosis, prognosis, and plan of care for the patient/client. Then, once the evaluation has been completed and all data have been analyzed, the diagnosis for the patient/client and the pattern(s) into which the patient/client fits are determined.

After a review of the prognosis statement, of the expected range of number of visits per episode, and of the factors that may modify the frequency of visits for the pattern in the *Guide*, the prognosis is determined. Mutually established outcomes and the interventions for the patient/client are determined.

In each case, the *Guide* has set the expected course of visits for the patient/client (see Expected Range of Number of Visits Per Episode of Care in each pattern in the *Guide*). This range should be appropriate for 80% of the population. Any additional impairment(s) found during the examination may or may not increase the number of expected visits. There are many factors that may modify the frequency or duration of visits. These may include: the patient's/client's adherence to the program set by the physical therapist, the type and amount of social support and caregiver expertise, the patient's/client's level of impairment, the patient's/client's health insurance plan, and the patient's/client's overall health status. Each patient/client must be looked at individually when determining the frequency and duration of visits.

INTERVENTIONS

Through all the information gathered in the examination and evaluation and with the diagnosis, prognosis, and plan of care in place, the specific interventions for this patient are selected. Whenever possible, interventions that have been shown to be effective through high-quality scientific research are utilized. At the end of all of the interventions is a composite section on anticipated goals and expected outcomes.

REEXAMINATION AND DISCHARGE

Reexamination will be performed throughout the episode of care, particularly as the setting of care changes. Discharge will occur when anticipated goals and expected outcomes have been attained.

PSYCHOLOGICAL ASPECTS

For each case, psychological aspects are important to consider when attempting to motivate patients/clients to comply with a long-range intervention program of exercise and functional training. Among these considerations for all patterns are:

- Behavior is governed by expectancies and incentives
- The likelihood that people adopt a health behavior depends on three perceptions:
  - The perception that health is threatened
  - The expectancy that their behavioral change will reduce the threat
  - The expectancy that they are competent to change the behavior

It is necessary for physical therapists to understand reasons for noncompliance and formulate intervention plans accordingly. The number one indicator of future noncompliance is past poor compliance. Any psychological considerations beyond these in a particular case will be further detailed in that case.

PATIENT/CLIENT SATISFACTION

And finally for each case, the patient/client satisfaction with the physical therapy management would be determined by using the standard Patient/Client Satisfaction Questionnaire found in the back of the *Guide*.

REFERENCES

1. American Physical Therapy Association. Guide to physical therapist practice. 2nd ed. *Phys Ther.* 2001;81:9-744.

CHAPTER ONE

Primary Prevention/Risk Reduction for Cardiovascular/ Pulmonary Disorders (Pattern A)

Donna Frownfelter, PT, DPT, MA, CCS, FCCP, RRT
Elizabeth Dean, PT, PhD
Jane L. Wetzel, PT, PhD

PREVENTION AND THE PROMOTION OF HEALTH, WELLNESS, AND FITNESS

Traditionally, physical therapists have treated patients or clients at the level of impairment (ie, those with medical and surgical conditions). Given health care trends, physical therapist practitioners now must consider with every patient/ client they see one or more of the following: the promotion of health and wellness, the prevention of disease and disease progression, and the elimination of unnecessary invasive care (ie, medical and surgical interventions).

The diseases of civilization, namely, ischemic heart disease (IHD), cancer, smoking-related conditions, hypertension (HTN), stroke, and diabetes, are our leading causes of morbidity and mortality. In addition, osteoporosis is highly linked to lifestyle factors and is similarly associated with considerable morbidity and (indirectly) mortality.

The efficacy of noninvasive interventions—including education, optimal nutrition, and exercise—is unequivocal in the prevention and management of the diseases of civilization. Physical therapists are uniquely positioned in the health care system to lead the assault on these conditions.[1] In terms of prevention, physical therapists can assess and address risk factors by prescribing aggressive interventions to reverse in some cases or at least modify the risk factors for these dis-

eases of civilization. In this way, significant morbidity and functional limitation that can progress to marked disability can be prevented or reduced. These are singularly important physical therapy outcomes.

TYPES OF PREVENTION

Physical therapists have a role in the three distinct levels of prevention, namely primary, secondary, and tertiary. Primary prevention refers to the prevention of a disease in a high-risk or suspected potentially high-risk person or population through general positive health promotion efforts. Secondary prevention strives to decrease the duration of illness or the severity of disease and its sequelae through early diagnoses and timely intervention early in the disease process. Finally, tertiary prevention attempts to decrease the degree of disability, to promote rehabilitation, and to restore function in patients with chronic, irreversible diseases.

To determine the goals of prevention the physical therapist systematically evaluates risk factors for the respective diseases of civilization. Physical therapists must include risk factor assessment in the examination of every patient/client regardless of the presenting diagnosis. The physical therapist may see a patient for an orthopedic or neurological impairment and during the history taking portion of the examination find cardiovascular, pulmonary, or endocrine risk

Table 1-1

MAJOR RISK FACTORS RELATED TO LIFESTYLE AND THEIR IMPACT ON HEALTH

Risk Factor	Cardiovascular (THD & Hypertension) and Peripheral Vascular Disease	Obstructive Lung Disease	Stroke	Diabetes	Cancer	Osteoporosis
Smoking	X	X	X	X	X (↑ risk of all-cause cancer*	X
Physical inactivity	X		X	X	X	X
Obesity	X	X	X	X	X	X
Nutrition	X		X	X	X	X
High blood pressure	X		X	X		
Dietary fat†/blood lipids	X		X	X	X	
Elevated glucose levels	X		X	X	X	
Alcohol‡	X		?	X	X	X

*Smoking is not only related to cancer of the nose, mouth, airways, and lungs, but smoking increases the risk of all-cause cancer.

†Partially saturated, saturated, and trans-fats are the most injurous to health.

‡Alcohol can be protective in moderate quantities, red wine in particularly.

Adapted from Frownfelter D, Dean E. *Cardiovacular and Pulmonary Physical Therapy: Evidence and Practice.* 4th ed. St. Louis, Mo: Mosby; 2005:6.

factors. These risk factors may indeed be more important than the presenting orthopedic or neurologic diagnosis in terms of the individual's health. Since patients/clients may not be aware of their risk factors and how to reduce them, an assessment of their knowledge about the risk factors and their reduction should be an inherent component of every examination. This holistic approach is consistent with health care trends today and with the World Health Organization's (WHO)[2] definition of health and health promotion with an emphasis on participation in life rather than a primary focus on impairment of a body part.

IMPORTANCE OF PREVENTION OF DISEASES OF CIVILIZATION

This past century has seen changes in health care priorities from prevention and management of acute infectious diseases to the diseases of civilization (IHD, smoking-related conditions, HTN, stroke, diabetes, and cancer). It is notable that most individuals will have one or more risk factors for one or more of these conditions. Entering the "health care system" is indicative, in part, of the failure of this system to provide motivation, strategies, and lifestyle choices to prevent risk and subsequent impairment. As a society and as physical therapists, a commitment must be made to reducing the number of patients rather than focus on treatment.

Physical therapists have unique educational backgrounds and experience to be leaders in contemporary health care and prevention.[1]

Lifestyle choices of individuals, often coupled with tobacco use, alcohol consumption, and stress, are the bases for the diseases of civilization in high-income countries, and they pose the greatest threats to public health.[3-7] Eight major risk factors related to lifestyle and their impact on health are shown in Table 1-1.

The current use of the terminology, "metabolic syndrome," encompasses insulin resistance diabetes, high blood pressure (BP), elevated triglycerides and cholesterol, and obesity. This condition has appeared in low-, middle-, and high-income countries.[8-10] The WHO has long proclaimed that the diseases of civilization are "largely" preventable.[5]

WHO defines health as emotional, spiritual, intellectual, and physical well-being, not merely the absence of disease and impairment.[2] This definition emphasizes the fact that health is multidimensional rather than just physical well-being alone, and therefore, other factors need to be examined and evaluated. When all factors are taken into account, the individual's capacity to perform functional activities and to be able to fully participate in life will be maximized.

Dean described a model of comprehensive physical therapy with a focus on patient education in which both the learner and the content are matched.[11] Components of the model include one's health beliefs, self-efficacy, and sense of perceived control. Such a model is useful in understanding how an individual's beliefs impact health and illness, and the response and reaction to them and their care.[12] Asking an individual some targeted questions enables the physical therapist to understand the patient's perceptions of risk factors and to prescribe preventive strategies. Interest has increased in the academic and clinical communities regarding the assessment of health awareness and comprehension of risk factors, self-efficacy, and readiness to effect sustained lifestyle behavioral changes. Lack of knowledge of risk factors and poor lifestyle choices have traditionally been addressed through educational sessions during therapeutic sessions. Today we know behavior change is multifactorial and compliance with recommended lifestyle changes requires innovative strategies to ensure new patterns of living are sustained.[13] Effecting these lifelong, sustainable, healthy lifestyle choices is a major challenge for physical therapy.

PREVENTION FOR EARLIEST YEARS

Risk factors for the diseases of civilization have their foundations in childhood. For example, IHD secondary to atherosclerosis is the leading cause of mortality in industrialized countries. Prevention of this condition needs to begin in childhood when lifestyle patterns are being established.[14-16] Smoking, diets high in refined carbohydrates and fats, and inactivity precipitate damage to the endothelial lining of the arteries and atherosclerotic deposition. Recently, these risk factors have been associated with increased levels of fibrinogen and C-reactive protein (CRP), an established marker of inflammation.[17] Inflammation has been implicated in many chronic conditions, including IHD, stroke, asthma, gastrointestinal ulcers, cirrhosis of the liver, Alzheimer's disease, cancer, and autoimmune conditions.[18,19] Diets high in refined carbohydrates and fats and inactivity have been identified as being pro-inflammatory, thus, possible contributors to the diseases of civilization through this mechanism.

Promoting healthy lifestyles early in life encourages children to be responsible for their health. Evidence of cardiovascular disease in children, such as HTN, Type 2 diabetes mellitus, obesity, and cardiac dysfunction is alarming. Children today may anticipate premature death and chronic diseases that can precipitate other sequelae or health complaints.[20] Actuaries and epidemiologists have predicted a leveling or lowering of life expectancy due to these factors. As a team member, the physical therapist needs to be knowledgeable about psychosocial determinants of health, so that lifelong health behavior change can be effected in all young clients and patients.

PREVENTION FOR ALL PATIENTS/CLIENTS

Consistent with the Hippocratic Oath, the overriding philosophical tenet of health care professionals is to promote wellness and prevent illness and disability. Should illness or disability occur, the least invasive interventions need to be used,[21] rather than intervening after invasive interventions.[22,23]

Given the abundance of knowledge related to the efficacy of noninvasive interventions in the prevention and management of the diseases of civilization, physical therapists have a primary responsibility for the translation of this knowledge in daily practice. This includes detecting cardiovascular, pulmonary, and endocrine risk factors and providing targeted education and personal, individualized prevention programs. When a patient has a physical impairment or problem, the timing of the risk factor reduction education may be optimal in terms of a teachable moment. For example, when a patient is seen in acute care for a total knee replacement secondary to osteoarthritis (OA) and has been inactive, is overweight, and has HTN, this can be a prime opportunity to provide not only acute care, but the concept of a long-term more active lifestyle to prevent further joint problems and decrease cardiovascular and other health-related manifestations. If this patient smokes, this is an optimal time to consider quitting, given the individual has likely not been smoking since before surgery to avoid problems, such as delayed wound healing, pulmonary complications, and delayed recovery. In addition, the physical therapist can institute smoking cessation based on recommendations endorsed by the American Physical Therapy Association (APTA) in conjunction with other resources (eg, American Lung Association and SmokEnders).[24]

Prevention Related to Aging and Psychosocial/Cultural Factors

Functional capacity has been estimated to decrease by 10% per decade of life. Half of this decline is due to sedentary living. As little as 30 minutes of moderately intense exercise most days of the week offsets the effects of inactivity and premature aging.[25] That aging can be somewhat offset with relatively minimal exercise daily is highly encouraging for individuals who are less inclined to exercise and for the physical therapist who advocates exercise and attempts to increase adherence to an exercise program.

Psychosocial and cultural issues play a major role in determining whether an individual exercises or is willing to consider an exercise program. In one study, the exercise levels of black American women were compared with levels recommended for health.[26] Only a small proportion of the sample of black American women exercised daily at a level consistent with those recommended for good health. They exercised less than the guidelines with respect to both the duration of exercise sessions and the number of exercise days in the week. The health of black American women is of particular concern to clinicians given they have a higher risk of cardiovascular disease and stroke than white American women. Prevention is a high priority for this high-risk group.[27] In terms of exercise barriers and facilitators, this group reported the need for a safe physical environment and the need for education about exercise and motivational considerations.

The health consequences of the lifestyles of black Seventh Day Adventists have been examined. Adventists promote spiritual well-being and a healthy diet and lifestyle. They have a significantly lower incidence of chronic disease compared with black Americans who are not Seventh Day Adventists.[28] In general, Mormons tend to be fitter and have fewer risk factors for IHD than other Americans.[29] These naturalistic observations are consistent with the unequivocal body of knowledge supporting the significant reduction of mortality with optimal nutrition, weight control, regular physical activity, and avoidance of smoking.[30]

Prevention Related to Ischemic Heart Disease

The risk factors for IHD are undisputed.[31] Nonmodifiable risk factors include age, family history, and gender. Modifiable risk factors include increased cholesterol, increased homocysteine, smoking, inactivity, HTN, diabetes, overweight, and stress.[32-34] CRP levels above 100 have recently been correlated with IHD and serve as a marker of inflammation. Sharing a lifestyle with someone with IHD[35] and having overweight parents[36] have been reported more recently as contributing risk factors. These factors place children at risk.

The specific effects of risk factor interventions are being better documented, which is essential for evaluating the validity of risk factor reduction as a physical therapy outcome. A 1% reduction in cholesterol, for example, reduces the risk of IHD by 3%, and a long-term diastolic BP reduction of 5 to 6 mmHg reduces the risk by 20% to 25%.[37] These findings support the concept that relatively small preventive changes in risk factors can translate into major health benefits.

Prevention Related to Hypertension and Stroke

HTN can be a function of lifestyle choices including smoking, reduced physical activity, stress, and diet (eg, salt intake). Stroke can result from high BP and thrombus formation from atherosclerosis. An individual with a stroke secondary to atherosclerosis should be viewed and monitored as an individual with cardiac risk factors, and appropriate prevention interventions should be instituted.

Prevention Related to Glucose Intolerance and Diabetes

Glucose intolerance is directly related to diabetes, inactivity, and dietary factors, including the consumption of refined foods and the addition of sugar to the diet. Glucose intolerance due to insulin insensitivity is the precursor for Type 2 diabetes and its deadly sequelae. These sequelae include angiopathy, cardiopathy, neuropathy, retinopathy, and renal disease. Angiopathy manifests itself as impaired perfusion to the tissues that may result in potential limb amputation, IHD, and renal disease. People with diabetes have an increase in IHD as compared with people without diabetes.[22] Prevention programs, including increasing aerobic exercise and diet control, will play a vital role in reducing risk for this population.

Prevention Related to Smoking Conditions

Smoking is a major risk factor for morbidity and mortality globally. The hazards of smoking are well publicized (eg, on cigarette packages, in the news, and in schools). Smoking is the leading cause of preventable death in the world.[38] For every cigarette smoked, an individual's life expectancy is estimated to be shortened by 11 minutes.[39] Smoking history needs to be documented in every patient and smoking cessation implemented.[40,41] Even for patients who have quit smoking, the duration that they smoked and the amount they smoked are crucial. Risk reduction is progressive, with some risks being reduced sooner and others later. Lung cancer, for example, can still emerge some decades after smoking cessation. Smoking is the primary cause of chronic obstructive pulmonary disease (COPD) and has been linked to cancer, heart disease, and asthma. The risks for IHD are cumulative with smoking and can also lead to stroke.[39] Active and passive smoking have been implicated in COPD and coronary heart disease (CHD). Environmental pollution from smoking influences the development of the respiratory system in children and results in low birth weight in babies whose mothers smoke.

In addition, smoking contributes to other conditions that are systemic and not just involving the respiratory system.[42] Other smoking-related conditions include peripheral vascular disease, HTN, osteoporosis, and cancer of multiple organs including the oral cavity, airways, and lungs.

Smoking in children is highly correlated with parental smoking. There is evidence that low birth weight and parental smoking are predictors of childhood asthma. Thus, the child's and the parents' smoking histories need to be a component of the pediatric assessment.[37] The effects of secondhand smoke are now well documented.

Although other risk factors can impair the cardiovascular and pulmonary systems, no other factor has such severe consequences that are so easily prevented with smoking cessation. Motivation to quit smoking can be promoted based on health and economic benefits.

ANATOMY

The cardiovascular and pulmonary systems consist of the heart, the vascular system, and the lungs.[42] The system is interdependent in providing optimal oxygen (O_2) transport to the tissues and excretion of carbon dioxide (CO_2) as an end product of metabolism. Any change or impairment in a unit of the cardiovascular and pulmonary system will interrupt O_2/CO_2 regulation and may result in dyspnea (the patient's perception of shortness of breath) and decreased exercise tolerance.

The oxygen transport system refers to the delivery of oxygenated blood through the lungs and heart to the tissues for cellular utilization and the return of partially desaturated blood to the lungs to be reoxygenated. The oxygen transport pathway consists of multiple steps from the atmosphere to the tissue level. It includes available oxygen, oxygen delivery, oxygen consumption, and oxygen extraction. An imbalance between supply and demand will produce signs and symptoms (eg, dyspnea, increased work of breathing, increased myocardial workload, and possible angina) that limit the patient during activity, leading to a decrease in function of the patient/client. This limitation may be short term, but if the imbalance is long term, it will have serious effects on other body systems.

The oxygen transport system can serve as a basis for the examination and evaluation of patients with cardiovascular and pulmonary impairments and their multisystem manifestations.[43-46] In addition to an analysis of impairment or dysfunction, the clinician must also base the decision on where to focus interventions in concert with the individual's goals with respect to participation in life and its composite activities. This philosophy is consistent with WHO's *Classification of Function*.[47]

PULMONARY SYSTEM

Thorax

The thorax consists of 12 ribs. The first seven are true ribs attaching to the sternum anteriorly and the vertebrae posteriorly. Ribs 8, 9, and 10 attach to the sternum through the cartilage of the 7th rib. Ribs 11 and 12 are floating ribs, which only attach posteriorly.

During normal development in the first 12 months of life, the thorax changes configuration from ribs that are horizontal forming a more circular chest wall to a more rectangular shape with ribs that rotate downward and inward. This results in a more elliptical chest configuration. The change in the shape of the chest wall is accomplished through the gravitational and muscular stresses applied as the child becomes more upright during sitting, standing, and walking during the first 12 to 15 months of life. Developing muscle tone and strength facilitate this development.

Sternum

The sternum consists of three parts: the manubrium, the body, and the xiphoid process. The sternal angle or Angle of Louis between the manubrium and body of the sternum is easily palpated by sliding the examining fingers down the sternum from the sternal notch. The level of the second rib, which attaches to the sternum at the sternal angle, marks the bifurcation of the main stem bronchi and the arch of the aorta. The heart is located below and to the left of the lower one-third of the sternum. The xiphoid process is attached to the body of the sternum by fibrocartilage that fuses with aging.

Movements of the Thorax

Movements of the thorax are determined by muscles acting on the ribs and chest wall. The first seven ribs have a primary rotation component and increase the superior dimension of the upper chest wall. The upper chest movement is often referred to as a pump handle movement. Ribs 8, 9, and 10 provide more lateral costal movement (up and out to the sides), sometimes referred to as bucket handle movement. During inspiration, the thorax moves in three planes: anterior-posterior, superior-inferior, and lateral (transverse). Inspiration is associated with trunk extension, and expiration is associated with trunk flexion.

Muscles of Respiration

Inspiration is an active movement facilitated primarily by the diaphragm and intercostal muscles during normal quiet breathing. The diaphragm contributes two-thirds of the inspiration effort at rest. With increased activity, the accessory muscles are recruited. Any muscle that attaches to the chest wall can function as an accessory or adjunct muscle of respiration. The accessory muscles may assist in either inspiration or expiration.

Normal respiratory mechanics and function depend on the interaction of the diaphragm, intercostal muscles, and abdominal muscles. Loss of any of these may impair respiration, increase shortness of breath, and decrease exercise tolerance.

Diaphragm

The diaphragm is a dome-shaped muscle, innervated by the phrenic nerve on each side, which divides the thoracic and abdominal cavities. The upper surface supports the pericardium, heart, pleurae, and lungs. The lower surface is almost covered by the peritoneum and lies over the liver, stomach, kidneys, supra renal glands, and spleen. The abdominal muscles form a support for the abdominal viscera, which maintains their position beneath the diaphragm. Loss of abdominal wall support leads to flattening of the diaphragm and decreases the efficiency of diaphragmatic movement. Three major vessels pass through the diaphragm, the aorta, the inferior vena cava, and the esophagus. Other structures that pass through are the vagus nerve trunks and branches of the gastric vessels.

The diaphragm descends as it contracts, and in doing so, displaces the abdominal viscera such that the abdomen protrudes correspondingly. As the central tendon of the diaphragm stabilizes, the lateral costal fibers contract and a lateral costal movement ensues, resulting in the bucket handle movement. During deep breathing, the upper chest is displaced superiorly.

Diaphragmatic movement can be controlled voluntarily in a concentric deeper slower inspiration and a controlled eccentric exhalation. Professional voice users such as singers, public speakers, and wind instrumentalists, and parents calling their children have learned the art of controlled exhalation and voice projection.

The role of the diaphragm acting not only as a breathing muscle but one of postural stability is now better understood. The so-called core of the trunk consists of the abdominal muscles, diaphragm, pelvic floor muscles, and back extensor muscles. If the work of breathing is overloaded and the diaphragm cannot support both breathing and posture, its role as a primary muscle of respiration takes priority.[48]

Intercostal Muscles

The intercostal muscles provide chest wall stability and serve as accessory muscles of respiration. There are 11 such muscles on each side of the chest wall that are active in both inspiration and expiration. Conditions, such as fractured ribs or in situ chest tubes, can lead to spasm of the intercostal muscles, which may affect rib mobility and ventilation.

Abdominal Muscles

The abdominal muscles (ie, rectus abdominus, internal and external obliques, and transversus abdominus) provide a firm yet flexible wall to maintain the position of the abdominal viscera. The compressive force of the abdominal muscles is important in coughing, defecation, urination, childbirth, vomiting, postural control, and core stability.

Accessory Muscles

Any muscle attaching to the chest wall (depending on the position of the body), may be recruited to increase inspiratory volume if it lifts the chest cage and to enhance forced expiration if it depresses the chest cage. The accessory muscles of inspiration include the levatores costarum, pectoralis major, pectoralis minor, rhomboids, scaleni, serratus anterior, sternocleidomastoid, thoracic erector spinae, and trapezius. The accessory muscles of expiration include the iliocostalis lumborum and the transversus thoracis (sternocostalis). Several muscles may be accessory muscles for either inspiration or expiration depending on whether their anterior or posterior muscle fibers contract (latissimus dorsi) or depending on which end of the muscle is fixed (quadratus lumborum and serratus posterior inferior).

Upper Airways

The upper airways consist of the nose and nasal pharynx and extend down to the larynx, which divides the upper and lower airways. The nose filters, warms, and humidifies the inspired air and contributes to vocal resonance along with other structures. The airways are lined with a mucous blanket consisting of pseudostratified columnar ciliated epithelium. As air passes from the nose to the alveoli, its temperature equilibrates to that of the body and becomes 100% saturated with water vapor. If the air is cold and dry, warming and humidification is provided by the airways. If humidification is inadequate, mucociliary clearance may be impaired.

The mucous blanket consists of two layers: a thin sol layer and a thick gel layer. The cilia beat rapidly in the sol layer in a cephalad direction, moving the gel layer and in turn debris, such as dust and excess secretions, to the upper airways, where they can be expelled with coughing or swallowing. Adequate hydration is essential because 90% of the mucous blanket is water. Patients who are dehydrated will have a deficit in airway clearance. Other factors associated with disruption of the so-called mucociliary escalator are smoking and anesthesia, which decrease or paralyze ciliary action.

Larynx and Vocal Folds

The larynx is composed of cartilage and muscle, which protect the lower airways and control exhalation during speech. Air passes the vocal folds (vocal cords), producing the characteristic sounds associated with speech. In addition, they have a role in the regulation of the intrathoracic and intra-abdominal pressures. For example, a patient with a tracheostomy may have difficulty with transfers or walking when the tracheostomy is open. A Passey Muir speaking valve allows for inspiration through the tracheostomy and closes on exhalation. Normal intrathoracic and intra-abdominal pressures can be maintained and, in turn, functional activity facilitated.

Lower Airways

The trachea lies anterior to the esophagus. It divides into the right and left main stem bronchi. Cartilagenous rings that are "C" shaped are open posteriorly to facilitate esophageal movement of liquids and food. The right main stem bronchus is more vertically positioned than the left one and consequently more often the site of aspiration of foreign material or secretions.

There are 23 generations of airways. The main, lobar, and segmental bronchi form the 1st to the 4th generations. The subsegmental bronchi make up the 5th to 7th generations. Up to about the 11th generation, there is cartilaginous support for the airways. The terminal bronchioles are at approximately the 12th to 16th generations, where now there is little to no cartilaginous structure. At this point, the terminal bronchioles are within the lung parenchyma and the traction on them from the lungs keeps them open and moving. The respiratory bronchioles from the 17th to the 19th generations provide a transition from the conducting airways to the alveoli. The alveolar ducts leading to the alveolar sacs form the 20th to the 23rd generations and are the areas where respiration takes place.

Between the alveolar sacs are the Pores of Kohn, which allow for collateral ventilation. Within the alveolar sacs are Type I and Type II cells that form the structure of the alveoli and produce surfactant, a phospholipid that decreases surface tension, thereby maintaining alveolar patency. Alveolar macrophage cells containing lysosomes kill bacteria and engulf foreign materials that enter the lungs. They are either then transported to the lymphatic system for removal or to the terminal bronchioles where they are expelled by the mucous blanket. In addition to these mechanisms, immunoglobin cells aid in fighting infection by attracting macrophages to the infection site.

Pleura

The lungs are covered by the visceral and parietal pleurae. A potential space between the pleurae can accumulate fluid (ie, pleural effusion) in conditions where lung water and fluid balance are disrupted (eg, tumor or pneumonia). This fluid can compress the lung parenchyma and limit ventilation.

CARDIOVASCULAR SYSTEM

The cardiac pump consists of four chambers, the right and left atria, and the right and left ventricles. The right atrium and right ventricle are separated by the tricuspid valve. The right atrium serves as a collecting chamber for deoxygenated blood returning through the superior and inferior venae cavae from the venous system draining the head and neck, and the rest of the body, respectively. The deoxygenated blood in the right atrium passes through the tricuspid valve into the right ventricle during ventricular relaxation, or diastole, when the valve opens. The pressure in the right ventricle ranges between 15 to 30 mmHg during systole and 0 to 8 mmHg during diastole.[49-52] Alterations in these pressures may signal cardiovascular pump dysfunction and explain activity-limiting signs and symptoms.[52] Blood entering the right ventricle accumulates until the right ventricular pressure matches the right atrial pressure causing the tricuspid valve to close.[53] During right ventricular contraction, or systole, deoxygenated blood passes through the pulmonic valve into the pulmonary circulation to the pulmonary capillary bed. Here, CO_2 and O_2 diffuse across the interstitium to and from the alveoli, where CO_2 is eliminated and the blood becomes oxygenated before returning to the left side of the heart.[54]

Oxygenated blood returning from the lungs empties into the left atrium from one of four pulmonary veins. The left atrium and left ventricle are separated by the mitral valve. During diastole, the pressure in the left ventricle is low and the mitral valve opens. Moving down its pressure gradient, the blood moves from the left atrium into the left ventricle until the pressure at the end of diastole exceeds the pressure in the left atrium. The mitral valve closes as left ventricular contraction begins. As the pressure rises, the aortic valve between the left ventricle and the aorta opens and blood is ejected into the systemic vasculature. At rest, a stroke volume (SV) of 70 mL of blood is ejected with each ventricular contraction.[53] Normal SV ranges between 50% to 70% of the end-diastolic volume (EDV). This percentage is referred to as the ejection fraction (EF=SV/EDV) and may be used to quantify the contractile state of the ventricle.[53] Pressure in

the left ventricle ranges between 100 to 140 mmHg during systole and 3 to 12 mmHg during diastole.[49-52] Left ventricular end-diastolic pressure (LVEDP) is a primary indicator of left ventricle performance.

Compared with the right ventricle, the greater pressure in the left ventricle increases the tension applied to the myocardium throughout much of the cardiac cycle. The left ventricle has a greater muscle mass and uses more energy because it ejects blood into the systemic vasculature, which has a larger cross sectional area than the pulmonary vasculature. The arterial system accepting the blood has an initial arterial pressure at the end of diastole that ranges from 60 to 90 mmHg, which elevates during left ventricle contraction, or systole. Normal arterial pressure during systole ranges from 90 to 140 mmHg. These pressures are readily measured with a BP cuff. The mean arterial pressure (MAP) ranges from 70 to 105 mmHg and is important for determining normal vasculature status, unimpaired by diseases or disorders. Vascular pressures contribute to myocardial wall tension and influence cardiac performance. Resting pressures are also influenced by the autonomic nervous system (sympathetic and parasympathetic), which generates a myogenic resting tone to the smooth muscle in the arterioles, directing blood flow in accordance with hormonal and neurotransmitter signals. Early signs of vascular diseases and disorders may be detected through simple BP measures. Elevations in BP may appear before the patient becomes symptomatic.

Conduction System

The rate, rhythm, and conduction of electrical signals are critical to cardiac function. Cardiac cells are self-excitatory, enabling the heart to contract rhythmically and automatically. The sinoatrial (SA) node is located in the posterior wall of the right atrium. It is the normal pacemaker of the heart, generating a rate of 60 to 100 bpm. The AV node in the floor of the right atrium serves as a pacemaker of the impulses delaying the wave of excitation to the ventricles, giving the atria time to fill and empty their contents into the ventricles. The AV node has an inherent rate of 40 to 60 bpm. From the AV node arises a fiber grouping known as the AV Bundle or Bundle of His, which then divides into the left and right bundle branches that divide into the Purkinje Fibers, where the wave of excitation is spread to the ventricles. The ventricles have an inherent rate of 40 bpm. The electrocardiogram (ECG) pattern demonstrates the electrical activity of the heart and is represented by the P-QRS-T wave, where the P wave indicates atrial depolarization, the QRS complex represents ventricular depolarization, and the T wave represents ventricular repolarization.

Nervous System Control

Activation of the sympathetic nervous system increases during exercise, resulting in the release of epinephrine from the adrenal medulla and norepinephrine from the cardiac plexus. Beta-adrenergic receptors on the ventricles signal myocardial contractility when stimulated by increases in epinephrine and norepinephrine. Together, Starling's law of the heart (which indicates that the force of the heartbeat is determined by the length of the cardiac muscle fibers, so that an increase in diastolic filling increases the force of the heartbeat) and these neurohormonal responses result in effective cardiac contraction and SV during activity. The SA node also responds sending a wave of depolarization through the conduction system. Heart rate (HR) increases. Cardiac output (CO) requirements for activity are met by the increases in HR and SV (CO=HRxSV).[53]

Coronary Arteries

Energy for myocardial muscle contraction is provided primarily by aerobic metabolism. Oxygen is carried in the blood to the myocardium via the coronary arteries. These arteries begin at the root of the aorta and travel outside the cardiac muscle and beneath a fibrous fluid-filled pericardial sac to various regions of the heart. The major coronary vessels are the left anterior descending (LAD), left circumflex artery (LCA), posterior descending artery (PDA), and the right coronary artery (RCA). The left main coronary artery bifurcates into the LAD and the circumflex branches. The anterior wall of the myocardium and the interventricular septum receive blood from the LAD and several diagonal branches. The LCA has several obtuse marginal branches that perfuse the lateral wall. The PDA comes off the RCA in 86% of the cases and perfuses the posterior or diaphragmatic wall and the AV node. The RCA supplies the right ventricular wall, the SA node in 60% of the cases, and the AV node in 80% of the cases.[55,56] Oxygenated blood travels through the coronary plexus that perfuses three layers of the heart—the epicardium, myocardium, and endocardium. The endocardium is the last portion of the heart to be perfused and is the most vulnerable to loss of coronary flow. Myocardial ischemia and infarctions may occur when coronary flow is limited.[55,56]

Peripheral Circulation

The peripheral circulation is as important as the central circulation in that the heart depends on the peripheral circulation to provide oxygenated blood to peripheral tissues and return deoxygenated blood to the central circulation for reoxygenation. The peripheral circulation consists of arteries, veins, and lymphatic vessels. Arteries are classified as large, medium, and small, and each has a unique anatomical structure to fulfill a unique physiologic function. Large arteries consist largely of elastin, the medium-sized arterioles consist predominantly of smooth muscles, and the small capillaries embedded in the tissues of the body, consist primarily of endothelium, one cell thick.

Veins are also classified as large, medium, and small. The small venules receive blood from the capillaries, which then flows into the medium-sized veins and then the large

veins—the superior and inferior venae cavae—that return deoxygenated blood to the right atrium. Unlike arteries that have to support high BP fluctuations, veins are thin walled as they accommodate blood at low pressure. Some venous beds (eg, the spleen and the gut) serve as reservoirs to store blood until it is needed. Some veins have such low pressure that they may be collapsed. These veins may distend when there is a back-up of blood and may constitute a pathologic sign, (eg, jugular venous distension).

The lymphatic system also consists of a system of large, medium, and small vessels. They are characteristically thin walled and slightly muscular to fulfill their role in maintaining fluid balance in the periphery. For further detail on the lymphatic system, see Pattern H: Impaired Circulation and Anthropometric Dimensions Associated With Lymphatic System Disorders.

PHYSIOLOGY

PULMONARY SYSTEM

The oxygen transport system is the pathway in which oxygen passes through the airways and lungs, diffuses through the pulmonary circulation into the blood to the heart, and is then transported in the blood through the peripheral circulation to the tissues for metabolism. At the tissue level, oxygen consumption is titrated to metabolic need, and carbon dioxide, a metabolic byproduct, is removed. In those cases when O_2 is not moving effectively or CO_2 is not being removed effectively, interventions need to be directed.

Formulas for minute ventilation (MV) and CO give a sense of "breath-to-breath" understanding of pulmonary physiology. MV is the product of the tidal volume (TV) times the respiratory rate (RR) (MV=TVxRR). TV is normal breathing at rest volume. With each breath, air in the tracheobronchial tree or anatomic dead space does not participate in gas exchange. The anatomic dead space is approximately equivalent to 1 cc per pound of body weight. Thus a 150-lbs person has approximately 150 cc of anatomic dead space. A typical tidal breath is 500 cc, and 350 cc of that reaches the alveoli for ventilation (air that passes to the alveoli to participate in gas exchange). The normal RR is between 12 and 20 bpm. If a person is breathing 16 bpm with a normal TV of 500 cc, the volume of the anatomic dead space will be 150 cc and alveolar ventilation will be 350 cc. If a person's breathing is excessively rapid and shallow, the TV will decrease. In this latter case, the anatomic dead space remains the same, but the effective alveolar ventilation is decreased. For example, the rapidly breathing patient may have a TV of only 400 cc with each breath. With a constant 150 cc of anatomic dead space, that means that there will be only 250 cc of alveolar ventilation. This example provides the rationale for instructing patients to breathe slowly and deeply. In contrast, if an individual is breathing deeply so that the TV is increased to 750 cc with each breath and with a constant 150 cc of anatomic dead space, alveolar ventilation will be 600 cc. The more effective the alveolar ventilation, the more optimal the oxygen delivery for overall oxygen transport.

VENTILATION/PERFUSION

Ventilation is the process of gases moving into and out of the lungs. Perfusion is the passage of fluid (eg, blood) through a specific organ or area of the body. Ventilation-Perfusion Matching is the matching of the movement of gases and the circulation of blood through the lungs (perfusion). Ideally there would be a one to one match of ventilation and perfusion. In reality gravity pulls blood to dependent areas based on position. In the upright position there is greater perfusion in the lower lung fields and greater ventilation in the upper lung fields. In the middle lung there is the most optimal ratio of ventilation to perfusion. To maintain optimal blood gases a ratio of four parts ventilation to five parts perfusion should exist. Many disease processes can cause a mismatching of ventilation and perfusion. Physiological shunting refers to perfusion in excess of ventilation as is found in atelectasis and pneumonia. Physiological dead space refers to ventilation in excess of perfusion as is found in pulmonary embolus.

ARTERIAL BLOOD GASES

Arterial blood gas analysis provides a profile of the pH, pCO_2, pO_2, and pulse oxygen saturation (SpO_2). The pH (normal range: 7.35 to 7.45) indicates the effectiveness of the acid base balance, identifies whether the patient has an acute or a chronic acid base problem, and indicates whether the person has an uncompensated, partially compensated, or compensated condition, The pCO_2 (normal range: 35 to 45 mmHg) is indicative of alveolar ventilation. If the pCO_2 is above 45 mmHg, the patient is said to be hypoventilating (blowing off less CO_2 than normal). If the pCO_2 is below 35 mmHg, the patient is said to be hyperventilating (blowing off more CO_2 than normal). The pO_2 (normal range: 80 to 100 mmHg, but lower in elderly people) is indicative of arterial oxygenation. SpO_2 of the hemoglobin (Hgb) at rest is normally 98%. Clinically, having a patient's SpO_2 greater than 90% at the start of exercise and preventing desaturation below this level are generally accepted clinical guidelines for safe and effective treatment. If the O_2 saturation falls below 90%, supplemental oxygen is indicated. Oxygen can be titrated 1 L at a time until the SpO_2 stabilizes at 90% or higher with exercise. If O_2 saturation decreases below 90%, limited O_2 will be available at the tissue level. Patients may exercise using anaerobic metabolism that may lead to leg cramps, shortness of breath, and an even greater decreases in O_2 saturation.

CARDIAC SYSTEM

The coronary vessels fill during diastole by utilizing a pressure gradient between the aorta and the distal coronary plexus, thus increasing coronary blood flow. If arterial BP or CO falls, due to cardiovascular pump dysfunction or failure or internal bleeding, the pressure gradient and coronary flow will be diminished. Additionally, if diastolic time is reduced, as occurs with the higher HRs observed during activity or with decreased BP, there is less time for coronary artery perfusion. In either case the oxygen available to the myocardium is limited and may result in ischemia.[57,58]

During activity, the cardiac muscle pump increases the force and rate of contraction to provide an enhanced CO. Arterial pressure rises during activity increasing the afterload against which the heart must work. At the same time increased venous return augments EDV, enhancing preload to optimize the length tension of the cardiac muscle, thereby taking advantage of the Frank Starling mechanism.[53,58] The overall tension in the heart is greater during exercise during both systole and diastole, thus challenging the coronary circulation to deliver adequate oxygen and nutrients for myocardial metabolism.

The heart extracts 75% of the oxygen in the coronary blood flow at rest and is therefore one of the most oxidative tissues in the body.[53,58] During activity, the metabolic demands of the heart are increased further requiring the myocardium to extract even more oxygen. Since oxygen extraction is almost fully enhanced at rest, any increase in myocardial oxygen supply is dependent on coronary flow that is influenced by the vascular anatomy and diastolic time (Figure 1-1).[58] There must be enough oxygen to support cardiac tissue metabolic requirements, or cardiac pump function will be disrupted. Myocardial oxygen demand is a linear function of HR, afterload, and contractile state, as influenced by neurohormonal controls and EDV or preload.[58-60] Any imbalance between myocardial oxygen supply and demand is likely to occur during activity when the metabolic needs are greatest. Cardiovascular signs (angina, shortness of breath, or overwhelming fatigue) or signs of abnormal physiologic responses (blunted or falling BP, ST segment changes, or arrhythmias) may appear indicating myocardial incompetence. As the HR, arterial pressure (afterload), and EDV approach their upper limits and as coronary flow state is fully enhanced, nearly all the oxygen in the blood within the coronary arteries is extracted. Therefore, an individual may function without signs or symptoms at rest or with low levels of activity. However, when myocardial metabolic needs are increased as HR and BP rises, unwanted signs and symptoms may appear indicating an inability of the coronary system to supply nutrients to meet metabolic demands in the myocardium.[58] Activities may need to be limited to avoid life-threatening cardiac events.

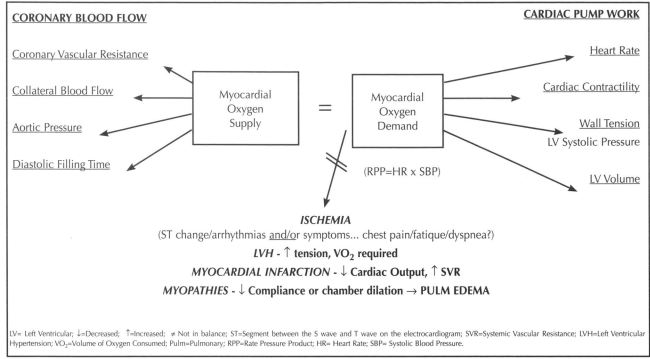

CORONARY BLOOD FLOW   **CARDIAC PUMP WORK**

Coronary Vascular Resistance   Heart Rate

Collateral Blood Flow   Myocardial   Cardiac Contractility
                               Oxygen   =   Myocardial
Aortic Pressure   Supply   Oxygen   Wall Tension
                                                      Demand   LV Systolic Pressure
Diastolic Filling Time
                                                                     LV Volume

                                    (RPP=HR x SBP)

                          ISCHEMIA
        (ST change/arrhythmias <u>and/or</u> symptoms... chest pain/fatique/dyspnea?)
              LVH - ↑ tension, VO₂ required
        MYOCARDIAL INFARCTION - ↓ Cardiac Output, ↑ SVR
     MYOPATHIES - ↓ Compliance or chamber dilation → PULM EDEMA

LV= Left Ventricular; ↓=Decreased; ↑=Increased; ≠ Not in balance; ST=Segment between the S wave and T wave on the electrocardiogram; SVR=Systemic Vascular Resistance; LVH=Left Ventricular Hypertension; VO₂=Volume of Oxygen Consumed; Pulm=Pulmonary; RPP=Rate Pressure Product; HR= Heart Rate; SBP= Systolic Blood Pressure.

Figure 1-1. Determinants of myocardial oxygen supply and demand. Adapted from Ellestad M. *Stress Testing. Principles and Practice.* 3rd ed. Philadelphia, Pa: FA Davis; 1986:24.

PATHOPHYSIOLOGY

OBESITY

Obesity is excess body fat for a given height and gender. It occurs when more calories are taken in than are burned up in a given period of time. Excess calories are stored as fat. Obesity tends to run in families. Obese children tend to be obese adults. This may be due to the family having similar diets and activity levels. Metabolic rate plays a role in obesity, as is evidenced by the fact that some people eating the same diet as others will gain weight more easily. Metabolic rate is fairly steady in an individual, but it is higher in physically active people. The diagnosis of obesity is made by calculating the individual's body mass index (BMI) (705 x body weight [lbs] divided by [height in inches x height in inches]) or by using a BMI chart. A BMI of 30 or greater is defined as obesity.[61]

Obesity has doubled over the last decade with approximately 61% of the American population being overweight. The complications related to obesity are wide ranging and include: IHD, cardiac myopathy, chronic heart failure, HTN, stroke, insulin insensitivity, Type 2 diabetes, gall bladder disease, dyslipedemia, OA, gout, and pulmonary diseases including alveolar hypoventilation and sleep apnea.[1]

Individuals who are obese tend to be less active and may be aerobically deconditioned. Consequently the work of breathing and cardiovascular work are increased with activity. It becomes a viscous cycle of increased shortness of breath, decreased activity, eating, less activity, decreased function, increased perception of exertion that results in overall decreased activity levels, and thus increased major health risks as a result of the sequelae of obesity.

CORONARY ARTERY DISEASE

Coronary artery disease (CAD) is the presence of an obstruction that limits coronary blood flow but does not significantly inhibit heart muscle function. This is differentiated from CHD, or coronary heart disease, where the presence of an obstruction led to permanent damage to the heart muscle fiber, thus impairing heart muscle function. The primary risk factors for CAD include HTN, cigarette smoking, and hyperlipidemia. Secondary risk factors include age, male gender, race, obesity, stress, and decreased activity levels. Factors that are modifiable are HTN, hyperlipidemia, smoking, obesity, abnormal glucose tolerance and diabetes, stress level, and activity level.[1]

CONGESTIVE HEART FAILURE

Congestive heart failure (CHF) results from impaired cardiac pumping caused by IHD. It may lead to myocardial infarction (MI) and potentially to cardiomyopathy. Failure of the ventricle to eject blood efficiently results in volume overload, chamber dilatation, and elevated intracardiac pressures. Retrograde transmission of increased hydrostatic pressure from the left heart can lead to pulmonary congestion, an elevated right heart pressure leading to systemic venous congestion, and peripheral edema. Pneumonia is a common occurrence secondary to CHF in older people.

IMAGING

Radiography or x-ray is the oldest and most widely available modality for imaging of the lungs. Plain chest x-rays are used to diagnose the site and progression or improvement of pneumonia of the lung. They are also used to ascertain the general size of the heart in relation to the thorax, the presence of hyperinflation of the lungs, and the position of the diaphragm. The usual view is an anteroposterior one.

Thallium imaging, which evaluates myocardial blood flow, may be used to indicate areas of the heart with relatively decreased perfusion or areas of infarction. Thallium exercise testing enhances the detection of myocardial ischemia.[62]

Echocardiography is used to assess valve integrity, the size of the ventricles, and cardiac muscle pump function.

Multigated acquisition (MUGA, also known as a radionuclide angiogram, or RNA scan) assesses ventricular size, ejection fraction, and therefore, cardiac muscle pump function.

Magnetic resonance imaging (MRI) may be used to detect significant coronary blockages. Cine computed tomography (or ultrafast CT scan, also called electron-beam CT) may be used to scan the heart at rest or during exercise and can detect myocardial thickening and can estimate CO. Positron emission tomography (PET scan) is able to assess myocardial blood flow.

PHARMACOLOGY

The following pharmacological agents may be utilized in the management of patients with community-acquired pneumonia:

♦ Antibiotics
  • Examples: Penicillins, cephalosporins, vancomycin, gentamicin
  • Actions: Inhibit bacterial growth
  • Administered: Oral or parenteral
  • Side effects:
    ▪ Hypersensitivity reactions, gastrointestinal upset, secondary infections, ototoxicity, and nephrotoxicity
    ▪ Ototoxicity and nephrotoxicity are rare

The following medications are often used to manage patients with CHF:

♦ Digoxin
  • Actions: Increases force of the heart by increasing $Ca++$ in heart cells; can control dysrhythmias by reducing the number of impulses from the SA node
  • Administered: Oral
  • Side effects:
    ▪ Nausea, loss of appetite, visual disturbances, and confusion
    ▪ Blood levels of digoxin must be monitored to prevent toxicity

♦ Lasix
  • Actions: Decrease amount of fluid by increasing amount of salt and water lost in urine
  • Administered: Oral
  • Side effects:
    ▪ Can reduce potassium levels
    ▪ Can increase blood sugar in diabetics
    ▪ May predispose one to osteoporosis, muscle cramps or weakness, irregular heartbeat, abdominal pain/diarrhea, low BP, headache, dizziness, numbness in feet, and easy bruising or bleeding

Calcium supplements may be given to patients to enhance bone density particularly if they are on drugs which may predispose them to osteoporosis.

♦ $Ca++$ supplement daily 1200 mg
  • Actions: May help prevent osteoporosis
  • Administered: Oral
  • Side effects:
    ▪ Constipation, intestinal bloating, and excess gas
    ▪ Possible increase risk of kidney stones

Case Study #1: Obesity-Related Shortness of Breath

Juan Martinez is a 12-year-old overweight male recently hospitalized for right lower lobe community acquired pneumonia and has shortness of breath.

PHYSICAL THERAPIST EXAMINATION

HISTORY

♦ General demographics: Juan is a 12-year-old male who has learned to speak and understand English and communicates fairly well. His parents speak little English. He is right-hand dominant.

♦ Social history: Juan and his family moved to Chicago from Mexico to improve their opportunities and provide him with better education.

♦ Employment/work: Both parents are employed in service jobs without health care benefits. Juan comes home from school and watches his younger brother and sister until his parents return from work.

♦ Living environment: The family currently lives in a basement apartment in a lower income neighborhood. There are eight steps into the apartment.

♦ General health status
- General health perception: The parents are concerned; they feel his health has been worse since they moved to the United States. Previously the weather was warmer and the air drier.
- Physical function: Juan has been discouraged that he cannot fully participate in gym and is tired at school while changing classes secondary to shortness of breath and fatigue.
- Psychological function: Juan is somewhat discouraged at his inability to physically keep up with his classmates in gym and after school activities.
- Role function: Student, son, babysitter.
- Social function: He tends to be somewhat isolated from the other students, often on the sideline of activities rather than participating in them.

♦ Social/health habits: He enjoys eating and has been excited about the vending machines in the school where he often spends his allowance on candy, soda, and snacks.

♦ Family history: His mother and father both smoke two to three packs per day. His father has a history of HTN and is currently on medication. His mother has diabetes that is not well controlled on oral medication.

♦ Medical/surgical history: Juan has had frequent colds but has not previously had visits to the emergency room or hospital.

♦ Prior hospitalizations: Juan was hospitalized 2 weeks ago for right lower lobe community-acquired pneumonia. He was in the hospital for 3 days, then at home for another week.

♦ Preexisting medical and other health-related conditions: None known. Juan has not had regular medical follow-up visits, only for illness.

♦ Current condition(s)/chief complaint(s): Juan's current complaint is congestion and shortness of breath with activity. He is having trouble in junior high school going from one classroom to the next and participating in physical education classes secondary to increased shortness of breath that limits his function.

♦ Functional status and activity level: Juan is quite sedentary with limited participation in physical education classes and no after school activities. When he comes home from school he watches TV.

♦ Medications: Juan is finishing his antibiotic prescription, and he takes no other medications.

♦ Other clinical tests: At time of his recent hospitalization, his chest x-ray indicated right lower lobe posterior segment pneumonia (serial x-rays have demonstrated improvement of the pneumonia).

SYSTEMS REVIEW

♦ Cardiovascular/pulmonary
- BP: 130/84 mmHg (normal for age: 85 to 114/50 to 85 mmHg)
- Edema: None
- HR: 100 bpm (normal for age: 75 to 110 bpm)
- RR: 20 bpm (normal for age: 16 to 22 bpm), which increases significantly with exertion, and he uses the accessory muscles even with minimal exertion

♦ Integumentary
- Presence of scar formation: None
- Skin color: Within normal limits (WNL)
- Skin integrity: WNL

♦ Musculoskeletal
- Gross range of motion: WNL
- Gross strength: Decreased in UE, LE, and trunk
- Gross symmetry: Symmetrical
- Height: 5' (1.52 m)
- Weight: 154 lbs (69.85 kg)

♦ Neuromuscular
- Balance: Difficulty with balance noted
- Locomotion, transfers, and transitions: WNL but slow to mobilize and tends to push up using the armrests of the chair when transferring from sit to stand

♦ Communication, affect, cognition, language, and learning style: WNL
- Communication, affect, and cognition: Alert and able to communicate, speaks well, follows directions, seems motivated to improve his health and ability to function in school and leisure activities
- Learning preferences: Visual learner

TESTS AND MEASURES

♦ Aerobic capacity/endurance
- 6-Minute Walk test
  - Juan walked 100 feet and complained of dyspnea
  - HR which was 100 bpm (high end of normal) at rest increased to 132 bpm after exertion
  - BP which was 130/84 mmHg (systolic is high for age and diastolic is at the very upper limit of normal for age) at rest increased to 138/84 mmHg
  - Use of visual analogue scale (10 cm) for perception of dyspnea revealed 2 cm at rest and 7 cm following the 6-Minute Walk test[63]

♦ Anthropometric characteristics
- BMI for his age=Weight (lbs) ÷ height (inches) ÷ height (inches) x 703
  - Juan's BMI was 30, which indicates that he is obese[61]
  - Truncal obesity

- ◆ Arousal, attention, and cognition
  - Alert and oriented x3
- ◆ Circulation
  - Auscultation
    - Heart sounds appear normal
    - HR at rest 100 bpm (high end of normal)
  - ECG: Normal sinus rhythm
- ◆ Ergonomics and body mechanics
  - Poor body mechanics during daily activities
  - Poor sitting posture
- ◆ Gait, locomotion, and balance
  - Unable to perform sit to stand without pushing with arms on armrests of chair
  - Able to stand on one foot for only 10 seconds
  - Complains of some problems with balance when stair climbing or when engaged in play activities
- ◆ Muscle performance
  - Decreased core muscle strength: 3+
  - Slight flaring of lower ribs
  - Manual muscle test (MMT) grades 4/5 for upper (UE) and lower extremity (LE) muscles
- ◆ Posture
  - Abdominal girth shifts center of mass anteriorly and thus shifts the center of gravity
  - Slightly forward head
  - Slight swayback
- ◆ Range of motion
  - Chest wall mobility decreased at mid and lower chest wall
  - Mid chest expansion (4th rib) using tape measure= 1 ½ inches
  - Lower chest expansion (7th rib/xiphoid) using tape measure=1 ⅞ inches
- ◆ Self-care and home management
  - Interview concerning ability to perform and perform safely self-care and home management actions, tasks, and activities revealed that Juan gets short of breath during his activities of daily living (ADL), taking care of his own room, and performing his chores in the house
- ◆ Ventilation and respiration/gas exchange
  - Auscultation: Decreased breath sounds right lower chest posteriorly, crackles, and expiratory wheezing
  - Breathing pattern: Juan tends to use accessory muscles of respiration, especially when he becomes dyspneic with activity
  - Cough: Moderately productive of thick yellow sputum
- ◆ Work, community, and leisure integration or reintegration

- Interview concerning ability to manage and to manage safely work, community, and leisure actions, tasks, and activities revealed that Juan gets short of breath in school and during leisure activities
- Juan would like to be more active in after school activities and in leisure time activities in their district park
  - He would like to try swimming since he feels it would be easier and more fun for him

EVALUATION

Juan is a 12-year-old overweight child, who is limited in his exercise and functional activities secondary to shortness of breath. He is currently mildly congested from a resolving pneumonia. He has significant risk factors for cardiovascular and pulmonary disease, as well as diabetes. His family history of smoking and lack of physical activity are major concerns that need to be addressed.

DIAGNOSIS

Juan is a client at risk of cardiovascular/pulmonary disease and diabetes. He has impaired aerobic capacity/endurance; anthropometric characteristics; ergonomics and body mechanics; gait, locomotion, and balance; muscle performance; posture; range of motion; and ventilation and respiration/gas exchange. He is functionally limited in self-care and in school, community, and leisure actions, tasks, and activities. These findings are consistent with placement in Pattern A: Primary Prevention/Risk Reduction for Cardiovascular/Pulmonary Disorders and secondarily in Pattern C: Impaired Ventilation, Respiration/Gas Exchange, and Aerobic Capacity/Endurance Associated With Airway Clearance Dysfunction. These impairments and functional limitations will be addressed in determining the prognosis and the plan of care.

PROGNOSIS AND PLAN OF CARE

Over the course of the visits, the following mutually established outcomes have been determined:

- ◆ Ability to perform self-care activities is improved
- ◆ Aerobic capacity and endurance is increased
- ◆ Balance is increased
- ◆ Energy expenditure per unit of work is decreased
- ◆ Fitness is improved
- ◆ Functional independence in ADL and instrumental activities of daily living (IADL) is increased
- ◆ Knowledge of behaviors that foster healthy habits, wellness, and prevention is increased
- ◆ Muscle performance is increased

- Physical capacity is improved
- Physical function is improved
- Posture is improved
- Range of motion (ROM) is improved
- Risk factors are reduced
- Risk of secondary impairment is reduced
- Self-management of symptoms is improved

To achieve these outcomes, the appropriate interventions for this patient are determined. These will include: coordination, communication, and documentation; patient/client-related instruction; therapeutic exercise; functional training in self-care and home management; functional training in work, community, and leisure integration or reintegration; and airway clearance techniques.

Based on the diagnosis and prognosis, Juan is expected to require between three and six visits over a 4- to 6-week period of time with follow-up visits at 3 and 6 months to ensure compliance and behavior changes for Juan and his family. The physical therapist will need to work with the family over a period of time to address risk factors and to assure that clear communication occurs and that community resources are available in Spanish (ie, smoking cessation, inexpensive means to increase physical activity, and improve nutrition). Time must allow for repetition and follow-up as parents understand risk factors and how they can be modified or ablated and how they can provide a more active personal and family life for Juan in order to improve his health status. It is essential that parental behaviors change relating to smoking, diet, and activity.[64] Juan's prognosis is good secondary to his motivation and the concern of parents to have his health improve and their dreams of opportunity and family improvement come to fruition. Finding resources available in Spanish and for low-income participants may be a challenge that will need to be overcome. Fortunately, in Illinois a program of AllKids[65] will provide examination and health care for children of low-income families. This will be a resource in which they will be encouraged to enroll for their children's health care. Additional benefits are available for families when children are enrolled in AllKids.

INTERVENTIONS

RATIONALE FOR SELECTED INTERVENTIONS

Patient/Client-Related Instruction

Juan has an improving pneumonia, and airway clearance techniques will be used to mobilize secretions in the right lower lobe. Juan will be shown how to independently perform postural drainage for his right lower lobe lateral and posterior segments.[66] Emphasis will also be placed on

hydration by drinking approximately eight glasses of water frequently per day. The color of his urine will be monitored to ensure that it is a pale yellow.

Therapeutic Exercise

Evidence exists that individual behaviors and lifestyle choices do influence the course of obesity, and incorporating healthy habits is essential to lessen the long-range burden upon society.[67]

The majority of obesity is due to lack of physical exercise and faulty diets, or in other words, an imbalance between the calories consumed and the calories expended.[68] Thus, exercise that requires caloric expenditure will be essential in Juan's obesity management. Therapeutic exercise for this patient will include aerobic/endurance training, strengthening, breathing exercises, and ventilatory strategies.

Juan has elevated BP that is common in children who are obese.[69] Adaptations of the cardiovascular system to aerobic conditioning are similar in individuals whether they are young or old.[70] Therefore, aerobic exercise, even low-impact and moderate intensity exercise, will enhance his aerobic fitness. Aerobic exercise will improve his blood pressure, cardiac output, stroke volume, VO_2 max, perceived exertion during submaximal exercise, and maximum heart rate.[71-73]

Walking is an ideal aerobic activity for the whole family, since it has been shown that family-based interventions in the pediatric population are essential. Parent and family behaviors need to be targeted if treating children with obesity is to be successful.[69] In addition to walking, a swimming program for aerobic conditioning may be an enjoyable exercise that will be easier on his joints and that he can share with friends.

Core strengthening will promote stronger abdominals and back muscles to improve the strength of the core to prevent injury with activity. As Juan loses weight his truncal obesity will decrease, which will also improve breathing and posture.[48] Postural exercises will help improve his forward head and swayback. Progressive strengthening of his upper and lower extremities will be incorporated into his program. since both aerobic exercise and resistance exercise help to reduce body fat, and progressive resistance strengthening exercises also appear to increase fat-free mass.[74]

Breathing exercises will increase alveolar ventilation in both lower lobes and will promote more efficient control of breathing.[66] Pursed lip breathing, emphasis on relaxation of the accessory muscles, and more focus on the diaphragm will promote breathing control.[66] Exercises to assist in secretion clearance will lead to improved ventilation and oxygenation.[75] Focus on bilateral lateral costal breathing will promote diaphragmatic breathing.

Ventilatory strategies will prevent breath holding with activity, since these strategies enable the patient to focus on breathing with activity. Breathing strategies will specifically pair trunk extension with inspiration and trunk flexion with exhalation to improve ventilation and oxygenation and reduce exertional dyspnea. These pairings are inherent with normal breathing, and they lead to a facilitation of breathing and movement and an elimination of breath holding with exertion.[76]

COORDINATION, COMMUNICATION, AND DOCUMENTATION

Communication will occur with Juan's parents to follow through on recommendations and behavioral changes including family activities. A referral will be made to a social worker or case manager so that the family can enroll in AllKids and so that Spanish resources may be obtained in the community for the parents' health concerns. A referral to a nutritionist through AllKids will be requested to help the family understand and restructure their nutrition and Juan's needs for weight reduction. A school physical education teacher will be contacted to serve as an ally for Juan to allow him to rest as needed and at the same time encourage more active participation in school sports activities at the junior high. All elements of the client's management will be documented.

PATIENT/CLIENT-RELATED INSTRUCTION

Juan and his family will be instructed to become more physically active individually and as a family. Instruction will be given to improve Juan's nutrition and hydration, and a referral will be made to a nutritionist as needed. The family will be provided information about the ways to participate in community health care resources for medical management and smoking cessation. Education will be provided to his parents in the steps necessary to enroll in AllKids for better medical follow-up and resources for the whole family.

THERAPEUTIC EXERCISE

- ◆ Aerobic capacity/endurance conditioning
  - Juan will progress to aerobic activities four to five times a week for 30 to 40 minutes
    - Initially he will start with what feels comfortable at a low level activity and slowly increase his time and effort (eg, start walking 10 minutes then increase to 15, 20, 25, and 30 minutes), and then he will progressively increase his speed to further increase his aerobic capacity
  - Use the 15-Count Breathlessness Score (also known as the Ventilatory Response Index) to monitor exertion[77]
    - Patient takes a deep breath and counts out loud to 15, which should take about 8 seconds
    - Count the number of breaths needed to complete the count, including the initial breath, so that the minimum score is one

- Living in the basement apartment, he can use the stairs for additional activity beginning with one repetition of up and down stopping as little as possible and gradually increasing repetitions building up to five of up and down without stopping
- Juan can put on music and dance around for continuous aerobic activity
- Videotapes of hip hop dancing/karate/kick boxing may be used as a fun means of providing aerobic conditioning

- ◆ Balance, coordination, and agility training
  - Standing on stable surface progressing to more dynamic standing balance
  - Modify base of support while balancing
  - Alter arm positions while maintaining balance
  - Tandem walking on a line
  - Stand on one foot with eyes open using support and increase time to 30 to 60 seconds, then eliminate support, and finally close eyes
  - Play games with siblings to see who can stand the longest on one foot and bat a balloon to each other standing on one foot (alternating feet)
  - Grapevine steps
  - Dancing the Electric Slide

- ◆ Body mechanics and postural stabilization
  - Body mechanics instruction while at home and school
  - Bridging, unilateral bridging, maintain bridge and add hip flexion right and then left, maintain bridge and add knee extension right and then left, decrease base of support
  - Prone glut sets
  - Prone arm raises unilateral and then bilateral, progressing to quadruped and then over the exercise ball
  - Leg raises unilateral prone, progressing to quadruped
  - Alternate opposite arm and leg
  - Incorporate the use of the foam roller and unstable surfaces like wobble board or foam rubber cushion in sitting and standing with bilateral and unilateral stance
  - Utilize ball for supine and prone exercises to strengthen core postural muscles
  - Bilateral leg raises while prone over the exercise ball
  - Challenge patient out of center of gravity/base of support
  - Utilize balance beam for standing on both legs, then one leg
  - Postural awareness training
    - Use of mirror for visual input of appropriate alignment

◆ Flexibility exercises
- Stretching exercises should be done after warming up, using a slow and steady stretch accompanied by deep breathing, and building hold up to 30 to 60 seconds
- Stretching to increase chest wall mobility to include trunk flexion and extension, lateral trunk flexion, and trunk rotation

◆ Gait and locomotion training
- Instruction in paced ambulation (using ratio of 1:2 for inspiration to expiration for breathing while ambulating)

◆ Relaxation
- Breathing strategies to increase relaxation (eg, pursed lip breathing, increasing the expiratory time)
- Breathing strategies to control dyspnea (eg, effective use of the diaphragm, decreased use and relaxation of accessory muscles, pursed lip breathing)

◆ Strength, power, and endurance training
- General strengthening exercises for LEs, including LE hip/knee flexion/extension, bridging, straight leg raises, terminal knee extension, and progressive weights
- Progress to 20 sit to stands without using his arms to push up
- UE progressive resistive strengthening program beginning with light weights (overhead press, upright rows, shoulder shrugs, shoulder flexion and abduction, elbow flexion and extension, wrist flexion and extension, chest flys, serratus, lat rows)
- Sit-ups leading to changing the lever arm and adding LE activity at the same time to increase the difficulty as Juan gets stronger
- Back extensor strengthening beginning with simple back extension leading up to changing the lever arm, doing modified push-ups, and using an exercise ball
- Breathing exercises to increase the strength of the diaphragm (eg, diaphragmatic weights, ventilatory muscle training device)
- Breathing exercises to increase lateral costal expansion using quick stretch to facilitate selective expansion and resistance to lateral rib cage to increase strength

FUNCTIONAL TRAINING IN SELF-CARE AND HOME MANAGEMENT

◆ IADL training: Instruction in ventilatory strategies (especially pursed lip breathing with 1:2 ratio of inspiration to expiration) with chores, such as vacuuming and bed making, since he complains of shortness of breath when performing these activities

◆ Injury prevention or reduction
- Juan was instructed in appropriate body mechanics and posture during activities
- Core strengthening for facilitating postural alignment

FUNCTIONAL TRAINING IN SCHOOL, COMMUNITY, AND LEISURE INTEGRATION OR REINTEGRATION

◆ IADL training: Juan will leave a book bag in his locker and only carry necessary books or consider a rolling back pack to help decrease previously experienced shortness of breath

◆ Leisure
- Juan and his family will be instructed to try to find time as a family to do activities (ie, a walk after dinner, go to a local park or pool, or mall walk)
- The parents should be encouraged to allow Juan to attend before school physical activities (eg, playground games)
- The parents should be encouraged to allow Juan to attend an after school sport by having a friend or family member watch the siblings so Juan can participate once or twice a week
- The family should be encouraged to look into park district programs to increase leisure physical activity
- Communicate with physical education teacher to help Juan increase physical activity incorporating appropriate rest breaks and using ventilatory strategies (eg, pursed lip breathing using 1:2 ratio)

AIRWAY CLEARANCE TECHNIQUES

◆ Breathing strategies
- Ventilatory strategies (eg, pursed lip breathing with 1:2 ratio) will be used to help Juan pace his breathing with movement and to enhance his breathing control[63]

◆ Manual/mechanical techniques
- Airway clearance techniques will include self-postural drainage
  - Juan will lie on the left side over his bean bag chair, take deep breaths, and self-percuss his right chest wall[62]
- Instruction will be given in the use of the Flutter device for airway clearance two to three times per day until secretions are no longer a problem[61]

◆ Positioning
- Juan will be instructed in the postural drainage position for the right lower lobe lateral and posterior segments

ANTICIPATED GOALS AND EXPECTED OUTCOMES

♦ Impact on pathology/pathophysiology
  - Pneumonia is resolved.
  - Tissue perfusion and oxygenation are enhanced.

♦ Impact on impairments
  - Aerobic capacity is increased to 20 minutes of walking without dyspnea in 4 weeks.
  - Balance is improved and movement and posture are more efficient at school while using a rolling backpack.
  - Chest wall expansion at the middle chest (4th rib) is increased to 2 inches, and expansion at the lower chest (7th rib/xiphoid) is increased to 2 3/8 inches.
  - Endurance in increased, to enable him to participate in school and after school activities with less dyspnea.
  - Energy expenditure per unit of work is decreased.
  - Muscle performance is increased with core muscles increasing to 4+/5 and extremity muscles increasing to 5/5.
  - Participation is increased in physical education classes with decreased dyspnea.
  - Relaxation is increased.
  - ROM of the chest wall is WNL.
  - Ventilation and respiration/gas exchange are improved.
  - Work of breathing is decreased.

♦ Impact on functional limitations
  - Ability to perform physical actions, tasks, and activities related to self-care, school, community, and leisure is improved in 4 to 6 weeks.
  - Enjoyment is found with increased activity, and participation is increased in school, physical education, and community activities.

♦ Risk reduction/prevention
  - Cardiovascular and pulmonary risk behaviors are reduced for the whole family (smoking cessation, improved nutrition and hydration, increased physical activity).
  - Parents will cooperate with no smoking around the children to prevent the effects of secondhand smoke until they are able to quit smoking.
  - Understanding is increased regarding the need for hydration in order to promote airway/normal mucociliary clearance to prevent further infections.

♦ Impact on health, wellness, and fitness
  - Client will help the siblings and parents to become more active as a family unit and to adopt increasingly healthy lifestyle choices to promote lifelong health as the primary goal.
  - Health status is improved through cessation of smoking, good nutrition, weight control, physical activity, and optimal hydration to maintain optimal mucociliary clearance and prevent further infection.
  - Physical capacity is increased.
  - Physical function is improved.

♦ Patient/client satisfaction
  - Sense of well-being is improved.

REEXAMINATION

Reexamination is performed throughout the episode of care.

DISCHARGE

Juan is discharged from physical therapy after a total of 6 physical therapy sessions, 4 following the hospitalization and 1 session each at 3 and 6 months to give time for behavior change and compliance and attainment of his goals and expectations. These sessions have covered his entire episode of care. He is discharged because he has achieved his goals and expected outcomes.

PSYCHOLOGICAL ASPECTS

The family's income is low, and they have needed Juan to help care for siblings. This has reduced Juan's ability to participate in park or school activities. The parents may be tired, and it may be difficult to motivate them to get the entire family more active (eg, walk after dinner, walk in the mall, participate in park activities). They may also have difficulty quitting smoking, especially since initially they may not be motivated to stop. It is imperative that the parents understand the risk factors, and repeated discussions may be necessary to make sure they are clear and understood.

Juan needs to take personal responsibility for his health. At this age, he can be treated like a responsible person making his own choices toward achieving a healthy lifestyle. This is a teachable moment, as Juan has been having more and more colds and now a recent bout with pneumonia. He is short of breath and wants to feel better and not have this recur. The fact that he was discouraged about his health can be a motivator for change, so education can play a major role in enhancing a healthier lifestyle.

Case Study #2: Shortness of Breath and Post-Debridement of Right Knee

Mr. Philip Jameson is a 29-year-old male postright knee arthroscopic debridement, who is a "weekend warrior."

PHYSICAL THERAPIST EXAMINATION

HISTORY

♦ General demographics: Mr. Jameson is a 29-year-old white male high school graduate, whose primary language is English. He is right-hand dominant.

♦ Social history: He was recently divorced and has no children. He cooks infrequently and often relies on buying fast food on the way to and from work.

♦ Employment/work: He is a long distance truck driver. He reports that it is a stressful job; however, the pay and benefits are good.

♦ Living environment: He lives on the second floor of an apartment building with an elevator, which he uses on a regular basis.

♦ General health status
  • General health perception: Mr. Jameson feels that his health is "OK." He understands that he is overweight and needs to stop smoking and probably should "eat better" and indicates he is ready to institute change.
  • Physical function: He does not exercise during the week, but engages in sport activities on occasional weekends.
  • Psychological function: Normal, although he states that he is saddened about his divorce, but reports he is "moving on."
  • Role function: Truck driver, son, brother, and friend.
  • Social function: He socializes with friends and plays football and basketball occasionally on the weekends. He also enjoys playing on the computer and reading. He attends church on Sundays.

♦ Social/health habits: Mr. Jameson has had a 30-packs-a-year smoking history. He has tried to quit "cold turkey," but states he has not succeeded beyond a few days. He eats many meals outside the home, usually opting for fast food.

♦ Family history: His father, who was a heavy smoker, died of a massive heart attack at 40 years of age. Recently, his mother, who is 48 years of age and a nonsmoker, was diagnosed with CAD. Two weeks ago, his 32-year-old brother underwent an exercise stress test to evaluate complaints of chest pain. Further testing is scheduled. Mr. Jameson expressed concern that his brother may also have had a heart attack as did his father.

♦ Medical/surgical history: Mr. Jameson's medical history is unremarkable. Prior to this injury, he had visited a doctor only once and that was for a chest infection. He has not had any prior hospitalizations or previous surgeries until this episode.

♦ Preexisting medical and other health-related conditions: He has had a history of frequent colds, and last year he required antibiotics for pneumonia. He reports having heartburn about three to four times weekly. His bowel habits are normal.

♦ Current condition(s)/chief complaint(s): Mr. Jameson was injured during a basketball game with friends 3 weeks ago. He underwent arthroscopic surgery for debridement of his right knee. His postarthroscopic course was uneventful. He is motivated to return to work, as his sick time is limited.

♦ Functional status and activity level: Mr. Jameson was an avid sports participant during all of his junior and senior high school years. After that, he participated in sports activities less and less, as he worked more and more. Currently, he participates occasionally in a weekend game of basketball or football, but has been experiencing more shortness of breath, since he has put on 40 lbs since graduation from high school. He is able to complete all ADL; however, he performs them slowly and with mild shortness of breath. He is concerned about his return to work.

♦ Medications: He is currently taking Tylenol PM at night so he can sleep, and he takes Tylenol as needed during the day for pain relief. When he has heartburn, he will take an antacid.

♦ Other clinical tests: Resting and postprandial blood sugars are within the high normal range.

SYSTEMS REVIEW

♦ Cardiovascular/pulmonary
  • BP: 140/84 mmHg
  • Edema: Right knee is mildly edematous
  • HR: 80 bpm
  • RR: 16 bpm
♦ Integumentary
  • Presence of scar formation: Portals appear to be healing well
  • Skin color: Good
  • Skin integrity: WNL

- Musculoskeletal
  - Gross range of motion: WNL except right knee decreased flexion/extension
  - Gross strength: WNL except right knee
  - Gross symmetry: Symmetrical
  - Height: 5'10" (1.78 m)
  - Weight: 210 lbs (95.26 kg)
- Neuromuscular
  - Balance: Within functional limits (WFL), slightly altered as a result of arthroscopic debridement
  - Locomotion, transfers, and transitions: Movement at times appears a little uncomfortable
- Communication, affect, cognition, language, and learning style: WNL
  - Learning preferences: Hands-on active learning style and a tactile learner

TESTS AND MEASURES

- Aerobic capacity/endurance
  - 6-Minute Walk test
    - He was only able to walk 1200 feet (365.8 m) in 6 minutes because of his knee problem
      - Range is reported to be from 1312 to 2297 feet (400 to 700 m) in healthy adults, and approximately 1903 feet (580 m) for healthy men
      - Gender specific reference equations for the 6-minute walk distance for men=(7.57 x heigh_{cm}) – (5.02 x age) – (1.76 x weight_{kg}) – 309 m, and for women=(2.11 x height_{cm}) – (2.29 x weight_{kg}) (5.78 x age) + 667 m[78]
    - HR at rest was 80 bpm and rose to 102 bpm after walk
    - BP at rest was 140/84 mmHg and rose to 158/86 mmHg after walk
    - Recovery time was 5 minutes
    - Right knee pain increased from 1/10 at rest to 3/10 at termination of 6-Minute Walk test using the numeric pain rating scale (NPR) where 0=no pain and 10=worst possible pain[79]
- Anthropometric characteristics
  - His BMI=30.2, which indicates that he is obese[61]
  - Waist to hip ratio
    - His waist girth=39 inches (measured the waist at the smaller circumference of the natural waist)
    - His hip girth=39 inches (measured the circumference of the hips at the widest part of the buttocks)
    - His body shape is "apple shaped," which indicates he has more weight around his waist and has the potential for more health risks

- His waist to hip ratio is 1.00, which appears to indicate an increased risk for metabolic syndrome, heart disease, and diabetes[80]
- Arousal, attention, and cognition
  - He is alert, oriented, and motivated for rehabilitation and return to work
- Circulation
  - Normal reperfusion time
  - Capillary refill time: Slowed bilaterally in the LEs (R>L)
  - Auscultation revealed both S1 and S2, but no S3 or S4
- Ergonomics and body mechanics
  - He uses the armrests of the chair to assist in going from sit to stand primarily due to his obesity
  - Poor body mechanics during daily activities
  - Poor sitting posture, including slumped posture with forward head and rounded back
- Gait, locomotion, and balance
  - He ambulates independently
  - His steps are slightly unequal, and he demonstrates a slightly shortened stride length
  - He has decreased heel/toe on right
  - He has slight difficulty balancing unsupported on right lower extremity (RLE)
- Muscle performance
  - Both UEs and left lower extremity (LLE): WNL
  - Right knee flexion: 4/5
  - Right knee extension: 4-/5
  - Trunk flexors and extensors: WNL
- Pain
  - His resting pain was graded as 1/10 on the NPR (ranging from 0=no pain to 10=worst possible pain)[71]
  - Pain increases to 3/10 on exertion, transition activities, and during ADL
- Posture
  - His posture is habitually slumped in sitting and standing
  - He has a slightly increased thoracic curve and a slightly forward head and neck
- Range of motion
  - Overall ROM of UEs and LEs: WNL, except right knee
  - Right knee extension: -10 degrees
  - Right knee flexion: -10 to 95 degrees
- Self-care and home management
  - Interview reveals that he performs all ADL independently

- Since his debridement, he reports some difficulty and more shortness of breath with climbing stairs, but he does not require assistance
- He has microwave meals in the freezer and buys fast food when he goes out

♦ Ventilation and respiration/gas exchange
- Auscultation revealed coarse breath sounds somewhat decreased at bases
- Dyspnea noted and appears to be related to deconditioning

♦ Work, community, and leisure integration or reintegration
- Interview revealed that Mr. Jameson is concerned about returning to his job as a truck driver because he relies on his right knee to move from the accelerator to the brake, which has residual limited range and decreased muscle strength
- His shortness of breath is a further concern, as he is feeling more fatigued than usual
- He is unable to participate in previous sport activities at this time (eg, basketball and football)

EVALUATION

Mr. Jameson is a 29-year-old obese male, who is 4 weeks status/post arthroscopic debridement of his right knee and has residual decreased ROM of the right knee with pain, which increases with exertion, with transition activities, and during ADL. He is experiencing dyspnea with moderate exertion. He has several modifiable risk factors for cardiovascular and pulmonary disease and diabetes including smoking, poor nutrition, being overweight, and inactivity. Although he is ambulating independently using a straight cane, his gait is abnormal (increased sway) with asymmetrical stride length, and his oxygen consumption is correspondingly increased.

DIAGNOSIS

Mr. Jameson is an obese occasional weekend athlete, who has undergone an arthroscopic debridement of his right knee, has slight knee pain, and is at risk for cardiovascular and pulmonary disease. He has impaired: aerobic capacity/ endurance; anthropometric characteristics; circulation; ergonomics and body mechanics; gait, locomotion, and balance; muscle performance; posture; range of motion; and ventilation and respiration/gas exchange. He is functionally limited in self-care and home management and in work, community, and leisure actions, tasks, and activities. These findings are consistent with placement in Pattern A: Primary Prevention/ Risk Reduction for Cardiovascular/Pulmonary Disorders and in Musculoskeletal Pattern I: Impaired Joint Mobility,

Motor Function, Muscle Performance, and Range of Motion Associated With Bony or Soft Tissue Surgery.[81] These impairments and functional limitations will be addressed in determining the prognosis and the plan of care.

PROGNOSIS AND PLAN OF CARE

Over the course of the visits, the following mutually established outcomes have been determined:
♦ Ability to perform ADL is improved
♦ Aerobic capacity is increased
♦ Endurance is increased
♦ Energy expenditure per unit of work is decreased
♦ Gait, locomotion, and balance are improved
♦ Muscle performance is increased
♦ Pain is decreased
♦ Physical capacity is improved
♦ Posture is improved
♦ Risk factors are reduced
♦ ROM is increased
♦ Targeted behavior change strategies are adopted
♦ Understanding of risk factors for cardiovascular and pulmonary disease and diabetes is increased

To achieve these outcomes, the appropriate interventions for this patient are determined. These will include: coordination, communication, and documentation; patient/client-related instruction; therapeutic exercise; functional training in self-care and home management; and functional training in work, community, and leisure integration or reintegration.

Based on the diagnosis and prognosis, Mr. Jameson is expected to require between 12 to 18 visits over a 6-month period of time. Six months of reinforcement is recommended to develop new behavior patterns consistent with a healthier lifestyle. In this example, Mr. Jameson has good social support, is motivated, and will follow through with his home exercise program. He is not severely impaired and is generally healthy.

INTERVENTIONS

RATIONALE FOR SELECTED INTERVENTIONS

Individuals are referred to physical therapists for primary musculoskeletal, neuromuscular, and integumentary diseases, disorders, and conditions and at the same time may have risk factors or existing comorbidities affecting the cardiovascular and pulmonary systems. During the examination and evaluation of any of the other systems, the cardiovascular and pulmonary risk factors must be identified and appropriate interventions planned to prevent or improve them. Prevention of diseases due to lack of exercise, poor diet, and smoking related conditions are essential in today's health services environment. Often individuals know that they should practice a healthy lifestyle and make good food choices, yet do not follow through and make the necessary changes.[13] Physical therapists need to increasingly focus on moving individuals to daily regimes of healthy lifestyles and fitness.

When an individual has a surgical procedure (as with this case), the short-term interventions for the musculoskeletal system will rectify any impairments that result from the original injury and follow-up surgery. However, if risk factors that may have long-term ramifications for cardiovascular and pulmonary dysfunction are identified, they must be addressed for long-term health. A modest reduction in cardiac risk factors through lifestyle changes may reduce the risk of cardiovascular disease and prevent metabolic syndrome.[9,22] Adopting healthy practices will also ease the many burdens of chronic disease on society.[82]

Patient/Client-Related Instruction

A sedentary lifestyle and poor nutritional choices in combination with stress, tobacco use, and excessive alcohol consumption are the causes of the "diseases of civilization" in high-income countries. They pose a great threat to public health, because they result in increased cardiovascular disease, peripheral vascular disease, COPD, stroke, diabetes, cancer, and osteoporosis.[3] Yet with moderate lifestyle changes, significant risk factor reduction and improved quality of life have been noted.[38] Mr. Jameson will need education about risk factor reduction and how to fit these changes into his life and work. Understanding the benefits of physical activity for his short-term rehabilitation program for his knee and for his long-term risk reduction program will promote a more healthy lifestyle.[25] Evidence exists that when physical therapists counsel their clients about risk reduction, they are more likely to change poor health habits, leading to a healthier lifestyle.[83]

Therapeutic Exercise

Exercise is the key intervention for strengthening and endurance in conjunction with smoking cessation, optimal nutrition, weight control, and stress management.[25] The health benefits of regular exercise are innumerable. Mortality and age-related morbidity are decreased, function and quality of life are enhanced, and cardiovascular/pulmonary, musculoskeletal, neuromuscular including neurocognitive function, and endocrine functions are improved.[84,85] The regular participation in aerobic conditioning and strength training exercise programs has been shown to increase levels of functional capabilities, facilitate maintenance of independence, and therefore, improve quality of life.[86]

Aerobic conditioning/endurance training improves cardiovascular/pulmonary function in multiple ways. It increases: CO, SV, maximum heart rate (MHR),[87] VO_2 max, max O_2 pulse, systolic BP,[88,89] endurance,[90] anaerobic threshold,[91] arterial flow capacity, the caliber of the arterial vessels,[92] systemic arterial compliance, left ventricular performance,[93] lipid profiles,[84] and tonic vagal modulation of the cardiac period.[94] It decreases HR and perceived exertion during exercise.[88]

Aerobic conditioning activities, such as running, rowing, and walking, and resistance strength training exercises have been shown to be inversely associated with the risk of CHD.[95] Performing paced breathing during aerobic conditioning may augment endurance. Strength training programs increase endurance performance and decrease BP in hypertensive individuals.[96,97] Both aerobic conditioning/endurance exercises and resistance strength training exercises appear to be beneficial in reducing body fat, and resistance exercises also appear to increase fat-free mass.[74]

While studies have shown that the changes in respiratory function are less profound than cardiac function,[87] exercise training increases ventilation.[88]

Postural exercises will also be incorporated into his exercise program. Postural slumping may contribute to shortness of breath since it rounds the posterior chest wall, decreasing its ability to provide stability and in turn decreasing the ability of the anterior chest to be sufficiently mobile to facilitate breathing. Core strengthening exercises for the abdominals and back extensor muscles will be utilized to improve posture, endurance, and breathing.[48]

Currently, the Centers for Disease Control and Prevention (CDC) and the American College of Sports Medicine (ACSM) recommend engaging in at least 30 minutes of physical activity 5 days a week. The physical activity for Mr. Jameson will incorporate these guidelines and will include: moderate-intensity aerobic conditioning/endurance training at a frequency of 3 to 5 days/week with each session having a duration of at least 30 minutes; strength training/resistance exercises done 2 to 3 days/week; and flexibility/stretching exercises done daily.[98,99]

Thus, optimal outcomes will be reached by combining the short-term rehabilitation program for Mr. Jameson's knee with the long-term lifestyle changes that incorporate physiological monitoring of exercise and activity to promote long-term gains.[44]

COORDINATION, COMMUNICATION, AND DOCUMENTATION

Communication will occur with Mr. Jameson and his family regarding all components of his program to engender support for his program. Mr. Jameson will be advised to see his physician for his elevated BP. A referral will be made to a nutritionist for weight control and for a heart healthy diet. All elements of the client's management will be documented.

PATIENT/CLIENT-RELATED INSTRUCTION

Mr. Jameson will be instructed in the risk factors for cardiovascular and pulmonary disease and diabetes.[3,9,15,16,22] In addition, he will be provided with information regarding the importance of strength and endurance exercises, the necessity of smoking cessation, and the need for diet and activity changes. Several options will be presented to him for cigarette cessation, including the use of nicotine patches, gum, spray, group support, Smoke Enders, or online/telephone support. Instruction will also be provided in ways to deal with his stressful job. The food pyramid will be reviewed with Mr. Jameson, and methods will be found to wean him off refined foods, salt, and sugar. He will also be given instructions as to how to read food labels. He will be instructed to maintain a physical activity and exercise log and to complete the entries on a regular basis (eg, weight and waist girth; type, intensity, and duration of physical activity and exercise).

THERAPEUTIC EXERCISE

- ◆ Aerobic capacity/endurance conditioning
  - • Progressive walking program with a goal of moderate-intensity activity 30 minutes at least five times per week
- ◆ Parameters for aerobic capacity/endurance conditioning[91]
  - • Mode
    - ▪ Aerobic
    - ▪ Use of large muscles
    - ▪ Continuous or for prolonged period
    - ▪ Examples: Walking, treadmill, bicycle, climbing machine, elliptical trainer, hiking
  - • Duration
    - ▪ Minimum of 20 to 30 minutes before any other parameters are altered
    - ▪ Increase duration progressively
    - ▪ Goal is a minimum of 40 to 50 minutes
  - • Intensity
    - ▪ Determine the training intensity—for example, usually 60%, 70%, or 80%, but may be much lower depending on his fitness level
    - ▪ Determine the MHR=220 minus the age
    - ▪ Determine the target heart rate (THR): THR=MHR minus the resting resting heart rate (RHR) times the training intensity (%) + RHR
    - ▪ Teach client to count pulse at rest and during exercise
    - ▪ Determine appropriate perceived exertion
      - ▸ Perceived exertion—Borg Scale (linear scale)[100]
        - ○ Borg 15-point linear scale
        - ○ 6
        - ○ 7=Very, very light
        - ○ 8
        - ○ 9=Very light
        - ○ 10
        - ○ 11=Fairly light
        - ○ 12
        - ○ 13=Moderately hard
        - ○ 14
        - ○ 15=Hard
        - ○ 16
        - ○ 17=Very hard
        - ○ 18
        - ○ 19=Very, very hard
        - ○ 20=Exhaustion
  - • Frequency
    - ▪ Start with three to four times per week unless period of exercise is less than 15 minutes
    - ▪ Progress to six times a week (ideally)
    - ▪ If walking program is selected, strive for 3 miles in 45 minutes, 5 to 6 days a week
    - ▪ Swimming or walking in a therapeutic pool for at least 30 minutes is another option for increasing aerobic capacity in light of his arthroscopic debridement
- ◆ Balance, coordination, and agility training
  - • Challenge the client's center of gravity and give him improved body awareness and proprioception for position in space through balance and proprioceptive activities
  - • Equipment may include the use of foam rubber mats, a balance board, or a mini-trampoline
  - • Tossing a ball or providing resistance may be added while performing balance activities
- ◆ Body mechanics and postural stabilization
  - • Body mechanics training
    - ▪ Since postural slumping may be the cause of some of his dyspnea, Phillip will be instructed in more effective posture and the relationship of posture to improved breathing
    - ▪ Instruct patient to keep chin and stomach in, and pinch lower scapula borders pinched together
    - ▪ Instructions in sitting, standing, ADL, and IADL, especially bending and lifting
    - ▪ Instructions for sitting while truck driving
    - ▪ Energy conservation techniques will be reviewed
  - • Postural control training and postural stabilization exercises: Axial extension of head, slight scapula retraction, and abdominal contraction to improve posture, endurance, and breathing
    - ▪ Elbow press back: Sitting, standing against wall

- Elbow press down: Supine with forearms up
- Abdominal strengthening: Isometrics, on Styrofoam rollers building to core stabilization coordinated with arm and leg movements, sitting knees up and 1/2 lower downs (eccentric contractions)
- Bridging: Add leg movement
- Quadruped: Neutral spine, coordinate with arm and leg movements
- Prone: On elbows, press up
- Prone: Plank position, modified push-ups
- Sitting: Stomach in; chin in; arms up; elbow press back; pectoralis stretch
- Exercise ball: Arm and leg exercises with trunk stabilization
- Standing: Posture, arm pull-downs
- Standing: "W" position of arms, wall slide
- Postural alignment during gait, may use a book or pillow on top of head to facilitate alignment
- Posture awareness training
  - Notes all around home, car, truck
  - Use mirror for visual input of appropriate alignment

- Flexibility exercises
  - Stretching exercises should be done after warming up, using a slow and steady stretch accompanied by deep breathing, and building hold up to 30 to 60 seconds
  - Knee wall slides
    - Client supine with the feet against the wall and with the hips and knees flexed to 90 degrees
    - Slide foot toward floor to increase knee flexion
  - Quad sets to increase knee extension
  - Corner stretch for stretch anterior chest
  - Trunk ROM
  - A bicycle will be used to gain knee ROM peddling both forward and backward
  - Sport-specific stretching program prior to return to participation in basketball and football activities (eg, hamstrings, gastroc/soleus, quadriceps, hip flexors, low back)

- Gait and locomotion training
  - Ambulation training full weightbearing with corrections for any gait deviations

- Relaxation
  - Phillip will be instructed to take time out to purposely relax and breathe to improve overall relaxation during the day, rather than waiting until feeling stressed
  - He will learn to be aware of the stress in his neck and shoulders and be able to do shoulder shrugs, shoulder rolls, and neck stretches to relieve the tension, thus incorporating relaxation into his lifestyle
  - Visualization and imagery may also be used to induce total relaxation
  - Instruction in Jacobson's relaxation techniques with emphasis on breathing may also be incorporated into his relaxation training

- Strength, power, and endurance training
  - Exercises for knee will include quad sets, straight leg raises, closed kinetic chain exercises, stairs, and use of the StairMaster to increase strength, power, and endurance
  - Breathing exercises using an inspiratory training device to increase strength and endurance of the respiratory muscles
  - Begin with mat progressive resistive exercises with free weights or elastic bands (arm press-ups, flys, overheads, scapula adduction and depression) for UE and trunk strengthening
  - UE weight training program with free weights, elastic bands, or machines (eg, overhead press, upright row, shoulder shrugs, shoulder flexion, shoulder abduction, shoulder extension [latissimus], elbow flexion and extension, wrist flexion and extension)
  - LE weight training program with free weights, elastic bands, or machines (eg, squats, lunges, hip flexion, hip extension, hip abduction, hip adduction, hip external and internal rotation, heel rises)
  - Sport-specific training as his knee improves so that he can return to basketball and football: Carioca, lateral movements, "Z" runs, shuttle runs, simulation of throwing activities progressing to weighted balls

FUNCTIONAL TRAINING IN SELF-CARE AND HOME MANAGEMENT

- Self-care
  - Awareness of posture and chest wall mobility during all ADL
  - Use breathing strategies (eg, pursed lip breathing with 1:2 ratio of inspiration to expiration to pace breathing with activities) to perform activities that make him dyspneic

- Home management
  - Stocking and maintaining healthy food choices at home that can be easily prepared
  - Climb stairs instead of using elevator
  - Walk to market whenever possible and carry loads equally weighted in both hands
  - Purchase home exercise equipment (eg, stationary bicycle or treadmill, free weights)

FUNCTIONAL TRAINING IN WORK, COMMUNITY, AND LEISURE INTEGRATION OR REINTEGRATION

- ◆ Work
  - Make healthy food choices at work and limit fast food consumption
  - Review postural alignment and postural changes to perform when driving the truck and encourage use of a lumbar support pillow
  - Perform isometric exercises (eg, elbow press backs, quad sets) in truck when stopped at a traffic light
  - Stop driving the truck after 1 hour and perform ROM and strengthening exercise for the LEs and walk 5 to 10 minutes
  - Have a jump rope in the truck so he can either walk or jump rope for aerobic conditioning while on overnight runs
- ◆ Leisure
  - Mr. Jameson must find leisure activities that are more aerobically conditioning than his usual activities of basketball and football (eg, walking, bicycling, swimming)
  - Schedule endurance activity so he performs the activity 5 days a week
  - Identify friends with interests in health promotion with whom to share these activities and build socializing around fitness activities
  - Return to normal leisure activities (eg, basketball and football) when fully conditioned to do so

ANTICIPATED GOALS AND EXPECTED OUTCOMES

- ◆ Impact on pathology/pathophysiology
  - Physiological response to increased oxygen demand is improved.
  - Symptoms associated with increased oxygen demand are decreased.
- ◆ Impact on impairments
  - Balance is improved so patient can stand unsupported on RLE.
  - Endurance is increased, and Mr. Jameson is able to walk 1900 feet within 6 minutes.
  - Muscle performance is increased so that knee flexion and extension are WNL.
  - Posture is improved.
  - ROM is increased in knee flexion/extension so that he is able to return to work safely.
  - Shortness of breath with activity is lessened after smoking cessation and weight loss.
  - Weightbearing status is improved so that patient no longer requires an assistive device.
- ◆ Impact on functional limitations
  - All ADL are performed with minimal dyspnea.
  - All physical activities needed for work and home management are resumed.
  - Gait is improved without the use of an assistive device.
- ◆ Risk reduction/prevention
  - Healthy lifestyle behaviors are adopted and maintained to prevent cardiovascular and pulmonary disease and diabetes.
  - Risk factors are understood and reduced for cardiovascular and pulmonary diseases and diabetes.
  - Weekend activities are safely performed as a result of increased LE strength and stretching prior to and after engaging in sport activities.
- ◆ Impact on health, wellness, and fitness
  - Exercise and increased activity are incorporated into his daily routine.
  - Fitness and health are improved.
  - Physical capacity is improved.
  - Physical function is improved and will continue to improve.
  - Targeted behavioral changes are adopted including quitting smoking, improved nutrition, optimal weight, and increased activity.
- ◆ Patient/client satisfaction
  - Sense of well-being is improved.
  - Stress is decreased and managed more effectively.

REEXAMINATION

Reexamination is performed throughout the episode of care.

DISCHARGE

Mr. Jameson is discharged from physical therapy after a total of 14 physical therapy sessions and attainment of his goals and expectations. These sessions have covered his entire episode of care. He is discharged because he has achieved goals and expected outcomes.

PSYCHOLOGICAL ASPECTS

Healthy lifestyle behaviors will be adopted as Mr. Jameson is concerned that he may have a heart condition like his father, mother, and now brother. He understands the risk factors and wants to be healthy and to decrease his health risk. He is motivated and believes he can change his behaviors and make a difference.

Case Study #3: Congestive Heart Failure and Pneumonia-Related Shortness of Breath

Mrs. Sarah Wilson is a 72-year-old female with dyspnea posthospitalization for acute congestive heart failure and pneumonia.

PHYSICAL THERAPIST EXAMINATION

HISTORY

♦ General demographics: Mrs. Wilson is a 72-year-old black American female. She is right-hand dominant.

♦ Social history: She is a widow, who has three children and seven grandchildren. Two of her sons live in other states. Her daughter lives 10 minutes away and visits her mother once every couple of weeks. Her husband died 2 months ago.

♦ Employment/work: She is a retired librarian, who had a books-on-wheels program in her seniors' community and managed the in-house library.

♦ Living environment: Mrs. Wilson has lived in a seniors' community in the assisted living section for the last 5 years.

♦ General health status
  • General health perception: She considers herself to be in poor to fair health at this time.
  • Physical function: Mrs. Wilson is unable to walk to meals secondary to dyspnea and weakness. She needs assistance with dressing and meals. She is now using a cane all the time.
  • Psychological function: Adjusting to her husband's death has been difficult for her. She admits to feeling "down," depressed, and quite alone and isolated since her husband's death 2 months ago. She states that she doesn't feel like doing anything and wishes people would just leave her alone.
  • Role function: Mother, grandmother, librarian, friend.
  • Social function: She had been quite active in her assisted living community and was responsible for managing the library. She had a books-on-wheels program for the residents, who were physically unable to come to the library. Socially she and her husband participated in most activities together as a couple. She has many acquaintances in the community but few friends.

♦ Social/health habits: She had a 120-pack-a-year smoking history, but she quit 2 years ago. She drinks an occasional glass of wine (one to two times per week).

♦ Family history: Her father died of an MI at 75 years of age. Her mother died at 80 due to complications of a single pin open reduction and internal fixation of a hip fracture.

♦ Medical/surgical history: Mrs. Wilson was diagnosed with COPD 5 years ago and has been seeing her pulmonologist once a year. Her general practitioner has been monitoring her during the interim times. Two years ago she had a MI. Her cardiac status was well controlled until 2 months ago, when her husband died, and she indicated that she had been "forgetting" to take her medications. Over the past 2 months prior to the hospitalization she experienced increased dyspnea and had decreased her activities. She gained 10 pounds in the last week. One week ago she was hospitalized and diagnosed with acute CHF. She is now being followed by home care after this hospitalization for acute CHF and pneumonia.

♦ Prior hospitalizations: She was hospitalized for the birth of each of her children. Thirty years ago she had an appendectomy. She was hospitalized 3 years ago for pneumonia, and 2 years ago when she sustained her MI.

♦ Preexisting medical and other health-related conditions: She has COPD and a history of a MI. She reported having diarrhea weekly and complains of urinary urgency with some dribbling. Mrs. Wilson wears bifocal eyeglasses, and her hearing is WNL.

♦ Current condition(s)/chief complaint(s): Mrs. Wilson is experiencing dyspnea during low intensity activity. She is using her cane more frequently because she feels weaker and less confident when walking. She reports feeling "down" and that it is hard to get motivated to do anything.

♦ Functional status and activity level: She has exercised minimally in the past 2 months. She had enjoyed spending time with her grandchildren, who reside close by, but lately they have had to come to her apartment because she chooses to go out less. She reports that she is less able to actively play with them. The home care agency is sending an aide to her home three times per week to assist with bathing. Her daughter has hired a companion to stay with her mother for a few weeks to help with dressing, meals, and observation for safety, as well as to socialize. She is unable to walk to meals secondary to dyspnea and weakness. Mrs. Wilson is now using a cane all the time. Prior to the hospitalization she only used it for longer walks in the community and in the shopping mall. She has little interest in participating in activities in the retirement community.

♦ Medications: She is currently on digoxin, lasix, and antibiotics.

♦ Other clinical tests:

- Pulmonary function tests: FEV_1=65% predicted, FVC= 88% predicted, and FEV_1/FVC=80 % predicted

- Arterial blood gases: Indicate compensated respiratory acidosis

  - pH=7.33 (normal: 7.35 to 7.45)
  - pCO_2=48 mmHg (normal: 35 to 45 mmHg)
  - pO_2=76 mmHg (normal: 80 to 100 mmHg)
  - Base excess/base deficit (BE/BD)=-2 mEq/L (normal: -2 to +2),
  - Hematocrit (Hct)=48% (normal: 37% to 47%)
  - White blood cell count (WBC)=4.0 (normal: 4.2 to 5.4 million/mm³)
  - Hgb=11 g/dl (normal: 12 to 16 g/dL)
  - SpO2 at rest=92% (normal: 95% to 100%)

- DEXA test: Done 2 years ago indicated osteopenia (T score=-1.75, normal T score: Better than -1)

SYSTEMS REVIEW

♦ Cardiovascular/pulmonary

- BP: 110/70 mmHg
- Edema: Mild ankle edema bilaterally
- HR: 110 bpm
- RR: 20 bpm

♦ Integumentary

- Presence of scar formation: Old appendectomy scar
- Skin color: WNL
- Skin integrity: Intact

♦ Musculoskeletal

- Gross range of motion: WFL, slightly decreased shoulder flexion bilaterally
- Gross strength: Generalized weakness in both UE and LE
- Gross symmetry: Symmetrical
- Height: 5'3" (1.6 m)
- Weight: 106 lbs (48.09 kg)

♦ Neuromuscular

- Balance: WFL
- Locomotion, transfers, and transitions: WFL but is unsteady when turning

♦ Communication, affect, cognition, language, and learning style:

- Communication, affect, and cognition: Affect rather flat, communication WNL, and cognition WNL
- Learning preferences: Visual learner

TESTS AND MEASURES

♦ Aerobic capacity/endurance

- 6-Minute Walk test
  - Walked 70 feet (21.35 m) with dyspnea on Borg Scale that increased from 8/19 at rest to 13/19 after walk (range is reported to be from 1312 to 2297 feet [400 to 700 m] in healthy adults, and approximately 1640 feet [500 m] for healthy women)[78]
  - HR at rest was 110 bpm and increased to 132 bpm after walk
  - BP was 110/70 mmHg at rest and increased to 122/72 mmHg after walk
  - Vital signs recovery time after walk to baseline was 12 minutes

♦ Anthropometric characteristics

- BMI=weight (lbs) ÷ height (inches) ÷ height (inches) x 703)[61]
- BMI=18.8 (normal: 18.5 to 24.9)

♦ Arousal, attention, and cognition

- Alert and oriented x3
- Motivation poor at this time

♦ Ergonomics and body mechanics

- Observation revealed poor body mechanics during ADL and during ambulation

♦ Circulation

- Pulse exam=110 at rest, which is considered tachycardia
- Pulse is regular
- Auscultation of heart
  - S1 and S2 heard at rest
  - No S3 or S4
- LE dorsalis pedis pulses slightly diminished

♦ Gait, locomotion, and balance

- Observation of gait, locomotion, and balance revealed:
  - Short stride
  - Short arm swing
  - Somewhat unsteady and catches herself on turns
  - Holds on to furniture to walk around her apartment
  - Tends to hold rail in the hallway, which she claims is a "habit" developed lately not for balance, but because she is just "tired"

♦ Muscle performance

- Strength: Overall 4-/5

♦ Posture

- Forward head and neck
- Kyphotic posture

- Slight barrel chest
- Slightly flexed hips and knees
♦ Range of motion
  - Decreased lateral costal chest wall mobility
  - Decreased hip joint extension (-8 degrees), knee joint extension (-5 degrees), and shoulder joint flexion (-10 degrees) bilaterally
♦ Self-care and home management
  - Mrs. Wilson needs minimal help with dressing and meals
  - She also must be observed to ensure safety during ADL and IADL
  - She is unable to walk to meals secondary to dyspnea and weakness and lack of endurance since the dining room is 600 feet from her room
♦ Work, community, and leisure integration or reintegration
  - She is no longer active in her assisted living community, where she had been responsible for managing the library and also for providing a books-on-wheels program for the physically challenged residents
♦ Ventilation and respiration/gas exchange
  - Auscultation of lungs
    - Crackles heard bilaterally at both lower lobes 1/3 way up posterior lung fields, but now resolving
  - Breathing pattern: Primarily upper chest breathing using accessory muscles
  - Cough: Productive of small amount of clear mucus

EVALUATION

Mrs. Wilson has COPD and had sustained a MI. She is deconditioned secondary to lack of activity over the past 2 months, which has been compounded by 5 days of hospitalization. She had gained 10 pounds in the past week. One week ago she was diagnosed with acute CHF. Dyspnea and weakness limit her function. She appears depressed, lacks motivation, and has withdrawn from her usual activities in the retirement community, where she previously reported feeling valued.

DIAGNOSIS

Mrs. Wilson has COPD, CHF, and sustained a MI. She has impaired: aerobic capacity/endurance; anthropometric characteristics; gait, locomotion, and balance; muscle performance; posture; range of motion; and ventilation and respiration/gas exchange. She is functionally limited in self-care and home management and in work, community, and leisure actions, tasks, and activities. These findings are consistent with placement in Pattern A: Primary Prevention/Risk Reduction for Cardiovascular and Pulmonary Disorders and

secondarily in Pattern C: Impaired Ventilation, Respiration/Gas Exchange, and Aerobic Capacity/Endurance Associated With Airway Clearance Dysfunction and Pattern D: Impaired Aerobic Capacity/Endurance Associated With Cardiovascular Pump Dysfunction or Failure. These impairments and functional limitations will be addressed in determining the prognosis and the plan of care.

PROGNOSIS AND PLAN OF CARE

Over the course of the visits, the following mutually established outcomes have been determined:

♦ Affect is improved, and community and family roles are resumed
♦ Awareness of risk factors is improved
♦ Endurance is improved
♦ Gait, locomotion, and balance are improved, and independent ambulation in the building and use of the cane for community ambulation are achieved
♦ Independence in ADL and IADL is achieved
♦ Mrs. Wilson will be able to resume going to meals (eg, 600 feet to the dining area)
♦ Muscle performance is increased
♦ Nutrition and hydration status are improved
♦ Physical and psychological status will be improved

To achieve these outcomes, the appropriate interventions for this patient are determined. These will include: coordination, communication, and documentation; patient/client-related instruction; therapeutic exercise; functional training in self-care and home management; and functional training in work, community, and leisure integration or reintegration.

Based on the diagnosis and prognosis, Mrs. Wilson is expected to require between 10 to 18 visits over an 8-week period of time (twice a week for 4 weeks, then once a week for several weeks). She has been depressed and has co-morbidities that may affect the prognosis.

INTERVENTIONS

RATIONALE FOR SELECTED INTERVENTIONS

About one-fourth of the US population lives with some form of cardiovascular disease, including CHF.[101] Many changes may occur in the heart with age including decreases in the: heart muscle strength, heart size, left ventricular internal diastolic and systolic dimensions, EDVs, pacemaker cells in the sinus node, compliance of the large arteries in the cardiothoracic circulation, CO, SV, peak HR, maximum oxygen consumption, secretion and release of catecholamines, sympathetic nerve activation, receptor sensitivity, tonic vagal modulation of the cardiac period, and cardiovagal baroreflex sensitivity. Increases may occur in the: left ventricular mass and wall thickness, ventricular after-loading, and epicardial fat. The atrial septum and leaflets of the valvular structures thicken. The left atrium and aortic root become dilated.[87,102-106]

The pulmonary system also undergoes changes including decreases in the: ROM of the rib cage articulations, respiratory muscle strength, gas exchange of oxygen and carbon dioxide, elastic fibers, elastic recoil, overall surface area of the alveoli, number of alveoli, alveolar vascularity, rate and quantity of gas exchange, vital capacity, TV, peak airflow, and gas exchange. Increases may occur in the: size of the alveolar ducts, residual volume, ventilation-perfusion imbalance, and breathing frequency.[87,107-112]

Managing risk factors for cardiovascular/pulmonary deconditioning in the elderly is challenging secondary to other comorbidities (eg, COPD and CHF), motivation, and emotional issues (eg, loss of her spouse and her social network and role in the community). Yet promotion of increased activity and a healthy lifestyle can make positive changes in decreasing risk factors in the elderly.[33] Secondary prevention plays a major role in decreasing or slowing the disease progression.[16] In addition, Woo found an improved quality of life in the elderly with more active and healthy lifestyles.[30]

Therapeutic Exercise

Even for individuals with chronic diseases, evidence supports the use of regular exercise consisting of aerobic conditioning and resistance strength training to increase functional capabilities, facilitate maintenance of independence, and improve quality of life.[86,113] The rationale detailed in Case Study #2 provides support for the use of exercise for this client's deconditioning. Of note is the finding that a high-velocity resistance training program increased strength and peak power more than a low-velocity resistance training program in older women.[114]

In addition, gait velocity was improved significantly in older persons who performed postural control exercises and resistance training to fatigue for knee extension, hip abduction, ankle dorsiflexion, hip extension, and knee flexion.[115] For older women, gait velocity and other related gait parameters were increased with LE muscle strength training programs.[116,117] Programs using both strength and endurance training were also shown to result in increased gait velocity in older women.[118]

Even low intensity strength training was observed to result in increased gait stability and especially in mediolateral steadiness in older individuals who were disabled, and gait performance was improved even when only moderate strength gains were achieved.[119]

The exercise prescription for this individual should be based upon the examination results and should be individually specific with appropriate intensity and duration to physically challenge her.[87] The exercise prescription for this individual should incorporate straightforward and fun aerobic conditioning/endurance training, balance training, flexibility exercises, and progressive strength training. The exercise prescription should also be aimed at her health needs, goals, and beliefs.[85] It has been recommended that the exercise prescription for individuals like Mrs. Wilson emphasize gradually progressive activities that are of low to moderate intensity, are low-impact, and avoid heavy static-dynamic lifting. The prescribed training HR for aerobic endurance training is 40% to 80% of MHR reserve (as compared to 50% to 85% of MHR reserve that has been recommended for young and middle-aged individuals).[120]

Mrs. Wilson's exercise programs may be prescribed in a variety of formats from individually performed programs at home to programs in the fitness facility or community center. Community-based programs have been shown to result in improved function and enhanced well-being.[121] Even the use of a videotaped strength training program for use at home was shown to result in increased strength, social functioning, and perceived vigor, and in control of perceived tension and anger.[122]

The frequency of the exercise prescription has also been investigated for individuals of Mrs. Wilson's age. One study had three different groups of elderly women (60 to 75 years of age) exercise for 1 hour over a 12-week period of time once, twice, or three times/week. A fourth group served as the control group. While all three groups had significant increases in muscular endurance, sit and reach flexibility, balance, and coordination, the improvement found in each of the three exercise groups was proportional to the frequency of the program.[123]

Congestive Heart Failure

In addition, data increasingly support the benefits of exercise and increased physical fitness for patients with CHF. Exercise training for patients with CHF has led to significant improvements in maximal, submaximal, and endurance exercise capacity.[124] It also improved systemic arterial compliance in patients with CHF.[125] In addition, exercise for these patients has also been shown to increase quality of life and decrease mortality.[126]

A combination of aerobic exercise and circuit weight training for patients with CHF resulted in increased muscle strength, peak exercise oxygen uptake, exercise test duration, and ventilatory threshold and in a decrease in submaximal exercise HR and rate pressure product.[127] The significant changes in exercise capacity of patients with CHF may be the result of several factors, including increases in CO, skeletal muscle metabolism, peak blood flow to the exercising limb due to the vascular resistance reduction,[128] and arterial function.[125]

Chronic Obstructive Pulmonary Disease

Progressive exercise training and physical activity for patients with COPD improves exercise tolerance and decreases dyspnea, but also enhances functional improvements in ADL and health-related quality of life.[129]

Data indicate that strength training programs for these patients significantly increase their strength, endurance training programs significantly increase their submaximal exercise capacity, while using a program of both strength training and endurance training significantly increases both parameters. Significant improvements were also noted in breathlessness scores and in dyspnea with combined programs of strength and endurance training.[130]

Combined programs of endurance training and progressive resistance strength training for these patients were shown to improve their functional outcomes,[131] their muscle function, and their treadmill walking endurance.[132]

Mental Health

Exercise has been shown to have many positive benefits on mental health particularly in elderly individuals. Aerobic endurance exercise programs have been shown to significantly reduce depressive symptoms in older individuals,[133] and progressive resistance strength training programs have also been shown to be an effective antidepressant in depressed elders.[134,135]

COORDINATION, COMMUNICATION, AND DOCUMENTATION

Mrs. Wilson requires a complete work-up by the team with an integrated management strategy. Her low BMI and heart condition require dietary recommendations from the nutritionist. Dietary information will be reinforced by the physical therapist, who will prescribe a regular physical activity program and a structured exercise program. Mrs. Wilson's medications and their effectiveness are to be reviewed by her physician, and their efficacy will be monitored by the physical therapist as her physical activity increases. Referrals will be made to both a social worker for assessment of her depression and need for further consultation and to a retirement community nutritionist for instruction in ways of maintaining a low sodium diet and a heart healthy diet and in ways to monitor her weight to assess the stability of her CHF management. With Mrs. Wilson's permission, her case will be discussed with the home care nurse and the nurse for the retirement community.

Discussions will occur with the team to ascertain the possible need for skilled care versus assisted living if Mrs. Wilson does not progress sufficiently and if there is inadequate control of the progression of her cardiac and pulmonary manifestations. All elements of the client's management will be documented.

PATIENT/CLIENT-RELATED INSTRUCTION

Mrs. Wilson will be instructed regarding the importance of following her home exercise program and becoming more active in the social and physical activities in the residence. She will understand her medications and the importance of monitoring her diet, weight, and level of dyspnea to maintain control of her CHF.

THERAPEUTIC EXERCISE

- ♦ Aerobic capacity/endurance conditioning
  - During all aerobic/endurance training, vital signs will be monitored and perceived exertion will be determined using the Borg Scale of Perceived Exertion[100]
    - Borg 10-point nonlinear scale
      - 0=Nothing at all
      - 0.5=Very, very light/weak (just noticeable)
      - 1=Very light/weak
      - 2=Light/weak
      - 3=Moderate
      - 4=Somewhat heavy/strong
      - 5=Heavy/strong
      - 6
      - 7=Very heavy/strong
      - 8
      - 9
      - 10=Extremely heavy/strong (almost maximal) *Maximal
    - Borg 15-point linear scale
      - 6
      - 7=Very, very light
      - 8
      - 9=Very light
      - 10
      - 11=Fairly light
      - 12
      - 13=Moderately hard
      - 14
      - 15=Hard
      - 16
      - 17=Very hard
      - 18
      - 19=Very, very hard
      - 20=Exhaustion
  - She will start with a low-impact walking program progressing from low to moderate intensity. Her prescribed training HR for aerobic endurance training will begin at 40% of MHR reserve and progress as her endurance improves

- Walking will progress to walking to one meal, then two, then all three meals and walking to activities and resuming her library cart service
- Mrs. Wilson expressed interest in joining a new dance class to enhance her aerobic capacity

◆ Balance, coordination, and agility training
  - Balance exercise both static and dynamic
    ▪ Standing on one leg
    ▪ Standing and balancing on foam surface
    ▪ Marching in place
    ▪ Side stepping down hallway with light touch on handrail progressing to no support of rail
    ▪ Tandem walking with one hand support on handrail progressing to no rail

◆ Body mechanics and postural stabilization
  - Body mechanics training
    ▪ Appropriate sitting posture for work and leisure activities
    ▪ Appropriate use of body mechanics while working in the library
    ▪ Appropriate lifting and carrying instructions
    ▪ Appropriate bending instructions
  - Postural control training
    ▪ Proper alignment of head, cervical and thoracic spines, shoulders, pelvis, hips, and knees
    ▪ Axial extension
    ▪ Scapula retraction and depression
    ▪ Chicken wing position (hands behind head, horizontal abduction of shoulders)
    ▪ Transition of position from supine to sitting, standing, and walking
    ▪ Transition of position to functional activities during the day
  - Postural stabilization activities
    ▪ Axial extension starting in supine and progressing to sitting and upright
    ▪ Maintenance of axial extension position with bilateral arm raises
    ▪ Maintenance of axial extension position with arm raises with addition of weights, starting, for example, with 1 lb for 8 to 12 reps and increasing accordingly
    ▪ Glut sets
    ▪ Bridging
    ▪ Utilize ball for core stability training
    ▪ Unilateral LE extension in quadruped
    ▪ Incorporate the use of the foam roller and unstable surfaces like foam rubber cushion in standing with bilateral and unilateral stance
  - Postural awareness training

    ▪ Use of mirror for visual input of appropriate alignment
    ▪ Notes all around home

◆ Flexibility exercises
  - Stretching exercises should be done after warming up, using a slow and steady stretch accompanied by deep breathing, and building hold up to 15 to 30 seconds
  - Done two to three times a day, at least two to three repetitions
  - Cervical ROM in all directions
  - Shoulder ROM in all directions
  - Scapula ROM in all directions including diagonals
  - Chest mobility exercises including trunk extension, lateral flexion, and rotation
  - Hip and knee ROM in all directions

◆ Gait and locomotion training
  - Ambulation program with progressive increase in the endurance component
  - Progress to independent walking in the facility and to restricted cane use during community ambulation

◆ Relaxation
  - Pursed lip breathing and pacing to be able to increase her endurance with more controlled breathing
  - Relaxation of accessory muscles of respiration (eg, biofeedback, visual imagery, Jacobsen's techniques) with diaphragmatic breathing
  - Rapid breathing techniques with body relaxation to control bouts of dyspnea

◆ Strength, power, and endurance training
  - During all strength training, vital signs should be monitored and perceived exertion determined using the Borg scale[100]
  - Appropriate breathing techniques will be used to avoid any Valsalva maneuver
  - UE and LE strength training beginning with low weights or light elastic bands and progressing in accordance with Mrs. Wilson's capabilities
  - Breathing exercises to increase the strength of the diaphragm (eg, ventilatory muscle training device)
  - General strengthening and endurance exercises in the resident's daily exercise program, such as group exercise programs, social activities, walking to meals, and resuming her role actively as the residence librarian

FUNCTIONAL TRAINING IN SELF-CARE AND HOME MANAGEMENT

◆ Self-care
  - Mrs. Wilson will be instructed in the performance of all of her self-care activities in her apartment using energy saving techniques (eg, using a terry cloth bathrobe when getting out of the shower)

♦ Home management
  ● She will be able to do basic chores in her apartment with support of the cleaning service from the residence
  ● She will be instructed to sit during as many ADL as feasible
  ● She will be instructed in energy conservation techniques (eg, placing regularly used pots on an easily accessible shelf, using a rolling cart in the kitchen to move things from place to place)

FUNCTIONAL TRAINING IN WORK, COMMUNITY, AND LEISURE INTEGRATION OR REINTEGRATION

♦ Leisure
  ● Mrs. Wilson will participate in increasing leisure activities in the retirement community and with her family
    ▪ Group outings
    ▪ Social events of her choosing
    ▪ Her activities as librarian
    ▪ Participation in family outings and activities with her grandchildren
    ▪ Opportunities to volunteer with other residents to feel more connected and participative in the community
    ▪ Participation in dance classes that have begun in her assisted living community

ANTICIPATED GOALS AND EXPECTED OUTCOMES

♦ Impact on pathology/pathophysiology
  ● Physiological response to increased oxygen demand is improved.
  ● Symptoms associated with increased oxygen demand are decreased.
♦ Impact on impairments
  ● All physical activities needed for work and home management are resumed.
  ● Endurance is increased, and Mrs. Wilson will progressively increase the distance she walks from one meal to three meals per day.
  ● Gait is improved without the use of an assistive device in her apartment and use of a cane for long walks and in the community.
  ● Muscle performance is increased to WFL.
  ● Posture is improved.
  ● Shortness of breath with activity is lessened with ventilatory strategies and energy conservation techniques.

♦ Impact on functional limitations
  ● All ADL are performed with minimal dyspnea.
♦ Risk reduction/prevention
  ● Healthy lifestyle behaviors are adopted and maintained to prevent further cardiovascular and pulmonary disease.
  ● Risk factors are understood and reduced for cardiovascular and pulmonary disease.
  ● Activities are safely performed as a result of increased LE strength.
♦ Impact on health, wellness, and fitness
  ● Exercise and increased activity are incorporated in her daily routine.
  ● Fitness and health are improved.
  ● Physical capacity is improved.
  ● Physical function is improved and will continue to improve.
  ● Targeted behavioral changes are adopted including improved nutrition, optimal weight, and increased activity.
♦ Patient/client satisfaction
  ● Sense of well-being is improved.
  ● A more positive attitude and ability to pursue more social relationships and inclusion into the community will be optimized.

REEXAMINATION

Reexamination is performed throughout the episode of care.

DISCHARGE

Mrs. Wilson is discharged from physical therapy after a total of 12 physical therapy sessions over 8 weeks of home care and attainment of her goals and expectations. These sessions have covered her entire episode of service. She is discharged because she has achieved her goals and expected outcomes.

PSYCHOLOGICAL ASPECTS

Mrs. Wilson has experienced not only the loss of her husband but of his social significance. A social service consult or discussion with the staff may be beneficial to try to get her to verbalize and plan strategies to make more social friendships in the facility and to be more active and participate with residents in meals. She enjoyed her role as librarian, and it gave her a social outlet, so that getting back to that role may help her feelings of being down and give more meaning to her life.

Gaining strength, balance, and endurance will help her feel more independent and confident in her environment. The family can help support her activities and encourage her participation with the grandchildren and her friends in the community.

Family and staff can look for natural connections in the community (eg, other widows) that may help support Mrs. Wilson during this time of transition following her husband's death and her hospitalization.

References

1. Dean E. Epidemiology as a basis for physical therapy. In: Frownfelter DL, Dean E, eds. *Cardiovascular and Pulmonary Physical Therapy: Evidence and Practice.* 4th ed. St. Louis, Mo: Mosby Elsevier; 2006.

2. World Health Organization. *Definition of Health.* Available online at: www.who.int/about/definition. Accessed November 2005.

3. Bijnen FC, Caspersen CJ, Mosterd WL. Physical inactivity as a risk factor for coronary artery disease: a WHO and International Society and Federation of Cardiology position statement. *Bulletin World Health Organization.* 1994;72:1-4.

4. Musaiger AO. Diet and prevention of coronary heart disease in the Arab Middle East countries. *Med Princ Pract.* 2002;11(Suppl 2):9-16.

5. World Health Organization. *Technical report series.* 2003;916: i-vii, 1-149.

6. Heart and Stroke Foundation Canada (2005). Available at: www.heartandstroke.ca. Accessed November 2005.

7. Bradberry JC. Peripheral arterial disease: pathophysiology, risk factors, and role of antithrombotic therapy. *J Am Pharm Assoc.* 2004;44(2 Suppl 1):S37-S44.

8. Charkoudian N, Joyner MJ. Physiologic considerations for exercise performance in women. *Clin Chest Med.* 2004;25:247-255.

9. Cheng A, Braunstein JB, Dennison C, et al. Reducing global risk for cardiovascular disease: using lifestyle changes and pharmacotherapy. *Clin Cardiol.* 2002;25:205-212.

10. Ebrahim S, Smith GD. Exporting failure? Coronary heart disease and stroke in developing countries. *Int J Epidemiol.* 2001;30:201-205.

11. Dean E. A psychobiologic adaptation model of physical therapy practice. *Phys Ther.* 1985;65:158-161.

12. Stretcher VJR, Rosenstock IM. The health belief model. In: Glantz K, Lewis FM, Rimer BK, eds. *Health Behavior and Health Education: Theory, Research and Practice.* San Francisco, Calif: Jossey-Bass; 1997.

13. Steptoe A, Wardle J, Cui W, et al. Trends in smoking, diet, physical exercise, and attitudes toward health in European university students from 13 countries, 1990-2000. *Prev Med.* 2002;35:97-104.

14. McCrindle BW. Cardiovascular risk factors in adolescents: relevance, detection, and intervention. *Adolesc Med.* 2001;12:147-162.

15. Misra A. Risk factors for atherosclerosis in young individuals. *J Cardiovasc Risk.* 2000;7:215-229.

16. Zafari AM, Wenger NK. Secondary prevention of coronary heart disease. *Arch Phys Med Rehabil.* 1998;79:1006-1017.

17. Sakakibara H, Fujii C, Naito M. Plasma fibrinogen and its association with cardiovascular risk factors in apparently healthy Japanese students. *Heart Vessels.* 2004;19:144-148.

18. Anonymous. Your heart attack risk: inflammation counts. *Harvard Women's Health Watch.* 2003;10:1-3.

19. Brod SA. Unregulated inflammation shorts human functional longevity. *Inflammation Res.* 2000;49:561-570.

20. Katz D. The basic (care) and feeding of homosapiens, consensus, controversy, and cluelessness. Proceedings of the Canadian Cardiovascular Congress, Toronto, ON, 2003 (A).

21. Svendsen A. Heart failure: an overview of consensus guidelines and nursing implications. *Can J Cardiovasc Nurs.* 2003; 13:30-34.

22. Scott CL. Diagnosis, prevention, and interventions for the metabolic syndrome. *Am J Cardiol.* 2003;92:35-42.

23. Doyle J, Creager MA. Pharmacotherapy and behavioral intervention for peripheral arterial disease. *Rev Cardiovasc Med.* 2003;4:18-24.

24. AHCPR Supported Clinical Practice Guidelines 2002. Smoking cessation brief clinical interventions. Available at: www.ncbi.nlm.nih.gov. Accessed January 2005.

25. Varo Cenarruzabeita JJ, Martinez Hernandez JA, Martinez-Gonzalez MA. Benefits of physical activity and harms of inactivity. *Medl Clin (Barc).* 2003;121:665-672. (Abstract).

26. Whitt M, Kumanyika S, Bellamy S. Amount and bouts of physical activity in a sample of African-American women. *Med Sci Sport Exerc.* 2003;35:1887-1893.

27. Wilbur J, Chandler PJ, Dancy B, Lee H. Correlates of physical activity in urban Midwestern Latinas. *Am J Prev Med.* 2003b;25:69-76.

28. Nyenhuis DL, Gorelick PB, Easley C, et al. The Black Seventh-Day Adventist exploratory health study. *Ethnicity Dis.* 2003;13:208-212.

29. LaMonte MJ, Eisenman PA, Adams TD, et al. Cardiorespiratory fitness and coronary heart disease risk factors: the LDS Hospital Fitness Institute cohort. *Circulation.* 2000;102:1623-1628.

30. Woo J, Ho SC, Yu AL. Lifestyle factors and health outcomes in elderly Hong Kong Chinese aged 70 years and over. *Gerontology.* 2002;48:234-240.

31. Williams MA, Fleg J, Ades PA, et al. Secondary prevention of coronary heart disease in the elderly (with emphasis on patients > or=75 years of age): an American Heart Association scientific statement from the Council on Clinical Cardiology Subcommittee on Exercise, Cardiac Rehabilitation, and Prevention. *Circulation.* 2002;105:1735-1743.

32. Keller C, Fleury J, Mujezinovic-Womack M. Managing cardiovascular risk reduction in elderly adults. By promoting and monitoring healthy lifestyle changes, health care providers can help older adults improve their cardiovascular health. *J Gerontol Nurs.* 2003;29:18-23.

33. Shapiro JS. Primary prevention of coronary artery disease in women through diet and lifestyle. *N Engl J Med.* 2000;343:16-22.

34. Twisk JW, Kemper HC, van Mechelen W, Post GB. Which lifestyle parameters discriminate high- from low-risk participants for coronary heart disease risk factors. Longitudinal analysis covering adolescence and young adulthood. *J Cardiovasc Risk.* 1997;4:393-400.

35. Macken LC, Yates B, Blancher S. Concordance of risk factors in female spouses of male patients with coronary artery disease. *J Cardiopulm Rehabil.* 2000;20:361-368.

36. Paterno CA. Coronary risk factors in adolescence. The FRICELA study. *Revista Espanda de Cardiologia.* 2003;56:452-458. (English abstract).

37. Sleight P. Cardiovascular risk factors and the effects of intervention. *Am Heart J.* 1991;121:990-994.

38. Mokdad AH, Marks JS, Stroup DF, Gerberding JL. Actual causes of death in the United States, 2000. *JAMA.* 2004;291:1238-1245.

39. Shaw M, Mitchell R, Dorling D. Time for a smoke? One cigarette reduces your life my 11 minutes. *BMJ.* 2000;36:297-298.

40. Yohannes AM, Hardy CC. Treatment of chronic obstructive pulmonary disease in older patients: a practical guide. *Drugs Aging.* 2003;20:209-228.

41. Mozaffarian D, Fried LP, Burk GL, et al. Lifestyles of older adults: can we influence cardiovascular risk in older adults? *Am J Geriatr Cardiol.* 2004;13:153-160.

42. Dean E. Cardiopulmonary anatomy. Cardiopulmonary physiology. In: Frownfelter D, Dean E, eds. *Cardiopulmonary Physical Therapy: Evidence and Practice.* St. Louis, Mo: Mosby Elsevier; 2006.

43. Dean E. Oxygen transport: a physiologically-based conceptual framework for the practice of cardiopulmonary physiotherapy. *Physiother.* 1994;80:347-359.

44. Ross J, Dean E. Integrating physiological principles into the comprehensive management of cardiopulmonary dysfunction. *Phys Ther.* 1989;69:255-259.

45. Dean E, Ross J. Discordance between cardiopulmonary physiology and physical therapy. *Chest.* 1992a;101:1694-1698.

46. Dean E, Ross J. Oxygen transport. The basis for contemporary cardiopulmonary physical therapy and its optimization with body positioning and mobilization. *Phys Ther Pract.* 1992b;1:34-44.

47. World Health Organization. International Classification of Functioning, Disability and Health. (2002). Available at: www.sustainable-design.ie/arch/ICIDH-2PFDec-2000.pdf. Accessed November 2005.

48. Hodges PW, Gandevia SC. Postural activity of the diaphragm is reduced in humans when respiratory demand increases. *J Physiology.* 2001;537:999-1008.

49. Ceisla ND, Murdock KR. Lines, tubes, catheters, and physiological monitoring in the ICU. *Cardiopul Phys Ther.* 2000;11(1):16-25.

50. Hillegass EA. Cardiovasculascular diagnostic tests and procedures. In: Hillegass EA, Sadowsky HS, eds. *Essentials of Cardiopulmonary Physical Therapy.* 2nd ed. Philadelphia, Pa: WB Saunders Co; 2001:336-377.

51. Sadowsky HS. Monitoring and life-support equipment. In: Hillegass EA, Sadowsky HS, eds. *Essentials of Cardiopulmonary Physical Therapy.* 2nd ed. Philadelphia, Pa: WB Saunders Co; 2001:509-534.

52. Watchie J. Cardiology. In: Watchie J, ed. *Cardiopulmonary Physical Therapy. A Clinical Manual.* Philadelphia, Pa: WB Saunders Co; 1995:22-23.

53. Widmaier EP, Raff H, Strang KT. Cardiovascular Physiology. In: Widmaier EP, Raff H, Strang KT, eds. *Vander's Human Physiology. The Mechanisms of Body Function.* 10th ed. Boston, Mass: The McGraw Hill Co; 2006:387-458

54. Widmaier EP, Raff H, Strang KT. Respiratory physiology. In: Widmaier EP, Raff H, Strang KT, eds. *Vander's Human Physiology. The Mechanisms of Body Function.* 10th ed. Boston, Mass: The McGraw Hill Co; 2006:477-500.

55. Laird RJ, Irwin S. Cardiovascular structure and function. In: Irwin S, Tecklin JS, eds. *Cardiopulmonary Physical Therapy. A Guide to Practice.* 4th ed. St. Louis, Mo: Mosby; 2004:20-27.

56. Moore KL. *Clinically Oriented Anatomy.* 4th ed. Baltimore, Md: Lippincott, Williams & Wilkins; 1999:123-135.

57. Ellestad M. Cardiovascular and pulmonary responses to exercise. In: Ellestad M, ed. *Stress Testing. Principles and Practice.* 3rd ed. Philadelphia, Pa: FA Davis; 1986:9.

58. Cahalin L. Cardiac muscle dysfunction. In: Hillegass EA, Sadowsky HS, eds. *Essentials of Cardiopulmonary Physical Therapy.* 2nd ed. Philadelphia, Pa: WB Saunders Co; 2001:106-181.

59. Skloven ZD. Hemodynamics. In: Irwin S, Tecklin JS, eds. *Cardiopulmonary Physical Therapy.* 3rd ed. St. Louis, Mo: Mosby; 1995:22-33.

60. Kitzman KM, Beech BM. Family based interventions for pediatric obesity: methodological and conceptual challenge from family psychology. *J Fam Psychol.* 2005;20(2):175-189.

61. Howley ET, Franks BD. *Health Fitness Instructor's Handbook.* 3rd ed. Champaign, Ill: Human Kinetics: 1997.

62. Dilsizian V, Rocco TP, Freedman NM, et al. Enhanced detection of ischemic but viable myocardium by the reinjection of thallium after stress-redistribution imaging. *N Engl J Med.* 1990;323(3):141-146.

63. American Association of Cardiovascular and Pulmonary Rehabilitation. *Guidelines for Pulmonary Rehabilitation Programs.* 2nd ed. Champaign Ill: Human Kinetics; 1998.

64. McCool FD, Rosen MJ. Nonpharmacologic airway clearance therapies: ACCP evidence based clinical practice guidelines. *Chest.* 2006;129:250S-259S.

65. State of Illinois AllKids. Website. Available at: http://www.allkidscovered.com. Accessed August 2006.

66. Frownfelter DL, Massery M. Facilitating ventilation patterns and breathing strategies. In: Frownfelter DL, Dean E, eds. *Cardiovascular and Pulmonary Physical Therapy: Evidence and Practice.* St. Louis, Mo: Mosby Elsevier; 2006.

67. US Department of Health and Human Services. Prevention makes common "cents." Available at: http://aspe.hhs.gov/health/prevention. Accessed December 2006.

68. Flegal KM, Carroll MD, Ogden CL, et al. Prevalence and trends in obesity among US adults, 1999-2000. *JAMA.* 2002;288(14):1723-1727.

69. Schiel R, Beltschikow W, Stein G. Overweight, obesity and elevated blood pressure in children and adolescents. *Eur J Med Res.* 2006;11(3):97-101.

70. Hagberg JM, Graves JE, Limacher M, et al. Cardiovascular responses of 70- to 79-yr-old men and women to exercise training. *J Appl Physiol.* 1989;66(6):2589-94.

71. Guyton AC, Hall JE. *Medical Physiology.* 10th ed. Philadelphia Pa: WB Saunders, 2000.

72. LeMura LM, von Duvillard SP. *Clinical Exercise Physiloigy.* Philadelphia Pa: Lippincot Williams & Wilkins; 2004.

73. McArdle WD, Katch FI, Kaatch VL. *Exercise Physiology: Energy, Nutrition, & Human Performance.* Baltimore Md: Lippincott Williams & Wilkins; 2007.

74. Toth MJ, Beckett T, Poehlman ET. Physical activity and the progressive change in body composition with aging: current evidence and research issues. *Med Sci Sports Exerc.* 1999;31(11 Suppl):S590-S596.

75. Downs AM. Chapter 21 Clinical Applications of Airway Clearance Techniques in Frownfelter DL, Dean E. *Cardiovascular and Pulmonary Physical Therapy: Evidence and Practice.* St. Louis Mo: Mosby Elsevier; 2006.

76. Gandevia SC, Butler JE, Hodges PW, Taylor JL, Balancing acts: respiratory sensations, motor control and human posture. *Clin Exp Pharmacol Physiol.* 2002;29:118-21.

77. Prasad SA, Randall SD, Balfour-Lynn IM. Fifteen-count breathlessness score: an objective measurement for children. *Pediatr Pulmonol.* 2000;30(1):56-62.

78. Enright PL, Sherrill DL. Reference equations for the six-minute walk in healthy adults. *Am J Respir Crit Care Med.* 1998; 158(5):1384-1387.

79. Jensen MP, Karoly P, Braver S. The measurement of clinical pain intensity: a comparison of six methods. *Pain.* 1986;27(1): 117-126.

80. Rimm EB, Stampfer MJ, Givanucci E, et al. Body size and fat distribution as predictors of coronary heart disease among middle-aged and old US men. *Am J Epidem.* 1995; 141(12):1117-1127.

81. Moffat M, Rosen E, Rusnak-Smith S, eds. Impaired joint mobility, motor function, muscle performance, and range of motion associated with bony or soft tissue surgery (pattern I). *Musculoskeletal Essentials: Applying the Preferred Physical Therapist Practice Patterns.* Thorofare, NJ: SLACK Incorporated; 2006:345-348.

82. US Department of Health and Human Services. Prevention makes common "cents." Available at: http://aspe.hhs.gov/health/prevention. Accessed July 2006.

83. RRTC Health & Wellness Consortium. Available at: http://www.healthwellness.org/archive/research/study5.htm. Accessed March 2006.

84. Kushi LH, Fee RM, Fulsom AR, et al. Physical activity and mortality in postmenopausal women. *JAMA.* 1997;277(16):1287-1292.

85. Nied RJ, Franklin B. Promoting and prescribing exercise for the elderly. Am Fam Physician. 2002;65(3):419-426.

86. Ellingson T, Conn VS. Exercise and quality of life in elderly individuals. J Gerontol Nurs. 2000;26(3):17-25.

87. Landin RJ, Linnemeier TJ, Rothbau DA, et al. Exercise testing and training of the elderly patient. *Cardiovasc Clin.* 1985; 15(2):201-218.

88. Hagberg JM, Graves JE, Limacher M, et al. Cardiovascular responses of 70- to 79-yr-old men and women to exercise training. *J Appl Physiol.* 1989;66(6):2589-2594.

89. Malbut KE, Dinan S, Young A, et al. Aerobic training in the 'oldest old': the effect of 24 weeks of training. *Age Ageing.* 2002;31(4):255-260.

90. Mazzeo RS, Tanaka H. Exercise prescription for the elderly: current recommendations. *Sports Med.* 2001;31(11):809-818.

91. Blumenthal JA, Emery CF, Madden DJ, et al. Cardiovascular and behavioral effects of aerobic exercise training in healthy older men and women. *J Gerontol.* 1989;44(5):M147-M157.

92. Prior BM, Lloyd PG, Yang HT, et al. Exercise-induced vascular remodeling. *Exerc Sport Sci Rev.* 2003;31(1):26-33.

93. Seals DR, Taylor JA, Ng AV, et al. Exercise and aging: autonomic control of the circulation. *Med Sci Sports Exerc.* 1994; 26(5):568-576.

94. Innvista. Cardiovascular changes in aging. Available at: http://www.innvista.com/health/anatomy/cardage.htm. Accessed April 2006.

95. Tanasescu M, Leitzmann MF, Rimm EB, et al. Exercise type and intensity in relation to coronary heart disease in men. *JAMA.* 2002;288(16):1994-2000.

96. Hurley BF, Roth SM. Strength training in the elderly: effects on risk factors for age-related diseases. *Sports Med.* 2000; 30(4):249-268.

97. Martel GF, Hurlbut DE, Loh ME, et al. Strength training normalizes resting blood pressure in 65- to 73-year-old men and women with high normal blood pressure. *J Am Geriatr Soc.* 1999; 47(10):1215-1221.

98. Department of Health and Human Services. Physical activity for everyone: Recommendations: Are there special recommendations for older adults? Available at: http://www.cdc.gov/nccdphp/dnpa/physical/recommendations/older_adults.htm. Accessed June 2006.

99. American College of Sports Medicine. *Guidelines for Exercise Testing and Prescription.* 7th ed. Philadelphia, Pa: Lippincott Williams & Wilkins; 2005.

100. Borg G. *Borg's Perceived Exertion and Pain Scales.* Champaign Ill: Human Kinetics; 1998.

101. National Center for Chronic Disease Prevention and Health Promotion, Centers for Disease Control and Prevention. *Preventing Heart Disease and Stroke: Addressing the Nation's Leading Killers.* Atlanta, Ga: CDC; 2002.

102. Kitzman DW. Normal age-related changes in the heart: relevance to echocardiography in the elderly. *Amer J Ger Cardiology.* 2000;9(6):311-320.

103. Niinimaa V, Shephard RJ. Training and oxygen conductance in the elderly. II. The cardiovascular system. *J Gerontol.* 1978; 33:362-367.

104. Tate CA, Hyek MF, Taffet GE. Mechanisms for the response of cardiac muscle to physical activity in old age. *Med Sci Sports Exerc.* 1994;26:561-567.

105. Seals DR. Habitual exercise and the age-associated decline in large artery compliance. *Exerc Sport Sci Rev.* 2003;31(2):68-72.

106. Seals DR, Monahan KD, Bell C, et al. The aging cardiovascular system: changes in autonomic function at rest and in response to exercise. *Int J Sport Nutr Exerc Metab.* 2001;11(Suppl): S189-S195.

107. Krumpe PE, Knudson RJ, Parsons G, et al. The aging respiratory system. *Clin Geriatr Med.* 1985;1:143-175.

108. Crapo RO. The aging lung. In: Mahler DA, ed. *Pulmonary Disease in the Elderly Patient.* New York, NY: Marcel Dekker; 1993.

109. Verbeken E, Cauberghs M, Mertens I, et al. The senile lung. comparisons with normal and emphysematous lungs. I. Structural aspects. *Chest.* 1992;101:793-799.

110. D'Errico A, Scarani P, Colosimo E, et al. Changes in alveolar connective tissue of the aging lung. An immunohistochemical study. *Virchows Archiv.* 1989;415:137-144.

111. Gillooly M, Lamb D. Airspace size in lungs of lifelong non-smokers: effect of age and sex. *Thorax.* 1993;48:39-43.

112. Merck. Effects of aging. Available at: http://www.merck.com/mmhe/sec04/ch038/ch038g.html. Accessed April 19, 2006.

113. Morey MC, Pieper CF, Crowley GM. Exercise adherence and 10-year mortality in chronically ill older adults. *J Am Geriatr Soc*. 2002;50(12):1929-1233.

114. Fielding RA, LeBrasseur NK, Cuoco A, et al. High-velocity resistance training increases skeletal muscle peak power in older women. *J Am Geriatr Soc*. 2002;50(4):655-662.

115. Judge JO, Underwood M, Gennosa T. Exercise to improve gait velocity in older persons. *Arch Phys Med Rehabil*. 1993;74(4):400-406.

116. Hunter GR, Treuth MS, Weinsier RL, et al. The effects of strength conditioning on older women's ability to perform daily tasks. *J Am Geriatr Soc*. 1995;43(7):756-760.

117. Lord SR, Lloyd DG, Nirui M, et al. The effect of exercise on gait patterns in older women: a randomized controlled trial. *J Gerontol A Biol Sci Med Sci*. 1996;51(2):M64-M70.

118. Sipila S, Multanen J, Kallinen M, et al. Effects of strength and endurance training on isometric muscle strength and walking speed in elderly women. *Acta Physiol Scand*. 1996;156(4):457-464.

119. Krebs DE, Jette AM, Assmann S. Moderate exercise improves gait stability in disabled elders. *Arch Phys Med Rehabil*. 1998;79(12):1489-1495.

120. Pollock ML, Graves JE, Swart DL, et al. Exercise training and prescription for the elderly. *South Med J*. 1994;87(5):S88-S95.

121. King AC, Pruitt LA, Phillips W, et al. Comparative effects of two physical activity programs on measured and perceived physical functioning and other health-related quality of life outcomes in older adults. *J Gerontol A Biol Sci Med Sci*. 2000;55(2):M74-M83.

122. Jette AM, Harris BA, Sleeper L, et al. A home-based exercise program for nondisabled older adults. *J Am Geriatr Soc*. 1996;44(6):644-649.

123. Ourania M, Yvoni H, Christos K, et al. Effects of a physical activity program. The study of selected physical abilities among elderly women. *J Gerontol Nurs*. 2003;29(7):50-55.

124. Larsen AI, Aarsland T, Kristiansen M, et al. Assessing the effect of exercise training in men with heart failure; comparison of maximal, submaximal and endurance exercise protocols. *Eur Heart J*. 2001;22(8):684-692.

125. Parnell MM, Holst DP, Kaye DM. Exercise training increases arterial compliance in patients with congestive heart failure. *Clin Sci (Lond)*. 2002;102(1):1-7.

126. Lloyd-Williams F, Mair FS, Leitner M. Exercise training and heart failure: a systematic review of current evidence. *Br J Gen Pract*. 2002;52(474):47-55.

127. Maiorana A, O'Driscoll G, Cheetham C, et al. Combined aerobic and resistance exercise training improves functional capacity and strength in CHF. *J Appl Physiol*. 2000;88(5):1565-1570.

128. Aronow WS. Exercise therapy for older persons with cardiovascular disease. *Am J Geriatr Cardiol*. 2001;10(5):245-249.

129. Hirata K, Okamoto T, Shiraishi S, et al. The efficacy and practice of exercise training in patients with chronic obstructive pulmonary disease (COPD). *Nippon Rinsho*. 1999;57(9):2041-2045.

130. Ortega F, Toral J, Cejudo P, et al. Comparison of effects of strength and endurance training in patients with chronic obstructive pulmonary disease. *Am J Respir Crit Care Med*. 2002;166(5):669-674.

131. Panton LB, Golden J, Broeder CE, et al. The effects of resistance training on functional outcomes in patients with chronic obstructive pulmonary disease. *Eur J Appl Physiol*. 2004;91(4):443-449.

132. Clark CJ, Cochrane LM, Mackay E, et al. Skeletal muscle strength and endurance in patients with mild COPD and the effects of weight training. *Eur Respir J*. 2000;15(1):92-97.

133. Penninx BW, Rejeski WJ, Pandaya J, et al. Exercise and depressive symptoms: a comparison of aerobic and resistance exercise effects on emotional and physical function in older persons with high and low depressive symptomatology. *J Gerontol B Psychol Sci Soc Sci*. 2002;57(2):P124-P132.

134. Singh MA, Clements KM, Fiatarone MA. A randomized controlled trial of progressive resistance training in depressed elders. *J Gerontol A Biol Sci Med Sci*. 1997;52(1):M27-M35.

135. Singh MA, Clements KM, Fiatarone MA. A randomized controlled trial of the effect of exercise on sleep. *Sleep*. 1997;20(2):95-101.

CHAPTER TWO

Impaired Aerobic Capacity/ Endurance Associated With Deconditioning (Pattern B)

Elizabeth Dean, PT, PhD

INTRODUCTION

Aerobic deconditioning in patient populations is a function of two principal mechanisms: 1) the removal of gravitational stress, and 2) the removal of exercise stress. This chapter briefly describes the related integrative system anatomy and physiology and the associated pathophysiology that can lead to aerobic (ie, oxygen [O_2] transport) deconditioning. Such deconditioning results either from threats to O_2 transport or from dysfunction of one or more steps in the O_2 transport pathway by one or both of the principal mechanisms.[1,2]

ANATOMY

Oxygen transport is the process by which O_2 is carried in the blood and supplied to the tissues of the body to meet metabolic demands (Figure 2-1). The steps in the O_2 transport pathway include the airways; lungs; pulmonary circulation; blood (volume and constituents including proteins); heart (electrical activity, electromechanical coupling, and mechanical activity); peripheral circulation (arterial, venous, and lymphatic); and oxidative metabolism at the tissue level (the biochemical processes and oxidative enzymes support-

ing the functions of the Krebs cycle and the electron transfer chain) (see Pattern A: Primary Prevention/Risk Reduction for Cardiovascular/Pulmonary Disorders and the article by Dean[1] for detailed review of the anatomy of the cardiovascular/pulmonary systems).

PHYSIOLOGY

The determinants of oxygen delivery (DO_2) and consumption (VO_2) are shown in Figure 2-2. The DO_2 are precisely titrated to meet VO_2. Normally, a person's capacity to deliver O_2 exceeds the demand, which ensures sufficient O_2 transport reserve in times of increased O_2 demand in health and illness.[3] However, people who have severely compromised O_2 transport and are unable to meet even resting metabolic demands, rely increasingly on anaerobic metabolism, which results in increased levels of lactate.[4] Although this mechanism is adaptive in the short term, when lactate levels are sustained and not adequately biodegraded in patients who are severely ill, multisystem consequences can contribute to further multiorgan system dysfunction and failure. See Pattern A: Primary Prevention/Risk Reduction for Cardiovascular/Pulmonary Disorders for a detailed review of the physiology of the cardiovascular/pulmonary systems.

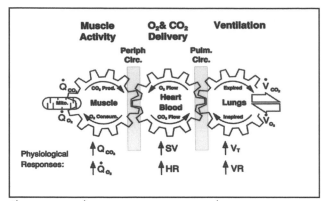

Figure 2-1. The oxygen transport pathway.

PATHOPHYSIOLOGY

DECONDITIONING

The factors that threaten and impair O_2 transport have been well documented and previously described in detail.[2,5] They include extrinsic factors related to the patient's care (eg, medications and surgery), intrinsic factors related to the patient, the underlying pathophysiology, recumbency, and restricted mobility. When patients are hospitalized, VO_2 is threatened or compromised by recumbency secondary to bed rest and to restricted mobility. Both recumbency and restricted mobility contribute to bed rest deconditioning.[6,7] The role of recumbency in bed rest deconditioning is often less well appreciated by clinicians compared with the more apparent effects of restricted mobility. The hemodynamic effects of prolonged recumbency, however, are thought to contribute equally or even more to bed rest deconditioning than restricted movement. Being physiologically distinct in terms of their effects, recumbency and restricted mobility are assessed and managed differently by the physical therapist.

The negative multisystem sequelae of bed rest are well documented and are undisputed.[8-13] The classic study by Saltin and colleagues[14] demonstrated marked multisystem deterioration with 3 weeks of bed rest in five healthy young men and then documented the recovery of aerobic capacity with strenuous training. When these subjects were followed 30 years later,[15,16] all had an age-related decrement in aerobic power. Comparatively, however, bed rest had a more profound impact on their physical work capacity than 30 years of aging.

The recumbent, immobile position associated with bed rest adversely affects organ system function as a result of hemodynamic fluid shifts and down-regulation of the O_2 transport system.[17,18] Clinically, this is important in patient management because of the direct relationship between how sick the patient is and the amount of time she or he is confined to bed. Virtually all organ systems are adversely affected

including the musculoskeletal, neurological, gastrointestinal, genitourinary, and endocrine/metabolic systems, in addition to the person's psychological health and well-being. Deconditioning associated with bed rest reduces VO_2peak and O_2 transport reserve that is needed for an individual to perform work and respond effectively to changing metabolic requirements.[19] The time needed to recondition exceeds that to decondition. Thus, preventing or minimizing O_2 transport deconditioning is a physical therapy priority with a view to returning the individual to optimal health, functional activity, and social participation consistent with the International Classification of Function (Figure 2-3).[20]

CARDIOVASCULAR AND HEMODYNAMIC EFFECTS

The cardiovascular deconditioning that results from bed rest blunts the capacity for volume and pressure regulation and also elicits a cephalad (ie, head ward) fluid shift from the extravascular to the intravascular compartment and from the peripheral to central areas, which then stimulates diuresis and thus the loss of plasma volume.[21-26] In turn, the hematocrit is increased, and the individual is at risk of developing deep vein thromboses and thromboemboli. These risks are augmented by stasis of venous blood and increased blood viscosity due to increased platelet count, platelet stickiness, and plasma fibrinogen.[27] Orthostatic intolerance is a primary manifestation of adverse fluid shifts and losses associated with recumbency. The hemodynamic consequences

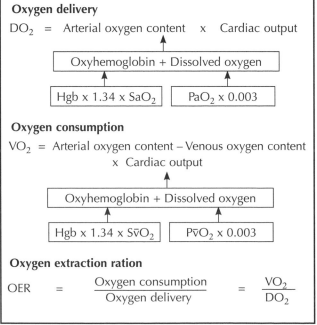

Figure 2-2. The determinants of oxygen delivery (DO_2) and oxygen consumption (VO_2).[2,3]

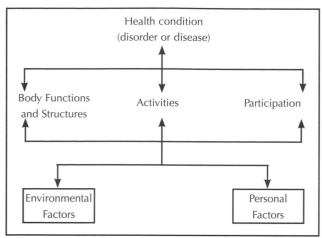

Health condition
(disorder or disease)

Body Functions
and Structures

Activities

Participation

Environmental
Factors

Personal
Factors

Figure 2-3. International Classification of Function (World Health Organization, 2002).[20]

of recumbency that contribute to bed rest deconditioning are preventable. Although investigators have recognized for more than 40 years the benefits of nursing acutely ill patients in chairs rather than beds,[28] bed rest nursing continues to prevail.

Venous thromboembolic disease that is primarily associated with recumbency and inactivity is preventable with conservative management (including exercise, body positioning, and compression garments and devices) and prophylactic anticoagulation in some instances.[29] Other risk factors for venous thromboembolic disease include being elderly and a smoker. Conditions that are associated with risk include previous thromboembolus, cardiovascular disease, pulmonary disease, cancer, obesity, and paralysis.[30] Patients with neuromuscular dysfunction and paresis are particularly prone to pulmonary aspiration and reflux, both of which are major O_2 transport risk factors. The work of the heart can be increased in a patient who is immobile and recumbent, as can the work of breathing due to O_2 kinetic inefficiency and cardiopulmonary biomechanical factors. The work of the heart is greater as a result of the increased cardiac filling pressures, HR associated with recumbency, and increased blood viscosity. The work of breathing is increased as a result of reduced lung volumes and impaired expiratory flow rates secondary to encroachment of the viscera on the underside of the diaphragm; increased intrathoracic blood volume; restricted chest wall motion; and compressive effect that the heart and lungs have on each other and the adjacent mediastinal structures. Even though the role of bed rest-related atrophy in impairing smooth muscle and cardiac muscle function has been less well described as compared with the descriptions of bed rest-related atrophy of skeletal muscle that constitutes the respiratory and peripheral muscles, the impact of deconditioning of these smooth and cardiac muscle types can be anticipated to have direct and profound hemodynamic consequences.

The blood vessels of the muscle and splanchnic circulations dilate during recumbency. With prolonged bed rest, they may lose both their capacity (ie, their sensitivity to stimuli) and their ability to constrict (ie, reduced smooth muscle fiber mass). The capacity of these vessels to constrict prevents blood pooling, maintains circulating blood volume when the patient is gravitationally challenged as in assuming the upright position, and distributes blood flow to organs commensurate with metabolic need. Because of these fluid shifts even after a short period of recumbent bed rest (24 hours), a patient may feel lightheaded and faint (ie, orthostatic intolerance) and have poor balance. Individuals differ with respect to their susceptibility to orthostatic intolerance, thus this needs to be specifically assessed based on serial monitoring of fluid and electrolyte balance and hemodynamics, and management must be instituted accordingly.[22,23]

The implications of recumbency and bed rest (even short periods) on O_2 transport are profound. The only countermeasure to aerobic deconditioning secondary to reduced gravitational stress is gravitational stress as an intervention, and the only countermeasure to deconditioning secondary to reduced exercise stress is exercise. Even vigorous exercise when performed during recumbency fails to offset the hemodynamic effects of deconditioning resulting from the loss of gravitational stress in that position. Thus, bed exercises even if rigorous, such as intense recumbent LE cycling, do not address the primary etiological determinant of bed rest deconditioning associated with recumbency.

HEMATOLOGIC EFFECTS

Long-term exercise training increases blood volume and modifies blood constituents and rheology to adjust to those exercise demands.[31-33] Blood volume changes have implications for cardiac output, which is singularly important in the DO_2 equation shown in Figure 2-2. The number of red blood cells increases to augment the amount of hemoglobin, which is also fundamental to DO_2. In addition, platelet stickiness is reduced with long-term exercise, which in turn reduces resistance to blood flow through the vasculature, hence, decreases the work of the heart.

PULMONARY EFFECTS

Recumbency reduces all lung volumes and capacities with the exception of the closing volume of the dependent airways, which is increased (see review Dean[6]). This increase is associated with reduced functional residual capacity, in particular, and arterial desaturation.

Hospitalized patients often breathe at low lung volumes and are prone to atelectasis, a risk that is increased in older people and smokers. This is complicated by reduced surfactant production and distribution as a result of reduced lung expansion, which is the primary stimulant for surfactant production and distribution. Impaired mucociliary clearance, particularly in older people and smokers, can lead to retention of airway secretions and airway obstruction. These changes can increase airway resistance, reduce lung compliance, and increase the work of breathing. The effects of breathing at low lung volumes may be compounded with pain, sedation, general anesthesia, and existing or new cardiopulmonary dysfunction. A patient's functional residual capacity may take 1 to 2 weeks to recover completely from general anesthesia. Reduced functional residual capacity is associated with increased airway closure of the dependent airways and arterial desaturation. If the patient is exposed to an infective microorganism, bacteria may colonize and pneumonia may ensue. Hospital-acquired pneumonias are associated with more morbidity and mortality than community-acquired pneumonias, thus, their prevention is a physical therapy priority.

The function of the heart and lungs is interdependent and for this reason these organs need to be considered as a unit. Respiratory function may be affected by cardiac insufficiency, which can lead to a back-up of fluid from the left to the right side of the heart and pulmonary edema. Conversely, cardiac function can be affected by respiratory insufficiency.[34]

MUSCULOSKELETAL EFFECTS

Muscle atrophy and impaired proprioception may be detected in a patient within days of bed rest, leading to weakness, incoordination, and imbalance.[14,35,36] These processes are likely initiated as soon as the stress of gravity and exercise are removed and occur at an undetectable genetic level reflecting the down-regulation of oxidative enzyme production, hence O_2 transport and metabolism.[37,38]

With progressive muscle weakness, ligaments and joints may be at greater risk of strain. Muscles and their inert structures are differentially affected. In the knee extensors, for example, tendon stiffness is reduced, and the hysteresis characteristics of the soft tissue become exaggerated, whereas these changes do not occur in the plantarflexors.[39] The limited positioning alternatives in bed may contribute to poor postural alignment, stiffness, and soreness. Weightbearing of various body parts not adapted for weightbearing occurs during bed rest and increases a patient's risk of skin abrasion and breakdown.

Inactive or immobile patients are at risk for bone demineralization, which is of particular importance in older populations, in patients with paresis and disabilities, in postmenopausal women, and in patients receiving steroid medication. Prevention of disuse osteoporosis is a primary aim because remineralization of bone, even with aggressive exercise, body positioning, electrical stimulation, and possible pharmaceutical agents, is unlikely.[40] In patients who are critically ill, cytokines have been implicated in inactivity-related inflammation and muscle injury and atrophy.[41] Activity is the critical countermeasure.

NEUROMUSCULAR EFFECTS

With a patient's increasing severity of acute illness, neuromuscular effects of deconditioning include critical illness myopathies and neuropathies that may result from reduced arousal, prolonged coma, generalized infection, restricted body positioning and movement, and pharmacotherapy. The physical therapist is responsible for monitoring patients for the manifestation of myopathies and neuropathies and preventing those associated with reduced arousal and limited body positions and movement. Other neuromuscular effects include those resulting from vascular dysfunction, including blood clots, HTN, and stroke-related effects.

Abnormal blood gases and fluid and electrolyte imbalances may produce neuromuscular signs and symptoms. These causes need to be identified in the examination and ongoing monitoring of acutely ill patients to avoid misattribution of these signs to a primary neuromuscular etiology, particularly when illness is prolonged. With medical remediation of these imbalances, their neuromuscular manifestations should resolve.

GASTROINTESTINAL EFFECTS

Medical and surgical patients are at risk of gastrointestinal dysfunction with illness and hospitalization.[34] Such dysfunction is likely associated with altered nutrition, eating capacity, and physical activity. Recumbency and bed rest and the physical stress of illness may all have an impact on gastrointestinal function. Surgical patients, for example, are prone to disruption of fluid compartmentalization, both as a direct and indirect result of surgery. First, hemodynamics are disrupted due to recumbency, medications, anesthesia, breathing at low lung volumes, pain, and the surgical insult. Cardiovascular and thoracic surgeries have the greatest impact on fluid balance and distribution. In addition, fluid accumulation in potential spaces in the gut and thorax (termed third spacing) may be a serious problem in maintaining and restoring normal fluid balance and hemodynamics. Thus, assessment of fluid and electrolyte balance is fundamental to the physical therapy examination, evaluation, and intervention planning and prescription. Electrolyte imbalances lead to disruption of cellular electrical conduction and homeostasis, thus, may be manifested as apparent problems in organ systems, such as in the cardiovascular (eg, dysrhythmias) and in the musculoskeletal and neuromuscular systems (eg, abnormal activity and responses of excitable tissue).

Another common clinical concern is paralytic ileus of the bowel due to anesthesia, sedation, fasting, recumbency, and restricted mobility. Avoidance of bowel obstruction and stress ulceration are primary medical goals of prevention. In addition, the physical therapist's role includes assessing these effects, considering them in the overall physical therapy management, and prescribing movement to offset their deleterious effects. Exercise stimulates normal movement of the bowel (ie, increased gastrointestinal transit time and renal drainage). Approximating normal nutritional habits and physical activity to the greatest extent possible during hospitalization will help normalize gastrointestinal and renal function.

Finally, the physical stress of illness may lead to stress ulceration and bleeding of the gut. Severely ill patients or patients with trauma or burns may be at risk and should have prescribed stress ulceration prophylaxis. Whether reducing a patient's anxiety through relaxation and reduction of sympathetic arousal has a role in minimizing this risk warrants detailed study.

GENITOURINARY EFFECTS

The kidneys also have an essential role in endocrine function, including the regulation of erythropoietin, adrenal function, and angiotension production. Disruption of kidney function impacts homeostasis as a whole. Renal manifestations of primary or secondary pathology are of considerable clinical concern and warrant a high level of surveillance and management by the physical therapist.

In the seriously ill patient, particularly one with hemodynamic insufficiency, perfusion of the kidneys and other vital organs may be compromised. Renal dysfunction is a serious complication in patients with cardiopulmonary dysfunction, diabetes, or both. Such dysfunction directly affects fluid and electrolyte balances, which influence each other. These imbalances may manifest themselves as reduced urinary output and precarious blood volume changes that have implications for hemodynamic status and physical therapy management.

Physical sexual dysfunction in men has been largely attributed to atherosclerosis, diabetes, and the side effects of many medications. Report of erectile dysfunction has important clinical implications for the physical therapist in that it may be an early sign of the systemic effects of atherosclerosis, diabetes, or both, or other factors, such as depression and the side effects of medication.

INTEGUMENTARY EFFECTS

Skin breakdown and pressure sores are largely preventable. Their prevention is a high priority given that a hospitalized patient likely has reduced O_2 transport reserve and reduced immunity resulting in a greater risk of infection with skin breakdown and a greater adverse effect on recovery. Skin breakdown may also limit body positioning alternatives and movement.

Skin breakdown most commonly occurs over bony prominences including the back of the head, scapulae, elbows, sacrum, trochanters, and heels. Risk factors for skin abrasion and pressure ulcers include age, prolonged hospitalization, restricted mobility, general debility, low body weight, low diastolic BP, and surgical intervention.[42] In addition, patients with preexisting weakness and paralysis are at greater risk.

Patients who have reduced capacity to move and be upright, particularly as they age, are at high risk for skin breakdown and opportunistic infection. Furthermore, healing and repair of tissue and immunological integrity are impaired in such patients, supporting the need for extreme vigilance with respect to prevention. All patients are at risk, but those who are smokers, are older, have diabetes, or have impaired immunity warrant particular vigilance.

ENDOCRINE AND METABOLIC EFFECTS

Gravitational and exercise stresses increase insulin sensitivity of metabolically active tissue. Their absence leads to insulin resistance and increased circulating insulin levels and glucose levels, both of which are toxic to cells.[43-45] The long-term reduction in insulin sensitivity is the basis of Type 2 diabetes and the associated increased insulin levels in the blood.[46] Stress of illness also may contribute to abnormal blood sugar levels, even in individuals who are not diabetic. High blood sugar levels are associated with increased risk of infection and bacteremia.

IMMUNOLOGICAL EFFECTS

The relationship between immunity and activity is becoming better recognized.[47-49] Physical activity has anti-inflammatory effects and is essential to maintain optimal immunity.[50-52] Restricted activity can impair immune function, and training can enhance it.[53] Conversely, overtraining, such as in athletes, can impair immunity.

PSYCHOLOGICAL EFFECTS

Hospitalization is associated with loss of personal control, loss of stimulation, disorientation, boredom, depression, and anxiety about one's future well-being.[54] Patients are deprived sensorily and may develop a psychoneurosis that is particularly prevalent in older people.[55] Bed rest has been associated with changes in the electroencephalogram (EEG) and behavior.[56] Health care professionals and the family are likely to view patients differently when they are upright and moving. In addition, patients may perceive themselves as less sick with a better prognosis when they are upright and moving versus recumbent and immobile. That a positive outlook influences health and well-being profoundly has been established even for people with chronic conditions. Whether this extends to people with acute conditions is compelling and warrants study.

PATHOPHYSIOLOGY

METABOLIC SYNDROME

Metabolic syndrome refers to a virulent and lethal group of atherosclerotic risk factors including high cholesterol, high triglycerides, HTN, obesity, and insulin resistance. It affects almost 50 million people in the United States.[57] The incidence of the syndrome is increasing and warrants aggressive noninvasive management. Insulin resistance is largely predicted by BMI, smoking, age, and daily physical activity. Warning signs of metabolic syndrome include a fasting blood glucose >115 mg/dL, a "beer belly," total cholesterol >240 mg/dL, triglycerides >160 mg/dL, and BP >140/90 mmHg.[58] These signs are associated with adverse health behavior choices, including reduced activity, deconditioning, and poor nutrition.

Diet and exercise are the cornerstones of the multifactorial approach to preventing, potentially reversing, and managing this lethal condition. Optimal nutrition and weight reduction can counter the effects of metabolic syndrome and its associated dyslipidemia, HTN, and obesity.[58] Physical activity further augments the dietary benefits by increasing insulin sensitivity of tissue membrane.[59,60]

Insulin resistance is a primary feature of metabolic syndrome and predisposes the individual to Type 2 diabetes. Type 2 diabetes is a life-threatening multisystem condition that is pandemic in Western countries and has physical and functional consequences, in addition to compromising perceived health status and quality of life.[61] Type 2 diabetes can no longer be termed adult-onset diabetes because it is being diagnosed in children, predisposing them to blindness, heart disease, stroke, vascular insufficiency, renal disease, autonomic dysfunction, and peripheral neuropathies.[62,63] Inositol is a poison that forms on the membranes of cells in the presence of high blood sugar and has been implicated in the deadly systemic consequences of diabetes. The primary consequences include pathology of the macro and micro vasculature and nerve endings. Impaired glucose tolerance and hemoglobin AIC (HbA1C) are markers for vascular complications of the large and small blood vessels independent of an individual's progression to diabetes. Early detection of glucose intolerance and insulin resistance allows for intensive dietary and exercise modification that can be more effective than drug therapy in normalizing postprandial glucose and inhibiting progression to diabetes.[64] Such intervention could help prevent more severe manifestations including metabolic syndrome and frank diabetes. Diabetic autonomic neuropathy as an independent risk factor for stroke may reflect increased vascular damage and may effect the regulation of cerebral blood flow in individuals with diabetes.[65]

Individuals with Type 2 diabetes mellitus have increased risk of cardiovascular disease compared with individuals without diabetes, thus strict control is essential. Moderate physical activity with a faster walking pace[66] along with weight loss is a powerful combination to reduce the risk of Type 2 diabetes as well as reverse it. These interventions with a balanced diet can reduce the risk of developing diabetes among those who are at high risk by 50% to 60%.[67] Cigarette smoking, an independent risk factor for Type 2 diabetes,[68] is particularly lethal for an individual with diabetes.[62]

The diseases of civilization including metabolic syndrome are the leading killers in North America, yet are largely preventable.[69] The multiple factors contributing to these diseases must be considered and addressed programmatically. Further information on the diseases of civilization may be found in Pattern A: Primary Prevention/Risk Reduction for Cardiovascular/Pulmonary Disorders.

IMAGING AND LABORATORY TESTS

DECONDITIONING AND METABOLIC SYNDROME

Imaging and laboratory tests, specifically those used to evaluate limitations of structure, function, and activity,[70] have value in evaluating deconditioning that results primarily from impairments of O_2 transport. Acute deconditioning associated with fluid losses with recumbency and reduced activity is best evaluated based on clinical measures of fluid and electrolyte balance, hemodynamics, and ECG. Indirectly, fluid and electrolyte imbalances may manifest themselves as cardiovascular, musculoskeletal, and neuromuscular impairments. Appropriate serial evaluation is necessary to ascertain whether impairments of these systems are secondary to fluid and electrolyte imbalances.

Imaging in patient populations is useful in detecting primary cardiac dysfunction or lung dysfunction. Chest x-rays (CXRs) are used to determine lung consolidations, atelectasis, unexpected pulmonary complications (ie, pneumothorax), and abnormal cardiac conditions (ie, hypertrophy, cor pulmonale). Imaging investigations may also include: nuclear scans that use thallium or technetium 99 stannous pyrophosphate to evaluate myocardial blood flow; MRI to evaluate wall thickening and whether tissue is healthy or infarcted; cine computed tomography (CT) or ultrafast CT scan to evaluate myocardial abnormalities and cardiac output; and positron emission tomography (PET scan) to evaluate myocardial blood flow.

Ultrasonogaphy or echocardiography, using 1, 2, and 3 dimensional techniques, is a noninvasive test that shows the size, shape, and motion of the cardiac structures.

Biochemical measures may identify creatine kinase levels that increase with catabolism of muscle associated with deterioration of the peripheral muscles as occurs in extreme deconditioned states. Biochemistry markers are used commonly for serial evaluation of cardiac enzymes and their normalization after MI or the identification of an evolving infarction during hospitalization. These markers may include the determination of the levels of the following enzymes: creatine kinase (CK), especially the isoenzyme CK-MB that indicates myocardial injury; aspartate aminotransferase (AST); serum lactic dehydrogenase (LDH); serum alpha-hydrokybutyrate dehydrogenase (SHBD); myoglobin; and troponin. Biomarkers for systemic inflammation are increasingly used clinically.

Exercise or its lack may have profound effects on blood biochemistry. Measures of high-density lipoprotein (HDL) and low-density lipoprotein (LDL) cholesterol, triglycerides, CRP, homocysteine, and HbA1C are important indices of improved aerobic conditioning and health behaviors including diet, smoking cessation, and reduced stress.

In acutely ill patients who have been recumbent, a standardized postural test can be done to assess hemodynamic response to the upright position. Ideally, patients simply participate in physically supporting themselves when being positioned upright. The muscle activity required for this test facilitates the action of the peripheral muscles and venous return, which is essential to prime the autonomic nervous system function and orthostatic tolerance. A tilt-table challenge test may be indicated in select cases, for example, when patients are less able to cooperate or are in need of more intensive care. The tilt-table challenge test, which takes the patient from supine to progressive elevation of the head on the table, is another test used to determine the patient's hemodynamic responses with positional changes including BP responses. If the tilt-table challenge test is used, the physical therapist must keep in mind that patients are more restricted, are potentially less able to activate peripheral muscles to maintain venous return and cardiac output, and are also less able to verbalize distress. Close hemodynamic monitoring is required in both tests, but particularly with use of the tilt-table challenge test.

For subacute and chronic patients, examination of deconditioning secondary to disuse (eg, reduced exercise capability) and prescription of interventions are based on stress testing. For these patients, exercise stress testing may range from submaximal tests to maximal VO_2 studies with or without invasive investigations.[71,72] Standard treadmill and cycle ergometer tests are usually the tests of choice for these patients. Tests have also been modified to allow testing of various patient populations and varied age groups. Ramped protocols that change the speed and/or grade, for example, every 20 seconds rather than every 3 minutes of testing, are useful means of gauging progressive exercise responses. Invasive investigations that can be performed concurrently include the injection of thallium, which enhances detection of myocardial ischemia.

Exercise testing may be done in conjunction with blood work and hemodynamic assessments, including cardiac output measures. Such laboratory tests include tests of the O_2 transport pathway and include:

♦ Airway and lung function: Pulmonary function tests

♦ Blood work: Including blood biochemistries (fluid and electrolytes) and fasting and postprandial blood sugar levels

♦ Heart (electrical and mechanical function): Including HR, BP, rate pressure product (HR x systolic BP), and ECG

♦ Peripheral vascular function: Including peripheral BPs and ultrasound pulse evaluation

♦ Tissue perfusion and metabolism: Including inspection and assessment of tissue oxygenation

PHARMACOLOGY

DECONDITIONING

Consistent with the values of primarily noninvasive practice, physical therapy's goal is to have the patient avoid the need for pharmacologic support. If medication is indicated, the physical therapy goal is to minimize its dosage if possible, and eventually enable the individual to be weaned from that medication. When medication at a minimal dose cannot be avoided and impacts physical therapy outcomes, the physical therapist has a role in monitoring the patient's responses to ensure that it is effective and its side effects minimal.

Some investigators have suggested the use of potent inotropes to preserve aerobic capacity in acutely ill patients, however, the results of such studies are largely of theoretical interest rather than of clinical benefit. The effects of pharmacological agents do not replace the systemic long-term benefits of the "physiologic body position," that is, being "upright and moving," even when prescribed at low intensity.

Certain medications are used to enhance physical performance and minimize exercise risk. These medications may include analgesics, bronchodilators, and coronary artery vasodilators.

♦ Analgesics
  - Acetaminophen (eg, Tylenol)
  - Nonsteroidal anti-inflammatory drugs (NSAIDs) (eg, aspirin, Motrin [ibuprofen], Aleve [naproxen sodium])
  - Corticosteroids (eg, prednisone, prednisolone, methylprednisolone)

♦ Bronchodilators
  - Beta-agonists
    - Short-acting inhaled: Proventil and Ventolin (albuterol), Maxair (pirbuterol), Alupent (metaproterenol)
    - Long-acting inhaled: Serevent (salmeterol), Foradil (formoterol)
  - Anticholinergics: Atrovent (ipratropium), Spiriva (tiotropium)
  - Combivent contains a short-acting beta-agonist (albuterol) and an anticholinergic (ipratropium)
  - Theophylline: Theo-dur, Slo-bid, Uniphyl, Uni-Dur

♦ Coronary artery vasodilators
  • Nitrates: Sublingual, chewable, or buccal (systemic)

METABOLIC SYNDROME

Some medications that are prescribed for patients with metabolic syndrome, such as bronchodilators, coronary artery vasodilators, and antihypertensives, can augment the patient's exercise responses and thereby aerobic capacity. Conversely, as aerobic conditioning improves, medications can often be eliminated or reduced.

The following generic pharmacological agents can be utilized in the management of patients with metabolic syndrome and its components (eg, HTN, glucose intolerance, Type 2 diabetes, hypercholesterolemia, elevated triglycerides, and often obesity).

♦ HTN
  • Diuretics
  • Beta blockers (eg, propranolol)
  • Calcium channel antagonists
  • Angiotensin converting enzyme (ACE) inhibitors
♦ Type 2 diabetes
  • Oral glycemic agents
  • Insulin
♦ Hypercholesterolemia
  • Cholesterol-lowering agents
♦ Elevated triglycerides
  • Triglyceride reducers
♦ Obesity-related complaints
  • Antacids
  • Laxatives
  • Analgesics for musculoskeletal stress that can compromise physical activity and exercise capacity

---

Case Study #1: Lifestyle-Related Cholecystitis and Deconditioning

Mrs. Marie Rodriguez, who has just been discharged from the hospital 3 days after elective open laparoscopic surgery for cholecystitis, is deconditioned due to perioperative complications that threatened her long-term health.

PHYSICAL THERAPIST EXAMINATION

HISTORY

♦ General demographics: Mrs. Rodriguez is a 45-year-old Mexican American. Her family moved from Mexico City to the United States when she was 13 years of age. She has reading, writing, and speaking literacy in both Spanish and English.

♦ Social history: She lives with her husband in a suburban neighborhood of a medium-sized city in Texas. Her two children are grown and attending college out of state. Her mother lives close by and relies on Mrs. Rodriguez and her family to help out given her deteriorating health and disability. She and her family are Catholic by faith.

♦ Employment/work: Mrs. Rodriguez is a qualified practicing engineer, who has worked full-time for the same company for 22 years (with the exception of 6 months off at each of the births of her two children). She is eligible for promotion in the company and has been working longer hours this past year, which has stressed both her and her family.

♦ Living environment: Mrs. Rodriguez and her husband live is a spacious two-story home with 14 steps to the top floor with a handrail.

♦ General health status
  • General health perception: Mrs. Rodriguez acknowledges that she has neglected her health over the years. She has been overweight since childhood and gained weight after the birth of each child. Mrs. Rodriguez has attempted a number of diets on her own, but none has had sustained success. In fact, she gained several more pounds after having lost some weight each time. She is aware that she cannot maintain the pace when walking with her colleagues. She believed there was a genetic component with respect to her gall bladder disease given that two aunts have had the same problem. Mrs. Rodriguez is at the contemplative stage of readiness to change her health behavior with respect to both weight control and more active lifestyle as defined by Prochaska and DiClemente.[73] Their model is called the Transtheoretical Model of Change and consists of five stages: 1) precontemplation—not intending to take action, 2) contemplation—intending to change in the next 6 months, 3) preparation—intending to take action usually within the next month, 4) action—made specific modifications in lifestyle within past 6 months, and 5) maintenance—work to prevent relapse. Mrs. Rodriguez believes she needs professional guidance to succeed.
  • Physical function: She would like to achieve an above average level of health and fitness that would enable her to be more physically active with her husband and with her future grandchildren.
  • Psychological function: Based on observation and the absence of any dysfunction reported by her general practitioner, Mrs. Rodriguez appears to be free from any significant pathology. However, she reports feeling unattractive to her husband and has in recent years avoided physical intimacy with him.

- Role function: Wife, mother, friend, daughter, daughter-in-law, colleague, youth counselor at her church.
- Social function: Mrs. Rodriguez enjoys socializing with her immediate and extended families and with her friendship network. She and her husband have a large house so they do most of the entertaining for family gatherings. Mrs. Rodriguez also enjoys socializing with colleagues and is only now (because her children are independent) spending more time with them outside work. She has served as a youth counselor at her church for 10 years and devotes one evening a week to this activity.

- Social/health habits: Mrs. Rodriguez has never smoked. She lived in her family home until the age of 22 years when she married. Her father smoked 2 packs per day, thus, she passively smoked until her early 20s when she left home. She is a social drinker. She reports never having used recreational drugs or performance-enhancing agents.

- Family history: Her father died of lung cancer 5 years ago. Her mother is obese and hypertensive, as is an aunt. Two aunts have gall bladder disease. Her maternal grandmother died of ovarian cancer. She has three living siblings who Mrs. Rodriguez reports are not under a physician's care.

- Medical/surgical history: Mrs. Rodriguez was diagnosed 8 years ago as having borderline HTN, and over the past 2 years she has had a fasting blood sugar in the high normal range. Her general practitioner suggested she "take less salt and sugar," and "walk more." There was no physical therapy referral at that time, and she had not been followed regarding the outcome of these recommendations. Mrs. Rodriguez has been overweight since childhood; her current BMI is 32.3 kg/m². Over the past 2 years, she has developed arthritic discomfort and pain in her hips with the right more severe than the left. This causes her to limp when she is on her feet for very long (approximately 20 to 30 minutes) or is physically active (walking up stairs or hills).

- Prior hospitalizations: She was hospitalized for the births of her two children.

- Preexisting medical and other health-related conditions: Mrs. Rodriguez is obese and has borderline HTN,[74] prediabetic blood sugar levels,[75] and arthritic pain in both hips (R>L). Mrs. Rodriguez's risks for IHD, peripheral vascular disease (PVD), blindness, and cancer are above average,[76] and she is also at increased risk of stroke and renal dysfunction due to her borderline HTN. She has no known allergies. Mrs. Rodriguez is menopausal. She does not report any unusual increase in thirst or weight gain, but experiences urgency and increased urinary frequency. She cannot say specifically that she has a change in orthostatic tolerance, sweating, and peripheral perfu-sion. Her thyroid function is normal. Mrs. Rodriguez has had a long history of peridontal disease and has her teeth cleaned every 6 months. Over the past 10 years, Mrs. Rodriguez had been conservatively medically managed for several previous bouts of cholecystitis that had been confirmed with ultrasound and other tests. Over the past 2 years, Mrs. Rodriguez's bouts of severe cholecystitis have been more frequent, more severe, and have taken longer to resolve, which has necessitated several absences from work. She has been controlling the symptoms by controlling the fat in her diet. Her prolonged exposure to passive smoke as a child until her young adulthood also predisposes Mrs. Rodriguez to pulmonary risk particularly given her apparent tendency toward bronchoconstriction and chest tightness. Mrs. Rodriguez also shows signs of osteopenia at three sites (lumbar spine and heads of femurs).

- Current condition(s)/chief complaint(s)
  - She complains of frequent bloating and difficult bowel movements. Her last bout of cholecystitis was 6 weeks ago. This patient's complaint may have been prevented with a healthier lifestyle and physical conditioning. Mrs. Rodriguez is obese and physically deconditioned predisposing her to one or more risk factors or manifestations of one or more diseases of civilization (see Dean[77]). Even if gall bladder dysfunction was not entirely preventable with better overall health and conditioning, less invasive surgery may have been indicated with less risk of perioperative complications, hastened recovery, reduced hospital stay, and hastened return to her ADL. Mrs. Rodriguez's lifestyle created both a medical and surgical condition. Normally, cholecystitis is simply managed with low risk. However, Mrs. Rodriguez's management was consistent with moderate to high perioperative risk. Minimally invasive laparoscopic surgery was not possible due to technical difficulties related to Mrs. Rodriguez's obesity and level of health. Therefore, she underwent open laparoscopic surgery.
  - She has arthritis in both hips, right more than left. She states she had cut back on stair climbing and hills, which has relieved her hip discomfort and shortness of breath associated with chest tightness.
  - She reports no sexual disturbance physically, but does acknowledge lack of libido in recent years. She reports urinary frequency and occasionally urgency, and stress incontinence when she sneezes or coughs. These complaints have worsened in recent years.
  - She reports disturbed sleep greater than 3 nights a week. On these nights, it takes Mrs. Rodriguez a couple of hours to fall asleep, and she is wakeful off and on throughout the night. This past year, she has

awoken more frequently feeling unrestored 4 or 5 mornings a week. Her husband is not aware of her snoring when sleeping.

♦ Functional status and activity level: Mrs. Rodriguez reports that she had been able to manage her ADL and home management. She has hired helpers to do the heavy work both indoors and out. She complains of fatigue and shortness of breath with minimal activity, and more vigorous activity aggravates her hip discomfort.

♦ Medications: Prior to this hospital admission, Mrs. Rodriguez was taking analgesics when her hip discomfort was severe. Eight years ago, she was prescribed a bronchodilator but does not use it anymore. She takes a daily multivitamin recommended by physician.

♦ Other clinical tests:
  - Arterial blood gases room air: WNL but with arterial oxygen saturation (SaO_2) of 96% (SpO_2—95%)
  - Pulmonary function tests
    ▪ FEV_1=85% predicted, FVC = 92%, FEV_1/FVC= 92% predicted, and PEFR=65% predicted
    ▪ Consistent with mild restrictive lung pathology
    ▪ Diffusing capacity and maximal inspiratory and expiratory pressure not tested
  - Total cholesterol: 200 mg/dL (desirable is <200 mg/dL)
  - LDL: 160 mg/dL
    ▪ Optimal level: <100 mg/dL
    ▪ Near optimal level: 100 to 129 mg/dL
    ▪ Borderline high level: 130 to 159 mg/dL
    ▪ High level: 160 to 189 mg/dL
    ▪ Very high level corresponding to highest increased risk of heart disease: >190 mg/dL
  - HDL: 40 mg/dL (normal for females is 40 to 85 mg/dL)
  - LDL/HDL: 4.0 (normal is <3.25)
  - Triglycerides: 278 mg/mL (normal for females is 35 to 135 mg/mL)
  - HbAIC: 7.0% (normal is 5% or less)
  - Homocysteine: 8.0 umol/L (normal is 5 to 15 umol/L)
  - CRP: 3 ug/mL (normal is <6 ug/mL)
  - Blood glucose: 110 mg/mL (fasting) and 170 mg/mL (postprandial) (normal fasting is 70 to 115 mg/100 mL and postprandial is <200 mg/dL)
  - Lab values: Other values were WNL
  - Postural tolerance test: HR, BP before, after at 1, 2, and 5 minutes were WNL
  - Chest x-ray
    ▪ Slightly enlarged heart with slight axis rotation
  - ECG: Normal sinus rhythm

  - Temperature: 98.6°F
  - Baseline preoperative Astrand-Rhyming ergometer test[72,78] to predict VO_2peak and to assess functional and aerobic capacity during nonweightbearing with relative control of hip discomfort: Results are summarized and interpreted on data sheet (Table 2-1)
  - Baseline preoperative 6-Minute Walk test to assess functional and aerobic capacity during weightbearing with potential limitation from hip discomfort: Results are summarized and interpreted on data sheet (Table 2-2)
  - DEXA 6 months ago revealed osteopenia in both femoral heads and lumbar spine

SYSTEMS REVIEW

♦ Cardiovascular/pulmonary
  - BP: 145/95 mmHg (Stage 1 HTN) (Normal= <120/<80; Pre-HTN=120 to 139/80 to 89; Stage 1 HTN=140 to 159/90 to 100; and Stage 2 HTN=at or over 160/at or over 100)[74]
  - Edema: Mild dependent edema of the ankles that is worse in evening
  - HR: 98 bpm
  - RR: 18 bpm

♦ Integumentary
  - Presence of scar formation: Surgical incision noted
  - Skin color: WNL
  - Skin integrity: No open sores or abrasions, surgical wound closed and minimal in appearance

♦ Musculoskeletal
  - Gross range of motion: WNL except for decreased ROM in both hips
  - Gross strength: Limited but WFL
  - Gross symmetry: Slightly kyphotic, mild lumbar scoliosis, and lordosis with protruding abdomen
  - Height: 5'4" (1.63 m)
  - Weight: 188 lbs (85.28 kg)

♦ Neuromuscular
  - Balance: WNL
  - Locomotion, transfers, and transitions: Right hip discomfort when standing up after prolonged sitting, and she experiences difficulty walking

♦ Communication, affect, cognition, language, and learning style
  - Communication, affect, and cognition: WNL
  - Learning preferences: Mrs. Rodriguez prefers reading and discussion as means of learning new material and is comfortable that written materials are presented in English rather than her mother tongue, Spanish
  - Uses glasses for reading

Table 2-1

MARIE'S DATA FOR CYCLE ERGOMETER TESTS—PREOPERATIVELY AND 2 MONTHS POSTPROGRAM AND TRAINING

Preoperative

Review of preexercise checklist √ (see Table 2-3)

Practice: 1 cycling session 48 h prior

Time of day: 9:00 am

Pulmonary function: See Table 2-3

Body weight (lb): 188

Height (in): 64

Body Mass Index (kg/m²): 32.3

Waist girth (in): 37

Waist-to-hip ratio: 1.0

Meds: Bronchodilator 10 min prior to exercise

Pulmonary function:

FEV$_1$: 85% predicted

FVC: 92% predicted

FEV$_1$/FVC: 92% predicted

PEFR: 65% predicted

SpO$_2$: 95%

Two Months Posttraining

Review of preexercise checklist √ (see Table 2-3)

1 cycling session 48 h prior

9:00 am

173

64

29.7

34

0.9

Bronchodilator 10 min prior to exercise

88% predicted

94% predicted

94% predicted

72% predicted

97%

Reason for test termination: 90% of age-predicted maximum heart rate—158 bts/min

Minute or stage	Watts 25 increments	RPM 50	METs predicted	Heart rate (bts/min) and EKG changes	Blood pressure (mmHg)	Rate pressure product (x10³)	SpO₂ (%)	Blood sugar (mg/dL)	Rating of perceived exertion or breathlessness (0-10)	Discomfort/pain (not anginal) (0-10)	Comments
0	0	0	1 / **1**	88 NSR / **80 NSR**	144/98 / **130/84**	12.7 / **10.4**	94 / **97**	100 / **95**	2 / **0.5**	1 / **1**	Discomfort right hip
0	0	0	1 / **1**	86 NSR / **79 NSR**	142/95 / **128/86**	12.2 / **10.1**	96 / **97**		2 / **0.5**	1 / **1**	
0	0	0	1 / **1**	88 NSR / **78 NSR**	144/96 / **133/88**	12.7 / **10.4**	96 / **98**		2 / **0.5**	1 / **1**	
1	50	50	3.8 / **3.9**								
2	50	50	3.8 / **3.9**	130 NSR / **120 NSR**	150/- / **138/-**	19.5 / **16.6**	95 / **97**		4 / **2**	1 / **0**	

*BOLD—responses at 2 months

continued

Table 2-1 (continued)

MARIE'S DATA FOR CYCLE ERGOMETER TESTS—PREOPERATIVELY AND 2 MONTHS POSTPROGRAM AND TRAINING

Minute or stage	Watts 25 Increments	RPM 50	METs predicted	Heart rate (bts/min) and EKG changes	Blood pressure (mmHg)	Rate pressure Product (x10³)	SpO₂ (%)	Blood sugar (mg/dL)	Rating of perceived exertion or breathlessness (0-10)	Discomfort/pain (not anginal) (0-10)	Comments
3	75	50	4.8								
			4.9								
4	75	50	4.8	133 NSR	158/-	21.0	94		5-6	1-2	Sweating
			4.9	**126 NSR**	**142/-**	**17.9**	**97**		**3**	**0**	
5	100	50	5.7								
			5.9								
6	100	50	5.7	148 NSR	164/-	25.5	94		6	2	
			5.9	**138 NSR**	**148/-**	**20.4**	**96**		**3-4**	**0.5**	
7	125	50	6.6								
			6.8								
8	125	50	6.6	158 NSR	172/-	27.2	93		7	2	1 PVC noted
			6.8	**144 NSR**	**155/-**	**22.3**	**95**		**4**	**0**	
9	50	50	3.8	148 NSR	160/-	23.7	93		6-7	1	
			3.9	**136 NSR**	**145/-**	**19.7**	**97**		**4**	**0.5**	
10	50	50	3.8	140 NSR	155/-	21.7	94		5	1	
			3.9	**128 NSR**	**138/-**	**17.7**	**98**		**3**	**0.5**	
11	0	0	1	120 NSR	148/-	17.8	94		4	1	
			1	**105 NSR**	**134/-**	**14.1**	**98**		**1**	**0**	
12	0	0	1	116 NSR	146/-	16.9	95		3	1	
			1	**98 NSR**	**136/-**	**13.3**	**98**		**1**	**0**	
13	0	0	1	100 NSR	144/-	14.4	96		3	0	
			1	**85 NSR**	**134/-**	**11.4**	**98**		**0.5**	**0**	
14	0	0	1	90 NSR	146/-	13.1	96		2	0	
			1	**78 NSR**	**132/-**	**10.3**	**98**		**0**	**0**	
15	0	0	1	85 NSR	144/-	12.2	97	86	1-2	0	
			1	**75 NSR**	**130/-**	**9.8**	**98**		**0**	**0**	
16	0	0	1	88 NSR	142/-	12.5	97		1	0	
			1	**75 NSR**	**132/-**	**9.9**	**98**	**84**	**0**	**0**	

*BOLD—responses at 2 months

continued

Table 2-1 (continued)
MARIE'S DATA FOR CYCLE ERGOMETER TESTS—PREOPERATIVELY AND 2 MONTHS POSTPROGRAM AND TRAINING

Interpretation of Data

Preoperatively: Initial Baseline Test

Weight Classification: Obesity Class I[66]

6.6 MET load achieved at 90% at age-predicted maximum heart rate

Rest: Relatively high resting physiologic variables

Warm-up: Prolonged responses to given work rate change

Peak: Disproportionately high physiologic responses for the peak work rate consistent with deconditioning

Cool-down: Prolonged cool-down for each cool-down work rate

Recovery: Recovery took 5 minutes for parameters to lower within 5% of baseline; remained elevated

Overall: Test well tolerated

Exercise prescription:

    Type: Cycle ergometry

    Intensity: 70 to 85% age-predicted maximum heart rate

    Frequency: 3 to 5x/wk

    Duration: 3 bouts of 10 minutes with 2 min rest between

Course: Retest in 2 months

Retest: 2 Months Posttraining

Weight Classification: Overweight[66]

Rest: Lower resting metabolic variables; less work of the heart at rest

Warm-up: Responded appropriately to incremental exercise

Peak: More rapid physiologic adjustment to a given work rate compared with baseline test

Cool-down: More rapid physiologic return to pretest measures and plateaud at those values

Recovery: Recovered within 3 to 4 minutes of exercise cessation

Overall: Test well tolerated

Exercise prescription:

    Type: Cycle ergometer

    Intensity: 70 to 85% age-predicted maximum heart rate

    Frequency: 3 to 5x/wk

    Duration: 30 to 40 min continuously

Retest indicated (see Table 2-6)

TESTS AND MEASURES

♦ Aerobic capacity/endurance
  • Prior to exercise testing, a check should be performed to ensure that testing may be done (see Table 2-3 for items to be checked)
  • Baseline preoperative tests served as the basis for postoperative comparisons (see History, Other Clinical Tests: Astrand-Rhyming ergometer test, 6-Minute Walk test, and cycle ergometer test)
  • Baseline average steps/day (pedometer reading): 2500 (sedentary lifestyle category)[79]

♦ Anthropometric characteristics
  • Skin fold measurement (seven sites): 33% body fat
  • Waist girth: 37 inches
  • Waist-to-hip ratio: 1.0
  • BMI (kg /m^2)=32.3, Class I obesity[80,81]

♦ Arousal, attention, and cognition
  • Alert, oriented x3
  • Mrs. Rodriguez reports no psychological or psychiatric condition, which is supported by the interview, history, and referral from her general practitioner

♦ Assistive and adaptive devices
  • Mrs. Rodriguez uses orthotics in her daily foot wear because of fallen arches

♦ Circulation
  • Auscultation
    ▪ Heart sounds appear normal
  • Pulse quality
    ▪ Peripheral pulses are blunted (likely due to excess adipose tissue)
  • ECG
    ▪ Normal sinus rhythm
  • Hemodynamic response to postural test
    ▪ Normal HR and BP responses after standardized test (15 minutes supine)
    ▪ HR and BP measured immediately on assuming sitting upright position and at 1 minute, 2 minutes, and 5 minutes: WNL
  • Peripheral perfusion: Capillary refill test
    ▪ Filling time prolonged in both hands and feet (high end of the normal range [10 to 12 seconds])
  • RPPrest (10^3): 14.2

♦ Integumentary integrity
  • Skin redness on tuberosities and bony prominences with prolonged recumbency (ie, 2 hours)
  • Extremities: No apparent disease
  • Incision is healed

♦ Motor function
  • Generally WNL

• Postoperative gag and swallowing reflexes slightly impaired

♦ Muscle performance (based on Oxford Manual Muscle Testing grading system 0 to 5)
  • Baseline manual muscle test grades
    ▪ Peripheral muscles: 3+/5 to 4-/5
    ▪ Abdominal muscles: 2+/5
    ▪ Back extensor muscles: 3/5
  • Respiratory muscles not tested

♦ Pain
  • Pain at rest: 0 for abdomen and hips (on 0 to 10 modified Borg scale)[82,83] (Table 2-4)
  • Pain with movement was between 2 and 3
  • Mrs. Rodriguez believes her discomfort and pain are manageable

♦ Posture
  • Standing posture reveals moderate lordosis
  • Slightly kyphotic
  • Mild lumbar scoliosis

♦ Range of motion
  • Reduced lower chest wall expansion: 1¾ at xiphoid
  • All joints WNL except:
    ▪ 80% of normal for right hip flexion and extension
    ▪ 60% right hip abduction
    ▪ 90% for left hip flexion, extension, and abduction
    ▪ 80% hip rotation bilaterally
    ▪ Spinal flexion, extension, and rotation decreased by 10%

♦ Self-care and home management
  • Short Form 36[84] score of 80 (0 to 100 scale) indicated Mrs. Rodriguez has been independent in self-care and home management (light housework)
  • She has hired help, but she and husband share light household and yard work

♦ Ventilation and respiration/gas exchange
  • Auscultation
    ▪ Apices difficult to auscultate
    ▪ Distant breath sounds consistent with excess thoracic adiposity
    ▪ Fine crackles to bases, right more than left
    ▪ End-expiratory wheezing
    ▪ Minimal detectable change with body position change or movement
  • Ventilatory pattern
    ▪ Breathing at low lung volumes
    ▪ Rapid shallow breathing
  • SaO$_2$ or SpO$_2$: 90% at rest increasing to 94% to 96% with deep breathing in 75-degree sitting

Table 2-2

MARIE'S DATA FOR 6-MINUTE WALK TESTS—PREOPERATIVELY AND 2 MONTHS POSTTRAINING

Preoperative

Review of preexercise checklist √ (see Table 2-3)

Practice: 1 test the day prior

Time of day: 9:00 am

Body weight (lb): 188

Height (in): 64

Body Mass Index (kg/m²): 32.3

Waist (in): 37

Waist-to-hip ratio: 1.0

Meds: Bronchodilator 10 min prior to exercise

Pulmonary function:

FEV$_1$: 85% predicted

FVC: 92% predicted

FEV$_1$/FVC: 92% predicted

PEFR: 65% predicted

SpO$_2$: 95%

Reason for test termination: Test terminated at predetermined time (ie, 6 minutes)

Two Months Posttraining

Review of preexercise checklist √ (see Table 2-3)

1 test 2 days prior

9:30 am

173

64

29

34

0.9

Bronchodilator 10 min prior to exercise

88% predicted

94% predicted

94% predicted

72% predicted

97%

Minute	Heart rate (bts/min) and ECG changes	Blood pressure (mmHg)	Rate pressure product (x10³)	SpO$_2$ (%)	Blood sugar (mg/dL)	Rating of perceived exertion or breathlessness (0-10)	Discomfort/ pain (not anginal) (0-10)	Comments
0	88 NSR	144/98	12.7	94	100	2	3	
	77	**130/84**	**10.0**	**97**	**90**	**0.5**	**1**	
0	86	142/95	12.2	96		2	3	
	79	**128/86**	**10.1**	**97**		**0.5**	**1**	
0	88	144/96	12.7	96		2	2	
	78	**133/88**	**10.4**	**98**		**0.5**	**1**	
1	98			95				
	82			**97**				
2	110			94		5-6	3	
	88			**97**		**3**	**0**	

*BOLD—responses at 2 months

continued

Table 2-2 (continued)

Marie's Data for 6-Minute Walk Tests—Preoperatively and 2 Months Posttraining

Minute	Heart rate (bts/min) and ECG changes	Blood pressure (mmHg)	Rate pressure Product ($\times 10^3$)	SpO_2 (%)	Blood sugar (mg/dL)	Rating of perceived exertion or breathlessness (0-10)	Discomfort/ pain (not anginal) (0-10)	Comments
3	114 **94**			94 **96**				
4	120 **110**			93 **95**		7 **4**	3 **0**	
5	132 **122**			92 **95**				
6	148 **130**	184/- **168/-**	27.2 **21.8**	92 **95**		8-9 **6**	3-4 **0**	Feeling tired
7	110 NSR **90 NSR**	160/- **145/-**	17.6 **13.1**	93 **97**				
8	100 NSR **85 NSR**	155/- **138/-**	15.5 **11.7**	94 **98**		5 **3**	5 **0.5**	
9	90 NSR **82 NSR**	148/- **134/-**	13.3 **11.0**	94 **98**				
10	88 NSR **77 NSR**	146/- **136/-**	12.8 **10.5**	95 **98**		3 **1**	2-3 **0**	Hip feels good
11	86 NSR **75 NSR**	144/- **134/-**	12.4 **10.1**	96 **98**				
12	88 NSR **75 NSR**	146/- **132/-**	12.8 **9.9**	96 **98**	85 **84**	2 **0**	2 **0**	

*BOLD—responses at 2 months

continued

Table 2-2 (continued)

MARIE'S DATA FOR 6-MINUTE WALK TESTS—PREOPERATIVELY AND 2 MONTHS POSTTRAINING

Interpretation of Data

Preoperatively: Initial Baseline Test

Distance walked: 1262 ft (no rest periods)

Average speed: 2.4 mph

Weight Classification: Obesity Class I[66]

Rest: Relatively high resting physiologic variables

Peak: Disproportionately high physiologic responses for the peak work rate consistent with deconditioning

Recovery: Recovery took 5 minutes for parameters to lower within 5% of baseline; remained elevated

Subjective responses: Discomfort/pain peaked at 3 to 4, and reduced to 2 after 6 to 7 minutes of exercise cessation

Exercise prescription implications: Minimize discomfort to maximize Marie's walking exercise capacity

Retest: 2 Months Posttraining

Distance walked: 1849 ft (no rest periods)

Average speed: 3.5 mph

Weight Classification: Overweight[66]

Rest: Lower resting metabolic variables; less work of the heart at rest

Peak: More rapid physiologic adjustment to a given work rate compared with baseline test

Recovery: Recovered within 3 to 4 minutes of exercise cessation

Subjective responses: Discomfort/pain reduced to low levels

Exercise prescription implications: Continue to minimize discomfort to maximize Marie's walking exercise capacity, and potential for musculoskeletal stress

Table 2-3
CHECKLIST BEFORE EXERCISE TESTING OR TRAINING SESSION

Client: _____

Date: _____

- ☐   Feeling well over the past 48 hours
- ☐   No infections (eg, upper respiratory tract infection) or influenza
- ☐   No temperature
- ☐   No unaccustomed muscle or joint discomfort or pain
- ☐   No chest tightness or pain
- ☐   No unaccustomed breathing difficulty or fatigue
- ☐   Adequate night's sleep
- ☐   Has not eaten heavily within past 3 hours
- ☐   No smoking within past 3 hours (patients who are smokers)
- ☐   Best time of day which is standardized across tests
- ☐   Wearing or using orthoses, walking aids, and devices
- ☐   Clothing appropriate for exercise conditions (indoors or outdoors)
- ☐   Appropriate socks and footwear that is comfortable, well-fitting, and has secured laces (double-knotted)
- ☐   Has water within easy access
- ☐   Taken preexercise medications at specified time
- ☐   Has nitroglycerine within reach (patients with cardiac dysfunction)
- ☐   Has inhaler within reach (patients with pulmonary dysfunction)
- ☐   Has sugar supply within reach (patients with diabetes)
- ☐   Standardize and record the use of orthotics and walking aids
- ☐   Other specifics for a given client or patient

♦ Work, community, and leisure integration or reintegration
   - Work-related sedentary activities present no problems other than right hip upon standing up after prolonged standing and walking
   - Mrs. Rodriguez requires no assistance to function in the community
   - She appears limited to ADL with a VO$_2$peak energy cost of less than 6.6 METs at 90% of age-predicted MHR

EVALUATION

Her history and findings are consistent with a chronic history of cholecystitis and deconditioning secondary to reduced exercise stress. Mrs. Rodriguez is obese (about 33% over her ideal BMI and 33% over her body fat composition even recognizing the limitations of body fold measures) and has borderline HTN. Prior to surgery, Mrs. Rodriguez reported shortness of breath on minimal exertion and required ongoing rests to complete tasks. Her aerobic capacity was poor to fair. Her functional capacity was limited by hip pain, rather than exertion. Her sedentary lifestyle and aerobic deconditioning are associated with reduced circulating blood volume, down-regulation of O$_2$ transport capacity, and reduced aerobic reserve capacity.

DIAGNOSIS

Mrs. Rodriguez is an obese patient who is 3 days postoperative open laparoscopic surgery for cholecystitis, has significant health risk factors, and also has pain. She has impaired aerobic conditioning/endurance; anthropometric characteristics; circulation; muscle performance; posture; range of motion; and ventilation and respiration/gas exchange. She is also functionally limited in work, community, and leisure actions, tasks, and activities. She is at risk for deconditioning because of her sedentary lifestyle, obesity, poor nutrition, high body fat, and obesity-related restrictive lung pathology. In addition, as a Mexican immigrant to the United States, she has additional risk factors due to exposure to the traditional Western diet and sedentary lifestyle.[85] These findings are consistent with placement in Pattern B: Impaired Aerobic Capacity/Endurance Associated With Deconditioning. These impairments and functional limitations will be addressed in determining the prognosis and the plan of care.

	Discomfort/Pain	Perceived Exertion	Breathlessness	Fatigue
		Table 2-4		

MODIFIED BORG SCALE FOR SUBJECTIVE RESPONSES FOR PAIN ASSESSMENT
(ALSO INCLUDED ARE THE SCALES FOR PERCEIVED EXERTION, BREATHLESSNESS, AND FATIGUE)

	Discomfort/Pain	Perceived Exertion	Breathlessness	Fatigue
0	Nothing at all	Nothing at all	Nothing at all	Nothing at all
0.5	Very very light	Very very weak	Very very light	Very very light
1	Very weak	Very weak	Very light	Very light
2	Weak	Weak	Light	Light
3	Moderate	Moderate	Moderate	Moderate
4	Somewhat strong	Somewhat strong	Somewhat hard	Somewhat hard
5	Strong	Strong	Hard	Hard
6				
7	Very strong	Very strong	Very heavy	Very heavy
8				
9				
10	Very very strong	Very very strong	Very very hard	Very very hard
	Maximal	Maximal	Maximal	Maximal

*Based on the Borg rating of perceived exertion scale[82,83]

PROGNOSIS AND PLAN OF CARE

Over the course of several months, the following mutually established outcomes have been determined:

♦ Ability to perform work, community, and leisure activities is improved

♦ Aerobic capacity and endurance are increased

♦ Increased empowerment to effect positive health behavior changes for herself and her family is achieved

♦ Lifelong health is enhanced with a reduction of her risk factors for the "diseases of civilization"

♦ Muscle performance is increased

♦ Physical function is improved

♦ Weight loss is achieved

To achieve these outcomes, the interventions will include: coordination, communication, and documentation; patient/client-related instruction; therapeutic exercise; functional training in work, community, and leisure integration or reintegration; and prescription, application, and, as appropriate, fabrication of devices and equipment.

Based on the diagnosis and prognosis, Mrs. Rodriguez is expected to require twice a week physical therapist visits for 8 weeks, at which time she will be reevaluated. At that time, a determination will be made as to additional visits. Mrs. Rodriguez has a good prognosis; however, this is contingent on her daily adherence to the implementation of the plan and follow-up by the physical therapist and the team in the months ahead.

INTERVENTIONS

RATIONALE FOR SELECTED INTERVENTIONS

An aggressive program of improved nutrition, weight loss, increased physical activity, and a long-term structured exercise program is essential for Mrs. Rodriguez to reduce her risk factors in a dose-dependent manner.[86,87]

Therapeutic Exercise

Mrs. Rodriguez's most important indicators for exercise are related to her aerobic deconditioning and health risk. Aerobic deconditioning is a premorbid concern (reduced exercise stress) and is identified postsurgically (reduced gravitational stress and reduced exercise stress).

The most important guidelines for defining activity and exercise parameters include hemodynamic response, blood sugar responses, discomfort/pain, and the avoidance of musculoskeletal complaints. Logistical issues include making health a priority for Mrs. Rodriguez and the need to build a program into her busy lifestyle and to develop this within the context of a health-conducive environment, that is, minimal barriers and maximal facilitators including social support and access. Personal factors include Mrs. Rodriguez's need for social support, for exercising with a friend, and for program variety as she finds repeated exercise programs monotonous and loses interest quickly.

The progression of early mobilization primes the O_2 transport and is the basis for early functional return.[7] Early mobilization is targeted at both the aerobic dysfunction and prevention of further problems. Note that enhanced mucociliary transport is but one potential goal of mobilization.[7] Mrs. Rodriguez's rapid early mobilization and progression through the postoperative period (Figure 2-4) to counter the deficits in and threats to her O_2 transport are shown in Table 2-5. Table 2-5 is included to illustrate the progression of mobilization and exercise as means of remediating her perioperative problems, and the continuum of aerobic conditioning and its prescription from the acute to the subacute and chronic phases of Mrs. Rodriguez's care. The parameters of this early mobilization were based on her responses to intervention. This program of early intervention enabled Mrs. Rodriguez to be discharged home on day 3, at which time this episode of care began.

A health-promoting exercise program should include prescribed resistance muscle training as well as aerobic exercise.[87] However, the prescriptive parameters of a resistance muscle training program to augment aerobic capacity consist of lower resistance and increased repetitions compared with strength training. In addition, movement and exercise that requires greater core stabilization are associated with greater hemodynamic stress (eg, UE exercise and trunk exercise) and thus should be prescribed judiciously.[88,89]

Increased physical activity and structured exercise are important components of programs to reduce weight, control HTN, normalize glucose sensitivity, and condition the cardiovascular system (see Review Dean[7]).

COORDINATION, COMMUNICATION, AND DOCUMENTATION

Communication is fundamental to patient-focused care and management. Mrs. Rodriguez will be updated and informed as will her family in accordance with her wishes. She will be consulted with respect to each intervention. The team establishes jointly how best the mutually established goals may be achieved and the parameters for the various components of her lifelong health program. Information exchange is essential for lifelong health. All elements of the patient's management, including examination, evaluation, diagnosis, prognosis, and interventions will be documented.

Mrs. Rodriguez's education will be targeted and tailored to her specific needs in the following areas:

♦ The effects of passive smoking will be discussed with members of her extended family as it affects Mrs. Rodriguez's airway sensitivity

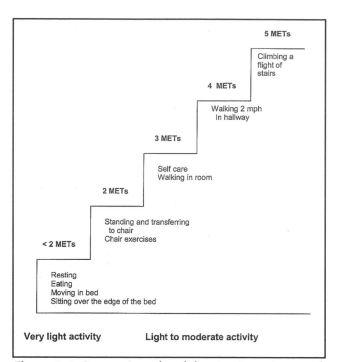

Figure 2-4. Progression of mobilization in patients with acute and medical and surgical conditions based on a consideration of METs. (Adapted from Woods SL. *Cardiac Nursing.* 5th ed. Philadelphia, PA: Lippincott, Williams & Williams; 2004.)

♦ The need for healthy, nonfad approach to nutrition and weight control that will include a review of the food pyramid[90] and advice to join Weight Watchers®

♦ The appropriate use of a bronchodilator prior to exercise and recording of its use

♦ The need for and recording of regular physical activity that will include a review of the activity pyramid[91] and the use of a pedometer

♦ The importance of a structured exercise program (three to five times a week) designed initially by the physical therapist that will eventually progress to a community program, such as Curves or a Tai Chi program[92,93] for an approach to fitness and for the incorporation of exercise in a social environment

♦ The necessity of quality sleep and relaxation and stress management that may include relaxation tapes and music

♦ The adoption of a lifelong approach to good health and sense of well-being that will enable her to fully participate with her family and provide service to her church

Mrs. Rodriguez will be referred to a nutritionist, who will provide information concerning her dietary needs and healthy eating both for her and her family. A Mexican American nutritionist will be particularly helpful and

Table 2-5

BACKGROUND DATA ON MARIE'S PERIOPERATIVE COURSE: BASELINE, PRESCRIPTIVE PARAMETERS (SET BY MARIA'S RESPONSES—TOLERATED WELL AND SAFELY), RESPONSES, AND PROGRESSION

Goal: Prescriptive "upright and moving"* to normalize fluid shifts and address bed rest deconditioning

	Preop	Postop: Day 1	Postop: Day 2	Postop: Day 3	Postop: Day 3 Discharge
Serial Assessment	On-going	→	→	Discharge outcomes attained	Health program designed
Education	Information about Sx related to PT goals and outcomes Mobilization Body positioning BC and C maneuvers Positions of comfort	Reinforce preop teaching during treatment Marie is reluctant to move and has reduced arousal; getting Marie moving is a high priority to avoid deterioration, complications, and prolonged hospital stay	Continue to reinforce preop teaching and extend to longer term goals		Marie's goals with team established Readiness to change determined Community resources reviewed Self-monitoring taught: *Exercise responses* *Log book recording* Nutritionist consult Psychology consult (weight loss) Follow-up plan with PT in consultation with team
Mobilization: *Aerobic* Sit up over the edge of bed	Review of postop mobilization coupled with BC and C	In accordance with responses and tolerance	In accordance with responses and tolerance	Self-initiated walks and activity continued Most time walking or in chair vs in bed	Physical activity prescribed Pedometer use
Transfer to chair		q4h	q2h		Structure exercise program
Stand, walk in place or walk		q4h x1 (shift weight in place)	q2h for 2 to 4 h q2h for 5 min		See text
Mobilization: *Strengthening*		Chest wall mobility exercise (forward flexion, side flexion, extension, rotation) ROM UE and LE	Encourage self-initiated walks and activity		
Body positioning	Review of postop body positioning coupled with BC and C	↑Head of bed 20° to 60° with feet dependent when not up and about	N/A	N/A	N/A
Breathing control and coughing maneuvers	Review of BC and C maneuvers	→	→	↑	BC integrated into relaxation strategies

Legend:
* parameters set by Marie's responses (tolerated well and safely)
BC=breathing control; C=coughing; UE=upper extremities; LE=lower extremities; N/A=not applicable at this stage

knowledgeable about traditional foods and the appropriate modifications to reduce fat, salt, and sugar contents and increase vegetable content. The physical therapist will review and provide a copy of the food pyramid[90] and will have Mrs. Rodriguez keep a weekly record of her food intake.

The health care team will continually review Mrs. Rodriguez's programs and make modifications as indicated.

PATIENT/CLIENT-RELATED INSTRUCTION

Patient education is recognized as a complex process that extends beyond conventional unidirectional knowledge transfer from the health care provider to the patient in the form of instructions or a brochure of information. Although many programs are prescribed for people with health risks, few prescribe programs to ensure sustainability.[94-96] Thus, ensuring appropriate follow-up is crucial for sustainable program effects. The physical therapist must recognize and value the need for education, must identify the specific indications for education and its content, and must evaluate the learner.

Identification of the patient's stage of readiness to implement health behavior change helps the physical therapist to determine when to intervene and at what level. The physical therapist must have highly developed expertise as a health educator to develop education materials and tailor them to each learner. Most importantly, yet often least implemented, is the need for long-term follow-up and support of the patient. To reverse adverse health behaviors that are the result of lifelong patterns and habits and develop sustained healthy lifestyles may take months or years to implement successfully. Follow-up will increase the probability of sustained avoidance of health risk. Prevention is by far the best physical therapist intervention.

The learner and the gaps in the learner's knowledge must be assessed. Readiness to participate in health behavior change also must be established to assess the individual's commitment to health behavior change at this time (see Physical Therapist Examination, General Health Status, General Health Perception for the Transtheoretical Model of Change). Although an individual may be at the precontemplative stage, that is, not considering or interested in changing behavior at this time, health education may still be imparted commensurate with the needs and stage of readiness to change. In addition, the physical therapist may serve as a resource and be available when the patient is ready to institute health behavior change. In Mrs. Rodriguez's case, there are distinct cultural considerations that must be addressed, that is, Mexican heritage that will influence her beliefs and lifestyle behaviors related to health. Mexican culture tends to be collectivistic versus individualistic. The degree to which Mrs. Rodriguez has collectivistic orientation will determine the extent to which she requires strong social support to implement her program and how she will integrate knowledge regarding risk factor reduction. In addition, although highly proficient in English, her first language is Spanish, which may influence how the health information is delivered. Further, this orientation will determine the degree to which Mrs. Rodriguez's program focuses on her capacity to help herself or emphasizes how her optimal health will enhance her contribution to the family.

Mrs. Rodriguez's instructional program will include the following elements:

- Clarification of her self-knowledge of the current pathophysiology responsible for producing symptoms that limit function and social participation and her needs and wants as a learner
- Definition of her personal goals and how to monitor outcomes and systematic recording of these in a log book
- Knowledge of blood sugar responses to meals and exercise, and how to measure these with a gluco-meter
- Knowledge of guidelines for monitoring sleep and sleep adequacy and for improving sleep quality so that it is optimally restorative
- Knowledge of untoward responses, eg, pain control, unusual exercise responses, and musculoskeletal complaints that could suggest aggravation of existing arthritic problems in her hips or new problems
- Understanding of the need to involve her family

Because Mrs. Rodriguez believes that health education sessions in her church, which is very community-oriented, would be beneficial, she has requested that the physical therapist provide an educational program to her youth group. This presentation is very important for expanding the concepts of lifelong healthy living to the Mexican American community.

THERAPEUTIC EXERCISE

- Aerobic capacity/endurance conditioning
  - Parameters for endurance conditioning
    - Mode
      - Use of large muscles and natural movements (eg, increased walking with the use a pedometer and cycling ergometer)
      - Walking will become a greater focus of her exercise program once she loses some weight and her hip pain resolves
      - Variable modes using tasks related to ADL to apply specificity and motor learning principles
    - Intensity
      - See Table 2-2
    - Duration
      - See Table 2-2
    - Frequency
      - See Table 2-2

- Course and progression
  - See Table 2-2
  - Within a prescription, progression is based on increasing exercise intervals and reducing rest periods
  - Load changes are made after conditioning evidence from a retest
- Flexibility exercises
  - Stretching exercises should be done after warming up, using a slow and steady stretch accompanied by deep breathing, and building hold up to 30 to 60 seconds
  - Slow active full ROM coordinated with deep breathing for: hip flexion, extension, abduction, and rotation; and spinal flexion, extension, and rotation
  - Whole body (daily routine) including limbs and chest wall
- Relaxation
  - Breathing relaxation strategies for stress reduction
  - Mrs. Rodriguez will experiment with various strategies such as yoga two times a week
- Strength, power, and endurance training
  - Diaphragmatic breathing exercises
  - Yoga breathing maneuvers beginning with upper chest, middle chest, lower chest, and total expansion
  - Abdominal and back extensor muscle training coordinated with breathing, for example:
    - Elbow press backs
    - Pelvic tilts with single leg raises
  - Weight training
    - Be careful to avoid Valsalva maneuver
    - Type: Light weights (dumbbells for UEs and cuff weights for LEs) beginning with maximum weight that patient can tolerate for 8 to 12 repetitions
    - Intensity: 8 to 12 repetitions, and she should feel that it was all should could life for the 8 to 12 repetitions
    - Build to 20% to 40% 1RM; 3- to 5-minute rest between sets for all major muscle groups
    - Frequency: three to five times a week

FUNCTIONAL TRAINING IN SELF-CARE AND HOME MANAGEMENT

Although Mrs. Rodriguez reported no significant limitation in terms of her ADL and IADL, she has in fact made modifications to her life. She had arranged for people to assist her in activities that she should be able to perform herself.

- Self-care and home management
  - Review all activities and postural alignment for self-care and home management
  - Provide information of correct ergonomics and alignment at home (easy chairs and bed) to minimize biomechanical hip stress that limits her aerobic capacity
- Injury prevention education during self-care and home management
  - Safety during activities
  - Ensure that work areas at home are ergonomically sound

FUNCTIONAL TRAINING IN WORK, COMMUNITY, AND LEISURE INTEGRATION OR REINTEGRATION

Mrs. Rodriguez is not particularly limited with respect to her work, but would like to enjoy a higher level of health and endurance to participate more fully in family and work-related activities.

- Work
  - Review all activities and postural alignment for work activities
  - Provide information on correct alignment at Mrs. Rodriguez's work station
  - Ensure that work areas are ergonomically sound
- Community
  - Safety awareness training during community activities
- Leisure
  - Safety awareness training
  - Facilitate ability to hike and engage in activities with her family
  - Ensure ability to be actively involved with her children's lives and their families after they marry

PRESCRIPTION, APPLICATION, AND, AS APPROPRIATE, FABRICATION OF DEVICES AND EQUIPMENT

For Mrs. Rodriguez to fully participate in her lifelong health plan, she needs the tools to self-monitor, record her findings regularly in a log book, and strengthen her sense of self-mastery.

- Revision of orthotics and education about replacing them particularly now since she is increasing her volume of exercise and weightbearing activities
- HR monitor
- Glucometer

ANTICIPATED GOALS AND EXPECTED OUTCOMES

- Impact on pathology/pathophysiology
  - Indicators of O_2 transport are improved.

- Self-mastery of her symptoms and physiologic responses to physical activity and exercise is increased.

♦ Impact on impairments
- Aerobic capacity is increased as evidenced by decreased resting HR, BP, and RR and enhanced submaximal exercise responses for a given work rate.
- Endurance is increased by increasing number of steps daily from baseline of 2500 to 3500 using a pedometer log.
- Muscle strength is increased to 4/5 to 5/5.
- Optimal BMI, waist circumference (<33 inches[97,98]), waist-to-hip ratio (<0.8), and body fat are improved by decreasing daily calories from fat from 35% to 22% to 25%, decreasing salt and sugar intake, and decreasing weight by 1 to 2 lbs per week.
- ROM is increased to normal in hips and spine.
- Stress incontinence is decreased based on Mrs. Rodriguez's self-report (fewer number of reported episodes of urgency, and urinary frequency has been reduced now to only once every 2 to 4 hours).

♦ Impact on functional limitations
- Capacity to enjoy physical activity with her family is increased.
- Endurance at work is increased.
- Functional work capacity is increased.
- Stamina for work-related social events is increased.

♦ Risk reduction/prevention
- Health risks associated with HTN, stroke, IHD, pulmonary dysfunction, diabetes, and osteoporosis are reduced.
- Risks are reduced by normalization of the following: BP <120/80 mmHg;[74] total cholesterol <200 mg/dL; LDL <100 mg/dL; HDL >35 mg/dL; ratio of LDL to HDL <3.25; triglycerides=40 to 150 mg/dL; glucose (fasting)=70 to 115 mg/dL; and glucose (postprandial) <200 mg/dL.
- Risks for IHD, respiratory dysfunction, HTN, stroke, renal disease, obesity, cancer, and diabetes are reduced.

♦ Impact on health, wellness, and fitness
- Behaviors that promote healthy nutrition, physical activity, and wellness are acquired.
- Fitness is improved.
- Health status is improved.
- Need for bronchodilator therapy is reduced.
- Physical capacity is increased.
- Physical function is improved.

♦ Impact on societal resources
- Documentation occurs throughout patient management and follows APTA's *Guidelines for Physical Therapy Documentation*.[99]

♦ Patient/client satisfaction
- Better balance between her work and personal life is achieved.
- Care is coordinated with family and other professionals.
- Patient's and family's knowledge and awareness of the diagnosis, prognosis, interventions, and understanding of anticipated goals and expected outcomes are increased.
- Sense of well-being is improved.
- Sleep and capacity to relax are improved.
- Stressors are decreased.

REEXAMINATION

Reexamination is performed throughout the episode of care. It is anticipated that patients placed in this pattern will require multiple episodes of care over the lifetime. Periodic reexamination and initiation of new episodes of care should occur as the patient's functional limitations or disability changes.

The recommended time for formal retesting to evaluate the effect of the aerobic and lifestyle training programs is 8 weeks. At this time, two submaximal retests will be conducted. The anticipated results are shown in boldface in Table 2-1 for the submaximal ergometer test and in Table 2-2 for the 6-Minute Walk test. The retest on the ergometer with a higher initial start work rate is shown in Table 2-6. The improvement in aerobic capacity on the 6-Minute Walk test and the ergometer test indicated the need for a second ergometer test with the higher initial work rate. This latter test provided the basis for modifying the exercise prescription for the next 8 weeks. The revised exercise prescription is outlined in Table 2-6.

DISCHARGE

Mrs. Rodriguez was discharged from this episode of physical therapy care that included her course of physical therapy and a home program based on her predischarge evaluation and exercise test after a total of 24 physical therapy sessions over 8 weeks. These sessions have covered her entire episode of care. She is discharged because she has achieved her goals and expected outcomes.

PSYCHOLOGICAL ASPECTS

Mrs. Rodriguez has experienced some anxiety about her health as she thought that her abdominal complaints may have been cancer since her grandmother died of ovarian cancer. She has shifted from the contemplative to preparation stage in terms of readiness to change to more positive health behaviors with respect to her weight and physical activity.

Table 2-6

MARIE'S DATA FOR CYCLE ERGOMETER TEST—RETEST AT 2 MONTHS FOR REVISION OF EXERCISE PRESCRIPTION

Preoperative

Review of preexercise checklist √ (see Table 2-3)
Practice: 1 cycling session 48 h prior
Time of day: 9:00 am
Pulmonary function: See Table 2-1
Meds: Bronchodilator 10 min prior to exercise
Reason for test termination: 90% of age-predicted maximal heart rate—158 bts/min

Two Months Posttraining

Review of preexercise checklist √ (see Table 2-3)
1 cycling session 48 h prior
9:00 am
See Table 2-1
Bronchodilator 10 min prior to exercise

Minute or stage	Watts 25 increments	RPM 50	METs predicted	Heart rate (bts/min) and ECG changes	Blood pressure (mmHg)*	Rate pressure product (x10³)	SpO₂ (%)	Blood sugar (mg/dL)	Rating of perceived exertion or breathlessness (0-10)	Discomfort/pain (not anginal) (0-10)	Comments
0	0	0	1	80	130/84	10.4	97	95	0.5	1	
0	0	0	1	79	128/86	10.1	97		0.5	1	
0	0	0	1	78	133/88	10.4	98		0.5	1	
1	50	50	4.0	114							
2	50	50	4.0	110	148/-*	16.3	97		2	0	
3	75	50	5.0	124							
4	75	50	5.0	122	152/-	18.5	97		3	0	
5	100	50	6.0	126							
6	100	50	6.0	128	158/-	20.2	96		3-4	0.5	
7	125	50	6.9	136							
8	125	50	6.9	132	165/-	21.8	95		4	0	
9	150	50	7.9	138							
10	150	50	7.9	138	169/-	23.3	95		5	0	
11	175	50	8.9	142							
12	175	50	8.9	144	172/-	24.8	95		6	0	
13	200	50	9.8	154						0.5	Tightness right calf muscle
14	200	50	9.8	158	176/-	27.8	97		4		
15	75	50	5.0	130			98		3	0.5	
16	75	50	5.0	125	154/-	19.4	98		1	0	
17	50	50	4.0	105			98		1	0	Feels lightheaded

continued

Table 2-6 (continued)

MARIE'S DATA FOR CYCLE ERGOMETER TEST—RETEST AT 2 MONTHS FOR REVISION OF EXERCISE PRESCRIPTION

Minute or stage	Watts 25 increments	RPM 50	METs predicted	Heart rate (bts/min) and ECG changes	Blood pressure (mmHg)*	Rate pressure product (x103)	SpO$_2$ (%)	Blood sugar (mg/dL)	Rating of perceived exertion or breathlessness (0-10)	Discomfort/ pain (not anginal) (0-10)	Comments
18	50	50	4.0	100	144/-	14.4	98		0.5	0	
19	0	0	1	95			98		0	0	
20	0	0	1	90	138/-	12.4	99			0	
21	0	0	1	88			98		0		
22	0	0	1	82	134/-	11.0	99			0	
23	0	0	1	84			98		0	0	
24	0	0	1	83	133/-	11.0	98	82	0	0	

Interpretation of Data

Retest: 2 Months Posttraining

9.8 MET load achieved at 90% at age-predicted maximum heart rate

Weight classification: Overweight[66]

Rest: Lower resting metabolic variables; less work of the heart at rest

Warm-up: Responded appropriately to incremental exercise

Peak: More rapid physiologic adjustment to a given work rate compared with baseline test

Cool-down: More rapid physiologic return to pretest measures and stabilized at those values

Recovery: Recovered within 3 to 4 minutes of exercise cessation

Overall: Test well tolerated

Exercise prescription modified:

    Type: Cycle ergometry

    Intensity: 70% to 85% age-predicted maximum heart rate

    Frequency: 3 to 5x/wk

    Duration: 3 bouts of 10 min with 2 min rest between (1st 3 wks) → 2 bouts of 15 min with 2 min rest between (2nd 3 wks)

Course: Retest in 8 wks

*Note: diastolic value not recorded during test.

In addition, she recognizes that her sleep has been deteriorating particularly at the onset of menopause. She further acknowledged the importance of the relationship between sleep and maximal function during the day. She reflected that *"Inadequate sleep probably affects my immune system as well."*

The diseases of civilization usually result after a lifetime of poor lifestyle choices. Change takes time and sustained change in choices when adopting a healthy lifestyle takes even longer. The patient and the physical therapist must consider building in a mechanism for sustained change over the years. The literature supports the concept that the continued involvement and support of a health care provider (eg, physical therapist) can help in the process of attaining lifelong health.[100]

Case Study #2: Metabolic Syndrome

Mr. Mark Smith is a 35-year-old male with marked aerobic deconditioning and the emerging signs of metabolic syndrome.

PHYSICAL THERAPIST EXAMINATION

HISTORY

♦ General demographics: Mr. Smith is a 35-year-old white male. He completed high school and 2 years of college before taking bus driver training. He is literate in English and adheres to no particular religious faith.

♦ Social history: Mr. Smith is separated from his wife. Their children, a 13-year-old girl and an 11-year-old boy, spend equal time between the two households.

♦ Employment/work: Mr. Smith has been a bus driver for 10 years. He previously worked in a paint factory for 3 years while putting himself through college.

♦ Living environment: He lives in a single-story home in a suburb of the city.

♦ General health status
  • General health perception: Mr. Smith believes that the absence of illness is equivalent to health. He is feeling more vulnerable since his father had died at the age of 54, and his brother was diagnosed with dysrhythmia 4 months ago. Prior to his father's death, Mr. Smith rated himself at the precontemplative stage with respect to readiness to change his health behavior. Mr. Smith would like to reduce his weight and weight-associated risk factors. He is also aware that he is under a great deal of stress due to work and his family problems. Mr. Smith is

also disgruntled that the bus company for whom he works has deemed him medically unsafe to resume his duties as a result of his chronic back problem and obesity. He has been suspended for 6 months, and his health risk factors will be reevaluated at that time for return to work.

  • Physical function: Mr. Smith states he is able to perform all his ADL independently, but he does have some difficulty as a result of his chronic low back problem.

  • Psychological function: He reports that he is depressed due to the stress of family, separation from his wife and from work, and sexual dysfunction. The employee assistance office at work is presently seeing him. The Beck Depression Scale was administered by the psychologist at his work-place and confirmed moderate to severe depression. Prior to all of this, he stated that he had generally good mental health. He had never been under the care of a counselor (other than when he was in high school), psychologist, or psychiatrist.

  • Role function: Estranged husband, father, son, friend, employee.

  • Social function: Mr. Smith enjoys having family and friends to his family home for social gatherings on weekends. He attends his children's activities at school when he is not working the night shift. He is the captain of the bus company's bowling league. He bowls once a week and more often during competition.

  • Social/health habits
    ▪ Mr. Smith has smoked one pack per day since 13 years of age. Over the past several months, this has increased to one-and-a-half packs per day because of the stress of his job suspension. Mr. Smith has attempted to quit smoking twice but only for a few days each time (the first time 15 years ago and the second time 5 years ago).
    ▪ He enjoys drinking beer after bowling and on weekends with his friends, who come over to watch sports.
    ▪ With respect to nutrition, Mr. Smith does not like vegetables and only eats fruit occasionally when it is mixed with something else. He eats fast food when on the job.

♦ The questionnaire Risk Factor Assessment for the Diseases of Civilization[76] revealed that Mr. Smith's risks for IHD and cancer and for other smoking-related conditions were very high. He is also hypertensive, thus increasing his risk of IHD, stroke, and renal disease, he is markedly over his ideal BMI, and his blood sugars are consistent with diabetes. His profile is consistent with metabolic syndrome.[58]

- Family history: Both his father and uncle died in their 50s of IHD. His mother left the family when he was 5 years old, so he has no knowledge of his maternal family history. His brother, who is 3 years older than he is, had a diagnosis of dysrhythmia 4 months ago.

- Medical/surgical history: Mr. Smith has had a history of HTN for 14 years and insulin resistance for 9 years (diagnosed as prediabetic). He has gastroesophageal reflux and indigestion. He has had a chronic low back problem which began about 8 years ago with an acute episode. He has had a history of obesity since childhood. He has no surgical history.

- Prior hospitalizations: None.

- Preexisting medical and other health-related conditions: Mr. Smith indicated that he has heartburn and indigestion after eating heavy meals, but these symptoms are alleviated with antacids. He also has chronic constipation with infrequent bowel movements (one time every 3 to 4 days). He also reports that he has had sexual dysfunction, in particular, erectile dysfunction for 5½ years. His urinary function is normal; however, his urine has shown high glucose levels. He also has periodontal disease, but visits the dentist infrequently. He has had a productive cough for a month or two over the course of a year, and this pattern has persisted for several years. Mr. Smith sleeps well on an average of 7 to 8 hours a night, and he reports feeling restored in the morning 4 to 5 out of 7 days. He has been told that he snores and breathes erratically at night. Mr. Smith has had blurred vision periodically (one time every 6 weeks) that he states is from being overtired.

- Current condition(s)/chief complaint(s): Mr. Smith indicated that his only symptom is shortness of breath on exertion. He has recovered from his latest exacerbation of low back pain, which occurred 6 weeks ago, but he is considered at high risk of recurrence by his physical therapist based on his deconditioning and obesity. The bus company is concerned about his obesity and back condition in terms of his return to work. He is to be reevaluated by the company physician for return to work in 6 months.

- Functional status and activity level: Prior to his last low back pain episode, Mr. Smith was able to do routine ADL and drive a city bus for 10 hour shifts. He does not exercise formally other than bowling 1 night a week and more during tournaments. He reports some breathlessness, but states this would go away if he didn't smoke.

- Medications: He is taking diuretics for HTN. He estimates that he takes his medication daily 75% of the time. During his last bout of acute back pain, he was taking painkillers but no longer needs these. He takes antacids as needed.

- Other clinical tests:
  - Abnormal values reported only:
    - Total cholesterol: 250 mg/dL (desirable is <200 mg/dL)
    - LDL: 250 mg/dL
      - Optimal level: <100 mg/dL
      - Near optimal level: 100 to 129 mg/dL
      - Borderline high level: 130 to 159 mg/dL
      - High level: 160 to 189 mg/dL
      - Very high level corresponding to highest increased risk of heart disease: >190 mg/dL
    - HDL: 40 mg/dL (normal for males is 40 to 60 mg/dL)
    - Ratio: 6.25 (normal is <3.25)
    - Triglycerides: 425 mg/dL (normal for males is 40 to 150 mg/mL)
    - Glucose (fasting): 200 mg/dL (normal is 70 to 115 mg/dL)
    - Glucose (postprandial): 260 mg/dL (normal is <200 mg/dL)
    - HbA1C: 9.8% (normal is 5% or less)
    - Homocysteine: 12 umol/L (normal is 5 to 15 umol/L)
    - CRP: 6 ug/mL (normal is <6 ug/mL)
  - ECG: Normal sinus rhythm
  - Pulmonary function tests: FEV_1=65% predicted, FVC=80% predicted, FEV_1/FVC=81% predicted, and PEFR=45% predicted
  - SpO_2 at rest: 95% and during exercise=88% (both measured 2 hours after last cigarette), which indicated desaturation during exercise[101]
  - Temperature: 98.6°F

SYSTEMS REVIEW

- Cardiovascular/pulmonary
  - BP: 160/98 mmHg (Stage 2 HTN)[74]
  - Edema: Dependent edema at the end of the day after driving for a 10-hour shift
  - HR: 85 bpm
  - RR: 16 bpm

- Integumentary
  - Presence of scar formation: None present
  - Skin color: Normal
  - Skin integrity: Dry skin, minimal LE hair, and absence of toe hair

- Musculoskeletal
  - Gross range of motion: WNL
  - Gross strength: WNL except for trunk flexors and extensors
  - Gross symmetry: WNL

- Height: 5'10" (1.78 m)
- Weight: 250 lbs (113.4 kg)
- ◆ Neuromuscular
  - Balance: WNL
  - Locomotion, transfers, and transitions: WNL
- ◆ Communication, affect, cognition, language, and learning style
  - Communication, affect, cognition, and language: Alert and oriented x3
  - Appears anxious
  - Learning preferences: Concrete experiential

TESTS AND MEASURES

- ◆ Aerobic capacity/endurance
  - Prior to exercise testing, a check should be performed to ensure that testing may be done (see Table 2-3 for items to be checked)
  - Astrand-Ryhming cycle ergometer test:[78] Results showed him to be <10th percentile or poor aerobic capacity based on prediction[101]
  - Treadmill walking test: See Table 2-7 for results of submaximal exercise test results
  - Steps/day: 1581 (severely sedentary category)[79]
  - Poor breathing control during activity
- ◆ Anthropometric characteristics
  - BMI (kg/m²): 36.3, which places him in Obesity Class II[80,81]
  - Body fat (%): 39.4%
  - Skin fold measurement (seven sites): 39.6% body fat
  - Waist girth: 49 inches
  - Waist-to-hip ratio: 1.2
- ◆ Arousal, attention, and cognition
  - Alert and oriented x 3
- ◆ Assistive and adaptive devices
  - None used
- ◆ Circulation
  - Pulse quality: Normal
  - ECG: Normal sinus rhythm
- ◆ Ergonomics and body mechanics
  - Poor body mechanics when lifting
  - Poor sitting posture and tolerance to sitting when driving his bus
- ◆ Gait, locomotion, and balance
  - Ambulates independently without assistive devices, but does become short of breath after three or four blocks
  - Balance: WNL
- ◆ Muscle performance (based on Oxford Manual Muscle Testing grading system 0 to 5)

- Peripheral muscles: 4/5 to 5/5
- Abdominal muscles: 2/5
- Back extensor muscles: 3/5
- ◆ Orthotic, protective, and supportive devices
  - Occasional shoe orthotics when feet hurt (two times a month)
- ◆ Pain
  - Back pain is resolved
  - Avoids body positions and activities that exacerbate symptoms
- ◆ Posture
  - Moderate kyphosis standing
  - Mild kyphotic sitting posture
  - Abdominal girth shifts center of gravity anteriorly
- ◆ Range of motion
  - Extremities: WNL
  - Decreased middle and lower chest wall expansion with rigidity
    - At level of 4th rib: 1¾ inches
    - At level of 7th rib/xiphoid: 2 inches
- ◆ Self-care and home management
  - Mr. Smith reports that he is capable of all self-care and home management
  - His outdoor work around the home has been limited due to his low back pain and obesity
- ◆ Sensory integrity
  - Sensation generally normal; however, slightly diminished sensation to light touch on the plantar surfaces of both feet
- ◆ Ventilation and respiration/gas exchange
  - Auscultation
    - Clear lung fields with distant sounds consistent with chest wall adiposity
    - Smoker's cough in the morning on arising and stimulated with exercise but no apparent bronchospasm or pulmonary secretion retention
  - Breathing pattern
    - Upper chest breathing due to thoracic and abdominal mass and chest wall compression
  - Cough productive of tenacious clear/white secretions on awaking in the morning; coughing lessens after having been up and about for 45 minutes to an hour
  - SaO_2 or SpO_2: 95% at rest and decreases with minimal to moderate levels of exertion
- ◆ Work, community, and leisure integration or reintegration
  - Mr. Smith can function adequately in the community with activities within 5 METs

Table 2-7
Mark's Data for Treadmill Walking Test: Baseline and at 2 Months Postprogram and Training*

Pretest Baseline

Review of preexercise checklist √ (see Table 2-3)

Practice: 2 treadmill walks 48 h prior to test

Time of day: 9:00 am

Body weight (lb): 250.5

Body Mass Index (kg/m2): 36.3

Waist girth (in): 49

Waist-to-hip ratio: 1.2

Medications: Cholesterol lowering medication, oral hypoglycemic, antihypertensive

Pulmonary function:

FEV_1: 65% predicted

FVC: 80% predicted

FEV_1/FVC: 81% predicted

PEFR: 45% predicted

SpO_2: 95%

Reasons for test:

Assessment of aerobic conditioning

Exercise prescription

Assessment of exercise safety and risk

Modality: Treadmill walking protocol

Level of handrail support: N/A ☐   Yes √   Level: Light two-finger support side rail √

Use of orthotics and types: N/A ☐   Yes √   Type: Insoles

Criteria for test termination: 90% of age-predicted maximal heart rate—167 bts/min

Two Months Posttraining

Review of preexercise checklist √ (see Table 2-3)

2 treadmill walks 48 h prior to test

10:00 am

236.5

34

44

1.0

70% predicted

81% predicted

86% predicted

54% predicted

Minute or stage	Speed mph	Grade (%)	METs predicted	Heart rate (bts/min) and ECG changes	Blood pressure (mmHg)*	Rate pressure product (x103)	SpO2 (%)	Blood sugar (mg/dL)	Rating of perceived exertion or breathlessness (0-10)	Discomfort/pain (not anginal) (0-10)	Comments
0	0	0		96 NSR	160/96	15.4	94	120	3	0	NSR throughout
				85 NSR	**138/86**	**11.7**	**98**	**105**	**1**	**0**	
0	0	0		100	155/98	15.5	95		3		
				86	**140/88**	**12.0**	**98**		**1**		

BOLD – responses at 2 months

continued

Table 2-7 (continued)

Mark's Data for Treadmill Walking Test: Baseline and at 2 Months Postprogram and Training*

Minute or stage	Speed mph	Grade (%)	METs predicted	Heart rate (bts/min) and ECG changes	Blood pressure (mmHg)*	Rate pressure product (x103)	SpO₂ (%)	Blood sugar (mg/dL)	Rating of perceived exertion or breathlessness (0-10)	Discomfort/pain (not anginal) (0-10)	Comments
0	0	0		98 / **85**	157/99 / **137/82**	15.4 / **11.6**	94 / **96**		3 / **1**		
1	2.5	0	2.9	108 / **96**			91 / **96**		5 / **3**		
2	2.5	0	2.9	115 / **98**	178/- / **148/-**	20.5 / **14.5**	90 / **95**		5 / **3-4**		
3	3.0	0	3.3	128 / **100**			88 / **94**		6-7 / **4**		
4	3.0	0	3.3	134 / **126**	184/- / **156/-**	24.7 / **19.7**	87 / **92**		7 / **4**		
5	3.0	2.5	4.3	140 / **132**			88 / **91**		8 / **5**		
6	3.0	2.5	4.3	136 / **126**	188/- / **160/-**	25.6 / **20.2**	87 / **91**		8 / **5**		
7	3.0	5.0	5.4	142 / **132**			90 / **94**		5 / **2-3**		
8	3.0	5.0	5.4	148 / **138**	178/- / **166/-**	26.3 / **22.9**	90 / **95**		5 / **1-2**		
9	3.0	7.5	6.4	158 / **144**			90 / **95**		6 / **3**		
10	3.0	7.5	6.4	154 / **142**	184/- / **175/-**	28.3 / **24.9**	91 / **95**		7 / **4-5**	0.5 / **0**	Groin feels pulled left side
11	3.0	10	7.4	160 / **148**			90 / **95**		7-8 / **6**	0 / **0**	
12	3.0	10	7.4	156 / **144**	168/- / **150/-**	26.2 / **21.6**	93 / **94**		8 / **6**		

BOLD – responses at 2 months
*Note: diastolic value not recorded during test.

continued

Table 2-7 (continued)

Mark's Data for Treadmill Walking Test: Baseline and at 2 Months Postprogram and Training*

Minute or stage	Speed mph	Grade (%)	METs predicted	Heart rate (bts/min) and ECG changes	Blood pressure (mmHg)*	Rate pressure product (x10³)	SpO₂ (%)	Blood sugar (mg/dL)	Rating of perceived exertion or breathlessness (0-10)	Discomfort/ pain (not anginal) (0-10)	Comments
13	3	12.5	8.5	168 **150**			94 **94**		9 **7**		
14	3	12.5	8.5	169 **148**	184/- **155/-**	31.1 **22.9**	88 **93**		9 **7**		
15	2.5	0	2.9	106 **94**			95 **94**		5 **3**		
16	2.5	0	2.9	105 **94**	164/97 **134/79**	17.2 **12.6**	95 **95**		4 **2**	0 **0**	
17	0	0	1	100 **88**			96 **95**		2 **1**	0 **0**	
18	0	0	1	102 **86**	155/92 **138/88**	15.8 **11.9**	97 **96**		2 **1**	0 **0**	
19	0	0	1	98 **84**	142/90 **133/78**	13.9 **11.2**	96 **97**		2 **0**	0 **0**	
20	0	0	1	95 **82**	144/98 **134/90**	13.7 **11.0**	97 **97**		1-2 **0**	0 **0**	
21	0	0	1	96 **84**	144/96 **132/86**	13.8 **11.1**	97 **97**	100 **90**	2 **0**	0 **0**	

continued

BOLD – responses at 2 months
*Note: diastolic value not recorded during test.

Table 2-7 (continued)
MARK'S DATA FOR TREADMILL WALKING TEST: BASELINE AND AT 2 MONTHS POSTPROGRAM AND TRAINING*

Interpretation

Baseline Test

Weight classification:[109] Obesity class II

Overall: Test tolerated well

Load achieved: 8.5 MET load achieved at 90% at age-predicted maximum heart rate

Rest: Relatively high resting physiologic variables

Warm-up: Prolonged responses to given work rate change

Peak: Disproportionately high physiologic responses for the peak work rate consistent with deconditioning

Cool-down: Prolonged cool-down for each cool-down work rate

Recovery: Recovery took 5 minutes for parameters to lower within 5% of baseline; remained elevated

Exercise prescription:

   Type: Treadmill walking

   Intensity: 60 to 80% of age-predicted maximal heart rate

   Duration: 4 to 8 min bouts with 2 min rest between (1st 3 wks) → 2 to 15 min bouts with 2 min rest between (2nd 3 wks)

   Frequency: 3 to 5x/wk

   Course: Retest in 8 wks

Retest 2 Months Posttraining

Weight classification: Obesity class I[66]

Overall: Test tolerated well

Load achieved: 8.5 MET load achieved at 80% age-predicted maximum heart rate

Rest: Lower resting metabolic variables; less work of the heart at rest

Warm-up: Responded appropriately to incremental exercise

Peak: More rapid physiologic adjustment to a given work rate compared with baseline test

Cool-down: More rapid physiologic return to pretest measures and stabilized at those values

Recovery: Recovered within 3 to 4 minutes of exercise cessation

Exercise prescription modification:

   Retest indicated with an increased start speed—see protocol and results in Table 2-8.

- Exercise limitation due to breathlessness and coughing at times
- He has managed to get to work, driving for a 10-hour shift prior to being deemed unsafe to work
- His leisure activities consist of walking, bowling, and activities with his children

EVALUATION

Mr. Smith's history and findings are consistent with a diagnosis of disuse deconditioning. In addition, his BP is classified as Stage 2 HTN[74] and his obesity as Class II.[80] Based on pulmonary pathology guidelines for pulmonary function test results, Mr. Smith would be considered having a mixed pattern of pathology (ie, mild restrictive and obstructive lung dysfunction). Although this would not itself warrant management, the fact that this pattern is found in combination with obesity and metabolic syndrome makes it a clinical concern. His aerobic capacity is classified as poor based on a submaximal treadmill walking exercise test and established norms for his age and gender.

Overall, Mr. Smith has significant risk factors, however, these have not been managed previously in an overall coordinated manner by his health care team. Collectively, his presentation is consistent with severe life-threatening pathology related to metabolic syndrome, warranting immediate intervention. In addition, Mr. Smith's depression needs to be addressed. Improvement in depression alone can improve functional capacity.

DIAGNOSIS

Mr. Smith is a patient with metabolic syndrome. He has impaired: aerobic capacity/endurance; anthropometric characteristics; ergonomics and body mechanics; muscle performance; posture; range of motion; sensory integrity; and ventilation and respiration/gas exchange. He is functionally limited in work, community, and leisure actions, tasks, and activities. These findings are consistent with placement in Pattern B: Impaired Aerobic Capacity/Endurance Associated With Deconditioning. The identified impairments and functional limitations will be addressed in determining the prognosis and the plan of care.

PROGNOSIS AND PLAN OF CARE

Over the course of the visits, the following mutually established outcomes have been determined:

- Aerobic capacity is increased
- Biomechanical efficiency of the LEs is increased
- Breathing during activity is controlled
- Care is coordinated with patient, family, and other professionals

- Case is managed throughout episode of care
- Ergonomics and body mechanics are improved
- Functional work capacity is increased
- Integumentary integrity is improved
- Knowledge of behaviors that foster healthy habits is gained
- Movement economy with training is improved
- Muscle performance is improved
- Patient adheres to smoking cessation program
- Patient and family adhere to dietary recommendations for weight loss
- Risk factors are reduced
- Risk of secondary impairment is reduced
- ROM is increased
- Sitting tolerance is increased in his bus seat with better ergonomics
- Stress is decreased

To achieve these outcomes, the appropriate interventions for this patient are determined. These will include: coordination, communication, and documentation; patient/client-related instruction; therapeutic exercise; functional training in work, community, and leisure integration or reintegration; prescription, application, and, as appropriate, fabrication of devices and equipment; and airway clearance techniques.

Mr. Smith is expected to require between 6 and 30 visits over a 6- to 12-week period of time. He has multiple system involvement and has limited aerobic capacity. Mr. Smith's readiness to commit to a program of health behavior change[73] and whether he has different stages of readiness for different health behaviors will affect the frequency and duration of visits and treatment outcomes. Because of his multiple co-morbidities, severity of risk factors to his health and life, and his social situation, Mr. Smith's episode of care is likely to be prolonged and may require a new episode of care or modification of the number of visits or increasing the duration of this episode of care to 24 months.

INTERVENTIONS

RATIONALE FOR SELECTED INTERVENTIONS

A comprehensive program is indicated for Mr. Smith. First, the degree to which he is interested in being committed to health behavior change at this juncture and whether there are differences in his priorities regarding his risky health behaviors, must be established. Mr. Smith has multiple lifestyle behaviors that need to be priorities; however, it would be overwhelming for Mr. Smith to initiate several drastic changes at once. Therefore, priorities need to be established and a plan of action instituted gradually over a prolonged period. In this way, changes will be introduced safely and with a greater probability of being sustained.

Given the major health behavior changes indicated, the question arises as to whether these health behavior changes are addressed concurrently or sequentially (based on priority). Health education including smoking cessation is the number one priority[102] in that smoking is the leading cause of death in the United States.[103] In addition, weight and inactivity rival smoking as a health risk. Thus, optimal nutrition, weight loss, physical activity, structured exercise, and stress management are clinical priorities.

Therapeutic Exercise

The aerobic benefits of exercise have been well established in relation to metabolic syndrome and overall health and well-being (see review reference[7]). Aerobic conditioning primes the successive steps in the O_2 transport pathway to optimize its delivery of O_2 and removal of CO_2 and other metabolic waste products. The plasticity of the O_2 transport system enables it to compensate for limited steps. For example, a person with cardiac insufficiency and suboptimal CO may compensate for those insufficiencies by increasing the capacity to extract O_2 at the tissue level. Another adaptation may include increased red blood cell count in people with chronic hypoxemia secondary to chronic lung disease. The increased metabolic demand that aerobic exercise will impose on Mr. Smith will increase his health and well-being, improve his insulin sensitivity, and normalize his cholesterol and triglyceride metabolism. Further, this exercise stimulus will increase his metabolic demand overall and reduce his weight. Exercise to address his metabolic dysfunction constitutes both resistance muscle training and aerobic exercise for their peripheral aerobic effects,[86] and both exercise prescriptions will yield dose-dependent benefits.[86,87]

Initially, nonstraining exercise (ie, avoiding the Valsalva maneuver) is recommended to avoid undue work of the heart and unduly increased BP.[104] Resistance exercise, isometric exercise, and exercise requiring postural control must be done carefully. Alternatively, aerobic type exercise is recommended involving large muscle groups and performed in a rhythmic, repetitive manner. Exercise requiring marked core stabilization is minimized at this point because of its disproportionate hemodynamic responses.[87,88] UE exercise should be modified to reduce any hemodynamic hypertensive response, and therefore, HR and BP should be continuously recorded to monitor the work of the heart.

COORDINATION, COMMUNICATION, AND DOCUMENTATION

Communication will occur with Mr. Smith regarding all components of his care. Documentation following APTA's *Guidelines for Physical Therapy Documentation*[99] will occur including: changes in impairments and functional limitations, changes in interventions, all elements of patient management, and outcomes of interventions. The plan of care will be discussed with the patient and his family. He will be consulted with respect to each intervention. A psychologist through his employee assistance program will be consulted regarding a smoking cessation program in conjunction with other health and physical therapy recommendations.[102,105] A conservative nonpharmacologic approach will be instituted first with close supervision and support.

A stress management program will also be recommended. A referral to a nutritionist/dietitian for weight control guidelines will be made to ensure an appropriate diet and weight loss program. The DASH (Dietary Approaches to Stop Hypertension) Diet is recommended for its antihypertensive benefit and because it warrants only minimal modification to change his blood sugar.[106-108] Guidelines for monitoring blood sugar during Mr. Smith's progressive health program will be outlined by the physical therapist to the health care team.

Mr. Smith will be referred to vocational rehabilitation for counseling to help him retool for a career change. He will be evaluated for outdoor work with the city that is moderately physically demanding.

Close communication will be maintained among the team to monitor his progress and provide support if he backslides.[94-96] The physical therapist will provide the outcomes of physical therapy to the team, that is, the degree of social participation (quality of life), return to work activities, and changes in structure and function (physiological impairments).[70]

Criteria for discharge from care will be reviewed along with the mechanism for ensuring sustainability of positive health changes.

PATIENT/CLIENT-RELATED INSTRUCTION

Patient education is recognized as a complex process that extends beyond the traditional unidirectional knowledge transfer, that is, from the health care provider to the patient with little attention to individualization and prescription. Readiness to institute health behavior change must be established for each of the health behaviors indicated that warrant change. Mr. Smith's beliefs about health and wellness in relation to his lifestyle behaviors related to health must be considered. Education regarding Mr. Smith's current condition, impairments, and functional limitations will be discussed. Risk factors concerning weight management, smoking cessation, and decreased aerobic capacity will be discussed.

Mr. Smith will be instructed in regular self-monitoring and recording of his HR, BP, rating of perceived exertion (RPE), discomfort/pain, and blood sugar levels (with the use of a glucometer). He will be instructed to maintain a log book that will be reviewed by his physical therapist.

Mr. Smith's children will be involved with their father's program, and they will be instructed about the impact of diet and exercise on health.

Mr. Smith's education will be tailored to his many specific needs and will be targeted at the following areas:

♦ Smoking cessation: The Agency for Health Care Policy and Research Supported Clinical Practice Guidelines[102] (adopted by the APTA) provide clear statements related to smoking cessation that can be used by physical therapists with their patients

♦ Healthy nutrition that will include instruction in the following areas:
  ● The food pyramid[90] and the nutrition rainbow[109] provide general guidelines for basic nutritional counseling by the physical therapist (addressing special needs and specific menu planning are usually in the domain of the dietitian)
    ▪ Food pyramid: The pyramid was redesigned in 2005 with vertical lines that provide guidelines of how much to eat, how to avoid fatty and other harmful foods, and how to make one's diet well rounded
      ▸ Grains: 3 oz every day of whole grain cereals, breads, crackers, rice, and pasta; 6 oz in total every day
      ▸ Vegetables: 2½ cups every day to include more dark green and orange vegetables and more dry beans and peas
      ▸ Fruits: 2 cups every day to include a variety
      ▸ Milk: 3 cups every day to include low-fat or fat-free milk products
      ▸ Meat and beans: 5½ oz every day to include low-fat or lean meats and poultry
    ▪ Nutrition rainbow: The concept of the rainbow is to remind individuals to eat a variety of fruits and vegetables of all colors because they are excellent sources of antioxidants, minerals, vitamins, and dietary fiber
      ▸ Red/pink fruits and vegetables: Contain lycopene, an antioxidant
      ▸ Red, blue, and purple fruits and vegetables: Contain athocyanin, a flavonoid and antioxidant
      ▸ Orange/yellow fruits and vegetables: Contain carotenoids, an antioxidant, which is converted to vitamin A; also contain folate and vitamin C
      ▸ Dark green leafy vegetables: Contain iron and calcium
      ▸ White fruits and vegetables: Contain antioxidants and indole
  ● Food shopping, preparing, and cooking

● Restriction of salt, sugar, and saturated and trans fats
● Inclusion of high fiber foods, multiple servings of vegetables and fruits daily, and generally low oil consumption
● Adoption of the DASH diet for its antihypertensive benefit and the fact that it warrants only minimal modification to positively alter his blood sugar[104-106]
● Knowledge of the caloric content of alcohol, particularly beer, and the need to monitor his alcohol intake until his current health crisis is under control and the possible benefit of a support group

♦ Weight control and normalization of blood sugar (with recommendations for low glycemic foods and small frequent snacks rather than infrequent large meals)

♦ Need for regular physical activity: The physical activity pyramid will be reviewed and a personalized copy added to his log book[91]

♦ Need for sleep quality and relaxation (stress management)

THERAPEUTIC EXERCISE

Blood glucose, vital signs (HR, BP, RPE), and symptoms are to be monitored pre- and postexercise programs. Initially Mr. Smith's blood glucose will be recorded during the rest periods of aerobic exercise to ensure no untoward changes. Mr. Smith will also record the type, intensity, duration, and frequency of his activities.

♦ Aerobic capacity/endurance conditioning
  ● Type
    ▪ Initially walking or cycling program
    ▪ Build to treadmill walking at his employer's health and fitness facility
  ● Mode: Walking, cycling, treadmill, swimming, or aquacize
  ● Intensity: 60% to 80% age-predicted HR maximum (RPE between 4 and 6)
    ▪ Walking program begins with 1500 steps a day for the first 2 weeks, and then progresses to 2000 and 2500 steps over the next 2 to 4 weeks with the use of a pedometer and glucometer and progression in accordance with tolerance and no adverse effects, particularly musculoskeletal injuries
    ▪ Walking program progresses from low to moderate intensity, beginning with whatever time he can tolerate, 7 days a week with appropriate rest given when needed
    ▪ Cycling program begins with 75 W at 50 rpm for 15 minutes and is repeated three times with 3-minute rest intervals between each 15 minutes
    ▪ When able, treadmill program begins at 3 mph with a 2.5% to 5% grade for 3 to 10 minutes with

2 minutes of rest and progresses within 4 weeks to 20 to 40 minutes of treadmill walking and no rest

- Frequency: five to seven times a week

♦ Body mechanics and postural control

- Body mechanics instruction for his computer set up at home, his car, and truck
- Body position instruction for strength and aerobic training
- Instruction in proper body mechanics while lifting
- Body mechanics training
  - Appropriate sitting posture for computer use and car and truck driving
  - Appropriate lifting and carrying instructions
- Postural control training
  - Proper alignment of head and cervical, thoracic, and lumbar spines
  - Axial extension
  - Scapula retraction and depression
  - Proper postural position during transitions from supine to sitting, standing, and walking
- Postural stabilization activities
  - Axial extension starting in supine and progressing to sitting and upright
  - Gluteal contractions
  - Bridging
  - On all fours alternate opposite arm and leg
  - Prone gluteal contractions
  - Incorporate use of the ball, foam roller, and unstable surfaces in sitting and standing with bilateral and unilateral stance
- Postural awareness training
  - Use of mirror for visual input of appropriate alignment
  - Reminder notes to prompt postural correction around his home and in his car and truck

♦ Flexibility exercises

- Stretching exercises should be done after warming up, using a slow and steady stretch accompanied by deep breathing, and building hold up to 30 to 60 seconds
- Type:
  - Active range of motion (AROM) for the spine including flexion (forward and side to side), extension, and rotation all coordinated with breathing control
  - Range of motion exercises for the peripheral joints
- Frequency: Once daily prior to exercise

♦ Relaxation

- Use of various relaxation techniques including deep breathing exercises and quiet meditation at night

- Nighttime walk with his children as a form of relaxation
- Use of music to enhance relaxation during walking and other activities

♦ Strength, power, and endurance training

- Diaphragmatic breathing exercises that may include use of inspiratory training device to increase strength and endurance
- Yoga breathing maneuvers beginning with upper chest, middle chest, lower chest, and total expansion
- Avoid Valsalva maneuver with exercises coordinated with rhythmic breathing and no breath holding[104]
- Abdominal and back extensor muscle training coordinated with breathing
  - Elbow press backs
  - Pelvic tilts with single leg raises
- Weight training
  - Type: Light weights (dumbbells for UEs and cuff weights for LEs) beginning with maximum that patient can tolerate for 8 to 12 repetitions
  - Intensity: 8 to 12 repetitions and may build to two to three sets or one set to maximum
  - Build to 20% to 40% 1RM; 3- to 5-minute rest between sets for all major muscle groups
  - Frequency: three to five times a week

FUNCTIONAL TRAINING IN SELF-CARE AND HOME MANAGEMENT

Although Mr. Smith reported no limitation in terms of his ADL and IADL, he had in fact made modifications given limitations in what he can do around home and the yard.

♦ Self-care and home management

- Provide information of correct ergonomics and alignment for self-care and home management
- Injury prevention education during self-care and home management

FUNCTIONAL TRAINING IN WORK, COMMUNITY, AND LEISURE INTEGRATION OR REINTEGRATION

♦ Work

- Mr. Smith's return to work is a primary goal, however, he believes that bus driving is not conducive to good health and is considering retraining to a more active type of occupation (he has always enjoyed forestry and is considering whether he could become an outdoor worker with the city or a forest ranger)
- Safety during activities
- Ensure that work areas at work are ergonomically sound

- Task-specific performance training (new vocation)
♦ Community
  - Safety awareness training during community activities
  - Participation in support group for single parents for social support
♦ Leisure
  - Safety awareness training (including self-monitoring)
  - Continue bowling
  - Participation in more active leisure activities (eg, walking, bicycling, water aerobics) rather than television watching and video games

ANTICIPATED GOALS AND EXPECTED OUTCOMES

♦ Impact on pathology/pathophysiology
  - Energy expenditure per unit of work is decreased.
  - Insulin sensitivity of tissue is improved.
  - O_2 transport is improved.
♦ Impact on impairments
  - Aerobic capacity with a VO_2peak of 12 METs is increased.
  - Daily steps are increased from baseline of 1581 steps a day to 2500 steps a day.
  - Endurance is increased.
  - Muscle performance (strength, power, and endurance) is increased.
  - Sexual function, specifically erectile function, is improved.
  - Submaximal exercise responses for a given work rate are reduced.
  - Work of breathing is decreased.
♦ Impact on functional limitations
  - Ability to assume or resume required work, community, and leisure roles is improved.
  - Ability to perform physical actions, tasks, and activities related to self-care and home management is increased.
  - Functional work capacity is increased to >10 METs, which is <10th percentile for aerobic capacity men between 30 and 39 years of age.[101]
♦ Risk reduction/prevention
  - Risk factors for diseases of civilization (IHD, smoking-related conditions, HTN and stroke, metabolic syndrome, and cancer) are reduced.
  - Risk of secondary impairment is reduced.
  - Safety is improved.
  - Self-management of symptoms is improved.
♦ Impact on health, wellness, and fitness

- Cigarette smoking is reduced from one pack per day to less than half a pack per day in the next month under guidance of employee psychologist and physical therapist.
- Consequences of Type 2 diabetes (HbA1C monitoring), IHD, cancer, HTN, and stroke are reduced.
- Fitness is improved.
- General health at home is improved.
- Health behaviors (cigarettes smoked, regular blood sugar levels before and after meals and exercise, nutrition records, daily steps walked daily, and structured exercise volume) are monitored and logged.
- Medication (oral hypoglycemic agents) need is decreased or at least the effective dose is minimized.
- Mental health is improved.
- Nutrition program of DASH[106-108] diet is successfully implemented.
- Nutritionist-directed health plan is consistent with the food pyramid guidelines and optimal diabetic nutrition plan.
- Physical capacity is increased.
- Physical function is improved.
- Sustained lifelong health is achieved.
- Weight loss goal of 1 to 1½ lb per week is achieved.
♦ Impact on societal resources
  - Health care costs are decreased.
  - Social and economic burden of disease is decreased.
  - Visits to the physician, clinic, and hospital are reduced.
  - Patient/client satisfaction
  - Capacity to enjoy physical activity with his family is increased.
  - Health-related quality of life and subjective sense of well-being is increased.
  - Quality of life is improved.
  - Sleep and capacity to relax are improved.

REEXAMINATION

Reexamination is performed throughout the episode of care. With optimal support and follow-up, patients placed in this pattern may require no further management or could benefit from periodic follow-up, which will depend on the needs of the patient. Mr. Smith has responded well to his initial program as evidenced by his having reached outcomes for that episode of care (see retests sub max and retest at higher starting point, Tables 2-7 and 2-8, respectively).

DISCHARGE

Mr. Smith is discharged from physical therapy with a home program based on his last examination and exercise test

Table 2-8

MARK'S DATA FOR TREADMILL WALKING RETEST TO MODIFY EXERCISE PRESCRIPTION (WITH HIGHER INITIAL START SPEED)

Pretest

Review of preexercise checklist √ (see Table 2-3)

Practice: 2 treadmill walks 48 h prior to test

Time of day: 9:00 am

Pulmonary function: See Table 2-7

Reason for test:

    Assessment of aerobic conditioning

    Exercise prescription

    Assessment of exercise safety and risk

Type of test: Treadmill walking protocol

Medications and timing in relation to test: Cholesterol lowering medication, oral hypoglycemic, antihypertensive

Level of handrail support: N/A ☐   Yes √   Level: Light two-finger support side rail √

Use of orthotics and types: N/A ☐   Yes √   Type: Insoles

Reason for test termination: 90% of age-predicted maximal heart rate—167 bts/min

Two Months Posttraining

Review of preexercise checklist √ (see Table 2-3)

2 treadmill walks 48 h prior

9:00 am

Minute or stage	Speed (mph)	Grade	METs predicted	Heart rate (bts/min) and ECG changes	Blood pressure (mmHg)*	Rate pressure product (x10^3)	SpO$_2$ (%)	Blood sugar (mg/dL)	Rating of perceived exertion or breathlessness (0-10)	Discomfort/pain (not anginal) (0-10)	Comments
0	0	0	1	85 NSR	136/84	11.6	98	104	1	0	
0	0	0	1	80	138/90	11.0	98		1		
0	0	0	1	84	137/82	11.5	98		1	0	
1	3.0	0	3.3	99			97		2		
2	3.0	0	3.3	101	147/-	14.8	97		2	0	
3	3.0	2.5	4.3	111			97		2		Sweating
4	3.0	2.5	4.3	115	155/-	17.8	95		2	0	
5	3.0	5.0	5.4	122			96		2-3	0	
6	3.0	5.0	5.4	120	162/-	19.4	95		3	0	
7	3.0	7.5	6.4	126			94		4		
8	3.0	7.5	6.4	132	164/-	21.6	94		4	0	
9	3.0	10	7.4	140			93		5		
10	3.0	10	7.4	144	174/-	25.1	93		5	0	

*Note: diastolic value not recorded during test.

continued

Table 2-8 (continued)

MARK'S DATA FOR TREADMILL WALKING RETEST TO MODIFY EXERCISE PRESCRIPTION (WITH HIGHER INITIAL START SPEED)

Minute or stage	Speed mph	Grade	METs predicted	Heart rate (bts/min) and ECG changes	Blood pressure (mmHg)*	Rate pressure product (x10³)	SpO₂ (%)	Blood sugar (mg/dL)	Rating of perceived exertion or breathlessness (0-10)	Discomfort/pain (not anginal) (0-10)	Comments
11	3.0	12.5	8.5	146			93		5-6		
12	3.0	12.5	8.5	148	178/-	26.3	93		6	0	
13	3.0	15	9.5	154			92		7		
14	3.0	15	9.5	156	185/-	28.9	92		7	0	
15	3.0	17.5	10.5	167			92		7-8		
16	3.0	17.5	10.5	166	188/98	31.2	92		8	0	
17	2.5	0	1	133			94		3		
18	2.5	0	1	122	145/89	17.7	94		3	0	
19	0	0	1	112			96		4		
20	0	0	1	99	140/88	13.9	97		3	0	
21	0	0	1	89			97		2		
22	0	0	1	85	138/88	11.7	98		1	0	
23	0	0	1	88			98	88	1		NSR throughout test

Interpretation of Data

Test tolerated well.

Compared with pretest:

Load achieved: 10.5 MET load achieved at 90% at age-predicted maximum heart rate

Rest: Lower resting metabolic variables; less work of the heart at rest

Warm-up: Responded appropriately to incremental exercise

Peak: More rapid physiologic adjustment to a given work rate compared with baseline test

Cool-down: More rapid physiologic return to pretest measures and plateaued at those values

Recovery: Recovered within 3 to 4 minutes of exercise cessation

Exercise prescription modified:

Type: Treadmill walking

Intensity: 60% to 80% of age-predicted maximal heart rate

Duration: 3- to 10-min bouts with 2-min rest between (1st 3 wks) → 2- to 15-min bouts with 2-min rest between (2nd 3 wks)

Frequency: 3 to 5x/wk

Course: Retest in 8 wks

*Note: diastolic value not recorded during test.

after a total of 28 physical therapy sessions and attainment of his goals and expectations. A long and carefully supervised rehabilitation period will be required (24 months) after this episode: to reduce his body weight; to optimize his waist-to-hip girth; to increase his aerobic capacity, strength, endurance, and functional status; and to ensure that his health benefits are sustained and that he has adopted a pattern of lifelong health behaviors.

PSYCHOLOGICAL ASPECTS

Mr. Smith initially experienced anxiety about his health particularly when his employer was reluctant to have him return to work. At that time, he was at the contemplative stage in terms of readiness to change to more positive health behaviors[73] and shifted readily to preparation and action.

Mr. Smith's entry into the health care delivery system is wake-up call. The goal is to develop sustained lifelong health and wellness and keep him out of the doctor's office and the hospital and to reduce his risk factor categorization on several health behaviors and that of others in the sphere of his influence (ie, his children).

The diseases of civilization usually result after a lifetime of poor lifestyle choices. Every patient will differ in how well long-term change is effected and sustained beyond short-term gains. This is a critical point. Short-term gains can be achieved relatively easily with good adherence by the patient. However, building in a mechanism for sustained change over the years is another issue and must be considered by the patient and the physical therapist alike. The physical therapist needs to establish optimal follow-up over time and to provide sustained support to monitor the achievement of his goals and progress his program as appropriate.

The physical therapist may facilitate the implementation of social support services by recognizing the signs of depression and extreme stress, which are beyond the capability of the physical therapy intervention, and making referrals to the appropriate mental health professionals (eg, social worker, psychiatrist, psychologist).

REFERENCES

1. Dean E. Oxygen transport: a physiologically-based conceptual framework for the practice of cardiopulmonary physiotherapy. *Physiother.* 1994;80:347-355.
2. Dean E. Oxygen transport: the basis for cardiopulmonary physical therapy. In: Frownfelter DL, Dean E, eds. *Cardiovascular and Pulmonary Physical Therapy: Evidence and Practice.* Philadelphia, Pa: Elsevier; 2006.
3. Epstein CD, Henning RJ. Oxygen transport variables in the identification and treatment of tissue hypoxia. *Heart & Lung.* 1993;22:328-348.
4. Phang PT, Russell JA. When does VO$_2$ depend on DO$_2$? *Resp Care.* 1993;38:618-630.
5. Dean E. Optimizing outcomes: relating interventions to an individual's needs. In: Frownfelter DL, Dean E, eds. *Cardiovascular and Pulmonary Physical Therapy: Evidence and Practice.* Philadelphia, Pa: Elsevier; 2006.
6. Dean E. Body positioning. In: Frownfelter DL, Dean E, eds. *Cardiovascular and Pulmonary Physical Therapy: Evidence and Practice.* Philadelphia, Pa: Elsevier; 2006.
7. Dean E. Mobilization and exercise. In: Frownfelter DL, Dean E, eds. *Cardiovascular and Pulmonary Physical Therapy: Evidence and Practice.* Philadelphia, Pa: Elsevier; 2006.
8. Allen C, Glasziou P, Del Mar C. Bed rest: a potentially harmful treatment needing more careful evaluation. *Lancet.* 1999;354:1229-1233.
9. Bassey EJ, Fentem PH. Extent of deterioration in physical condition during postoperative bed rest and its reversal by rehabilitation. *BMJ.* 1974;4:194-196.
10. Chobanian AV, Lille RD, Tercyak A, Blevins P. The metabolic and hemodynamic effects of prolonged bed rest in normal subjects. *Circulation.* 1974;49:551-559.
11. Dean E, Ross J. Discordance between cardiopulmonary physiology and physical therapy. Toward a rational basis for practice. *Chest.* 1992;101:1694-1698.
12. Dock W. The evil sequelae of complete bed rest. *JAMA.* 1944;125:1083-1085.
13. Ross J, Dean E. Integrating physiologic principles in the comprehensive management of cardiorespiratory dysfunction. *Phys Ther.* 1989;69:255-259.
14. Saltin B, Blomqvist G, Mitchell JH, et al. Response to exercise after bed rest and after training. *Circulation.*1968;38(VII):S1-S78.
15. McGuire DK, Levine BD, Williamson JW, et al. A 30-year follow-up of the Dallas Bedrest and Training Study: I. Effect of age on the cardiovascular response to exercise. *Circulation.* 2001;104:1350-1357.
16. McGuire DK, Levine BD, Williamson JW, et al. A 30-year follow-up of the Dallas Bedrest and Training Study: II. Effect of age on cardiovascular adaptation to exercise training. *Circulation.* 2001;104:1358-1366.
17. Ferretti G, Girardis M, Moia C, Antonutto G. Effects of prolonged bed rest on cardiovascular oxygen transport during submaximal exercise in humans. *Eur J Appl Physiol Occup Physiol.* 1998;78:398-402.
18. Sjostrand T. Determination of changes in the intrathoracic blood volume in man. *Acta Physiol Scand.* 1951;22:116-128.
19. Convertino VA. Cardiovascular consequences of bed rest: effect on maximal oxygen uptake. *Med Sci Sports Exerc.* 1997; 2:191-196.
20. World Health Organization. International Classification of Functioning, Disability and Health. (2002). Available at: www.sustainable-design.ie/arch/ICIDH-2PFDec-2000.pdf. Accessed February 2007.
21. Convertino VA, Bloomfield SA, Greenleaf JE. An overview of the issues: physiological effects of bed rest and restricted physical activity. *Med Sci Sports Exerc.* 2003;29:187-190.
22. Grenon SM, Hurwitz S, Sheynberg N, et al. Role of individual predisposition in orthostatic intolerance before and after simulated microgravity. *J Appl Physiol.* 2004;96:1714-1722.
23. Grenon SM, Sheynberg N, Hurwitz S, et al. Renal, endocrine, and cardiovascular responses to bed rest in male subjects on a constant diet. *J Invest Med.* 2004;52:117-128.

24. Hasser EM, Moffitt JA. Regulation of sympathetic nervous system function after cardiovascular deconditioning. *Ann NY Acad Sci.* 2001;940:454-468.

25. Hirayanagi K, Iwase S, Kamiya A, Sasaki T, Mano T, Yajima K. Functional changes in autonomic nervous system and baroreceptor reflex induced by 14 days of 6 degrees head-down bed rest. *Eur J Appl Physiol.* 2004;92:160-167.

26. Hirayanagi K, Kamiya A, Iwase S, et al. Autonomic cardiovascular changes during and after 14 days of head-down bed rest. *Autonom Neurosci.* 2004;27:110,121-128.

27. Wang JS, Jen CJ, Chen HI. Effects of exercise training and deconditioning on platelet function in men. *Arterioscler Thromb.* 1995;15:1668-1674.

28. Levin SA, Lown B. Armchair treatment of acute coronary thrombosis. *JAMA.* 1952;148:1365-1369.

29. Jacobs LG. Prophylactic anticoagulation for venous thromboembolic disease in geriatric patients. *J Am Geriatr Soc.* 2003;51:1472-1478.

30. Harvey RL. Prevention of venous thromboembolism after stroke. *Top Stroke Rehabil.* 2003;10:61-69.

31. Szygula Z. Erythrocytic system under the influence of physical exercise and training. *Sports Med.* 1990;10:181-197.

32. Svanberg L. Influence of position on the lung volumes, ventilation and circulation in normals. *Scand J Clin Lab Invest.* 1957;25:1-195.

33. El-Sayed MS. Effects of exercise and training on blood rheology. *Sports Med.* 1998;26:281-292.

34. Dean E. Oxygen transport deficits in systemic disease and implications for physical therapy. *Phys Ther.* 1997;77:187-202.

35. Bloomfield SA. Changes in musculoskeletal structure and function with prolonged bed rest. *Med Sci Sports Exerc.* 1997;29:197-206.

36. Lentz M. Selected aspects of deconditioning secondary to immobilization. *Nurs Clin North Am.* 1981;16:729-737.

37. Mettauer B, Zoll J, Sanchez H, et al. Links oxidative capacity of skeletal muscle in heart failure patients versus sedentary or active control subjects. *J Am Coll Cardiol.* 2001;38:947-954.

38. Tartaglia MC, Chen JT, Caramanos Z, et al. Muscle phosphorus magnetic resonance spectroscopy oxidative indices correlate with physical activity. *Muscle Nerve.* 2000;23:175-181.

39. Kubo K, Akima H, Ushiyama J, et al. Effects of 20 days of bed rest on the viscoelastic properties of tendon structures in lower limb muscles. *Brit J Sports Med.* 2004;38:324-330.

40. Takata S, Yasui N. Disuse osteoporosis. *J Med Invest.* 2001; 48:147-156.

41. Winkelman C. Inactivity and inflammation: selected cytokines as biologic mediators in muscle dysfunction during critical illness. *AACN Clinical Issues.* 2004;15:74-82.

42. Lindgren M, Unosson M, Fredrikson M, Ek AC. Immobility—a major risk factor for development of pressure ulcers among adult hospitalized patients: a prospective study. *Scand J Car Sci.* 2004;18:57-64.

43. Mendenhall LA, Swanson SC, Habash DL, Coggan AR. Ten days of exercise training reduces glucose production and utilization during moderate-intensity exercise. *Am J Physiol.* 1994;266:E136-E143.

44. Mikines KJ, Richter EA, Dela F, Galbo H. Seven days of bed rest decrease insulin action on glucose uptake in leg and whole body. *J Appl Physiol.* 1991;70:1245-1254.

45. Smorawinski J, Kaciuba-Uscilko H, Nazar K, et al. Comparison of changes in glucose tolerance and insulin secretion induced by three-day bed rest in sedentary subjects and endurance or strength trained athletes. *J Gravit Physiol.* 1998;5:P103-P104.

46. Sato Y. Diabetes and life-styles: role of physical exercise for primary prevention. *Brit J Nutr.* 2000;84(Suppl):S187-S190.

47. Ahlinder S, Birke G, Norberg R, et al. Metabolism and distribution of IgG in patients confined to prolonged strict bed rest. *Acta Med Scand.* 1970;187:267-270.

48. Pyne DB. Regulation of neutrophil function during exercise. *Sports Med.* 1994;17:245-258.

49. Pyne DB, Gleeson M, McDonald WA, et al. Training strategies to maintain immunocompetence in athletes. *Int J Sports Med.* 2000;21(Suppl 1):S51-S60.

50. Mascitelli L, Pezzetta F. Anti-inflammatory effects of physical exercise. *Arch Int Med.* 2003;163:1682-1688.

51. Nieman DC. Current perspective on exercise immunology. *Curr Sports Med Rev.* 2003;2:239-242.

52. Sonnfeld G. Space flight, microgravity, stress, and immune responses. *Adv Space Res.* 1999;23:1945-1953.

53. MacKinnon LT. Chronic exercise training: effects on immune function. *Med Sci Sports Exerc.* 2000;32:S369-S376.

54. Rubin M. The physiology of bed rest. *Am J Nurs.* 1988;88:50-56.

55. Ishizaki Y, Fukuoka H, Ishizaki T, et al. Evaluation of psychological effects due to bed rest. *J Gravit Physiol.* 2000; 7:183-184.

56. Zubeck JP, MacNeil M. Effects of immobilization: behavioural and EEG changes. *Can J Psych.* 1966;20:316-336.

57. Scott CL. Diagnosis, prevention, and interventions for the metabolic syndrome. *Am J Cardiol.* 2003;92:35-42.

58. Challem J, Berkson B, Smith MD. *Syndrome X. The Complete Nutritional Program to Prevent and Reverse Insulin Resistance.* New York, NY: John Wiley & Sons, Inc; 2000.

59. Straznicky NE, Lambert EA, Lambert GW, et al. Effects of dietary weight loss on sympathetic activity and cardiac risk factors associated with the metabolic syndrome. *J Clin Endocrinol Metab.* 2005 (Epub ahead of print).

60. Kottke FJ. The effects of limitation of activity upon the human body. *JAMA.* 1996;196:825-830.

61. Gregg EW, Mangione CM, Cauley JA, et al. Diabetes and incidence of functional disability in older women. *Diabetes Care.* 2002;25:61-67.

62. Abraham WT. Preventing cardiovascular events in patients with diabetes mellitus. *Am J Med.* 2004;116(Suppl 5A):39S-46S.

63. Ten S, MacLaren N. Insulin resistance syndrome in children. *J Clin Endocrin Metab.* 2004;89:2526-2539.

64. Singleton JR, Smith AG, Russell JW, Feldman EL. Microvascular complications of impaired glucose tolerance. *Diabetes.* 2003;52:2867-2873.

65. Cohen JA, Estacio RO, Lundgren RA, et al. Diabetic autonomic neuropathy is associated with an increased incidence of strokes. *Autonom Neurosci.* 2003;108:73-78.

66. Hu FB, Stampfer MJ, Solomon C, et al. Physical activity and risk for cardiovascular events in diabetic women. *Ann Int Med.* 2001;134:96-105.

67. Bauman AE. Updating the evidence that physical activity is good for health: an epidemiological review 2000-2003. *J Sci Med Sport.* 2004;7(1 Suppl):6-19.

68. Wannamethee SG, Shaper AG, Perry IJ. Smoking as a modifiable risk factor for type 2 diabetes in middle-aged men. *Diabetes Care*. 2001;24:1590-1595.

69. Annual Health Reports 1999-2004. Geneva, Switzerland: World Health Organization.

70. Dean E. Preferred practice patterns in cardiopulmonary physical therapy: a guide to physiologic measures. *CPTJ*. 1999;10:124-134.

71. Gylfadottir S, Dean E, Dallimore M. The six minute walk test for people with neuromuscular and musculoskeletal conditions: systematic review and rationale for evidence-based guideline update. Under review.

72. Noonan V, Dean E. Submaximal exercise testing: clinical application and interpretation. *Phys Ther*. 2001;80:782-807.

73. Prochaska JO, DiClemente CC. Transtheoretical therapy: toward a more integrative model of change. *Psychother Theory Res Pract*. 1982;9:276-288.

74. American Heart Association. Blood pressure guidelines. Available at: www.americanheart.org Accessed February 2007.

75. American Diabetes Association. Available at: http://www.diabetes.org/type-2-diabetes/treatment-conditions.jsp. Accessed February 2007.

76. Harvard University. School of Public Health. Health Risk Assessment. Available at: http://www.yourdiseaserisk.harvard.edu. Accessed February 2007.

77. Dean E. Epidemiology as a basis for contemporary physical therapy practice. In: Frownfelter DL, Dean E, eds. *Cardiovascular and Pulmonary Physical Therapy: Evidence and Practice*. Philadelphia, Pa: Elsevier; 2006.

78. Astrand P-O, Ryhming I. A nomogram for calculation of aerobic capacity from pulse rate during submaximal work. *J Appl Physiol*. 1954;7:218-221.

79. Tudor-Locke C, Bassett DR Jr. How many steps/day are enough? Preliminary pedometer indices for public health. *Sports Med*. 2004;34:1-8.

80. Executive summary of the clinical guidelines on the identification, evaluation, and treatment of overweight and obesity in adults. Expert panel. *Arch Int Med*. 1998;158:1855-1867.

81. WHO. *Consultation on Obesity*. Geneva, Switzerland: World Health Organization; 1997.

82. Borg G. Psychophysical basis of perceived exertion. *Med Sci Sports Exerc*. 1982;14:377-381.

83. Borg GAV. Psychophysiological bases of perceived exertion. *Scand J Rehabil Med*. 1970;2:92-98.

84. Devilly G. Short Form-36 Questionnaire. Available at: http://www.swin.edu.au/victims/resources/assessment/health/sf-36-questionnaire.html. Accessed January 3, 2007.

85. Goel MS, McCarthy EP, Phillips RS, Wee CC. Obesity among US immigrant subgroups by duration of residence. *JAMA*. 2004;292:2860-2867.

86. Oja P. Dose response between total volume of physical activity and health and fitness. *Med Sci Sports Exerc*. 2001;33(6 Suppl):S428-S437.

87. Izquierdo M, Hakkinen K, Ibanez J, et al. Effects of strength training on submaximal and maximal endurance performance capacity in middle-aged and older men. *J Strength Cond Res*. 2003;17:129-139.

88. Al-Obaidi S, Anthony J, Dean E, Al-Shuwai N. Cardiovascular responses to repetitive McKenzie lumbar spine exercise. *Phys Ther*. 2001;81:1524-1533.

89. Vincent KR, Vincent HK, Braith RW, et al. Strength training and hemodynamic responses to exercise. *Am J Geriatr Cardiol*. 2003;12:97-106.

90. United States Department of Health and Human Services. Consumer Information Center: The Food Guide Pyramid. http://www.mypyramid.gov/pyramid/index.html. Accessed February 2007.

91. United States Department of Agriculture. Consumer Information Center: My Pyramid. Available at: http://www.mypyramid.gov/pyramid/physical_activity.html. Accessed February 2007.

92. Jones AYM, Dean E, Scudds R. Effectiveness of a community-based t'ai chi program and implications for public health initiatives. *Arch Phys Med Rehabil*. 2005;86:619-625.

93. Tsai JC, Wang WH, Chan P, et al. The beneficial effects of Tai Chi Chuan on blood pressure and lipid profile and anxiety states in a randomized controlled clinical trial. *J Alt Comp Med*. 2003;9:747-754.

94. Lennon S, Quindry JC, Hamilton KL, et al. Loss of exercise-induced cardioprotection following cessation of exercise. *J Appl Physiol*. 2004;96:1299-1305.

95. Mujika I, Padilla S. Detraining: loss of training-induced physiological and performance adaptations. I. Short-term insufficient training stimulus. *Sports Med*. 2000;30:79-87.

96. Mujika I, Padilla S. Detraining: loss of training-induced physiological and performance adaptations. II. Long-term insufficient training stimulus. *Sports Med*. 2000;30:145-154.

97. Janssen I, Katzmarzyk PT, Ross R. Waist circumference and not body mass index explains obesity-related health risk. *Am J Clin Nutr*. 2004;79:379-384.

98. Zhu S, Wang Z, Heshka S, et al. Waist circumference and obesity-associated risk factors among whites in the third National Health and Nutrition Examination Survey: clinical action thresholds. *Am J Clin Nutr*. 2002;76:743-749.

99. American Physical Therapy Association. Guide to physical therapist practice. 2nd ed. *Phys Ther*. 2001;81:9-744.

100. Thomas RJ, Kottke TE, Brekke MJ, et al. Attempts at changing dietary and exercise habits to reduce risk of cardiovascular disease: who's doing what in the community? *Prev Cardiol*. 2002;5:102-108.

101. American College of Sports Medicine. *Guidelines for Exercise Testing and Prescription*. 7th ed. Philadelphia, Pa: Lippincott Williams & Wilkins; 2005.

102. AHHPR Smoking Cessation Guidelines. APTA Guideline Endorsement. *Phys Ther*. 1997.

103. Mokdad AH, Marks JS, Stroup DF, Gerberding JL. Actual causes of death in the United States, 2000. *JAMA*. 2004;291:1238-1245.

104. Fletcher BJ, Dunbar S, Coleman J, et al. Cardiac precautions for non-acute inpatient settings. *Am J Phys Med Rehabil*. 1993; 72:140-143.

105. AHCPR Supported Clinical Practice Guidelines. Smoking cessation brief clinical interventions. Available at: www.ncbi.nlm.nih.gov. Accessed February 2007.

106. Conlin PR, Chow D, Miller ER, et al. The effect of dietary patterns on blood pressure control in hypertensive patients: results from the Dietary Approaches to Stop Hypertension (DASH) trial. *Am J Hypertension*. 2000;13:949-955.

107. Obarzanek E, Proschan MA, Vollmer WM, et al. Individual blood pressure responses to changes in salt intake: results from the DASH-Sodium trial. *Hypertension*. 2003;42:459-467.

108. Resnick LM, Oparil S, Chait A, et al. Factors affecting blood pressure responses to diet: the vanguard study. *Am J Hypertension.* 2000;13:956-965.

109. Health Canada. Office of Nutrition Policy and Promotion. Revision of Canada's Food Guide to Health Eating. Available at: www.hc-sc.gc.ca. Accessed February 2007.

CHAPTER THREE

Impaired Ventilation, Respiration/ Gas Exchange, and Aerobic Capacity/ Endurance Associated With Airway Clearance Dysfunction (Pattern C)

Dawn M. Stackowicz, PT, MS, CCS
Marilyn Moffat, PT, DPT, PhD, FAPTA, CSCS
Donna Frownfelter, PT, DPT, MA, CCS, FCCP, RRT
Susan M. Butler McNamara, PT, MMSc, CCS

ANATOMY AND PHYSIOLOGY

The pertinent anatomy and physiology of the cardiovascular and pulmonary systems needed for airway clearance will be reviewed. This review will be related to the structural and mechanical abilities of the thorax and the lungs, the processes and functional abilities needed to maintain normal respiration and cough, and the cough reflex. For a detailed review of the anatomy and physiology of the cardiovascular and pulmonary systems, see Pattern A: Primary Prevention/Risk Reduction for the Cardiovascular/Pulmonary Disorders.

THE THORAX AND LUNGS

The muscles and bones of the thoracic cavity provide the structural support and protection for the pulmonary system. The bones included are the thoracic vertebrae, the ribs, and the sternum. The different muscles of inspiration and expiration provide assistance for changes in volume during normal or forced respiration. The primary muscles of inspiration are the diaphragm and the intercostals. Accessory muscles of inspiration are activated with exertion, respiratory distress, and cardiopulmonary disease progression. The sternocleidomastoid, scalenes, serratus anterior, pectoralis major and minor, trapezius, and erector spinae are some of the accessory muscles of inspiration. Expiration is primarily a passive activity occurring when the diaphragm and intercostals relax. Accessory muscles of expiration are activated for the same reasons that the accessory muscles of inspiration are activated. The main accessory muscles of expiration are the rectus abdominis, internal and external obliques abdominis, transverse abdominis, and internal intercostals.

The mechanical ability of the lungs is dependent upon the ease of the distensibility of the lung on inspiration (compliance) and the elastic recoil on exhalation (elastance). During normal healthy respiration, the muscular thoracic wall (physical component) overcomes the elastic recoil of the lungs (physiological component) creating a smooth breathing pattern. The work of breathing is the amount of muscular effort required to overcome the compliance of the lungs and the thorax.[1] During restful breathing, the accessory muscles of respiration are normally quiet. With chronic lung disease, the accessory muscles can become the primary muscles activated at rest. When airway clearance dysfunction occurs, an increase in the use of the accessory muscles may be needed to expel secretions and may result in an increased work of breathing.

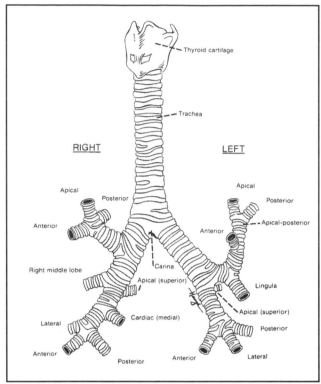

Figure 3-1. Tracheobronchial tree (a three-quarter view, rotated toward the right side). Reprinted from *Cardiovascular and Pulmonary Physical Therapy: Evidence and Practice.* 4th ed. Frownfelter D, Dean E. Page 62, 2005, with permission from Elsevier.

The work of breathing is described by the formula minute volume (MV) equals the tidal volume (TV) times the respiratory rate (RR) [MV = TV x RR].[2] When a patient increases his or her respiratory rate, the TV is decreased. Thus, there is more wasted ventilation that only moves in the dead space of the tracheobronchial tree. Less alveolar ventilation takes place and less oxygen is available. The effort of trying to take a deep breath and cough, in addition to a rapid respiratory rate just to breathe, exhausts the patient.

The upper and lower airways provide the structural support for the entry of air into the lungs. The upper airways consist of the nose, pharynx, and larynx. The nose warms the air, humidifies the air, and filters the air, thus protecting the lower airways from foreign particles. The pharynx is the area behind the nasal and oral cavities and extends to the top of the esophagus and larynx. The larynx is a complex structure similar to a sphincter valve. By closing, it protects the lower airways from food, liquids, and foreign objects. It also controls the airflow in and out that is needed for speaking and coughing. The lower airways include the trachea and bronchial tree. Separation between the trachea and bronchial tree is at the carina (Figure 3-1). The lungs are divided in five lobes, which are then in turn divided into bronchopulmona-

ry segments. The right lung has three lobes (upper, middle, and lower) and ten segments. The left lung has two lobes (upper and lower) and eight segments (Figure 3-2).

Gas exchange takes place via the oxygen transport pathway (see Pattern A: Primary Prevention/Risk Reduction for the Cardiovascular/Pulmonary Disorders). The pathway starts in the upper airways and flows through the pulmonary system to the tissue level. Adequate gas exchange depends on the processes of ventilation and respiration.

NORMAL RESPIRATION AND PULMONARY FUNCTION

First and foremost, respiration encompasses the entire process of the interchange of gases within the human body, and therefore includes the taking in of oxygen, the utilization of oxygen in the tissues, and the giving off of carbon dioxide. Five processes occur during respiration.[1] Understanding these processes can assist with differentiating between healthy and diseased breathing. These processes are ventilation, distribution, diffusion, perfusion, and circulation. Ventilation is simply the movement of air into and out of the lungs. Ventilation is often misunderstood for respiration; however, ventilation does not guarantee that the oxygen inhaled will combine with the blood in the lungs. Distribution is the passage of the air throughout the lungs to the alveoli. Adequate distribution occurs when the air reaches the areas of the lungs that have the most alveoli for gas exchange. In the normal upright lung, there are less alveoli in the upper or apical regions of the lung and a significant increase in alveoli in the lower regions or bases of the lungs. Diffusion is the passage

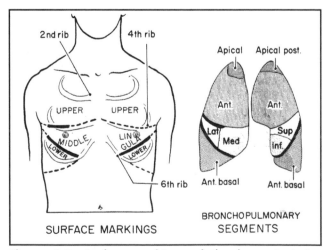

Figure 3-2. Surface markings of the lungs (anterior aspect). The underlying bronchopulmonary segments are also shown. Reprinted from *Cardiovascular and Pulmonary Physical Therapy: Evidence and Practice.* 4th ed. Frownfelter D, Dean E. Page 62, 2005, with permission from Elsevier.

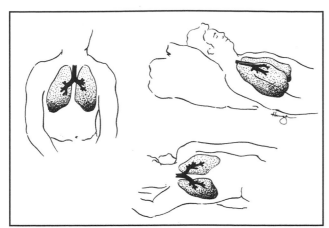

Figure 3-3. The effect of positioning on the perfusion of the lung. Note that gravity-dependent segments have the greatest amount of perfusion. Reprinted from *Cardiovascular and Pulmonary Physical Therapy: Evidence and Practice.* 4th ed. Frownfelter D, Dean E. Page 62, 2005, with permission from Elsevier.

of the gases between the alveoli and the blood. Adequate diffusion occurs with the exchange of oxygen and carbon dioxide in the pulmonary capillaries. Perfusion is the volume of blood pumped by the heart through the pulmonary capillaries (Figure 3-3). Perfusion is position dependent, similar to distribution. To assure adequate perfusion, an upright position is recommended as there is more blood flow to the bases of the lung to mix with the oxygen being distributed to the greater number of alveoli in the bases. The final process of respiration is circulation. Circulation is the movement of the blood from the pulmonary capillaries to the heart and the distribution of oxygenated blood throughout the body. A disturbance in the circulation pathway anywhere in the body impacts respiration as adequate oxygen does not reach the tissue. Retained secretions can result in mismatching of ventilation-perfusion and abnormalities in lung biomechanics.[3,4] Retained secretions due to the inability to produce a strong cough or aspiration can promote lung infections.[3,5]

Pulmonary function tests (PFTs) can identify impairments in mechanical ability that would affect a productive cough and determine if a disease process is obstructive or restrictive. Normal forced expiratory volume in 1 second (FEV_1) should be 75% of the forced vital capacity (FVC). Restrictive lung disease results in both decreased lung volumes and FVC; and obstructive lung disease results in larger lung volumes, but decreased FVC. Adequate vital capacity, inspiratory volume, and forced expiratory volume (FEV) are needed to assist in a productive cough. FEV_1 > 80% indicates restrictive disease and FEV_1 < 50% indicates obstructive disease. A minimal FEV_1 of 60% of actual vital capacity is a good predictor of adequate muscle strength for a productive cough.[6] This minimum should result in the ability to cough three to six times per expiratory flow.

Once adequate gas exchange is known and the thorax and lungs are providing sufficient air to expel secretions, the cough reflex mechanism should be evaluated. The cough reflex assists with removal of secretions from the upper respiratory tract at the level of the carina. Inability to remove secretions from the lower respiratory tract is where complications can arise and when infections can occur.[7] Many interventions focus on mobility of secretions from the lower to the upper respiratory tract for removal.

THE COUGH REFLEX

Normal airway clearance occurs via the mucociliary blanket and cough mechanism. The two layers of the mucous—the gel layer (upper) and the sol layer (lower)—lie beneath and communicate with the cilia (Figure 3-4). The cilia are fine, hair-like particles that line the airway and propel cells and other organisms from the lungs into the upper airways for expulsion. The two layers of the blanket consist of 90% water when a person is well hydrated. The mucociliary layer in the upper and lower respiratory tract assists with protecting the lungs from bacteria and infection. Causes of decreased mucociliary activity include, but are not limited to: dehydration, cigarette smoking, environmental and occupational pollutants, decreased humidity, age, pharmacological

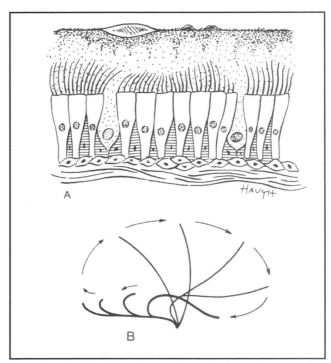

Figure 3-4. (A) The mucous consists of two layers—the gel layer (upper) and the sol layer (lower) that lies beneath and communicates with the cilia (B). Reprinted from *Cardiovascular and Pulmonary Physical Therapy: Evidence and Practice.* 4th ed. Frownfelter D, Dean E. Page 62, 2005, with permission from Elsevier.

agents (ie, inhaled anesthesia, narcotics, sedatives, high oxygen concentrations), suctioning, artificial airways, hypoxia, sleep, and lung transplant.[1]

A cough has been divided into four stages: 1) deep inspiration; 2) glottis closure; 3) generation of thoracoabdominal pressure; and 4) glottis opening and expulsion. During stage 1 or deep inspiration, one must be able to inspire enough air for a forceful and productive cough. An adequate inspiratory volume for a productive cough should be at least 60% of predicted vital capacity. During stage 2, the glottis (vocal fold) is closed to assist with the preparation of building thoracoabdominal pressure. During stage 3, the abdominal and intercostals muscles actively contract against the closed glottis. During stage 4, the glottis is opened and secretions are forcefully expelled as a result of the pressured air built up in the lower airways. By examining all of the stages of a patient's cough, problems can be identified and corrected to assist with airway clearance dysfunction.

PATHOPHYSIOLOGY

Inadequate airway clearance may be caused by medical or surgical conditions that cause impairment to adequately clear the airways. Some common reasons for a deficit in airway clearance include both primary and secondary reasons. Primary causes include pulmonary diseases, such as cystic fibrosis (CF) or COPD, where airway clearance deficit is a key impairment. Secondary deficits arise from neurological (such as, a cerebral vascular accident or spinal cord injury) or musculoskeletal (such as, severe kyphoscoliosis) impairments. In primary disease processes, increased or abnormal mucous production is the cause of airway obstruction and decreased airway clearance. For patients with secondary impairments, a decrease or imbalance in muscle strength and in the ability to change airway, intrathoracic, and intrabdominal pressures to cough may be the focus of concern.

Inclusion criteria into this practice pattern focuses on the impairment of oxygen transport related to the inability to remove secretions or mucous from the airways. There are many acute and chronic diseases that result in retained secretions or the inability to remove secretions.[3,4] Some risk factors or pathophysiological conditions that may be included in this practice pattern are: acute lung disorders; acute or chronic dependency on oxygen; organ, bone marrow, or stem cell transplants; cardiothoracic surgery; changes in baseline breath sounds and/or baseline chest radiograph; chronic obstructive pulmonary disease; frequent or recurring pulmonary infections; and tracheostomy or microtracheostomy.

Patients may have the following impairments, functional limitations, and/or disabilities: impaired gas exchange; impaired ventilatory forces and flow; impaired ventilatory volume; impaired airway clearance; impaired cough; and dyspnea at rest or with exertion that can result in inability to perform self-care and/or work tasks. The most important

area upon which to focus with airway clearance is where the impaired gas exchange is occurring in the oxygen transport pathway. For example, if secretions need removal, ventilatory forces, both flow and volume, should be addressed as they relate directly to airway clearance and cough. With chronic disease, such as bronchitis or cystic fibrosis, it is unknown if increased secretion production is part of the disease progression or is due to deterioration of respiratory function.[3,5,7]

Understanding the disease processes of CF and COPD can assist with the explanation of the pathophysiology of retained secretions and the need for airway clearance techniques.

CYSTIC FIBROSIS

CF is a complex multisystem clinical syndrome. It is an autosomal recessive trait and the most common and lethal genetic disease in the United States. The incidence is 1 in 3900 live white births.[8] The physiologic defect is cellular and involves the epithelial cells of the exocrine glands. Target organs include the sinuses, lungs, pancreas, intestines, biliary tracts, vas deferens, uterine cervix, and sweat glands. The pathophysiology is a defect in chloride ion transport. When the transport of sodium and chloride is disturbed, water is pulled back into the cell. This results in secretions that are drier and thicker. For the lungs, the mucociliary clearance mechanism is hindered,[9] and a breeding ground for bacteria is laid.[7] A vicious cycle of inflammation, infection, and destruction is created.[10] The normal anti-inflammatory response releases cytotoxins (ie, elastase, cytokines, etc) that cause further damage to the mucociliary clearance mechanism. In the other target organs, these thickened secretions lead to obstruction and malabsorption. For the sweat glands, the patient with CF has increased chloride levels when a sweat test is conducted. The initial hallmark symptom identified with CF is the saltiness noted by the mother upon kissing her newborn child.

CF is a chronic disease across the life span, even though it had been labeled as a pediatric disease. The median life span is 36.8 years.[8] The earlier the diagnosis occurs, the earlier the intensive intervention can begin. Diagnosis usually occurs by 15 months of age, though 10% of patients are diagnosed as adults. The most common criteria for diagnosis are:

♦ Meconium ileus at birth

♦ Failure to regain birth weight/failure to thrive

♦ Recurrent respiratory infections/chronic cough

♦ "Salty kiss"

CF care is best provided in specialized clinics that involve a multidisciplinary team approach. Members include a physician, nurse, social worker, nutritionist, physical therapist, and respiratory therapist. Management includes quarterly clinic visits at a minimum. Growth via height and weight is monitored in the pediatric population; only weight is monitored in the adult group. Physical examination is key, especially auscultation. Pulmonary function tests (PFTs) are performed at least annually, and spirometry (FVC, FEV_1) is performed at each visit. During clinic visits, trends are observed, and vitamin levels, complete blood counts (CBCs), and sputum cultures are checked. Chest x-rays and CT scans are also important tests used to assist in monitoring disease progress.

The improved life span in this patient population is due to the development of treatment options. These include pancreatic enzymes, supplemental vitamins, high caloric diets, airway clearance techniques, antibiotics, and mucolytic and bronchodilator medications. Research funded through the Cystic Fibrosis Foundation not only includes clinical studies (ie, medications), but also benchmark research involving correcting the underlying genetic defect through animal studies.

CHRONIC OBSTRUCTIVE PULMONARY DISEASE

Chronic pulmonary disease is usually divided into obstructive and restrictive disorders. Obstructive disorders are distinguished by an increase in airway resistance and resultant decrease in airflow during expiration. Restrictive disorders are distinguished by a decreased inspiratory capacity of the lungs. Only obstructive disorders will be the focus of this chapter. The most common obstructive disorders are asthma, bronchiectasis, chronic bronchitis, cystic fibrosis, and emphysema. A combination of chronic bronchitis, emphysema, and asthma is typical and is referred to as COPD.[1] Hyperinflated lungs, a flattened diaphragm, and an enlarged right ventricle of the heart due to increased pulmonary artery pressure are often seen on chest x-rays. COPD also results in abnormal pulmonary function tests, specifically, decreased vital capacity (VC), FEV_1, maximum voluntary ventilation, and diffusion capacity, and increased functional residual capacity and residual volume. Respiratory muscle weakness may also be found with moderate to severe COPD. Inspiratory muscle force is affected more than expiratory, and proximal upper extremity strength is affected more than distal upper extremity strength.[4]

COPD resulted in 1.5 million emergency department visits, 726,000 hospitalizations, and 119,000 deaths in the United States in 2000.[11] COPD treatment costs exceed $32 billion annually and caused $14 billion lost due to work absences in the US in 2002.[11]

Chronic bronchitis is characterized by a chronic cough lasting 2 years and producing sputum for at least 3 consecutive months each year. Long-term irritation to the tracheobronchial tree is believed to be the cause of chronic bronchitis. The most common cause of irritation is cigarette smoke; other causes are environmental and occupational irritants. Hypertrophy and hypersecretion of mucous in the tracheobronchial tree and decreased activity of the cilia lead to the chronic productive cough. Due to the increase in mucous production, an increase

in susceptibility to respiratory infections is common. As the disease progresses, recovery from the infections can be more difficult and can take longer periods of time.

Emphysema is characterized by permanent enlargement of the bronchioles and destructive changes in the alveoli. Loss of elastic recoil of the lung, excessive collapsing of airways upon exhalation, and chronic airflow obstruction are other changes noted with emphysema. There are different types of emphysema including panlobular (destruction with enlargement and loss of distinction between alveolar ducts and alveoli), centrilobular (destruction and enlargement of bronchioles), paraseptal (enlargement of air spaces under the pleura or along the septa), and irregular (due to scarring). The most common symptom of emphysema is dyspnea with little to no sputum production. Respiration is often rapid and shallow, and PLB may assist with controlling respiratory rates. The upper extremities are often typically and unconsciously placed in a stabilized position (standing with hands on the hips or sitting with forearms resting on knees) to enable more effective use of the accessory muscles of inspiration.

During acute COPD exacerbations, a multidisciplinary team approach that includes the physician, nurse, pharmacist, physical therapist, respiratory therapist, nutritionist, and social worker can achieve optimal treatment results. The goals of interventions include:

- Identifying and eliminating (if possible) the cause of the exacerbation
- Improving lung function with pharmacological agents, including bronchodilators and antibiotics
- Providing adequate oxygenation without the need for intubation
- Assuring secretion clearance
- Addressing nutrition needs, such as adequate hydration and caloric intake
- Reviewing risk factors and a healthy lifestyle, such as influenza and pneumonia vaccinations, smoking cessation, exercise rehabilitation, and proper use of medications (especially metered dose inhaler techniques)[11]

Hypoxemia often occurs during acute exacerbations and may cause tissue hypoxia. Care must be taken in administering oxygen therapy as the hypoxic drive can easily become hindered with COPD. A relatively low level of oxygen via a nasal cannula (up to 6L) may often correct the problem of hypoxemia. Smoking cessation is overwhelmingly the most important risk factor to address.[5]

IMAGING

The methods used to assess the anatomical structures of the lungs also focus on the surrounding tissue that may be interfering with the biomechanics and basic function of respiration.[1,12]

♦ Chest radiographs (CXRs or x-rays): CXRs continue to be the most common method to assess abnormalities in the chest. The difference between air, fat, water, tissue, and bone depend on their radiolucency or radiopacity. The density of the structure determines the "shadow" that is depicted on the resultant x-ray. CXRs are used to determine the area of consolidation of secretions/mucous in the lungs, atelectasis, unexpected pulmonary complications (ie, pneumothorax), and abnormal cardiac conditions (ie, hypertrophy, cor pulmonale).

♦ Computed tomography (CT): CT scans are summated digital x-rays used to obtain a more detailed view of the structure and tissue of the chest. They can also be used to assess the abdomen to rule out restrictive tissue or obstructive tissue/structures that could be interfering with one's ability to expand the lungs, rib cage, and/or diaphragm to take a deep breath for cough.

♦ Magnetic resonance imaging (MRI): MRIs, like CT scans, show a more detailed view of the structure and tissue of the chest. They may be indicated to show the detail of a nodule or mass or the thickness of the layers of the lung tissue that had been initially noted on a CXR. MRIs can be inconclusive in evaluating the lung parenchyma itself due to the active movement of air during imaging.

♦ Ventilation-perfusion (V/Q) scan: The V/Q scan is a combination of two separate imaging processes. The ventilation scan requires the inhalation of a radioactive gas, and the perfusion scan requires the injection of a radioactive tracer. Both scans are interpreted separately and compared if abnormalities are noted. V/Q scans are primarily indicated to rule out pulmonary emboli often due to the presence of a deep-vein thrombosis elsewhere in the body.

♦ Bronchoscopy: A bronchoscopy is a direct visualization of the trachea and bronchial tree via a fiber optic flexible tube inserted through the nose, mouth, or a tracheal tube. It can be used as a diagnostic or therapeutic intervention and is indicated when there is a need to assess for infection that cannot be determined from a sputum sample, to biopsy a nodule/mass for malignancy, or to remove severely viscous secretions that cannot be mobilized by the patient.

PHARMACOLOGY

The following pharmacological agents are utilized to assist in managing patients with airway clearance dysfunction:
♦ Mucolytic agents and expectorants
  • Mucolytic agents attempt to decrease the viscosity of secretions

  • Expectorants facilitate the production or expectoration of secretions
  • Both are used together to prevent the accumulation of thick secretions that clog the airways and prevent ventilation in the oxygen transport pathway
  • Both are used for acute conditions, as well as for the chronic diseases/disorders
  • While there has been some controversy reported regarding the long-term effectiveness of pharmacological agents to alter the progression of pulmonary disease, especially in the population with cystic fibrosis, there are new clinical studies underway to further appropriate use of these agents[11-17] Note: The Cystic Fibrosis Foundation has been a leader in partnering with pharmaceutical companies to further study any and all pharmacological agents that may enhance care of this patient population
  • Examples: Acetylcysteine (Mucomyst), DNase (Pulmozyme), hypertonic saline
  • Side effects: Chest tightness; wheezing, difficulty in breathing, clammy skin, fever, irritation of mouth, throat, or lungs
♦ Bronchodilators
  • Beta-adrenergic agonists
    ▪ Assist in relaxation of smooth muscle in the bronchioles and result in patent airways
    ▪ Can be administered orally, subcutaneously, or by inhalation
    ▪ Inhalation is the most common and effective method with the least amount of systemic side effects
    ▪ Nebulizers are preferred method of administration used for inpatients and metered dose inhalers (MDI) for outpatients
    ▪ The type of nebulizer used is key to the deposit of the medication in the airways
    ▪ Examples: Albuterol (Ventolin), Epinephrine HCL (Adrenalin)
    ▪ Side effects: Shakiness, tremor, headache, nosebleed, upset stomach, cough, dry mouth, throat irritation, rash
  • Anticholinergic agents
    ▪ Can be used in combination with beta-adrenergic agonists, may block reflex bronchoconstriction due to irritants, and is used to prevent wheezing and shortness of breath
    ▪ Can be administered by oral inhalation using open mouth technique (with mouthpiece 1 to 2 inches from mouth) or closed mouth technique (with mouthpiece well into mouth, past the front teeth, and with lips tightly closed): Slow deep breath as spray medication into mouth, hold breath for 5 to 10 seconds, remove inhaler, exhale slowly

- Example: Ipratropin bromide (Atrovent)
- Side effects: Dizziness, nervousness, drowsiness, headache, upset stomach, dry mouth, throat irritation, skin rash

♦ Antibiotics

- Indicated to treat respiratory tract infections that can cause increased secretion production and respiratory complications
- Can accelerate improvement of peak expiratory flow rates[15]
- Prophylactic treatment with chronic disease is not strongly supported by clinical trials and not recommended[11]
- Sensitivity and specificity of the cultured bacteria determines the antibiotic chosen (ie, *Staphylococcus Aureus* versus *Pseudomonas Aeroginosa*)
- Usually given via oral or intravenous administration but may be used in inhaled format
- Examples: Many to choose from[15]
  - Standard: Amoxicillin, tetracycline, doxycycline, trimethoprim-sulfamethoxazole, pipercillin, tobramycin, ceftazidime, imipenem
  - Modernized: Amoxicillin-clavulanate (Augmentin), Levofloxacin (Levaquin), Ciprofloxacin (Cipro), TOBI (inhaled tobramycin), Colistin
- Side effects: Diarrhea, headache, cough, stomach pain

♦ Others pharmacological agents that are controversial as to benefits of treatment[11]

- Corticosteroids
  - May assist with preventing airway inflammation and improving pulmonary function
  - Administered via inhalation
  - Examples: Flunisolide (AeorBid), FloVent, Methylpednisolone (Prednisone)
  - Side effects: Chest tightness, bruising, dizziness, white patches in mouth or throat, rash, stomach pain
- Decongestants
  - May assist with vasoconstriction of the mucosal layer in the nasal passages and dry up mucosal vasculature and congestion
  - Administered orally or nasally
  - Examples: Ephedrine (Primatene mist), Phenylpropanolamine (Triaminic), Pseudo-ephedrine (Sudafed)
  - Side effects: Fast heartbeat, headache, nervousness, coughing, dizziness

---

Case Study#1: Cystic Fibrosis

Melinda King is a 4-year-old female admitted with an acute exacerbation of cystic fibrosis and weight loss.

PHYSICAL THERAPIST EXAMINATION

HISTORY

♦ Demographic information: Melinda is a 4-year-old white female whose primary language is English. She is to start preschool.

♦ Social history: She is the first child of two married parents, who are both college graduates. Her mother has recently returned to work on a part-time basis.

♦ Play history: She rides her tricycle, plays soccer, and is starting ballet. She loves to play outdoors with the neighborhood children.

♦ Growth and development: Her current weight is 29 lbs (13.2 kg), which is 6.6 lbs (3 kg) less than her last CF clinic visit 2 months ago at which time she weighed 35.7 lbs (16.2 kg). She is right-hand dominant.

♦ Living environment: She lives with parents and 4-month-old brother in a two-level home in the suburban Philadelphia area.

♦ General health status

- Perception: Melinda is aware that she has cystic fibrosis. Her parents are fully aware of all aspects of the disease and appropriate treatment modalities. They are active in the Cystic Fibrosis Foundation's local chapter and the parent support group.
- Physical function: Until her recent illness, Melinda has been at an age appropriate level of functional activities.
- Psychological function: Her psychological function is age appropriate. She has been very excited about having a new younger brother.
- Role function: Daughter and sister in an intact family unit.
- Social function: Her social function includes age appropriate behaviors. Melinda will be starting preschool. She usually looks forward to playing with her two best friends.

♦ Health habits: With parental supervision, Melinda uses the Vest (High Frequency Chest Wall Oscillations and previously called the ThAIRapy Vest) for home airway clearance.

- Family history: No other immediate or extended family members have CF. Her 4-month-old brother does not have the disease.

- Medical/surgical history: Melinda was diagnosed with CF at 8 months of age. The diagnosis of CF was made based on her failure to regain her birth weight and chronic wheezing. She has had a recent weight loss of 6.6 lbs (3 kg). Her genotype is homozygous: delta F508/delta F508.

- Prior hospitalizations: She had a prior hospitalization at 8 months of age after her diagnosis for "Failure to Thrive."

- Preexisting medical and other health-related conditions: She has possible gastroesophageal reflux.

- Current condition(s)/chief complaint(s): She was admitted to the hospital with a 1-week history of productive cough, wheezing, and rhinorrhea. She has been on Keflex for 3 weeks and is gradually improving. She has demonstrated poor appetite and decreased level of physical activity. Her mother reports that Melinda has been less active and has shown no interest in going outdoors to play with her friends when they call on her. She has an intravenous line in place in the right brachial vein.

- Functional status and activity level: She has been functioning at age appropriate levels of functional and play activities.

- Medications: At time of admission she was on:
  - Flo Vent (110 micrograms): 2 puffs BID
  - Albuterol: 2.5 mg via nebulizer every 6 hours
  - Creon 10: With meals, 5 with snacks
  - ADEK (vitamins): 1 cc daily
  - LiquiE: 3cc daily
  - Vitamin K: 2.5 mg every 3 days

- Other clinical tests
  - Her chest x-ray revealed thickening of the bronchovascular markings in perihilar distribution, especially along markings for the right upper (RUL) and middle (RML) lobes and mild hyperinflation. An acute process/infiltrate is noted in the RUL.
  - Her Brasfield score, which is used to gauge lung disease, was 21/25. The chest x-ray is examined for: 1) air trapping; 2) increased pulmonary markings or scarring; 3) lobar lesions; 4) nodular cystic lesions; and 5) overall impression/general severity. The total score is 5 points for each category, or a total of 25, and points are subtracted for findings in each area.[18]
  - Sputum culture revealed the presence of *staphylococcus aureus*, which is sensitive to all antibiotics.
  - Bronchoscopic Alveolar Lavage (BAL) revealed no acid-fast bacilli and *staphylococcus aureus*.
  - A pH probe revealed no pathologic reflex.

SYSTEMS REVIEW

- Cardiovascular/pulmonary
  - BP: 97/60 mm Hg
  - Edema: None
  - HR: 120 bpm
  - RR: 40 bpm
- Integumentary
  - Presence of scar formation: None
  - Skin color: Pink
  - Skin integrity: Intact except for IV in right brachial vein
- Musculoskeletal
  - Gross ROM: Age appropriate
  - Gross strength: Age appropriate
  - Gross symmetry: Symmetrical
  - Height: 3' 4" (102 cm)
  - Weight: 29 lbs (13.2 kg)
- Neuromuscular
  - Balance: Age appropriate
  - Locomotion, transfers, and transitions: Age appropriate
- Communication, affect, cognition, language, and learning style: Age appropriate

TESTS AND MEASURES

- Aerobic capacity/endurance
  - She has been less active in play and exhibits decreased endurance while walking
  - During the 6-Minute Walk test, she was able to walk 1339 feet (408 meters)
    - Norms for children between 90 and 108 months (7.5 to 9 years) ranged from a 5th percentile rating of 1462 feet (446 meters) to a 90th percentile of 2030 feet (619 meters)[19]
    - Studies done on children with CF ranged from 1631 feet (497 meters) in children with better lung function[20] to 1335 feet (407 meters) in children with more severe lung disease.[21]
- Anthropometric characteristics
  - Body mass index (BMI) is 13.65 kg/m2 (59% BMI for age)[22]
- Arousal, attention, and cognition
  - She had shown decreased interest in playing with her friends prior to this episode
  - Usually she had been attentive and enjoyed playing with her friends
- Assistive and adaptive devices and equipment
  - Melinda has been using the Vest (HFCC) at home as a means of chest percussion and vibration for airway clearance

- ♦ Integumentary integrity
  - ● Disrupted at area of right brachial vein where IV has been inserted
- ♦ Motor function
  - ● Intact and age appropriate balance
- ♦ Muscle performance
  - ● Hand-held dynamometry revealed some weakness in hip flexion, knee extension, and ankle dorsiflexion strength
- ♦ Posture
  - ● Evidence of slightly forward head and slightly rounded thoracic spine
- ♦ Range of motion
  - ● Extremities: WNL
  - ● Decreased chest wall excursion at level of xiphoid
- ♦ Self-care and home management
  - ● At home, she had been able to perform all age-appropriate ADL
- ♦ Ventilation and respiration/gas exchange
  - ● Pulmonary signs of respiration/gas exchange
    - ■ Pulse oximetry: 98% (room air)
  - ● Pulmonary signs of ventilatory function
    - ■ Wet cough
    - ■ Diminished lung sounds throughout with crackles noted in the apical and posterior segments of the RUL and in the RML
    - ■ Her breathing pattern at this time exhibited increased use of the accessory muscles of respiration
- ♦ Work (job/school/play), community, and leisure integration or reintegration
  - ● Mother reports less active play
  - ● Melinda has shown no interest in going to soccer practice or playing outdoors

EVALUATION

Melinda is a 4-year-old female with a diagnosis of CF. She has been admitted to the hospital for the second time for an acute exacerbation of CF. This time she has had a 1-week history of a productive cough, wheezing, and rhinorrhea. Tests revealed thickening of the bronchovascular markings in perihilar distribution, especially along markings for right upper and middle lobes, and mild hyperinflation. A sputum culture revealed the presence of *staphylococcus aureus* with sensitivity to all antibiotics. She has been on Keflex for 3 weeks and is slowly improving. She has demonstrated poor appetite and weight loss. She demonstrates a wet cough, and abnormal and adventitious breath sounds. She has been less active in play activities.

DIAGNOSIS

Melinda King is a patient with a diagnosis of CF. She has impaired aerobic capacity/endurance, anthropometric characteristics, muscle performance, range of motion, and ventilation and respiration/gas exchange. She is functionally limited in play actions, tasks, and activities. These findings are consistent with placement in Pattern C: Impaired Ventilation, Respiration/Gas Exchange, and Aerobic Capacity/Endurance Associated With Airway Clearance Dysfunction. The identified impairments and functional limitations will then be addressed in determining the prognosis and the plan of care.

PROGNOSIS AND PLAN OF CARE

Over the course of the hospital visits, the following mutually established outcomes have been determined.

- ♦ Ability to perform physical activities related to play will be improved
- ♦ Aerobic conditioning/endurance will be improved
- ♦ Anthropometric characteristics will be improved
- ♦ Muscle performance will be increased
- ♦ Range of motion will be increased
- ♦ Ventilation and respiration/gas exchange will improve

To achieve these outcomes, the appropriate interventions for this patient are determined. These will include: coordination, communication, and documentation; patient/client-related instruction; therapeutic exercise; functional training in play actions, tasks, and activities; and airway clearance techniques.

Based on the diagnosis and the prognosis, Melinda is expected to be in the hospital for 10 days and then to be followed up in 2 weeks in the Outpatient Pediatric Cystic Fibrosis Clinic. She is expected to have quarterly follow-up visits in the clinic. Melinda's parents are highly motivated to prevent further hospitalizations, and they will follow through with her exercise and bronchial hygiene programs.

INTERVENTIONS

RATIONALE FOR SELECTED INTERVENTIONS

The interventions for children with CF have included therapeutic exercise, breathing techniques, and airway clearance techniques. Outpatient pulmonary rehabilitation programs usually include instruction in breathing techniques (pursed lip and diaphragmatic breathing); stretching; low impact strengthening exercises; and aerobic exercise on treadmills, arm ergometers, and bicycles.[23]

Therapeutic Exercise

In children with CF, peak exercise performance is reduced as a result of the decreased strength of their peripheral muscles,[24] their decreased pulmonary function,[25,26] and the alteration in their nutritional status.[27,28] Many studies have looked at the use of exercise to improve impaired performance in these children. While most of these studies have been uncontrolled, have used small numbers of subjects, and have been carried out over short periods of time, changes have been observed. In spite of the limitations, these studies have noted that exercise training results in increased strength,[29] increased peak exercise capacity with aerobic conditioning,[30-32] decreased shortness of breath,[33] enhanced ability to perform ADL,[32] and increased expectoration of sputum.[31,34-37] There is also an indication that exercise, including a swimming program, may improve or preserve lung volumes.[24,38-41] In addition to the physiological effects of exercise training for children with CF, it also leads to positive feelings about their self-worth and their physical appearance.[42] As with any exercise program, these programs for individuals with CF must be of adequate intensity to achieve the desired training effect, and greater improvement is achieved at higher work rates.[43]

Selvadurai and associates investigated the effects of aerobic training and resistance training in children with CF. They found on the one hand that aerobic training resulted in enhanced peak aerobic capacity, activity levels, and quality of life as compared to resistance training, while on the other hand resistance training resulted in increased weight gain, leg strength, and lung function. A combination of both aerobic and resistance training seems to be best for optimum results.[44]

Swisher and colleagues noted that while lung function is the primary factor in how well a child with CF performs on the 6-Minute Walk test, an intrinsic abnormality in muscle force production may also be influential in exercise performance, thus indicating the need for muscle strengthening with these children.[45,46]

Two long-term studies (one with children and adolescents and one with adults) have also supported the use of exercise with individuals with CF.[47,48] Schneiderman-Walker and colleagues investigated the effect of exercise in children over a 3-year timeframe in a randomized controlled study. They noted a slower rate of decline yearly in pulmonary function. Preservation of lung volumes (including a reduced decline in functional vital capacity) was found in the exercising group.[47]

Patients with CF have often had difficulty transferring exercises taught in rehabilitation programs to the community and sustaining them for a long period of time. Schneiderman-Walker's study provides data to support the importance of long-term exercise. Compliance with an exercise program was enhanced in adolescents when the exercise program was individually designed.[38]

Disease severity in CF is best objectively measured by pulmonary function test results (especially the FEV_1) and weight.[49,50] Therefore, any interventions that enhance or maintain pulmonary function in children with CF have major implications for long-term management of the disease, as well as for the individual's survival. Swimming and bicycling have been found to result in improved FEV_1. Weight training programs and general exercise have also been shown to result in improved FEV_1.[33,38,39] An interesting finding in the studies related to improvements gained from an exercise program is that these improvements often did not result in an increase in peak exercise testing in children and adolescents with CF.[47]

The addition of breathing techniques, like pursed lip breathing (PLB), can assist with controlling dyspnea that may occur during exercise. PLB increases rib cage and accessory muscle recruitment during inspiration and expiration; it also increases abdominal muscle activity during expiration.[51] PLB can promote a slower and deeper breathing pattern at rest and during exercise,[52] resulting in a decreased respiratory rate and decreased feeling of dyspnea.[23,53,54] Controlling dyspnea with exercise and at rest can enable patients, especially those with COPD, to increase their activity and exercise tolerance.

Overall, patients with acute pulmonary conditions may have low levels of tolerance to exercise and should begin slowly. Close monitoring of heart rate, blood pressure, respiratory rate, and oxygen saturation should be done for the patient with an acute condition. Teaching patients to monitor their own heart rate and tolerance to activity using perceived exertion (RPE) can also be beneficial.[54] Patients should be instructed to stop and cough out secretions during exercise when they feel they are loosened.

Airway Clearance Techniques

The indications for airway clearance (AC) are an impaired mucociliary transport, ineffective cough, overproduction of mucous, abnormal mucous, and dehydration.[56] Airway clearance is defined as the removal of mucous and foreign material from the airways.[6] The goal of AC is to improve oxygen transport. Historically, percussion and vibration with postural drainage (formerly known as chest physical therapy [CPT]) were the gold standard for treating AC dysfunction. With the advancement of technology and the creativeness of physical therapists, multiple devices and equipment have come along that are both as effective and not as effective as traditional CPT.[37,57,58]

When deciding which technique to utilize, effectiveness, efficiency, and adherence should be considered. Can the technique meet the goals of the treatment without complications? Is the treatment adaptable to any setting (ie, clinic, home, school, work)? Can the technique be performed independently or is assistance needed? Will the patient fatigue performing the technique? Is the technique comfortable and time-efficient? Is it cost effective for the patient? Is it the preferred technique of the patient/family and are they motivated to perform it? All of these factors should be discussed with the patient/family so the optimal treatment technique can be agreed upon between patient and therapist as it ultimately comes down to patient/family preference.[11,58-60]

The cough reflex assists with removal of secretions from the upper respiratory tract at the level of the carina. Inability to remove secretions from the lower respiratory tract is where complication can arise and when infection can occur.[6] Airway clearance techniques range from the former "gold standard of CPT," postural drainage, and manual techniques to current devices that may provide equal outcomes if patients/family are able and motivated to utilize them.[56,58] Many techniques focus on removal of secretions in the lower respiratory tract. The majority of techniques that have been researched relate to success with treatment of CF and bronchiectasis. They include but are not limited to: postural drainage, percussion and vibration, the active cycle of breathing technique with the forced expiratory technique, autogenic drainage, positive expiratory pressure (PEP) devices, high pressure chest wall oscillation, and exercise with breathing techniques.

Postural Drainage

Postural drainage (PD) is the basis of traditional CPT. PD is a series of gravity-assisted positions (typically head tilt down) that promotes mobilization of secretions from the bases of the lungs to the larger airways for expectoration. PD positions are related to the different segments in the lobes of the lungs (Figure 3-5). The positioning is based on the areas of consolidation heard with auscultation or seen on x-ray studies, with most patients tolerating the entire series of PD positions during a treatment if needed. PD can be contraindicated to those with acute head injuries, high intracranial pressure, or active hemorrhage in the brain.[1,62,63]

Patients who require intubation and mechanical ventilation can provide a challenge to the therapist desiring to perform PD. A more simplified version of the PD positions is recommended: supine, 45 degrees rotated toward prone with left side up, 45 degrees rotated toward prone with right side up, return to supine.[64]

Previously undetected/nondiagnosed gastroesophageal reflux has been reported in infants with CF. Sufficient evidence was obtained to warrant a change in the standard of practice put forth by the Cystic Fibrosis Foundation. As a result, the head down positions are no longer included in infant/toddler postural drainage positioning.[65,66]

Percussion and Vibration

Percussion and vibration (PV) are often teamed with PD and complete the traditional components of CPT. The goal of PV is to manually loosen secretions in the lower airways to move them toward the upper airways for expectoration. Percussion is a rhythmic clapping (cupped hand) on the chest wall over the area of consolidation during inspiration and

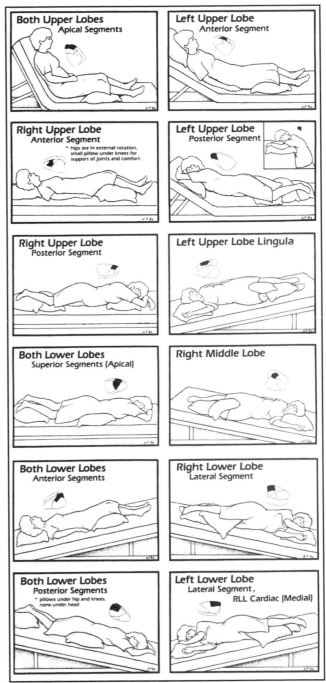

Figure 3-5. PD positions are related to the different segments in the lobes of the lungs. Reprinted from *Cardiovascular and Pulmonary Physical Therapy: Evidence and Practice.* 4th ed. Frownfelter D, Dean E. Page 342-343, 2005, with permission from Elsevier.

expiration. Vibration is a co-contracting of the muscles of the arms to create a high frequency vibratory force. The hands are placed on the chest wall over the area of consolidation to assist with loosening secretions during expiration. PD and PV can be time consuming, require the assistance of another person to perform the PV, and can have a delayed response in secretion expectoration anywhere from 30 minutes to 1 hour. Despite the limited evidence of the effectiveness of PD and PV, it is frequently used as the gold standard against which other techniques and devices are compared.[6]

Active Cycle of Breathing Technique

The active cycle of breathing technique (ACBT) is also used for airway clearance. Unlike PD and PV, ACBT encourages active participation by the patient. It includes a cyclic repetition of three phases: breathing control, thoracic expansion, and a forced expiratory technique (FET). Breathing control is diaphragmatic breathing at a normal tidal volume; thoracic expansion is deep inhalation with relaxed exhalation at vital capacity; and FET is a "huff" at mid- to low lung volume followed by a forced expiration with abdominal muscle contraction. The cycle consists of breathing control, then three to four thoracic expansions, then breathing control, followed by three to four thoracic expansions, then breathing control, followed by FET, and finally breathing control.

The ACBT has been shown to be an effective and efficient technique for the mobilization and clearance of excess bronchial secretions.[67,68] Lung function has been shown to improve following the initiation of the ACBT,[69] and hypoxemia is neither caused nor increased.[70] With an increase in lung volume that occurs with the ACBT, the resistance to airflow via the collateral channels is reduced.[71]

Orlik and Sands studied 80 children with CF over a span of 7 months and found a statistically significant increase in FEV_1, FVC, FEV_1/FVC, MEF 25% to 75%, and PEF in patients using the ACBT.[72] Phillips and colleagues found sputum weight, pulmonary function, and FVC to increase significantly with ACBT as compared with high frequency chest compressions.[73]

The ACBT can be paired with percussion during the thoracic expansions and can be done in PD positions for added expectoration.[11] The use of the sitting position alone for ACBT is effective and adherence to treatment is frequently better than with other positions.[74]

Studies using the ACBT have shown that it is not further improved by the addition of mechanical percussion,[75] positive expiratory pressure (PEP),[76] or the flutter.[77,78]

The ACBT has been shown to be effective with patients with CF,[11,67-74] as well as with other types of patients with COPD.[78-81] It has also been used as a gold standard of CPT with which sputum expectoration devices have been compared.[2,12,82,83]

Autogenic Drainage

Autogenic drainage (AD) mobilizes bronchial secretions during expiratory airflow. It is an active cycle of three phases that patients can perform independently. The three phases are: 1) the unsticking phase to loosen secretions in the smaller peripheral airways; 2) the collecting phase to mobilize the secretions to larger central airways; and 3) the evacuating phase to remove the secretions. AD requires a great deal of patience and concentration by the patient, not to mention proprioceptive, auditory, and tactile awareness of one's own secretions. These factors may make this technique difficult for children to learn. All three phases are performed with slow deep inspirations through the nose, a 2- to 3-second hold for collateral breathing to occur, and expiration through the mouth. Noting the vibration changes in the lungs during breathing is what cues the patient to progress through the phases. AD has been shown to be better tolerated by patients with CF and to result in less oxygen desaturation during the intervention when compared to PD and percussion.[84]

AD has been shown to be tolerated by patients with COPD and to be just as effective as ACBT in secretion clearance and improving pulmonary function.[85]

Of note are the findings that AD cleared mucus from the lungs faster than ACBT over the course of a given day; however, both methods improved ventilation. The pulmonary function test results for both techniques were the same, but improved forced expiratory flow from 25% to 75% was found in more patients using autogenic drainage, whereas improved forced vital capacity was greater in patients using ACBT.[85,86]

Positive Expiratory Pressure

Positive expiratory pressure (PEP) devices have become more popular with the invention of the Flutter® and the Acapella™. A PEP device promotes collateral ventilation by creating a backpressure into the airways and lungs during exhalation. This allows air pressure to build distal to the secretions and can force the secretions into the upper airways for expectoration. PEP devices can also prevent atelectasis and airway collapse and have been shown to improve oxygenation and exercise tolerance.[87] Overall, PEP devices have controversial evidence supporting their effectiveness over other forms of AC techniques.[88] Use of the devices is based primarily on patient preference.[12]

The Flutter® device is a hand-held pipe-like device with a steel ball that vibrates in a cone during exhalation to provide backpressure into the lungs. The level at which the device is held can provide high or low levels of pressure depending upon the needs of the patient (ie, the amount of secretions to expel vs. opening airways).[1] The use of the Flutter® device has resulted in improved pulmonary function tests (FVC and FEV_1) after 1 week of use and similar improvement in pulmonary function and exercise tolerance after 2 weeks of use compared to traditional CPT.[88] However, after 1 month the Flutter® device did not show improvement in pulmonary function compared to traditional CPT in pediatric patients with CF, but was the preferred method.[89] Other research has shown the Flutter® device to be just as effective as the ACBT in patients with non-CF bronchiectasis.[90]

The Acapella™ uses a counterweighted plug and magnet to create airflow oscillation, and a dial to adjust the expiratory pressure. Unlike the Flutter®, the Acapella™ comes in 2 models depending upon expiratory flow (>15 L/min and <15 L /min). The Acapella™ has been shown to be just as effective as the ACBT in secretion removal and may be considered more acceptable and user friendly by more patients than other AC techniques.[12] While the Acapella™ and Flutter® have similar intervention results, the Acapella™ may also be more user friendly than the Flutter®, as it is not position dependent and can be used with patients that have low expiratory flows.[92]

Patients can independently use PEP devices in the upright position. The devices can be used during acute or chronic phases of pulmonary illness and disease. They are used by a wide variety of patients with many different pulmonary conditions. The primary advantage of a PEP device is the ease of use and convenience in everyday life.

High Frequency Chest Wall Compression or Oscillation

High frequency chest wall compression or oscillation (HFCC) is a vest linked to an air-pulse generator that provides different frequencies of vibration/oscillation and levels of compression to the chest. The vest is donned in sitting, the air-pulse generator is turned on, and the compression and vibration are controlled by a foot pedal. Each frequency of vibration should last about 3 to 5 minutes, and the length of the intervention will depend upon the amount of secretions and the severity of the pulmonary condition. The patient can have continuous (during inhalation and exhalation) compression or intermittent (during inhalation only) compression. The patient should stop compressions and cough between each level of frequency.

Compared to traditional CPT, HFCC is supported in its consistency of compression and production of sputum because it is machine based.[3] It has also been shown to be as effective as PD and PV in hospitalized patients with CF and preferred by some patients with CF over traditional CPT.[6,93] However, it is not as effective as the ACBT in patients with infective exacerbation of CF.[15] Different waveform frequencies have been studied, and the triangle waveform produced more sputum than the sine waveform.[94,95]

HFCC is a technique that can be performed independently by the patient. The major disadvantage of the technique is the cost of the equipment (the air pulse generator and the vest). Most patients cannot afford to buy an air pulse generator outright, but some insurance companies may reimburse a monthly rental fee.

COORDINATION, COMMUNICATION, AND DOCUMENTATION

Interdisciplinary teamwork will include communication and collaboration with the nutritionist, social worker, physicians, nurses, and respiratory therapists. Coordination with nutritional services is needed to minimize energy output/caloric uptake associated with coughing. It will be important to ask for the meal and snack schedule in order to schedule airway clearance sessions around this schedule. Collaboration with physicians will occur regarding results of pH probe and existence of pathologic reflux. All elements of the patient's management will be documented.

PATIENT/CLIENT-RELATED INSTRUCTION

The parents will be educated about the strategies to use to incorporate physical activity into the family lifestyle and further identify games that will augment structured activities (ie, soccer and ballet/dance). Recommendations regarding the vest settings will be reviewed. Inclusion of play activities with blow toys and bubbles will be discussed and demonstrated. A review of manual techniques with modified postural drainage will be carried out to provide parents with an alternative to the vest treatments as needed. The education and instruction provided during the inpatient stay will be supplemented during outpatient visits in the Cystic Fibrosis Clinic.

THERAPEUTIC EXERCISE

- ◆ Aerobic capacity/endurance conditioning
  - • Since young children do best when exercise is incorporated into games and play activities, endurance activities will use that principle
  - • Activities for aerobic conditioning will include: walking on hospital grounds; stair climbing; crab soccer; playing tag; playing dodge ball
- ◆ Body mechanics and postural stabilization
  - • Work on postural alignment during games ("Simon Says" to stand up straight, pull elbows back)
  - • Perform wall slides with back and head flat against wall
  - • Strengthen core abdominals and back extensors using games (eg, wheelbarrow, bouncing on ball)
- ◆ Flexibility exercises
  - • Incorporate stretching into games (eg, trunk stretching while playing "Simon Says" to reach overhead, then bend to the sides, twist to right and left)
  - • Use exercise ball for side bending and upper back stretching
- ◆ Relaxation
  - • Paced breathing (ratio of 1:2 of inspiration to expiration) to enhance relaxation of accessory muscles
- ◆ Strength, power, and endurance training
  - • In the hospital, begin with gentle strengthening including:
    - ■ Ball activities/core stabilization:
      - ► Prone butterflies
      - ► Prone alternate arm and leg raises
      - ► Sitting alternate arm and leg raises
    - ■ Lower extremity strengthening

- ▸ March in place bring knees up to waist
- ▸ Walking on toes and heels
- ▸ Side stepping
  - ■ Breathing exercises to strengthen the muscles of respiration
    - ▸ Incentive spirometer
    - ▸ Blowing out through straws of decreasing diameter
    - ▸ Blowing ping pong ball across a table
    - ▸ Using pin wheels and other similar play objects to increase inspiration and expiration
- • When she progresses to the out-patient clinic, additional lower and upper extremity strengthening will be added and may include the addition of:
  - ■ Carioca
  - ■ Wall slides
  - ■ Wide balance beam walking
  - ■ Wheelbarrow races

FUNCTIONAL TRAINING IN PLAY INTEGRATION OR REINTEGRATION

- ♦ During her hospital stay, review with parents strategies for active play
- ♦ Identify activities that can involve all family members

AIRWAY CLEARANCE TECHNIQUES

- ♦ Breathing strategies
  - • Work on prolonging the expiratory phase of breathing using age-appropriate activities, such as blowing long streams of bubbles, using straw to blow paper objects across table, and other blow toys
- ♦ Manual/mechanical techniques
  - • Chest percussion, vibration, shaking and modified postural drainage (no head down positioning) to all lung fields
    - ■ Emphasis on RUL and RML
    - ■ Performed twice daily by physical therapy with 2 additional vest treatments
  - • Review of the vest settings
    - ■ Present settings are pressure of 5 with frequency settings of 5, 8, and 12 Hz for 7 minutes each
    - ■ Recommend change to use of 2 frequency settings at 8 and 12 Hz for 10 minutes each
    - ■ Vest will be used for 2 sessions per day while she is an inpatient
    - ■ Upon discharge, Melinda will continue to use the vest 3x/day
    - ■ The use of the vest 3x/day will be reassessed (for possible reduction to 2x/day) when Melinda is seen during the outpatient follow-up clinic visit

- • Coordination with albuterol nebulizer treatments to augment airway clearance techniques
- ♦ Positioning
  - • Modified postural drainage (no head down position) to avoid symptoms of gastroesophageal reflux)

ANTICIPATED GOALS AND EXPECTED OUTCOMES

- ♦ Impact on pathology/pathophysiology (disease, disorder, or condition)
  - • Her cough is nonproductive.
  - • Her pulmonary condition is improved as noted on her chest x-ray, and the acute RUL process/infiltrate is resolved.
  - • Wheezing is no longer present.
- ♦ Impact on impairments
  - • Melinda no longer demonstrates abnormal breath sounds.
  - • Melinda is able to participate in playing game of crab soccer for 15 minutes without rest.
  - • She can climb one flight of stairs without rest or leg fatigue.
  - • She has gained 3.3 lbs (1.5 kg) of weight during the hospital stay.
  - • The strength of her hip flexors, knee extensors, and ankle dorsiflexors have increased.
  - • Melinda is able to walk 1380 feet (421 meters).
- ♦ Impact on functional limitations
  - • Melinda is at preillness level of active play.
- ♦ Risk reduction/prevention
  - • Parents are aware of signs and symptoms of pulmonary problems.
  - • Parents have more strategies for airway clearance.
  - • The importance of airway clearance and physical activity for risk reduction is understood and will be continued upon discharge from the hospital.
- ♦ Impact on health, wellness, and fitness
  - • Melinda will be at age-appropriate level of physical fitness.
  - • Melinda's father will set aside time to actively play (eg, playing ball, taking walk, wheelbarrow walk) with her 3x/week.
  - • The family plans to start hiking together.
- ♦ Impact on societal resources
  - • Documentation occurs throughout the client management and follows APTA's *Guidelines for Physical Therapy Documentation.*
- ♦ Patient/client satisfaction
  - • Her parents will have knowledge and awareness of the diagnosis, interventions, and anticipatory strate-

gies for wellness that was demonstrated during treatment sessions.

- Her parents expressed awareness of the availability of the physical therapist for any questions or concerns that may arise during clinic visits.

REEXAMINATION

Reexamination is performed throughout the episode of care.

DISCHARGE

Melinda is discharged from physical therapy after a total of 10 days of physical therapy in the hospital and attainment of her goals and expectations. These sessions have covered her entire episode of care. She is discharged and will be checked in 2 weeks at the Outpatient Cystic Fibrosis Clinic and will be followed up quarterly thereafter.

Case Study #2: Cystic Fibrosis

Mr. John Deane is a 41-year-old male with CF and is hospitalized for hemoptysis and pulmonary exacerbation.

PHYSICAL THERAPIST EXAMINATION

HISTORY

- Demographics: John Deane is a 41-year-old white male whose primarily language is English. He is right hand dominant.

- Social history: John is married and lives in a suburban community in North Carolina. His wife is very supportive and has educated herself on CF care.

- Employment/work: He works full-time as an assembly line worker. His work schedule is 3 12-hour shifts per week.

- Living environment: John and his wife live in a two-story house with their bedroom on the ground floor.

- General health status
  - Perception: Considering his diagnosis, John perceives his health to be fair to good. He recognizes that he is at risk for pulmonary exacerbations if he does not follow his prescribed regimen.
  - Physical function: Until this episode, he has been working full-time and has been socially active through his bowling.

- Psychological function: John appears to be free from any significant pathology. However, he reports being concerned about his potential longevity considering his diagnosis.
  - Role function: Husband, friend, and colleague.
  - Social function: He socializes with friends and enjoys bowling.

- Social/health habits: John has never smoked, although his mother and father both smoked. He will have a glass of wine once in a while.

- Family history: John is one of two siblings, both of whom were diagnosed with CF. His older sibling died from CF over 20 years ago.

- Medical/surgical history: John was diagnosed with CF at the age of 6 months. He is pancreatic sufficient. There are no signs of cystic fibrosis related diabetes (CFRD).

- Prior hospitalizations: Although he had no known hospital stays as a child, he has had multiple prior hospitalizations for acute exacerbations as an adult.

- Current condition(s)/chief complaint(s): John was admitted to the hospital with hemoptysis and pulmonary exacerbation.

- Functional status and activity level: He reported increasing fatigue during the last week prior to admission, including decreased exercise tolerance. On his nonwork days, John's routine was to use his stair stepper for 20 minutes; he had not been able to follow through with his routine for over a week.

- Medications: John has been taking multivitamins, Advair 1 puff BID, Pulmozyme 2.5 mg via nebulizer, Bactrim daily, Albuterol via nebulizer, and Flonase. He is also on TOBI (inhaled tobramycin, which is cycled every 3 weeks) 300 mg via nebulizer.

- Other clinical tests:
  - Spirometry
    - Forced vital capacity (FVC)=2.89 L (58% predicted) and forced expiratory volume at one second (FEV_1)=2.01L (53% predicted).
  - Chest x-ray
    - His chest x-ray revealed increased interstitial markings and thickened bronchial walls that were more marked at right middle lobe.
    - His Brasfield score was 20/25.[18]
  - Sputum culture revealed methacillin resistant *staphylococcus aureus* (MRSA) and *pseudomonas fluoroescens*.
  - Bronchial artery embolization/cauterization was performed on day 1 of his admission to stop the hemoptysis. It was repeated on day 4 for reoccurrence of hemoptysis.

SYSTEMS REVIEW

- ◆ Cardiovascular/pulmonary
  - BP: 127/77 mm Hg
  - Edema: None
  - HR: 95 bpm
  - RR: 16 bpm
- ◆ Integumentary
  - Presence of scar formation: None
  - Skin color: WNL and pink
  - Skin integrity: Skin intact
- ◆ Musculoskeletal
  - Gross ROM: Decreased left shoulder range of motion to 90 degrees forward flexion and abduction from prior injury
  - Gross strength: WFL
  - Gross symmetry: Slightly kyphotic, mild lumbar scoliosis, and lordosis with protruding abdomen
  - Height: 5' 5" (1.65 m)
  - Weight: 143 lbs (65 kg)
- ◆ Neuromuscular
  - Balance: WNL
  - Locomotion, transfers, and transitions: No apparent problems
- ◆ Communication, affect, cognition, language, and learning style
  - Communication, affect, and cognition: WNL, alert, oriented x3, soft spoken
  - Learning style: Visual learner

TESTS AND MEASURES

- ◆ Aerobic capacity/endurance
  - 6-Minute Walk test
    - Performed 7 days after admission due to re-occurrence of hemoptysis (routinely scheduled on third day of hospital stay)
    - Resting: Heart rate=102 bpm, SpO_2=94% (room air), and rate of perceived exertion (RPE)=9 (Borg 6-20 scale)
      - ‣ Borg 15 point linear scale[96]
        - ∘ 6
        - ∘ 7 = Very, very light
        - ∘ 8
        - ∘ 9 = Very light
        - ∘ 10
        - ∘ 11 = Fairly light
        - ∘ 12
        - ∘ 13 = Moderately hard
        - ∘ 14
        - ∘ 15 = Hard
        - ∘ 16
        - ∘ 17 = Very hard
        - ∘ 18
        - ∘ 19 = Very, very hard
        - ∘ 20 = Exhaustion
  - Use of the visual analogue scale (0 to 10 cm) for perception of dyspnea revealed 2 cm at rest pre-test[96,97]
  - Peak exercise values: Heart rate=136 bpm, SpO_2=93%, RPE=15, and perception of dyspnea=7
  - Total distance walked in 6 minutes: 1235 feet
    - Range is reported to be from 1312 to 2297 feet (400 to 700 m) in healthy adults, and approximately 1903 feet (580 m) for healthy men
    - Gender specific reference equations for the 6-minute walk distance (6MWD) for men=(7.57 x $height_{cm}$) – (5.02 x age) – (1.76 x $weight_{kg}$) – 309 m, and for women=6MWD=(2.11 x $height_{cm}$) – (2.29 x $weight_{kg}$) (5.78 x age) + 667 m[98]
- ◆ Assistive and adaptive devices
  - John has not used any equipment to enhance his airway clearance
  - Airway clearance devices will be prescribed for this patient
- ◆ Circulation
  - Sinus rhythm
  - Adaptive blood pressure response to activity
- ◆ Muscle performance: WFL, however manual muscle tests revealed:
  - Hip flexor strength bilaterally: 4/5
  - Knee extensor strength bilaterally: 4-/5
  - Ankle dorsiflexion bilaterally: 4+/5
  - Shoulder flexion and abduction both to only 90 degrees: 4/5
  - Abdominals: 3+/5
  - Back extensors: 4/5
- ◆ Posture
  - Slight kyphosis
  - Mild lumbar scoliosis
  - Lumbar lordosis with protruding abdomen
  - Increased anteroposterior diameter of chest
- ◆ Range of motion
  - Decreased chest wall excursion, right greater than left, consistent with chest x-ray findings
  - Shoulder flexion and abduction limited to 90 degrees due to prior shoulder injury
- ◆ Self-care and home management
  - John is independent in all of his personal self-care activities
  - He usually helps with household chores

- His wife has been performing chest percussion with four modified postural drainage positions daily
♦ Ventilation and respiration/gas exchange
  - Observation revealed patient on 3 liters of O_2 per minute via nasal cannula
  - Pulse oximetry: 96% on 3 liters of O_2 per minute
  - Cough sequence/function
    - Assessment of cough revealed effective wet cough, productive of reddish tinged brown mucoid sputum
    - Increased work of breathing is noted postcoughing but no oxygen desaturation
  - Auscultation revealed diminished lung sounds throughout with scattered crackles especially in the posterior segments of the upper lobes, right greater than left, and in the right middle lobe
  - Currently, he is using more accessory muscles for respiration
♦ Work, community, and leisure integration or reintegration
  - John plans to return to work 2 weeks after his hospital discharge
  - His bowling season resumes in 2 months, and he wants to be ready to return to his leisure activity

EVALUATION

John Deane is a 41-year-old male with cystic fibrosis. He was admitted to the hospital with hemoptysis and acute pulmonary exacerbation. He had two hemoptic episodes in the week prior to admission. One episode occurred with increased exertion (moving furniture) and the second occurred with coughing during an airway clearance treatment. He has stopped exercising, but not his airway clearance prior to admission. He has decreased ability to walk a distance and has slightly diminished strength in his lower extremities. Prior to this admission, he has been working full time, three 12-hour shifts.

DIAGNOSIS

John Deane is a patient with a diagnosis of CF. He has impaired: aerobic capacity/endurance; circulation; muscle performance; posture; range of motion; and ventilation and respiration/gas exchange. He is functionally limited in self-care and home management and in work, community, and leisure actions, tasks, and activities as a result of this recent episode. He is in need of supportive devices and equipment. These findings are consistent with placement in Pattern C: Impaired Ventilation, Respiration/Gas Exchange, and Aerobic Capacity/Endurance Associated With Airway Clearance Dysfunction. The identified impairments, func-

tional limitations, and device and equipment needs will then be addressed in determining the prognosis and the plan of care.

PROGNOSIS AND PLAN OF CARE

Over the course of the physical therapy visits, the following mutually established outcomes have been determined.
♦ Ability to perform physical activities related to work is improved
♦ Aerobic conditioning/endurance is improved
♦ Muscle performance is increased
♦ Posture in improved
♦ Range of motion is increased
♦ Ventilation and respiration/gas exchange are improved

To achieve these outcomes, the appropriate interventions for this patient are determined. These will include: coordination, communication, and documentation; patient/client-related instruction; therapeutic exercise; functional training in self-care and home management; functional training in work, community, and leisure integration or reintegration; prescription, application, and as appropriate, fabrication of devices and equipment; and airway clearance techniques.

Based on the diagnosis and the prognosis, John is expected to be in the hospital for 14 days and then to be followed up in the Outpatient Adult Cystic Fibrosis Clinic. He is expected to be followed quarterly in the clinic. John has good social support, is motivated to get back to work, and will follow through with his exercise and pulmonary hygiene programs.

INTERVENTIONS

RATIONALE FOR SELECTED INTERVENTIONS

Therapeutic Exercise

The rationale for therapeutic exercise for this case is included in Rationale for Selected Interventions in Case Study #1. In addition, decreased bone mineral density has been observed in adults with CF despite normal vitamin D levels.[99] Fracture rates in adults with CF have been found to be two times as high as those found in normal individuals of comparable age.[100] Therefore, strengthening/resistance and weightbearing exercises will be extremely important for this population. In addition, Parasa found excessive kyphosis in 62% percent of his study patients with CF and back pain in 94% of this same population.[100] Exercise programs for adults with CF must address posture, trunk strengthening, and postural alignment during all ADL and IADL.

Of interest has been the demonstration by Hodges that every muscle of the trunk is both a postural muscle and a respiratory muscle.[101-104] If the respiratory muscles are overutilized (as they often are in patients with CF with excessive coughing and breathing), they will be compromised in their effectiveness as postural muscles. This is why excessive kyphosis and back pain are so frequently seen in these patients. Therefore, exercise must incorporate chest mobilization, strengthening of the core muscles in their correct postural positions so that their functions for respiratory and postural needs are normalized, and transferring normal alignment to work, community, and leisure actions, tasks, and activities.[105]

As with children with CF, short-term studies of the effects of exercise with adults have also shown similar benefits. Long-term compliance with exercise programs learned in rehabilitation programs is also a problem for the adult with CF. Better compliance was found by Bloomquist and associates in their study of individually determined exercise programs for adolescents over a 1-year period of time.[38] Sahl and colleagues[31] and Heijerman and coworkers[40] found that unsupervised exercise programs using cycle ergometry at home were better maintained by adults as opposed to rigidly designed exercise-training programs. Moorcroft and associates analyzed the effectiveness of an unsupervised home-based exercise program using lower/whole body aerobic exercise and upper body strength training exercise for adults with CF over a 1-year period of time. They found several beneficial effects, including reduced lactate levels, reduced heart rate, and a clear trend for preservation of pulmonary function.[48]

Since patients perceive that they have control over their exercise adherence (which may not always be the case with other aspects of the treatment of their disease), flexibility in program prescription should be one that is enthusiastically supported by staff so that exercise becomes a habit for these patients.[105]

Airway Clearance Techniques

The rationale for airway clearance techniques for this case is included in Rationale for Selected Interventions in Case # 1 above. In addition, of note is the fact that with hemoptysis, percussion is contraindicated until the incident has resolved. Alternative airway clearance techniques that may be used prior to resolution include the use of the Acapella™, the Flutter®, and/or the active cycle of breathing technique. Chatham and associates studied the effect of standard physical therapy (postural drainage and the ACBT) against resisted inspiratory maneuvers at 80% of maximum sustained inspiratory pressure during the first 4 days of exacerbation of respiratory symptoms in adult patients with CF. They found that short-term resistive inspiratory maneuvers treatment was more effective at clearing sputum and inflammatory mediators than standardized physical therapy.[107]

In addition, autogenic drainage was found to be as good as ACBT at clearing mucus in patients with CF and has been determined to be as effective for home treatment. Patients with CF should be assessed as to which method suits them best.[108]

COORDINATION, COMMUNICATION, AND DOCUMENTATION

Communication and collaboration across the interdisciplinary team are crucial with this patient due to the episodes of hemoptysis that required alteration in the plan of care, including change in the timing of the administration of the 6-Minute Walk test from day 3 to day 7 and the use of alternative airway clearance techniques.[107] All elements of the patient's management will be documented in the official record, including examination and evaluation findings, diagnosis, prognosis, interventions, and outcomes, as well as changes in ausculatory findings, sputum production, mode of airway clearance, results of the 6-Minute Walk test, and subsequent exercise prescription.

PATIENT/CLIENT-RELATED INSTRUCTION

John will be instructed in use of the Acapella™ device and the active cycle of breathing technique. A review of the rationale of using alternative methods of airway clearance will be done with John and his wife. Postural drainage positions will be reviewed to insure that trouble areas are emphasized at home. A discussion of the advantages of the use of the vest (HFCC) will be carried out using a videotape/DVD demonstration that will be given to the patient and his wife. A home exercise prescription will be given prior to discharge. John and his wife may contact the physical therapist via phone or e-mail should questions or concerns arise before next clinic visit. Further education will be provided during the outpatient clinic visits.

THERAPEUTIC EXERCISE

♦ Aerobic capacity/endurance conditioning
- Inpatient exercise training will incorporate use of the treadmill with attention to the following parameters
  - 5-minute warm-up at 2.2 mph
  - Intensity at least 3.0 mph, use incline as tolerated
  - Duration of 20 minute at peak intensity
  - 5-minute cool-down at 2.4 mph
  - Parameters
    ▸ Heart rate no greater than 130 bpm
    ▸ SpO_2 no less than 93%
    ▸ RPE no less than 13 and give copy of perceived exertion scale to John
    ▸ Dyspnea scale no greater than 8

- Instruct John in procedures for taking his own pulse
- During treadmill training, review how this exercise prescription can be applied to his stair stepper at home

♦ Body mechanics and postural stabilization
  ● Use of exercise ball for basic core stabilization routine
    ▪ Sitting upright with alternate leg raise
    ▪ Sitting upright with alternate arm and leg raise
    ▪ Lateral trunk flexion and rotation
    ▪ Abdominal and back extensor strengthening
  ● Normalization of interaction of core muscles for posture and respiration
  ● Review of back safety while on assembly line at work

♦ Flexibility exercises
  ● Exercises to increase the range of motion of the chest using sustained holds
    ▪ Extension, lateral flexion, and rotation

♦ Relaxation
  ● Use of relaxation techniques (eg, Jacobson's, Yoga techniques) to reduce use of accessory muscles of respiration

♦ Strength, power, and endurance training
  ● Upper and lower extremity and core strength training programs will be begun in the Outpatient Adult Cystic Fibrosis Clinic and all will be coordinated with breathing
    ▪ Upper extremity strengthening may use free weights or elastic bands and may incorporate overhead lifts, upright rows, shoulder shrugs, shoulder flexion, shoulder abduction, shoulder extension, elbow flexion and extension, and wrist flexion and extension
    ▪ Core strengthening of abdominals and back extensors may use active exercises, exercises on the ball, Yoga, Pilates, or any other trunk strengthening activities that John prefers
    ▪ Lower extremity strengthening may include wall slides, squats, rise up on toes, raise toes up, lower extremity leg weights or elastic bands for hip flexion, extension, abduction, adduction, and knee flexion and extension

FUNCTIONAL TRAINING IN SELF-CARE AND HOME MANAGEMENT

♦ Self-care and home management
  ● Coordination of inhaled medications (ie, Albuteral and Pulmozyme [dornase alpha]) with different methods of airway clearance will be incorporated into his daily self-care schedule to manage time more efficiently
  ● Instruction in energy conservation techniques during self-care will be provided (eg, use Terry cloth robe after showering)
  ● Incorporation of postural alignment during all ADL
  ● Instruction in incorporation of breathing exercises while performing self-care and home management actions, tasks, and activities

FUNCTIONAL TRAINING IN WORK, COMMUNITY, AND LEISURE INTEGRATION OR REINTEGRATION

♦ Work
  ● Resume three 12-hour shift work as soon as feasible
  ● Develop a schedule of exercises on nonworkdays to facilitate adherence
  ● Incorporation of postural alignment during all IADL
  ● Review incorporation of breathing exercises during workday (eg, stretch break raising arms up overhead coordinated with breathing)

♦ Community and leisure
  ● Resume bowling and instruct in how to coordinate with breathing
  ● Add activity of walking with wife in the evenings for additional aerobic conditioning

MANUAL MUSCLE TESTING

♦ Soft tissue mobilization techniques for trunk
♦ Mobilization of the rib cage and thoracic spine to increase chest mobility

PRESCRIPTION, APPLICATION, AND AS APPROPRIATE, FABRICATION OF DEVICES AND EQUIPMENT

♦ Assistive devices
  ● Positive airway pressure (PEP) device: Acapella™
    ▪ To promote collateral ventilation by creating a backpressure into the airways and lungs during exhalation, allowing air pressure to build distal to the secretions and forcing the secretions into the upper airways for expectoration
    ▪ This PEP device can also prevent atelectasis and airway collapse and improve oxygenation and exercise tolerance
  ● The Vest (HFCC)
    ▪ Use of this device will be discussed with John as a means of chest percussion and vibration to relieve his wife of the responsibility

© SLACK Incorporated 2007. Moffat M, Frownfelter D. *Cardiovascular/Pulmonary Essentials: Applying the Preferred Physical Therapist Practice Patterns.*SM

AIRWAY CLEARANCE TECHNIQUES

- ◆ Breathing strategies performed daily
  - Active cycle of breathing technique
    - Patient is sitting or lying down in relaxed comfortable position
    - He is then instructed with verbal and manual cues in initial breathing control (3 to 5 normal or tidal breaths), then he performs 3 to 4 thoracic expansions (3 to 5 deeper breaths with emphasis on thoracic expansion and therapist may use hands as tactile cue), then breathing control, followed by three to four thoracic expansions, then breathing control
    - This is repeated for multiple cycles until patient senses a need to clear secretions
    - Huff cough or FET is then performed
    - If patient does not sense a cough or has been nonproductive, a huff cough of FET can be performed at timed intervals of 5 minutes given ideal session is at least 15 minutes
  - Assisted cough techniques (eg, huffing technique, use of trunk flexion to facilitate cough)
  - Paced breathing
    - Timing breaths to conserve energy and accomplish desired tasks if increased dyspnea noted
    - Aim for ratio of inspiration to expiration of 1:2 (progress to 2:4, 3:6)
  - Repeated maximum inspirations against a fixed resistance
  - Stacked breathing
    - The patient takes two to four inspirations for each expiration to maximize inspiratory and expiratory volume
- ◆ Manual/mechanical techniques
  - Chest percussion, shaking, and vibration in combination with pulmonary postural drainage
  - Acapella™ device
    - Performed in comfortable sitting position or postural drainage position
    - Patient will exhale three to four times longer than inspiration (an inspiratory to expiratory ratio of 1:3 or 1:4)
    - Patient will perform 5 normal or tidal volume breaths alternating with 5 deeper breaths (diaphragmatic breathing instruction will precede this instruction)
    - Every 5 minutes, patient will initiate huff cough if coughing not stimulated through technique
    - May be performed concurrently with inhaled medications like bronchodilators or mucolytic agents, such as pulmozyme.

- ◆ Positioning
  - Positioning to alter work of breathing
    - Sitting to semi-fowler's positions provide best mechanical advantage to reduce work of breathing
    - Work of breathing is increased in supine position
  - Positioning to maximize ventilation and perfusion
  - Pulmonary postural drainage with emphasis on areas of retained secretions and decreased aeration

ANTICIPATED GOALS AND EXPECTED OUTCOMES

- ◆ Impact on pathology/pathophysiology
  - Hemoptysis is resolved.
  - Patient able to maintain pulse oximetry at 95% at rest and with activity.
  - Physiological responses to increased oxygen demand are improved.
  - Pre-illness level of sputum production is achieved.
  - Pre-illness lung sounds are achieved.
  - Pulmonary function tests are improved by no less than 5% predicted.
  - Supplemental oxygen no longer required.
- ◆ Impact on impairments
  - He is able to walk 10 minutes without fatigue prior to discharge.
  - Patient will understand and be able to demonstrate alternative modes of airway clearance, especially with the use of the Acapella™ device and the active cycle of breathing technique.
  - Posture is improved through improved self-awareness.
  - Preillness level of exercise tolerance is achieved.
  - Thoracic spine range of motion and chest mobility are improved.
  - Upper extremity, lower extremity, and core muscle strength have increased minimally in hospital phase.
- ◆ Impact on functional limitations
  - Ability to perform physical actions, tasks, or activities related to work, community, and leisure is improved.
  - Able to resume share of household activities (ie, vacuuming and grocery shopping).
  - Able to return to work for three 12-hour shifts.
- ◆ Risk reduction/prevention
  - Able to identify possible triggers for hemoptysis.
  - Patient is aware of potential signs and symptoms of pulmonary problems (eg, infection).
- ◆ Impact on health, wellness, and fitness
  - Patient has become more proactive in minimizing chance of reoccurrence of hemoptysis and pulmonary exacerbation.
  - Physical fitness is improved.

- Physical function is improved through use of usual and alternate methods for physical activity and airway clearance.
- ♦ Impact on societal resources
  - Documentation occurs throughout the client management and follows APTA's *Guidelines for Physical Therapy Documentation.*
- ♦ Patient/client satisfaction
  - John and his wife are active participants in the development of his inpatient and home program for airway clearance and physical activity.
  - Any concerns will be reviewed at follow-up during the outpatient clinic visits.

REEXAMINATION

Reexamination is performed throughout the episode of care. It will occur for any change in medical status, including new onset of hemoptysis or at 7 days to review progress and reassess present plan and specific interventions.

DISCHARGE

John is discharged from physical therapy after a total of 10 inpatient physical therapy sessions and attainment of his goals and expectations. These sessions have covered his entire episode of care in the hospital. He is discharged because he has achieved his goals and expected outcomes. Since patients with CF require life-long management, he will return to the Outpatient Adult Cystic Fibrosis Clinic for additional physical therapy consultation as part of his follow-up visit in 2 weeks.

Case Study #3: Bronchitis and Emphysema

Mr. Sylvester Mueller is a retired 67-year-old male admitted to the hospital with an acute exacerbation of chronic bronchitis, emphysema, and Organic Dust Toxic Syndrome (ODTS).

PHYSICAL THERAPIST EXAMINATION

HISTORY

- ♦ General demographics: Mr. Mueller is a 67-year-old English speaking white male with a high school education. He is right hand dominant.
- ♦ Social history: He has been married for 44 years, has 4 grown children (43-year-old son, 42-year-old daughter, 39-year-old daughter, and 30-year-old son), and 12 grandchildren.

- ♦ Employment/work: He has lived and worked on a grain farm for his entire life. Mr. Mueller retired from farming 2 years ago but continues to assist his oldest son around the farm.
- ♦ Living environment: Mr. Mueller and his wife live in a two-story home on the family farm where he grew up. There are 2 steps to enter the house with a handrail and one flight of stairs to the second floor with a handrail.
- ♦ General health status
  - Perception: He feels he is in fairly good health.
  - Physical function: He reports that his function is "good," except he has noted in the past few years increased difficulty and shortness of breath (SOB) going up and down stairs and increasing fatigue throughout the day.
  - Psychological function: Normal.
  - Role function: Farmer, husband, father, and grandfather.
  - Social function: He reports being active in the community and in local farming and agriculture youth groups.
- ♦ Social/health habits: He has been smoking since the age of 14, approximately 1 to 2 packs/day (53 to 106 pack years), and he is still smoking. He is a social drinker. He has limited water consumption throughout the day.
- ♦ Family history: His father died in a farming accident at 43 years of age, and his mother died of a stroke at 82 years of age. He is the oldest of 3 children (1 brother and 1 sister). He took over management and running of the family farm after the death of his father, and his own discharge from the service at 22 years of age.
- ♦ Medical/surgical history: Mr. Mueller was treated in and released from the emergency department (ED) three times in the past year due to difficulty breathing and unproductive cough and congestion.
- ♦ Preexisting medical and other health-related conditions: He has had a diagnosis of chronic obstructive pulmonary disease and possible ODTS.
- ♦ Current condition(s)/chief complaint(s): He was recently admitted to the hospital due to an acute exacerbation of COPD. It was speculated that he has ODTS that has progressed to Farmer's Hypersensitivity Pneumonitis (FHP), formerly known as Farmer's Lung Disease.[109,110] He wants to increase his ambulation distance and ability to assist with farm work without SOB and general fatigue.
- ♦ Functional status and activity level: He reports that he is independent with all ADL with noted increased difficulty going up a flight of stairs and walking around the barnyard (300 to 500 feet depending upon the day). He occasionally stops due to SOB.

◆ Medications: He reports no regular medications but prior to admission had finished a 2-week dose of antibiotics received during his recent ED visit.

◆ Other clinical tests: At time of admission
  ● Arterial blood gases (ABGs)[109,111]
    ▪ pH=7.32 (normal=7.35 to 7.45)
    ▪ PaO_2=75 mm Hg (normal=80 to 100 mm Hg)
    ▪ $PaCO_2$=47 mm Hg (normal=35 to 45 mm Hg)
    ▪ HCO_3-=28 mEq/L (normal=22 to 26 mEq/L)
    ▪ BE/BD (base excess/base deficit)=+2 mEq/L (normal=-2 to +2)
    ▪ SaO_2=88% (normal=95% to 100%)
    ▪ Interpreted as chronic respiratory acidosis.[112]
  ● Chest x-ray: Revealed consolidation in bilateral lower lobes (BLL) and right middle lobe (RML) and hyperinflation with depressed diaphragm
  ● Pulmonary function tests (PFTs)[3,12]
    ▪ Predicted vital capacity (VC)=[0.052 x height (cm)] – [0.022 x age (years)] – 3.60
      ▸ Mr. Mueller's predicted VC was (0.052 x 177.8 cm) – (0.022 x 67) – 3.60=4.1716 L
    ▪ 60% of predicted VC=2.50 L
    ▪ Actual forced VC=2.18 L
    ▪ FEV_1=1.02 L
    ▪ FEV_1/FVC=47%

SYSTEMS REVIEW

◆ Cardiovascular/pulmonary
  ● BP: 136/84 mmHg
  ● Edema: None noted
  ● HR: 93 bpm
  ● RR: 27 bpm
◆ Integumentary
  ● Presence of scar formation: None
  ● Skin color: Normal, appropriate blanch to touch and capillary refill
  ● Skin integrity: Intact
◆ Musculoskeletal
  ● Gross range of motion: WNL
  ● Gross strength: WNL
  ● Gross symmetry: Symmetrical
  ● Height: 5'10" (1.78 m)
  ● Weight: 180 pounds (81.65 kg)
◆ Neuromuscular
  ● Balance: Intact
  ● Locomotion, transfers, and transitions: WNL
◆ Communication, affect, cognition, language, and learning style
  ● All WNL

● Mr. Mueller is a quiet but well-spoken man and reports that he learns by "doing"

TESTS AND MEASURES

◆ Aerobic capacity/endurance
  ● Rating of Perceived Exertion (RPE)[55,96]
    ▪ Report of 15 or "hard" on Original Borg RPE scale of 6-20 while walking across the barnyard prior to admission
    ▪ 17 or "very hard" while walking in hospital hallway
  ● 15-Count Breathless Score (also known as the Ventilatory Response Index [VRI]) to monitor exertion[97]
    ▪ Level 2, which indicated that he must take two breaths in 8 seconds in order to complete counting aloud to 15
◆ Anthropometric characteristics
  ● BMI=25.8, which is considered overweight (25.0 – 29.9=overweight)[22]
◆ Environmental, home, and work barriers
  ● Mr. Mueller lives in a two-story home with the bedrooms on the second floor with 14 steps to the second floor, with a handrail
  ● He is retired but continues to assist with work around the farm with exposure to grain dust and dust due to dirt roads and driveways
  ● The barns are not air conditioned and are heated by oil furnaces
◆ Muscle performance
  ● Upper and lower extremity strength enable normal function, but testing reveals:
    ▪ Lower extremity strength: 4/5
    ▪ Upper extremity strength: 4/5
    ▪ Trunk flexor strength: 3+/5
    ▪ Trunk extensor strength: 4/5
◆ Posture
  ● Spine flexed with rounded shoulders in sitting and standing
◆ Range of motion
  ● Decreased lateral chest expansion
    ▪ Upper chest: 5 mm difference between resting breath and deep breath
    ▪ Lower chest: No difference between resting breath and deep breath
  ● Increased anteroposterior diameter of his chest
◆ Self-care and home management
  ● Prior to admission, Mr. Mueller was able to complete all of his self-care and home management actions, tasks, and activities but had to stop occasionally because of some dyspnea

- He noted increased difficulty climbing stairs
- ◆ Ventilation and respiration/gas exchange
  - Auscultation
    - Bilateral upper lobes: Rhonchi noted with air entry throughout
    - Right middle lobe: Rhonchi and expiratory wheeze
    - Bilateral lower lobes: Decreased to no breath sounds and expiratory wheeze
  - Decreased oxygen saturation (SpO_2)
    - Resting SpO_2: 90% to 93%
    - After ambulation SpO_2: 88%, rising to 92% after 2- to 3-minute rest
  - Breathing pattern
    - Occasionally leans forward with elbows on knees to assist with breathing or to catch his breath
    - Increased use of accessory muscles at this time
- ◆ Work, community, and leisure integration or reintegration
  - Mr. Mueller has noted increased difficulty walking around the barnyard (300 to 500 feet depending upon the day)
  - He occasionally stops his work activities due to SOB
  - He is anxious to get back to his community activities, especially his volunteer work with the local farming and agriculture youth groups

EVALUATION

Mr. Mueller is a 67-year-old male who has been diagnosed with chronic bronchitis and emphysema. He has been exposed to grain dust for his entire working life and has a 53-year history of smoking. He has acceptable vital signs, intact skin integrity, WNL ROM, symmetrical body alignment, and no abnormal neuromuscular findings. He has decreased strength in his upper and lower extremities and in his trunk. He has abnormal posture and severely decreased lateral chest excursion with resting and deep inspiration. His PFTs are below predicted values indicating obstructive pulmonary disease. He has abnormal and adventitious breath sounds in both lungs, and dyspnea and decreased oxygen saturation levels with ambulation.

DIAGNOSIS

Mr. Mueller is a patient with chronic bronchitis, emphysema, and ODTS. He has impaired: aerobic capacity/endurance, anthropometric characteristics, muscle performance, posture, and ventilation and respiration/gas exchange. He is functionally limited in self-care and home management and in work, community, and leisure actions, tasks, and

activities. He also has environmental, home, and work barriers. The findings also place him at risk for developing acute or chronic lung infections and future hospitalizations. These findings are consistent with placing him in Pattern C: Impaired Ventilation, Respiration/Gas Exchange, and Aerobic Capacity/Endurance Associated With Airway Clearance Dysfunction. These impairments will then be addressed in determining the prognosis and the plan of intervention.

PROGNOSIS AND PLAN OF CARE

Over the course of the hospital stay, the following mutually established outcomes have been determined:

- ◆ Ability to cough and clear secretions is attained
- ◆ Aerobic capacity and endurance is improved
- ◆ Awareness of environmental triggers and risk factors causing respiratory exacerbations is achieved
- ◆ Faulty posture is corrected
- ◆ Muscle strength is increased to within functional limits during 4 weeks
- ◆ Tolerance to physical activity is increased

To achieve these outcomes, the appropriate interventions for this patient are determined. These will include: coordination, communication, and documentation, patient/client-related instruction; therapeutic exercise; functional training in self-care and home management; functional training in work, community, and leisure integration or reintegration; and airway clearance techniques.

Based on the diagnosis and prognosis, Mr. Mueller is expected to be in the hospital for 5 days, and he will be followed up in the Pulmonary Clinic monthly. Mr. Mueller has good social support, is motivated, and will follow through with his exercise and pulmonary hygiene programs.

INTERVENTIONS

RATIONALE FOR SELECTED INTERVENTIONS

Therapeutic Exercise

Even for individuals with chronic diseases, evidence supports the use of regular exercise consisting of aerobic conditioning and resistance strength training to increase functional capabilities, facilitate maintenance of independence, and improve quality of life.[113,114] Progressive exercise training and physical activity for patients with COPD improves exercise tolerance and decreases dyspnea, but also enhances functional improvements in ADL and health-related quality of life.[115]

Data indicate that strength-training programs for these patients significantly increase their strength, endurance-training programs significantly increase their submaximal exercise capacity, while using a program of both strength training and endurance training significantly increases both parameters. Significant improvements were also noted in breathlessness scores and in dyspnea with combined programs of strength and endurance training.[116]

Combined programs of endurance training and progressive resistance strength training for these patients were shown to improve their functional outcomes,[117] their muscle function, and their treadmill walking endurance.[118]

Instruction in breathing exercises will be initiated to increase alveolar ventilation in both lower lobes and to promote more efficient control of breathing. PLB and emphasis on relaxation of the accessory muscles will be included.[119] These exercises will assist in secretion clearance and improved ventilation and oxygenation. The focus will be on bilateral lateral costal breathing.

Ventilatory strategies will include prevention of breath holding with activity. Breathing will be promoted that specifically pairs trunk extension with inspiration and trunk flexion with exhalation to improve ventilation and oxygenation and reduce exertional dyspnea.

Core strengthening will be started to promote stronger abdominals and back muscles to improve the strength of the core to prevent injury with activity. Postural exercises will also be performed to help improve his flexed posture. Progressive strengthening of his upper and lower extremities will be incorporated into his program since both aerobic exercise and resistance exercise help to reduce body fat, and progressive resistance strengthening exercises also appear to increase fat-free mass.[120]

Exercise and breathing techniques will be incorporated into his program to improve his tolerance to activity and to fulfill his desire to maintain his presence in the work aspects of his family farm. PLB will be taught to assist him in self-controlling his dyspnea with activity. See Rationale for Selected Interventions in Case Studies #1 and #2 for additional therapeutic exercise rationale.

Airway Clearance Techniques

The active cycle of breathing technique will be taught to Mr. Mueller. In addition, an Acapella™ device will be issued to him for use in everyday life as needed. See Rationale for Selected Interventions in Case Studies #1 and #2 for airway clearance techniques rationale.

COORDINATION, COMMUNICATION, AND DOCUMENTATION

Coordination of care and communication will occur with Mr. Mueller in an interdisciplinary team approach. The physician, nurse, physical therapist, and respiratory therapist will all focus on risk reduction, self-management of the disease process, and prevention of further hospital admissions. The

physical therapist will focus on airway clearance techniques and exercise to improve pulmonary function. All elements of the patient's management will be documented.

PATIENT/CLIENT-RELATED INSTRUCTION

Mr. Mueller will be instructed in the pathophysiology of COPD and ODTS, disease progression, and preventative actions he can take to care for himself. He will learn about healthy eating and consumption of 8 to 10 glasses of water or water-based fluids a day (excluding coffee, tea, and soda) to prevent dehydration and increase ease of secretion mobilization. He will learn about smoking cessation, respiratory protection devices, and limiting his exposure to grain dust during harvesting and other related agricultural activities. Mr. Mueller will be taught to recognize the signs and symptoms of respiratory distress (ie, shortness of breath, fatigue, bouts of coughing). He will also be taught energy conservation or symptom-modified activities to improve his tolerance to activity.

THERAPEUTIC EXERCISE

- ◆ Aerobic capacity/endurance conditioning or reconditioning
  - Mr. Mueller will be instructed in a daily walking program, monitoring his heart rate and RPE[55,96]
  - His inpatient walking program will use the following parameters:
    - 3-minute warm up at 2.0 mph
    - Intensity increase to 2.5 mph
    - Duration of 5 minutes, progressing as possible to 20 minutes
    - 5-minute cool-down at 2.2 mph
    - Parameters
      - ‣ Heart rate no greater than 130 bpm
      - ‣ SpO_2 no less than 90%
      - ‣ RPE no less than 11 to 13 and give copy of perceived exertion scale to Mr. Mueller
    - Instruct him in procedures for taking his own pulse
- ◆ Body mechanics and postural stabilization
  - Body mechanics training
    - Appropriate sitting posture for work and leisure activities
    - Appropriate use of body mechanics while working in the barn
    - Appropriate lifting and carrying instructions
    - Appropriate bending instructions
  - Postural control training
    - Proper alignment of head, cervical and thoracic spines, shoulders, pelvis, hips, and knees
      - ‣ Axial extension

- ▸ Scapula retraction and depression
- ▸ Chicken wing position (hands behind head, horizontal abduction of shoulders)
  - ▪ Transition of position from supine to sitting, standing, and walking
  - ▪ Transition of position to functional activities during the day
- Postural stabilization activities
  - ▪ Axial extension starting in supine and progressing to sitting and upright
  - ▪ Maintenance of axial extension position with bilateral arm raises, with progression to use of weights, starting, for example, with small weights for 8 to 12 reps and increasing accordingly
  - ▪ Gluteal sets
  - ▪ Bridging, with progression to abdominal contractions, and unilateral knee extension with bridging
  - ▪ Utilize ball for core stability training
  - ▪ Unilateral upper extremity elevation and lower extremity extension in quadruped
  - ▪ Incorporate the use of the foam roller and unstable surfaces like foam rubber cushion in standing with bilateral and unilateral stance
- Postural awareness training
  - ▪ Use of mirror for visual input of appropriate alignment
  - ▪ Notes all around home
- ◆ Flexibility exercises
  - Stretching exercises should be done after warming up, using a slow and steady stretch accompanied by deep breathing, and building hold up to 15 to 30 seconds
  - Done two to three times a day, at least 2 to 3 repetitions
    - ▪ Upper extremity range of motion exercises with deep breathing to increase his chest expansion and increase his shoulder flexion
    - ▪ Lateral flexion of the trunk with upper extremity abduction to increase the lateral expansion of the chest wall
    - ▪ Trunk rotation
    - ▪ Hands clasped behind back to open up anterior chest wall
- ◆ Relaxation
  - PLB to prevent air trapping in the lungs and enhance relaxation
  - Relaxation of accessory muscles of respiration (eg, biofeedback, visual imagery, Jacobsen's techniques)
  - Rapid breathing techniques with body relaxation to control bouts of dyspnea

- Slow paced breathing patterns during periods of rest
- ◆ Strength, power, and endurance training
  - During all strength training, vital signs should be monitored and perceived exertion determined using the Borg scale
  - Appropriate breathing techniques will be used to avoid any Valsalva maneuver
  - Hand-held weights or elastic band exercises for strengthening of upper and lower extremities beginning with low weights or resistance and progressing in accordance with his capabilities
  - Breathing exercises to increase the strength of the diaphragm (eg, ventilatory muscle training devices)

FUNCTIONAL TRAINING IN WORK, COMMUNITY, AND LEISURE INTEGRATION OR REINTEGRATION

- ◆ Mr. Mueller will be instructed in energy conservation techniques to use while he is working on the farm (eg, using wheeled cart instead of carrying farm objects)
- ◆ He will be instructed in injury prevention or reduction during work activities
  - Limit his exposure to grain dust during harvesting and other related agricultural activities
  - Use a respiratory protection mask device during that season
  - Drive in enclosed cab farm equipment with air-filtering systems

MANUAL TECHNIQUES

- ◆ Soft tissue mobilization
- ◆ Mobilization of the thoracic spine and rib cage

AIRWAY CLEARANCE TECHNIQUES

- ◆ Breathing strategies
  - Mr. Mueller will be instructed in assisted coughing/huff technique for a more productive and energy efficient cough
  - He will be instructed in ACBT to facilitate airway clearance
  - Mr. Mueller will be instructed in paced breathing that he can perform during more challenging and exhausting activities
  - Mr. Mueller will be instructed in PLB to prevent air trapping in the lungs/improve expiration and decrease respiratory distress
- ◆ Manual/mechanical techniques
  - Mr. Muller will be issued an Acapella™ PEP device to assist with secretion mobilization

♦ Positioning
  • Mr. Mueller will be instructed in positioning himself in a forward flexed position with his arms resting on his knees or a table to reduce the work of breathing and to enable him to control his respiratory rate during bouts of dyspnea

ANTICIPATED GOALS AND EXPECTED OUTCOMES

♦ Impact on pathology/pathophysiology (disease, disorder or condition)
  • His water based fluid intake (excluding beverages with caffeine like coffee, tea, and soda) is increased to 8 to 10 glasses/day.
  • Lungs are clear to auscultation due to his ability to effectively perform a productive cough.
  • Tissue perfusion and oxygenation shown with SpO_2 > 90 % are improved.

♦ Impact on impairments
  • Ambulation distance is increased as a result of increased tissue perfusion and oxygenation due to clear lungs.
  • Secretions are cleared with the ACBT and the huff technique.

♦ Impact on functional limitations
  • Agricultural chores are performed with the use of a respiratory protective device and/or enclosed cab farm equipment with air-filtering systems.
  • Respiratory rate and breathing are controlled with symptom-modified activity.
  • Walking is increased to 20 minutes without a rest break and with a RPE of 13 or "somewhat hard" on the original Borg scale within 6 weeks.

♦ Risk reduction/prevention
  • Ability to perform more tasks around the farm without signs/symptoms of respiratory distress is achieved.
  • Physical activity level is increased.
  • Self-management of his disease and reduction of his risk of respiratory (COPD and ODTS) exacerbations are realized by being aware of environmental triggers that he may encounter daily on the farm.

♦ Impact on health, wellness, and fitness
  • A walk program is begun upon discharge three to five times a week outside of farm-related activities.

♦ Impact on societal resources
  • By encouraging him to have active participation in his airway clearance and breathing exercises, secretions are self-mobilized and respiratory exacerbations and hospital readmissions are decreased.

• Future exacerbations that could result in returning to the doctor or hospital for care are prevented through awareness of his environmental triggers.

♦ Patient/client satisfaction
  • Awareness is achieved by Mr. Mueller and his family of environmental triggers that occur during harvesting and other daily chores around the farm.
  • Awareness of when he has the ability to continue with an activity or when he should rest is achieved.
  • Control of his disease process is achieved through self-management of his congestion and secretion mobilization with the ACBT and PEP devices.
  • Self-management of his activity level is increased.

REEXAMINATION

Reexamination occurred throughout the patient care interaction with goals and outcomes being updated and adjusted as needed.

DISCHARGE

Mr. Mueller is discharged from inpatient physical therapy after 5 treatments in 3 days. His acute exacerbation of COPD is resolving, he is independent with his breathing exercises, and he has a productive huff coughing technique. He will be followed up with pulmonary rehabilitation to continue improving his aerobic capacity, strength, and awareness of environmental triggers. He has agreed to stop smoking but fears returning to the habit as many of the family and others who work on the farm still smoke. He has an appointment with an outpatient counselor to assist him with this goal.

REFERENCES

1. Frownfelter D, Dean E. *Cardiovascular and Pulmonary Physical Therapy: Evidence and Practice.* 4th ed. St. Louis, Mo: Mosby/Elsevier, 2006.
2. Houtmeyers E, Gosselink R, et al. Regulation of mucociliary clearance in health and disease. *Eur Respir J.* 1999;13(5):1177-1188.
3. Dean E. Preferred practice patterns in cardiopulmonary physical therapy: A guide to physiological measures. *Cardiopulm Phys Ther J.* 1999;10(4):124-134.
4. Gosselink R, Troosters R, Decramer M: Distribution of muscle weakness in patients with stable chronic obstructive pulmonary disease. *J Cardiopulm Rehab.* 2000:20:353-360.
5. Weiss ST. Risk factors for COPD. Available at: www.uptodate.com. Accessed April 2005.
6. Hess DR. The evidence for secretion clearance technique. *Respir Care.* 2001;46(11):1276-1292.
7. Shah PL. Update on clinical trials in the treatment of pulmonary disease in patients in with cystic fibrosis. *Expir Opin Investig Drugs.* 1999;8(11):1917-1927.

8. Widerman E, Millner L, Sexauer W, et al. Health status and sociodemographic characteristics of adults receiving a cystic fibrosis diagnosis after age 18 years. *Chest*. 2000;118:427-433.

9. Puchelle E, Bajolet O, Abely M. Airway mucus in cystic fibrosis. *Paediatr Respir Rev*. 2002;3:115-119.

10. Chmiel JF, Davis PB. State of the art: why do the lungs with cystic fibrosis become infected and why can't they clear the infection? *Respir Res*. 2003:4:8.

11. Stoller JK. Overview of management of acute exacerbations of chronic obstructive pulmonary disease. Available at: www.uptodate.com. Accessed April 2005.

12. Hillegass EA, Sadowsky HS. *Essentials of Cardiopulmonary Physical Therapy*. 2nd Ed. Philadelphia, Pa: WB Saunders; 2001.

13. Ciccone C. Respiratory drugs. In: Ciccone CD. *Pharmacology in Rehabilitation*. 2nd Ed. Philadelphia, Pa: FA Davis; 1996.

14. King M, Dasgupta B, Tomkiewicz, et al. Rheology of cystic fibrosis sputum after in vitro treatment with hypertonic saline alone and in combination with recombinant human dexyribonuclease I. *Am J Respir Crit Care Med*. 1997;156(1): 173-177.

15. Isada C. Antimicrobial therapy for exacerbations of COPD. Available at: www.uptodate.com. Accessed April 2005.

16. Levy J. Antibiotic activity in sputum. *J Pediatr*.1986;108:841–846.

17. Döring G, Conway SP, Heijerman HGM, et al., for the Consensus Committee. Antibiotic therapy against Pseudomonas aeruginosa in cystic fibrosis: a European consensus. *Eur Respir J*. 2000;16:749–67.

18. Brasfield D, Hicks G, Soong S, Tiller RE. The chest roentgenogram in cystic fibrosis: a new scoring system. *Pediat*. 1979;63(1):24-29.

19. Roush J, Guy J, Purivs M. Reference values and relationship of the six minute walk test and body mass index in healthy third grade school children. *Internet J Allied Health Sci Pract*. 2006;4(3):1-6.

20. Moser C, Tirakitsoontorn R, Nussbaum E, et al. Muscle size and cardiorespiratory response to exercise in cystic fibrosis. *Am J Respir Crit Care Med*. 2000;162:1823-1827.

21. Nixon P, Joswiak M, Fricker F. A six-minute walk test for assessing exercise tolerance in severely ill children. *J Pediatrics*. 1996;129(3):362-366.

22. USDA Center for Nutrition Policy and Promotion. Body mass index and health. *Nutr Insight*. 2000;March.

23. Donado JR, Hill NS. Outpatient management. *Resp Care Clin N Am*. 1998;4:391-423.

24. Lands LC, Heigenhauser GJ, Jones NL. Analysis of factors limiting maximal exercise performance in cystic fibrosis. *Clin Sci*. 1992;83:391–397.

25. Godfrey S, Mearns M. Pulmonary function and response to exercise in cystic fibrosis. *Arch Dis Child*. 1971;46:144–151.

26. Cerny FJ, Pullano TP, Cropp, GJ. Cardiorespiratory adaptations to exercise in cystic fibrosis. *Am Rev Respir Dis*. 1982; 126:217–220.

27. Marcotte JE, Grisdale, RK, Levison H, et al. Multiple factors limit exercise apacity in cystic fibrosis. *Pediatr Pulmonol*. 1986; 2:274–281.

28. Coates AL, Boyce P, Muller D, et al. The role of nutritional status, airway obstruction, hypoxia, and abnormalities in serum lipid composition in limiting exercise tolerance in children with cystic fibrosis. *Acta Pediatr Scand*. 1980;69:353–358.

29. Strauss GD, Osher A, Wang CI, et al. Variable weight training in cystic fibrosis. *Chest*. 1987;92:273–276.

30. Orenstein DM, Franklin BA, Doershuk, et al. CF Exercise conditioning and cardiopulmonary fitness in cystic fibrosis. The effects of a three-month supervised running program. *Chest*. 1981;80:392–398.

31. Salh W, Bilton D, Dodd M, et al. Effect of exercise and physiotherapy in aiding sputum expectoration in adults with cystic fibrosis. *Thorax*. 1989;44:1006–1008.

32. de Jong W, Grevink RG, Roorda RJ, et al. Effect of a home exercise training program in patients with cystic fibrosis. *Chest*. 1994;105:463–468.

33. O'Neill PA, Dodds M, Phillips B, et al. Regular exercise and reduction of breathlessness in patients with cystic fibrosis. *Br J Dis Chest*. 1987;81:62–69.

34. McIlwaine MP, Davidson AG. Airway clearance techniques in the treatment of cystic fibrosis. *Curr Opin Pulm Med*. 1996; 2:447–451.

35. Oldenburg, FA, Dolovich, MB, Montgomery, JM, et al. Effects of postural drainage, exercise and cough on mucus clearance in chronic bronchitis. *Am Rev Respir Dis*. 1979;120,739-745.

36. Baldwin DR, Hill AL, Peckham DG, et al. Effect of addition of exercise to chest physiotherapy on sputum expectoration and lung function in adults with cystic fibrosis. *Respir Med*. 1994;88(1):49–53.

37. Bilton D, Dodd ME, Abbot JV, et al. The benefits of exercise combined with physiotherapy in the treatment of adults with cystic fibrosis. *Respir Med*. 1992;86(6):507-511.

38. Bloomquist M, Freyschuss U, Wiman LG, et al. Physical activity and self treatment in cystic fibrosis. *Arch Dis Child*. 1986;61:362–367.

39. Andreasson B, Jonson B, Kornfalt R, et al. Long-term effects of physical exercise on working capacity and pulmonary function in cystic fibrosis. *Acta Pediatr Scand*. 1987;76:70–75.

40. Heijerman HG, Bakker W, Sterk PJ, et al. Long-term effects of exercise training and hyperalimentation in adult cystic fibrosis patients with severe pulmonary dysfunction. *Int J Rehabil Res*. 1992;15:252–257.

41. Edlund LD, French RW, Herbst JJ, et al. Effects of a swimming program on children with cystic fibrosis. *Am J Dis Child*. 1986;140:80–83.

42. Gulmans VA, de Meer K, Brackel HJ, et al. Outpatient exercise training in children with cystic fibrosis: physiological effects, perceived competence, and acceptability. *Pediatr Pulmonol*. 1999;28:39–46.

43. Cassaburi R, Patessio A, Iolli F, et al. Reductions in exercise lactic acidosis and ventilation as a result of exercise training in patients with obstructive lung disease. *Am Rev Respir Dis*. 1991;143:9–18.

44. Selvadurai HC, Blimkie CJ, Meyers N, et al. Randomized controlled study of in-hospital exercise training programs in children with cystic fibrosis. *Pediatr Pulmonol*. 2002;33(3):194-200.

45. Swisher AK, Baer L, Moffett K, Yeater R. Influence of lean body mass and leg muscle strength on 6-Minute Walk test performance in children with cystic fibrosis. *Cardiopulm Phys Ther J*. 2005;16(3):5-9.

46. Swisher AK. Not just a lung disease: peripheral muscle abnormalities in cystic fibrosis and the role of exercise to address them. *Cardiopulm J*. 2006;17:9-14.

47. Schneiderman-Walker J, Pollock SL, Corey M, et al. A randomised controlled trial of a 3-year home exercise program in cystic fibrosis. *J Pediatr.* 2000;136:304–310.

48. Moorcroft AJ, Dodd ME, Morris J, et al. Individualised unsupervised exercise training in adults with cystic fibrosis: a 1 year randomized controlled trial. *Thorax.* 2004;59:1074-1080.

49. Mahadeva R, Webb K, Westerbeek RC, et al. Clinical outcome in relation to care in centres specialising in cystic fibrosis: cross-sectional study. *BMJ.* 1998;316:1771–1775.

50. Kerem E, Reisman J, Corey M, et al. Prediction of mortality in patients with cystic fibrosis. *NEJM.* 1992;326:1187–1191.

51. Breslin EH. The pattern of respiratory muscle recruitment during pursed-lips breathing in COPD. *Chest.* 1992;101:75–78.

52. Spahija J, de Marchie M, Grassino A. Effects of imposed pursed lips breathing on respiratory mechanics and dyspnea at rest and during exercise in COPD. *Chest.* 2005:128:640-650.

53. Dechman G, Wilson CR. Evidence underlying breathing retraining in people with obstructive pulmonary disease. *Phys Ther.* 2004;84(12):1189-1197.

54. Gigliotti F, Romagnoli I, Scano G. Breathing retraining and exercise conditioning in patients with chronic obstructive pulmonary disease: a physiological approach. *Respir Med.* 2003:97:197-204.

55. Scherer S, Cassady SL. Rating of perceived exertion: development and clinical applications for physical therapy exercise testing and prescription. *Cardiopulm Phys Ther J.* 1999; 10(4):143-147.

56. Cole P. Pathophysiology and treatment of airway mucociliary clearance. A moving tale. *Minerv Anestesiol.* 2001;67(4):206-209.

57. Main E, Prasad A, Schans C. Conventional chest physiotherapy compared to other airway clearance techniques for cystic fibrosis. *Cochrane Database Syst Rev.* 2005:25:CD002011. Review.

58. Butler SG, Sutherland RJ: Current airway clearance techniques. *NZ Med J.* 1998:111:183-86. Review.

59. McIlwaine, PM, Wong, LT, Peacock, D, et al. Long-term comparative trial of positive expiratory pressure versus oscillating positive expiratory pressure (flutter) physiotherapy in the treatment of cystic fibrosis. *J Pediatr.* 2001;138,845-850.

60. Prasad SA, Main E. Finding evidence to support airway clearance techniques in cystic fibrosis. *Disabil Rehabil.* 1998; 20:235–246

61. Prasad SA, Tannenbaum E, Mikelson C. Physiotherapy in cystic fibrosis. *J R Soc Med.* 2000;Suppl 38: 27-36.

62. Mavrocordatos P, Bissonnette B, Ravussin P. Effects of neck position and head elevation on intracranial pressure in anaesthetized neurosurgical patients: preliminary results. *J Neurosurg Anesth.* 2000;12:10-14.

63. Imle PC, Mars MP, Ciesla ND, et al. The effect of chest physical therapy on intracranial pressure and cerebral perfusion pressure. *Physiother Can.* 1997;49(1):48-55.

64. Fornataro-Clerici L, Roop TA. *Clinical Management of Adults Requiring Tracheostomy Tubes and Ventilators, A Reference Guide for Healthcare Practitioners.* Gaylord, Mich: Northern Speech Services; 1997.

65. Button BM Heine RG Catto-Smith AG et al. Postural drainage in cystic fibrosis: Is there a link with gastro-oesophageal reflux. *J Paediatr Child Health.* 1998;34:330-334.

66. Button BM, Heine RG, Catto-Smith AG, et al. Chest physiotherapy in infants with cystic fibrosis: to tip or not? A five-year study. *Pediatr Pulmonol.* 2003;35(3):208-213.

67. Pryor JA, Webber BA, Hodson ME, et al. Evaluation of the forced expiration technique as an adjunct to postural drainage in treatment of cystic fibrosis. *BMJ.* 1979;2:417-418.

68. Wilson GE, Baldwin AL, Walshaw MJ. A comparison of traditional chest physiotherapy with the active cycle of breathing in patients with chronic suppurative lung disease. *Eur Respir J.* 1995;8(Suppl 19):171S.

69. Webber BA, Hofmeyr JL, Morgan MDL, et al. Effects of postural drainage, incorporating the forced expiration technique, on pulmonary function in cystic fibrosis. *Brit J Dis Chest.* 1986;80;353-359.

70. Pryor JA, Webber BA, Hodson ME. Effect of chest physiotherapy on oxygen saturation in patients with cystic fibrosis. *Thorax.* 1990;45:77.

71. Menkes HA, Traystman RJ. Collateral ventilation. *Am Rev Respir Dis.* 1977;116:287-309.

72. Orlik T, Sands D. Long-term evaluation of effectiveness for selected chest physiotherapy methods used in the treatment of cystic fibrosis. *Med Wieku Rozwoj.* 2001;5(3):245-257.

73. Phillips GE, Pike SE, Jaffe A, et al. Comparison of active cycle of breathing and high-frequency oscillation jacket in children with cystic fibrosis. *Pediatr Pulmonol.* 2004;37(1):71-75.

74. Cecins NM, Jenkins SC, Pengelley J, et al. The active cycle of breathing techniques—to tip or not to tip? *Respir Med.* 1999;93:660-665.

75. Pryor JA, Parker RA, Webber BA. A comparison of mechanical and manual percussion as adjuncts to postural drainage in the treatment of cystic fibrosis in adolescents and adults. *Physiother.* 1981;67:140-141.

76. Hofmeyr JL, Webber BA, Hodson ME. Evaluation of positive expiratory pressure as an adjunct to chest physiotherapy in the treatment of cystic fibrosis. *Thorax.* 1986;41:951-954.

77. Pryor JA, Webber BA, Hodson ME, et al. The flutter VRP1 as an adjunct to chest physiotherapy in cystic fibrosis. *Respir Med.* 1994;88:677-681.

78. Pike SE, Machin AC, Dix KJ, et al. Comparison of flutter VRP1 and forced expirations (FE) with active cycle of breathing techniques (ACBT) in subjects with cystic fibrosis. *Netherlands J Med.* 1999;54(Suppl):S55.

79. van der Schans CP, Piers DA, Beekhuis H, et al. Effect of forced expirations on mucus clearance in patients with chronic airflow obstruction: effect of lung recoil pressure. *Thorax.* 1990;45:623-527.

80. Hasani A, Pavia D, Agnew JE, et al. Regional mucus transport following unproductive cough and forced expiration technique in patients with airways obstruction. *Chest.* 1994; 105:1420-1425.

81. Bellone A, Lascioli R, Raschi S, et al. Chest physical therapy in patients with acute exacerbation of chronic bronchitis: effectiveness of three methods. *Arch Phys Med Rehabil.* 2000;81:558-560,566.

82. Kim WD. Lung mucous: a clinician's view. *Eur Respir J.* 1997; 10(8):1914-1917.

83. Moreo K, Flume PK. New Directions in the Management of Cystic Fibrosis Disease. PRIME. 2003.

84. Giles DR, Wagener JS, Accurso FJ, et al. Short-term effects of postural drainage with clapping vs autogenic drainage on

oxygen saturation and sputum recovery in patients with cystic fibrosis. *Chest.* 1995;108:952-954.

85. Miller S, Hall DO, Clayton CB, et al. Chest physiotherapy in cystic fibrosis: a comparative study of autogenic drainage and the active cycle of breathing techniques with postural drainage. *Thorax.* 1995;50:165-169.

86. Savci S, Ince DI, Arikan H. A comparison of autogenic drainage and the active cycle of breathing techniques in patients with chronic obstructive pulmonary diseases. *J Cardiopuin Rehabil.* 2000; 20: 37-43.

87. Darbee JC, Ohtake PJ, Grant B, et al. Physiological evidence for the efficacy of positive expiratory pressure as an airway clearance technique in patients with cystic fibrosis. *Phys Ther.* 2004;84(6):524–537.

88. Elkins MR, Jones A, van der Schans C. Positive expiratory pressure physiotherapy for airway clearance in people with cystic fibrosis. Available at: http://www.cochrane.org/reviews/en/ab003147.html. Accessed February 13, 2007.

89. Gondor M, Nixon PA, Rebovich PJ, et al. A comparison of the flutter device and chest physical therapy in the treatment of cystic fibrosis pulmonary exacerbation [abstract]. *Pediatr Pulmonol.* 1996;22(suppl 13):307.

90. Padman R, Geouque DM, Engelhardt MT. Effects of the flutter device on pulmonary function studies among pediatric cystic fibrosis patients. *Del Med J.* 1999:71:13-18.

91. Thompson CS, Ashley J, Smith DL. Randomised crossover study of the flutter device and the active cycle of breathing technique in non-cystic fibrosis bronchiectasis. *Thorax.* 2002;57:446-448.

92. Volsko TA, DiFiore JM, Chatburn RL: Performance comparison of two oscillating positive expiratory pressure devices: Acapella versus flutter. *Respir Care.* 2003;48:124-130.

93. Mark JH, Hare KL et al. Pulmonary function and sputum production in patients with cystic fibrosis: a pilot study comparing the PercussiveTech HF device and standard chest physiotherapy. *Chest.* 2004;125(4):1507-1511.

94. Milla, CE, Hansen LG, Weber A, et al. High-frequency chest compression: effect of the third generation compression waveform. *Biomed Instrum Technol.* 2004;38(4):322-328.

95. Milla CE, Hansen LG, Warwick WJ. Different frequencies should be prescribed for different high frequency chest compression machines. *Biomed Instrum Technol.* 2006:40:319-324.

96. Borg G. *Borg's Perceived Exertion and Pain Scales.* Champaign, Ill: Human Kinetics; 1998.

97. Frownfelter D, Ryan J. Dyspnea: measurement and evaluation. *Cardiopulm Phys Ther J.* 1999;11(1):7-15.

98. Enright PL, Sherrill DL. Reference equations for the six-minute walk in healthy adults. *Am J Respir Crit Care Med.* 1998; 158(5):1384-1387.

99. Buntain HM, Greer RM, Schluter PJ, et al. Bone mineral density in Australian children, adolescents and adults with cystic fibrosis: a controlled cross sectional study. *Thorax.* 2004;59:149–155.

100. Parasa RB, Maffulli N. Musculoskeletal involvement in cystic fibrosis. *Bull Hosp Joint Dis.* 1999;58:37-44.

101. Hodges PW, Gandevia SC. Activation of the human diaphragm during a repetitive postural task. *J Physiol.* 2000;522: 165-175.

102. Hodges PW, Heijnen I, Gandevia SC. Postural activity of the diaphragm is reduced in humans when respiratory demand increases. *J Physiol.* 2001;537:999-1008.

103. Hodges PW, Gurfinkel VS, S. Brumagne, et al. Coexistence of stability and mobility in postural control; evidence from postural compensation for respiration. *Exp Brain Res.* 2002; 144:293-302.

104. Hodges P, Kaigle Holm A, Holm S, et al. Intervertebral stiffness of the spine is increased by evoked contraction of transversus abdominis and the diaphragm: in vivo porcine studies. *Spine.* 2003;28:2594-2601.

105. Massery M. Manual breathing and coughing aids. *Phys Med Rehab Clin N Amer.* 1996;7(2):407-422.

106. Abbott J, Dodd M, Bilton D, et al. Treatment compliance in adults with cystic fibrosis. *Thorax.* 1994;49:115–120.

107. Chatham K, Ionescu AA, Nixon LS, et al. A short-term comparison of two methods of sputum expectoration in cystic fibrosis. *Eur Respir J.* 2004;23:435-439

108. Orenstein D, Stern RC. *Treatment of the Hospitalized Cystic Fibrosis Patient.* New York NY: Marcel Dekke; 1998.

109. Centers for Disease Control and Prevention. Available at: http://www.cdc.gov/NASD/docs/d001001-d001100/d001027/d001027.htm Accessed January 20, 2007.

110. Kirkhorn SR. Agricultural respiratory hazards and disease, a primer for Wisconsin practitioners and health/safety professionals. Available at: www.worh.org/new_orh_docs/resre_farmershealth.asp. Accessed January 2006.

111. Comer S. *The ICU Quick Reference.* 2nd ed. Albany, NY: Delmar;1998.

112. Shapiro BA. *Clinical Application of Blood Gases.* Chicago, Ill: Year Book Medical Publishers; 1976.

113. Ellingson T, Conn VS. Exercise and quality of life in elderly individuals. *J Gerontol Nurs.* 2000;26(3):17-25.

114. Morey MC, Pieper CF, Crowley GM, et al. Exercise adherence and 10-year mortality in chronically ill older adults. *J Am Geriatr Soc.* 2002;50(12):1929-1933.

115. Hirata K, Okamoto T, Shiraishi S. The efficacy and practice of exercise training in patients with chronic obstructive pulmonary disease (COPD). *Nippon Rinsho.* 1999;57(9):2041-2045.

116. Ortega F, Toral J, Cejudo P, et al. Comparison of effects of strength and endurance training in patients with chronic obstructive pulmonary disease. *Am J Respir Crit Care Med.* 2002;166(5):669-674.

117. Panton LB, Golden J, Broeder CE, et al. The effects of resistance training on functional outcomes in patients with chronic obstructive pulmonary disease. *Eur J Appl Physiol.* 2004;91(4):443-449.

118. Clark CJ, Cochrane LM, Mackay E, et al. Skeletal muscle strength and endurance in patients with mild COPD and the effects of weight training. *Eur Respir J.* 2000;15(1):92-97.

119. Frownfelter DL. Massery M. Facilitating ventilation patterns and breathing strategies. In: Frownfelter DL, Dean E, eds. *Cardiovascular and Pulmonary Physical Therapy: Evidence and Practice:* St. Louis, Mo: Mosby Elsevier; 2006.

120. Toth MJ, Beckett T, Poehlman E. Physical activity and the progressive change in body composition with aging: current evidence and research issues. *Med Sci Sports Exerc.* 1999;31(11 Suppl):S590-596.

ADDITIONAL READINGS

American Association of Cardiovascular and Pulmonary Rehabilitation. *Guidelines for Pulmonary Rehabilitation Programs.* 2nd ed. Champaign, Ill: Human Kinetics, 1998.

Pryor JA, Webber BA. *Physiotherapy for Respiratory and Cardiac Problems.* New York, NY: Churchill and Livingstone; 1998.

Yankaskas JR, Knowles MR. *Cystic Fibrosis in Adults.* Philadelphia, Pa: Lippincott-Raven; 1999.

Impaired Aerobic Capacity/ Endurance Associated With Cardiovascular Pump Dysfunction or Failure (Pattern D)

Jane L. Wetzel, PT, PhD

ANATOMY AND PHYSIOLOGY

Pattern A details the anatomy and physiology of the healthy cardiac muscle pump. Various diseases and disorders may have an impact on the anatomy of the cardiovascular system causing a potential disruption in cardiac physiology. As mentioned in Pattern A, there may be an imbalance between the myocardial oxygen supply and demand that results in abnormal symptoms (angina, dizziness, fatigue) or abnormal physiologic measures (arrhythmias, ST-segment depression, falling or blunted BP responses during activity) (Figure 4-1).[1] The potential for imbalance between myocardial oxygen supply and demand is elevated during activity, especially for individuals with cardiovascular pathologies. This chapter begins with a discussion of pathological conditions contributing to cardiovascular pump dysfunction or failure. It introduces criteria for classifying the patient's cardiovascular pump function into failure or dysfunction by using clinical diagnostics and imaging, laboratory values, and physical examination findings at rest and during activity.

PATHOPHYSIOLOGY

HR, contractile state, and wall tension (ventricular pressure and ventricular volume) are determinants of myocardial oxygen demand.[1-3] Coronary blood flow and delivery of oxygen to the myocardium is influenced by coronary vascular resistance, collateral coronary blood flow, aortic pressure, and diastolic filling time (see Figure 4-1).[1] The appearance of cardiovascular signs and symptoms signal an imbalance between myocardial supply and demand that may be referred to as myocardial incompetence. Since oxygen extraction by the heart muscle is almost fully enhanced at rest, any increase in myocardial oxygen supply required during exercise is dependent on coronary flow.[1-2] Normally, coronary vascular resistance decreases during exercise to enhance blood flow, but the diseased coronary system may be fully dilated at rest making it more dependent on diastolic filling time and aortic pressure.[1] Small perturbations in HR and BP, as occurs with exercise, may cause individuals with cardiac pump dysfunction or failure to become symptomatic. Myocardial oxygen consumption (MVO_2) may be documented during symptomatic periods by using the HR-BP product or rate pressure product (RPP) and is represented by: $MVO_2 = HR \times BP$ (systolic).[3]

Coronary artery diseases may either occlude coronary flow, inhibiting oxygen supply to the heart, or cardiac disorders may increase the metabolic demand for oxygen to the cardiac pump. For example, conditions that cause an elevation in HR decrease the diastolic filling time and may limit myocardial oxygen supply. Similarly, cardiovascular pump disorders that limit the forward flow of blood to the systemic vasculature (aortic stenosis or HTN) may result in excessive pressure in the ventricles adding more tension to the myocardium, thereby increasing the metabolic oxygen requirement. As disease or cardiac conditions worsen, imbalance between

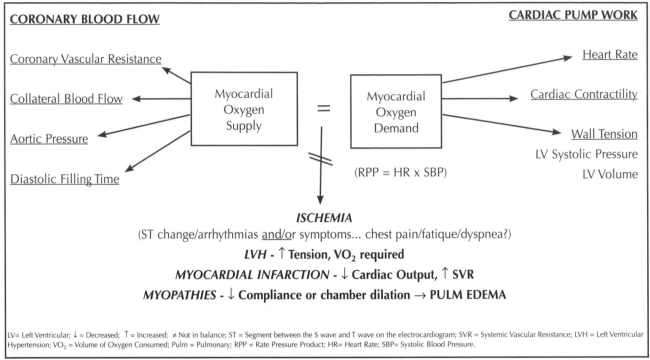

CORONARY BLOOD FLOW   **CARDIAC PUMP WORK**

Coronary Vascular Resistance — Myocardial Oxygen Supply = Myocardial Oxygen Demand — Heart Rate

Collateral Blood Flow

Aortic Pressure

Diastolic Filling Time

Cardiac Contractility

Wall Tension
LV Systolic Pressure
LV Volume

(RPP = HR x SBP)

ISCHEMIA
(ST change/arrhythmias and/or symptoms... chest pain/fatigue/dyspnea?)
LVH - ↑ Tension, VO$_2$ required
MYOCARDIAL INFARCTION **- ↓ Cardiac Output, ↑ SVR**
MYOPATHIES **- ↓ Compliance or chamber dilation → PULM EDEMA**

LV= Left Ventricular; ↓ = Decreased; ↑ = Increased; ≠ Not in balance; ST = Segment between the S wave and T wave on the electrocardiogram; SVR = Systemic Vascular Resistance; LVH = Left Ventricular Hypertension; VO$_2$ = Volume of Oxygen Consumed; Pulm = Pulmonary; RPP = Rate Pressure Product; HR= Heart Rate; SBP= Systolic Blood Pressure.

Figure 4-1. Determinants of myocardial oxygen supply and demand. Adapted from Ellestad M. *Stress Testing. Principles and Practice.* 3rd ed. Philadelphia, Pa: FA Davis; 1986:24.

myocardial oxygen supply and demand will occur at an earlier onset with lower activity states. Symptoms or abnormal physiologic measures also appear sooner, at lower activity states, and the RPP may be used to document worsening of cardiac performance. Some activities must be limited to prevent cardiac events and ensure patient/client safety.[2,4]

Cardiovascular pump dysfunction or failure occurs when there is an inability to maintain the CO required by the body to support aerobic metabolism.[4-6] An individual's aerobic capacity (VO$_{2max}$) depends on adequate myocardial contractility to support CO (SV x HR) and the ability to extract and use oxygen (a-vO$_2$ diff=arteriovenous oxygen difference) in the peripheral muscle (VO$_2$=CO x a-vO$_2$ diff).[7] According to the Social Security Administration, individuals who are unable to sustain 5 METs (1 MET=3.5 mL/kg/min) of activity are considered disabled.[8-10] Therefore, the *Guide to Physical Therapist Practice* stipulates that patients with cardiovascular pump dysfunction will have an aerobic capacity of at least 5 METs.[11] Additionally, the New York Heart Association (NYHA) classifies patients who have symptoms of excessive fatigue or dyspnea, palpitations, or angina during physical activity (5 to 6 METs)[12] as being limited by cardiac disease (NYHA Functional Class II) (Table 4-1).[13] The patient with cardiovascular pump dysfunction may benefit from therapeutic intervention or professional consultation, to improve cardiac performance for recreational, health-related, or fitness activities.[12-15]

Individuals with cardiovascular pump failure are intolerant or unsafe for many ADL, function below 5 METs, and would be classified as NYHA Functional Class III or IV.[12-14] According to the American Association of Cardiovascular and Pulmonary Rehabilitation (AACVPR), a patient with cardiac pump dysfunction who demonstrates signs and/or symptoms (including angina) at low levels of exercise (<5 METs) is high risk for complications during activity.[14] Frequent physiological monitoring and professional supervision during initial exercise training sessions is recommended.[12,14]

The patient with cardiovascular pump dysfunction or failure may have impaired aerobic capacity due to both central and peripheral impairments.[2,4] Most of the conditions contributing to cardiovascular pump dysfunction listed in Table 4-2 initially result in central impairments. Central impairments refer to the actual loss of SV and thus CO, while peripheral impairments refer to the decreased oxygen uptake or a-vO$_2$ diff in the peripheral muscle. Peripheral impairments may result from decreased blood flow to the extremities, which may be caused by a variety of possible factors, such as declining CO, increase in systemic vascular resistance (SVR), comorbidities (eg, atherosclerosis and HTN), an immune system response to disease, or as a side effect from medications (corticosteroids).[4] There may also be a loss of oxidative capacity in the peripheral muscle or deconditioning that occurs when activity is limited due to cardiovascular symptoms such as angina, palpitations, or dyspnea.[16]

Table 4-1

NEW YORK HEART ASSOCIATION FUNCTIONAL CLASSIFICATION OF HEART DISEASE

Functional Class	METs[12]	NYHA Definition[13]	Therapeutic Implication[13]
Normal/Class I	≥7	Patients with cardiac disease but without resulting limitations of physical activity. Ordinary physical activity does not cause undue fatigue, palpitations, dyspnea, or anginal pain.	Patients with cardiac disease whose physical activity need not be restricted.
Class II	5-6	Patients with cardiac disease that results in slight limitation of physical activity. Patients are comfortable at rest, but ordinary physical activity results in fatigue, palpitations, dyspnea, or anginal pain.	Patients with cardiac disease whose ordinary physical activity need not be restricted but who should be advised against severe or competitive efforts.
Class III	2-4	Patients with cardiac disease resulting in marked limitation of physical activity. Patients are comfortable at rest, but less than ordinary activity causes fatigue, palpitations, dyspnea, or anginal pain.	Patients with cardiac disease whose ordinary activities should be moderately restricted and whose more strenuous efforts should be discontinued.
Class IV	1	Patients with cardiac disease resulting in an inability to carry on any physical activity without discomfort. Fatigue, palpitations, dyspnea, or anginal pain may be present even at rest. If any physical activity is undertaken, symptoms increase.	Patients with cardiac disease whose ordinary activity should be markedly restricted or if medically unstable may need to be confined to bed or chair.

Definitions and therapeutic implications are adapted from Criteria Committee of the New York Heart Association. *Nomenclature and Criteria for Diagnosis of Diseases of the Heart and Great Vessels.* 9th ed. Boston, Mass: Little, Brown & Co; 1994:253-256. Metabolic equivalents estimation are reprinted with permission from American College of Sports Medicine. *Guidelines for Exercise Testing and Prescription.* 7th ed. Philadelphia, Pa: Lippincott Williams & Wilkins; 2006:100-101.

There are many diseases, disorders, and conditions that affect cardiac performance (see Table 4-2). Presence of these pathologic conditions may result in either an interruption of conduction of the impulse coordinating myocardial contraction (conduction blocks or arrhythmias) or impaired contractility of the ventricles [ischemia, MI, or myopathies].[2] Problems occurring in the left ventricle are the most common and typically result from poor perfusion and oxygen supply to the heart (atherosclerosis, CAD) imposing an imbalance between the myocardial oxygen supply and demand, resulting in a loss of SV and/or an onset of symptoms (angina, dyspnea, or overwhelming fatigue).[16] When a person develops significant atherosclerosis, both peripheral systemic arteries and coronary arteries have lesions that limit blood flow. Ischemia develops, resulting in a depression of the ST-segment of the ECG or causing pain in the affected tissue, claudication in the extremities, and angina in the heart (see Figure 4-1).[1,5,6,16] Prolonged ischemia in the heart

may result in decreased ventricular contractility and systolic dysfunction. Patients with autonomic nervous system dysfunction who do not feel ischemic pain may have extreme dyspnea, overwhelming fatigue, or diaphoresis as symptoms (anginal equivalents).[2,4,6,16,17]

Significant atherosclerosis in the systemic arteries may lead to HTN. The patient with HTN may acquire left ventricular hypertrophy (LVH) as a compensation to generate enough force and SV to overcome the increased afterload.[2,4,18] The heart may stiffen and lose its compliance. Diastolic dysfunction develops when the heart fails to relax completely for normal filling.[2,4,18] Additionally, the onset of HTN and/or LVH increases the myocardial oxygen demand by prolonging the isovolumic contractile period and elevating the LVEDP. Coronary flow may be inhibited as pressure rises, contributing to the onset of signs and symptoms of ischemia.[3] Early in the disease or disorder, signs and symptoms may be evident only during high exercise states, when the metabolic demands are extreme, and thus do not limit function. However, as the disease or condition worsens, signs and symptoms appear that may compromise the patient's safety and tolerance to everyday activity. Clinically, the myocardial oxygen requirement is estimated by the RPP, which is used to document the point where myocardial oxygen demand is greater than supply, causing the appearance of exercise-induced angina or producing angina equivalents.[16,19-21]

Severe imbalances between myocardial supply and demand (that result in a loss of contractility) and the ejection fraction (EF=SV/EDV) may be revealed clinically by decreases in systolic BP during activity. Chest pain may worsen with proportional changes in ST-segment depression and ischemia.[22] Ischemia may also lead to cardiac irritability and increase the risk of complex arrhythmias. A rise of the ST-segment above the isoelectric baseline on the ECG is a sign of myocardial cell injury and an impending infarction.[22,23] Chest pain will be intolerable, and the patient may lose consciousness as the event progresses to a cardiac arrest and MI or cell death. Infarction results in permanent scarring and loss of contractile function. Often, a significant Q wave may appear on the ECG indicating permanent myocardial cell death.[16,17,23] There may also be damage to the conduction system. Valve dysfunction may occur with abnormal contractility as EDV rises. This, in addition to abnormal blood flow through the ventricles, increases the risk for clot formation.

The size, type, and location of the infarction will determine the extent of myocardial tissue damage. Table 4-3 details the criteria for classification of cardiovascular pump function. A large anterior MI will impose greater myocardial compromise than a small necrotic area on the inferior wall. A transmural infarct, one that results in cell death across the myocardial wall, is more likely to develop dyskinesis or akinesis than a subendocardial infarct.[6,17,23] The greater the extent of damage, the greater the risk of a life-threatening event. If the patient survives, the myocardium may be irritable, develop arrhythmias, and have abnormal wall motion. Patients who have complications (see Table 4-3) in the first 48 hours post MI are at increased risk.[24] Recovery of injured myocardial tissue and cardiac function is influenced with good medical management and appropriate cardiac rehabilitation. Upon full recovery, if the EF falls between 35% to 40% or less, then cardiovascular pump failure is likely.[14,17,25] Risk for mortality increases.

The heart may lose contractile function either from conditions that introduce an increase in afterload (HTN, LVH, aortic stenosis) or from a loss of myocardium and systolic function (MI, stunned myocardium post cardiothoracic surgery, prolonged ischemia). Additionally, dysfunction in the heart (CHF, dilated myopathy, old MI, valve disorders, septal defects, post event sequelae) that results in inappropriate timing and sequencing between the cardiac chambers may disturb the myofibril length tension relationship[2,4] and impair contractility or cause abnormal blood flow currents

Table 4-2
PATHOLOGIC CONDITIONS CONTRIBUTING TO CARDIOVASCULAR PUMP DYSFUNCTION OR FAILURE

Disease, Disorder, or Condition

Atherosclerosis
Hypertension (HTN)
Left ventricular hypertrophy (LVH)
Coronary artery disease (CAD)
Myocardial infarction (MI)
Cardiomyopathies
- Dilated
- Hypertrophic
- Restrictive

Congestive heart failure (CHF)
- Acute or chronic
- Right, left, or biventricular
- Compensated or uncompensated

Valve disease/disorder
Conduction defect
Arrhythmia
- Malignant/complex
- Nonmalignant

Cardiothoracic surgeries/procedures
- Coronary artery bypass graft (CABG)
- Percutaneous transluminal coronary angioplasty (PTCA)
- Intracoronary stent, artherectomy
- Pacemaker insertion
- Valve repairs or replacement
- Aneurysm repair
- Cardiac transplantation
- Mechanical heart implant/support
  - Left ventricular assistive device (LVAD)
  - Right ventricular assistive device (RVAD)
  - Biventricular assistive device (BiVAD)
  - Extracorpeal membrane oxygenation (ECMO)

Postoperative or post cardiac event sequelae
- Cardiogenic shock
- Pericardial effusion
- Pericarditis
- Myocarditis
- Cardiac tamponade

Age
Renal failure
Diabetes
Pulmonary hypertension

increasing the risk of emboli and life-threatening arrhythmias. When these conditions worsen, a greater portion of the EDV will remain in the ventricle after systolic contraction causing the LVEDP to rise. The LVEDP is indirectly assessed by measurement of the pulmonary artery wedge pressure (PAWP) (see Imaging and Laboratory Tests) and is the most important indicator of left ventricle performance.[25-29]

Table 4-3

CRITERIA FOR CLASSIFICATION OF CARDIOVASCULAR PUMP FUNCTION

Condition or Disorder	Characteristics of Cardiovascular Pump Dysfunction	Characteristics of Cardiovascular Pump Failure
Hypertension[39]		**Systolic BP (mmHg)**	**Diastolic BP (mmHg)**	**For patients with HTN** Activity contraindicated if systolic is 200 mmHg or diastolic is 110 mmHg or greater. Activity should be terminated if systolic >250 mmHg and documented cardiovascular pump dysfunction or diastolic >115 mmHg[12]

Under Hypertension Dysfunction:

Pre-HTN: 120 to 139 / 80 to 89
Stage 1: 140 to 159 / 90 to 99
Stage 2: ≥160 / ≥100

Condition or Disorder	Characteristics of Cardiovascular Pump Dysfunction	Characteristics of Cardiovascular Pump Failure
MI[24]	**Uncomplicated MI** Patient does not display any of the characteristics of complicated MI in the first 48 hours post event	**Complicated MI[24] (Within first 48 hours post MI)** • V-tach or V-fib • Rapid SVT • Persistent tachycardia (>100 bpm) • 2nd (Mobitz II) or 3rd degree block • Persistent hypotension (<90 mmHg) • Pulmonary edema • Cardiogenic shock • Persistent angina or ↑ infarction • Lown grade arrhythmia ≥3[40]
MI CAD Cardiomyopathies Valve Disorder Acute CHF Postsurgical	• ↓ EF with exercise (30% to 50%)[11,38,51] • Exercise induced ischemia[12,14,38] (ST depression 1-2 mm) • Hypoadaptive BP response to increasing work on GXT[12,14] • Elevated HR for submax work • Early onset of dyspnea or extremity fatigue with activity • Aerobic capacity ≥5 METs or NYHA class I or II[11-14,38]	• ↓ EF with exercise (<30%)[11,38,51] • Exercise-induced ischemia[12,14,38] (ST depression >2 mm) • Blunted or falling BP (10 mmHg) with increasing work on GXT[12] • Severe dyspnea at rest or minimal exertion • Functional capacity <5 METs or NYHA class III or IV[11-14,38] • Poor chronotropic response • Diaphoresis, pallor, confusion[12] • Review labs: PTT for risk of bleeding, glucose levels, acidosis, electrolytes, cardiac enzymes for extension of MI[41] • Screen for lung/heart sounds and signs of acute CHF[4,44] (See below)
Arrhythmias[12,14,40]	• Frequent PVCs (6 to 10 per minute) • Presence of nonmalignant arrhythmias • Ventricular rate is controlled (<120 bpm at rest)	Activity contraindicated or ↑ risk if: • SVT or A-fib with uncontrolled ventricular rate (>120 bpm) • 2nd (Mobitz II) or 3rd degree block • Multifocal PVCs • Couplets or triplets • V-tach or V-fib • R on T

continued

Table 4-3 (continued)

CRITERIA FOR CLASSIFICATION OF CARDIOVASCULAR PUMP FUNCTION

Condition or Disorder	Characteristics of Cardiovascular Pump Dysfunction	Characteristics of Cardiovascular Pump Failure
Acute HF[4,51]	**Early signs and symptoms** • Hypoadaptive BP response to increasing work on exercise test • Elevated HR for submax work • Early onset of dyspnea or extremity fatigue with activity	All of the items listed for arrythmias *plus*: • Onset of bilateral lower lobe crackles that don't clear with cough at rest or after activity • Overnight weight gain 2 to 3 lbs • S_3 heart sound pre- or postexercise • Severe dyspnea at rest, paroxysmal nocturnal dyspnea • Jugular vein distention • Severe edema in periphery
Chronic CHF[2,4,14]	• Compensated at rest • Mild pulmonary edema • Abnormal PaO_2, SaO_2 at rest, ↓ below baseline but >90% SaO_2 with activity; no supplemental O_2 • RR <40 bpm with routine activity • Pulse pressure >10 mmHg	• Uncompensated at rest or decompensates with minimal activity • Severe pulmonary edema—flooding of alveoli in more than ½ lung fields, blood appearing in sputum • PaO_2, SaO_2, PaO_2 <90% without supplemental O_2 at rest • RR >40 bpm with minimal routine activity • >10 bpm ↓ HR with activity • Pulse pressure <10 mmHg • 2 pillow orthopnea

Adapted from: American Association of Cardiovascular and Pulmonary Rehabilitation. *Guidelines for Cardiac Rehabilitation and Secondary Prevention.* 4th ed. Champaign, Ill: Human Kinetics Books; 2004. American College of Sports Medicine. *Guidelines for Exercise Testing and Prescription.* 7th ed. Philadelphia, Pa: Lippincott Williams & Wilkins; 2006. American Physical Therapy Association. *Guide to Physical Therapist Practice.* Rev 2nd ed. Alexandria, Va: American Physical Therapy Association; 2003:505-520. Cahalin L. Cardiac muscle dysfunction. In: Hillegass EA, Sadowsky HS, eds. *Essentials of Cardiopulmonary Physical Therapy.* 2nd ed. Philadelphia, Pa: WB Saunders Co; 2001:106-181. Cahalin LP. Heart failure. *Physical Therapy.* 1996;76(5):516-534. Irwin S, Blessey RL. Patient evaluation. In: Irwin S, Tecklin JS, eds. *Cardiopulmonary Physical Therapy.* 3rd ed. St. Louis. Mo: Mosby; 1995:106-141. Lown B, Wolf M. Approaches to sudden death from coronary heart disease. *Circulation.* 1971;44:130-142. McNeer JF, Wallance AG, Wagner GS, et al. The course of acute myocardial infarction. Feasibility of early discharge of the uncomplicated patient. *Circulation.* 1975;51(3):410-413. Seventh Report of the Joint National Committee on Prevention, Detection, Evaluation, and Treatment of High Blood Pressure (JNC 7). NIH Publication No. 03-5231, May 2003. Available at: http//www.nhlbi.nih.gov. Accessed October 10, 2003.

Eventually, the left ventricle may become overwhelmed and forward flow so diminished that blood backs up, increasing the pressure in the left atria and the pulmonary artery, causing an increase in PAWP. This condition is referred to as backward failure.[4] Once pressure in the pulmonary circulation rises, the interstitial fluid increases and drives fluid into the lungs.[30,31] Pulmonary edema appears to varying degrees.[2] Mild pulmonary edema results in increased lymphatic flow and is tolerated without signs or symptoms, while severe pulmonary edema results in increased fluid in the lungs and damage to the pulmonary circulation.[2] Pressure and fluid increases in the pulmonary circulation may increase the tendency to cough. Left ventricular failure and/or hypoxic vasoconstriction associated with severe lung disease are common causes of pulmonary hypertension (PH). This increases the workload to the right ventricle. For patients with PH, blood may appear in the sputum (hemoptysis). Severe progressive exercise is contraindicated in patients with significant PH. However, submaximal steady state exercise may be permissible in those with milder forms of PH when managed by effective physiological monitoring.[32,33] The right ventricle may hypertrophy or develop signs of right ventriclar ischemia when pulmonary pressures are high. Conditions such as PH, cor pulmonale, tricuspid versus pulmonic valve dysfunction, or septal defects may contribute to increases in right ventriclar pressure. If the right ventricle does not maintain forward blood flow, then right atrial (RA) and central venous pressures (CVP) rise. Outwardly the patient may present with jugular vein distension (JVD), extremity edema, and abdominal pain due to liver engorgement. The patient then

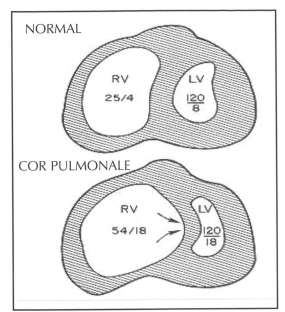

Figure 4-2. Interventricular interdependence: impact of right heart failure on left ventricle. Reprinted with permission from Marino PL. *The ICU Book*. Malvern, Pa: Lea & Febiger; 1991:161.

has right ventricular failure, or if both ventricles are involved, biventricular failure occurs (Figure 4-2).[29] Invasive lines are used to monitor cardiac chamber pressure changes for patients with cardiovascular pump dysfunction or failure. Excessive LVEDP is monitored by PAWP or pulmonary artery pressure (PAP), while dysfunction of the right ventricle or biventricular failure may be detected by measuring right atrial pressure or CVP. Both are routinely used along with the arterial line measures (BP and MAP) during therapeutic sessions (see Imaging and Laboratory Tests).[25-28]

Initially, when there is cardiovascular pump dysfunction or failure, CO may be maintained through the activation of compensatory mechanisms. Any decrease in BP signals sympathetic nervous system activation through the baroreceptor system.[2,18,34] The result is an increase in HR, myocardial contractility, rate of ventricular relaxation, and vasoconstriction in the peripheral vessels. Vasoconstriction limits flow to vital organs and increases the central BP and afterload to the heart. The kidney senses less blood flow and signals sodium retention in the arterial system. Water follows sodium and expands the extracellular volume. Preload increases may improve the Frank Starling mechanism in the patient with mild cardiovascular pump dysfunction, allowing forward flow to be maintained so activity can be tolerated.[2,4]

However, as blood volume increases preload in the patient with significant cardiac dysfunction, the heart may become overstretched. The ventricle fails and there is an increased stretch to the atria that signals the release of atrial natriuretic peptide (ANP).[2,18] Although ANP signals a diuresis, this

effort will be overshadowed by a further rise in LVEDP. Excessive fluid retention may result in further decline in SV in the patient with moderate to severe cardiovascular pump dysfunction. Tachycardia, cardiac chamber dilation, and pulmonary edema ensue and may be worsened with activity. An S_3 heart sound may be present.[2,4,25] Systolic BP may be hypoadaptive, flat, or fall with increasing exercise demand. Therefore, HR and BP limits are imposed to prevent the patient, who is compensated at rest, from decompensating with activity. The patient with significant pulmonary edema will complain of dyspnea, overwhelming fatigue, and have pulmonary crackles in dependent lung fields.[2,4]

For patients with chronic CHF, compensatory mechanisms, such as vasoconstriction and fluid retention, impose secondary disorders that impact on functional work capacity. The skeletal muscle may atrophy or develop type II fiber myopathies.[4,35] The patient may lose both contractile strength and endurance in skeletal muscle. Loss of skeletal muscle mass is known to be independently related to peak oxygen consumption and ventilatory responses in patients with chronic heart failure.[36] Vasoconstriction and increased blood volume adversely affect distal circulation in vital organs. Pancreatic secretion of insulin may become impaired. This, in addition to already elevated catecholamine levels, may lead to glucose intolerance.[2,18] Sympathetic nervous system activation and vasoconstriction may increase venous return and enhance cardiac contractility, but this also results in decreased blood flow in the peripheral vessels. Patients may lose blood flow in or suffer occlusions of distal vessels, leading to tissue ischemia and infarction. PVD or peripheral arterial disease (PAD) may also be present, resulting in claudication pain in the LEs that is often exacerbated during activity. Conditions such as retinopathies, neuropathies, and nephropathies develop or become worse.[37] Therefore, recommended activity HR and BP guidelines are more conservative in patients with these comorbidities (see American Diabetes Association Position Statement on Exercise and Diabetes).[37]

By reviewing pertinent medical information and noting physiological signs and symptoms at rest and with activity, the patient may be classified as having cardiovascular pump dysfunction or failure (see Table 4-3). When a patient has cardiovascular pump dysfunction, higher levels of activity (>5 METs) may result in abnormal or compensatory physiological responses to acute exercise. BP may be hyperadaptive or hypoadaptive during activity. Patients may have an elevated HR or ventilation appearing during activity as the body attempts to compensate in order to meet oxygen demands in the working muscle. A patient with cardiovascular pump dysfunction may have a decreased EF (30% to 50%) or may show signs of exercise-induced ischemia (1 to 2 mm ST-segment depression on ECG) indicating myocardial incompetence.[11,12,14,38] Elevated resting systolic and diastolic BP is also associated with the presence of heart disease and dysfunction.[20,21,23] Guidelines have been established by the

American Heart Association to assist in classification of resting BP to assist with medical and therapeutic management.[39]

A patient with cardiovascular pump failure will no longer be able to use compensatory mechanisms to supply CO for low levels of activity (<5 METs). This individual may have an extremely low left ventricular ejection fraction (LVEF) (<30%), exercise-induced ischemia (>2 mm ST), or be unsafe performing usual ADL.[11,12,14,38] There may be signs or symptoms that are contraindications to exercise (see Table 4-3). The patient with acute cardiovascular pump failure may also have signs of medical instability at rest. Limiting or modifying interventions may be necessary when there is an uncontrolled CO, either extremely hypotensive (<90 mmHg) or hypertensive (>200 mmHg) at rest or not adapting appropriately to exercise. Any episodes of inconsistent mentation, excessive respiratory rates (>40 bpm),[4] and life-threatening arrhythmias[40] may indicate instability and should be reported to the medical staff. Patients having signs of a complicated MI (see Table 4-3) will be at greater risk and are considered to have cardiovascular pump failure.[11,24,38]

IMAGING AND LABORATORY TESTS

Methods used to assess cardiovascular pump function include imaging performed at rest only and imaging during rest and exercise. Two purposes may be served by using imaging techniques. First, the medical team may learn whether pathologies affecting the cardiovascular pump interfere with CO necessary to support resting metabolism to maintain homeostasis and patient survival. Second, for imaging during exercise, the medical team may learn whether impairments to the cardiovascular pump limit CO during activity or provoke unsafe physiological responses.

Considering the extent to which a disease or condition may impact on function will be important. Therefore, information as to what activities the patient may or may not be able to tolerate safely is taken from the imaging obtained during exercise. Abnormalities detected by imaging at rest may be used to justify implementation of medical management and therapeutic strategies designed to prevent deterioration of patient status. Diagnostics include laboratory values that may be monitored prior to exercise to determine medical status for the purpose of selecting a safe level of therapeutic intervention. Review of laboratory and imaging may also explain signs and symptoms affecting activity intolerance.

Methods used to assess factors impacting on or defining cardiovascular pump function are listed below.[1,2,4,25-29,41-43] Those methods used to document cardiac performance during exercise are noted with an asterisk (*).

♦ Catheterization
  ● Invasive lines inserted into the vascular system (venous or arterial) may be advanced into various chambers of the heart to measure cardiac function or used to visualize pulmonary or coronary circulation
  ● Procedures and medications that may be applied during catheterization include:
    ■ Ergovine stimulation
    ■ Percutaneous transluminal coronary angioplasty (PTCA)/stent placement
    ■ Atherectomy
    ■ Percutaneous balloon valvotomy
    ■ Growth hormone infusion
    ■ Radiation
    ■ Laser applications
    ■ Intracardiac ultrasound
    ■ Transvenous pacing
  ● Radionucleotide angiogram (RNA) and ventriculogram (RNV)
    ■ RNA is used to determine patency in coronary arteries
    ■ RNV is used to identify abnormal wall motion or abnormal flow patterns associated with loss of contractility or valve dysfunction
      ► EF may be defined
    ■ Vascular and cardiac chamber pressures, the aortic, the ventricular systolic, and the end-diastolic pressures are taken
      ► Normally left ventricular pressure ranges between 100 to 140 mmHg for systole and 3 to 12 mmHg for end of diastole (LVEDP)[25,26,28]
      ► Differences in pressures between chambers may reveal extent of valve dysfunction

♦ Hemodynamic (HD) monitoring*
  ● Values may be observed during positional changes and during ADL
  ● Measures cardiac functions in real time through an invasive line placed in the vessels or a line advanced to a specific chamber of the heart or pulmonary circulation
  ● The readings are processed through a transducer and transmitted to an oscilloscope for visualization
  ● Arterial pressure (AP) or MAP: Invasive line inserted in an artery to measure mean arterial, systolic, or diastolic BP as an indication of systolic or diastolic load to the cardiovascular pump
    ■ Normal resting values[25,26,28]:
      ► 90 to 140 mmHg systolic
      ► 60 to 90 mmHg diastolic
      ► 70 to 105 mmHg=MAP
  ● CVP is a reading taken in the vena cava or right atria to detect fluid volume changes, right heart dysfunction, or excessive load
    ■ Normal values[25,26,28]: 0 to 8 mmHg

- Recommend <12 mmHg to initiate aerobic exercise in compensated CHF[2,4]
- PAPs: A balloon-tipped catheter (triple-lumen or pulmonary artery catheter) is advanced to the pulmonary artery
  - Normal values[25,26,28]=15 to 30 mmHg during systole or 3 to 12 mmHg in diastole; mean PAP=9 to 16 mmHg
    - If mean PAP >20 mmHg, patient will be symptomatic with activity, and may decompensate[25]
  - Elevation may indicate right ventricle stress, biventricular failure, or PH
- PAWP or pulmonary capillary wedge pressure (PCWP): Inflation of the balloon advances the pulmonary catheter further into the pulmonary artery for a wedge pressure reading to estimate left atrial pressure and indirectly LVEDP to detect left ventricle stress or left ventricular failure (LVF)
  - Normal values: 3 to 15 mmHg[25,26,28]
  - If >20 mmHg and dependent on intravenous (IV) inotrope and systolic BP <80 mmHg the patient may be a candidate for left ventricular assist device (LVAD)[38]
- Thermodilution catheter: Used to measure CO or cardiac index (CI)
  - Normal values[25,26,28]
    - CO=5 to 7 L/min rest
    - CI=2.6 to 4.2 L/min/m²

♦ Electrophysiologic testing (EPS)
  - A catheter that may either stimulate or record electrical activity in the heart[25,27]
  - Used to assess the conduction system in the heart
  - Ablation procedures may be performed via catheterization methods as electrical mapping procedures reveal abnormalities

♦ Echocardiography (ECHO)
  - Used to record cardiac tissue damage, valve function, wall motion, estimated EF, and inflammatory events[25,27,38]
  - Can detect coronary flow as well as items above
    - Modes
      - M-mode
      - Two-dimensional echo (2-D ECHO)
      - Doppler echo
      - Transesophageal echo (TEE)
      - Contrast echo

♦ ECG
  - Used to detect abnormal rhythms or ischemia
  - May also be visualized on the oscilloscope in the intensive care unit (ICU)
  - Resting 12 lead

- Telemetry*
  - Radio signal relay of ECG taken during activity
- Holter monitor*
  - Captures tape recording of ECG taken over 24 hours while patient/client participates in a typical day of activity, logging symptoms and tasks.

♦ Graded exercise test or stress test (GXT)*
  - An exercise test with a protocol that gradually increases in intensity and myocardial oxygen demand[27,38]
  - BP is documented and symptoms are monitored
  - May be combined with diagnostics (listed below) to provide different information regarding cardiovascular pump dysfunction
    - Standard test with ECG*
      - Provides information about ischemia and heart rhythms associated with physiologic responses
    - Thallium stress test* using thallium-201 or other radioactive nuclide perfusion for imaging
      - Used for detecting coronary artery perfusion problems and to detect reperfusion of cardiac tissue after exercise induced ischemia
    - Exercise ECHO*
      - Noninvasive method to visualize valve functioning and wall motion and to estimate EF and cardiac chamber pressures during exercise[44]
    - CPT or cardiopulmonary exercise testing (CP GXT)*
      - Metabolic gas analysis that provides information about oxygen consumption and energy utilization in the body tissues during exercise

♦ Pharmacologic stress test
  - Pharmacological agents (dypyridamole, adenosine, and dobutamine) are used to increase myocardial demand or accelerate coronary bloodflow when the patient cannot exercise. It may be combined with ECHO or another diagnostic tool[12,25,26]

♦ MUGA
  - Serial images of cardiovascular pump functions after infusion of radioactive dye are taken to capture one cardiac cycle

♦ CT scan
  - Used to detect masses, pericarditis, myocarditis, or aneurysms

♦ MRI
  - Used to examine cardiac contractility and blood flow

♦ Chest radiography
  - Used to detect cardiac enlargement, pulmonary edema, emboli, or HTN, as well as various lung disorders

♦ PET

- Used to measure metabolic functioning of the heart to demonstrate tissue viability and coronary flow
- ◆ Doppler
  - Vascular assessment used to detect deep vein thrombosis (DVT)
  - May be used to determine ankle brachial index (ABI) to detect restrictions in arterial blood flow in the peripheral arteries[44]
    - Doppler systolic BP of posterior tibial artery/dorsalis pedis on RLE or LLE ÷ Doppler systolic BP of brachial/radial artery on right upper extremity (RUE) or left upper extremity (LUE)
    - Normal ABI=Normal ratios range from 1.19 to 0.90[44]
- ◆ PFT[45]
  - Many patients with cardiovascular pump dysfunction are obese or smoke (see Patterns C and E)
  - FVC
    - Used to determine lung capacity and indirectly, respiratory muscle function
    - Important in CHF to detect changes in pulmonary edema[2]
  - FEV_1
    - Used to determine extent of lung flow disruption that may be impacted by years of smoking
  - PEFR
    - Used to determine airway reactivity to high flow states (ie, exercise) and the extent to which asthma may be impacting on lung volume flow
    - Used to determine when patient may safely exercise without exacerbation to evaluate the timing and effectiveness of the bronchodilator
- ◆ Respiratory muscle performance tests[2]
  - Maximal inspiratory pressure (MIP) and maximal expiratory pressure (MEP)
    - Used to determine the respiratory muscle strength in patients with CHF and pulmonary edema[2]
  - Maximal voluntary ventilation (MVV)
    - Used to determine the respiratory muscle endurance potential for patients with CHF or confounding pulmonary disorders associated with cardiac dysfunction[2]
- ◆ Blood tests
  - Blood lipids: Used to detect ongoing risk of CAD (see Pattern A)
    - Total cholesterol (Total Chol)
      - Normal value: Desirable <200 mg/dL
    - HDL
      - Normal value: 40 to 60 mg/dL

- LDL
  - Optimal level: <100 mg/dL
  - Near optimal level: 100 to 129 mg/dL
  - Borderline high level: 130 to 159 mg/dL
  - High level: 160 to 189 mg/dL
  - Very high level corresponding to highest increased risk of heart disease: >190 mg/dL
- Ratio (Total Chol/HDL)
  - Normal value: <3.25
- Triglycerides
  - Normal value: 40 to 150 mg/dL
- Blood factors: Used to detect ongoing risk of CAD (see Pattern A)
  - Homocysteine
    - Normal value: 5 to 15 umol/L
  - Lipoprotein a (LPa): Because of the variability associated with population characteristics, it has been recommended that each laboratory establish its own limits of normal[46]
    - Normal value for whites: 5.6 to 33.8 mg/dL
    - Normal values for blacks: 21.7 to 74.3 mg/dL
  - CRP
    - Normal value: <6 ug/mL
- Serum enzymes/diagnostic markers: Used to diagnose MI
  - CK[27,41]
    - Normal values:
      - ◆ 60 to 400 u/L males
      - ◆ 40 to 150 u/L females
    - Begins to rise 4 to 8 hours and peaks after 12 to 40 hours post MI[27,41]
  - Creatine kinase-myocardial band (CK-MB)
    - Normal values: 0 to 3% relative index[25,27,41]
    - An isoenzyme of CK specific to the myocardium
  - Lactate dehydrogenase (LDH)
    - There are five isoenzymes: LDH_1/LDH_2 >1= recent MI
    - Peaks 72 hours post MI
  - Aspartate aminotransferase (AST)
    - Normal values: 10 to 40 u/L for males[27,41] and 9 to 25 u/L for females
    - Peaks 24 hours post MI
  - Troponin 1
    - Normal values: <0 to 3 mg/mL[27,41]
    - Peaks at 24 hours post MI
  - Myoglobin
    - <100 ng/mL[27,41]
    - Peaks 3 to 25 hours post MI
  - Atrial Natriuretic Factor(ANF)/B-Type Peptide (BNP): BNP is diagnostic for CHF if elevated.

Used when patients present with shortness of breath to differentiate lung disease versus CHF when determining the cause of shortness of breath.[42,43]

> ▸ Normal ANF=20 to 77 pg/dL
> ▸ Normal BNP <100 pg/dL

- CBC: Used to detect anemia, infectious processes, and thrombocytopenia
  - ■ Hgb
    - ▸ Normal values[25,27,41]:
      - ○ 14 to 18 gm/dL males
      - ○ 13 to 16 gm/dL females
  - ■ Hct
    - ▸ Normal values[25,27,41]:
      - ○ 42% to 52% males
      - ○ 37% to 48% females
  - ■ WBC
    - ▸ Normal values: 4.3-10.8 x 10^{-3} cell per u/L[27,41]
  - ■ Platelets (Plts)
    - ▸ Normal values: 150-450 x 10^{-3} cell per u/L[27,41]
- Electrolytes
  - ■ Potassium (K^+)
    - ▸ Normal values: 3.5 to 5.1 mEq/L[27,41]
    - ▸ Abnormal values: Increased risk of arrhythmias
  - ■ Sodium (Na^+)
    - ▸ Normal values: 136 to 145 mEq/L[27,41]
  - ■ Chloride (Cl^-)
    - ▸ Normal values: 98 to 107 mEq/L[27,41]
- Glucose: Used to detect diabetes, hypo-, or hyperglycemia
  - ■ Fasting
    - ▸ Normal: 80 to 100 mg/dL[12,37]
    - ▸ Diabetes: 126 mg/dL[37]
  - ■ Random
    - ▸ 250 mg/dL with ketones or 300 mg/dL with no ketones=Exercise contraindicated[12,37]
- Coagulation: Measures used to evaluate the risk of bleeding
  - ■ Prothrombin time (PT)
    - ▸ Used to detect extrinsic pathway defects of coagulation
    - ▸ Normal values: 11.0 to 12.5 seconds
  - ■ Partial thromboplastin time (PTT)
    - ▸ Used to detect coagulation defects of the intrinsic system
    - ▸ Normal values: 21.5 to 34.1 sec
  - ■ International normalized ratio (INR)
    - ▸ Indicates what the PT would have been if using WHO's International Reference Reagent
    - ▸ Normal values: 1.5 to 2.5[41]

- Arterial blood gases: Used to detect metabolic or respiratory acidosis/alkalosis[45]
  - ■ pH: 7.35 to 7.45 (below 7.35=acidosis; above 7.45=alkalosis)
  - ■ PaO_2: 80 to 100 mmHg (below 80 mmHg= hypoxemia)
  - ■ $PaCO_2$: 35 to 45 mmHg (above 45 mmHg= hypercapnea; below 35 mmHg=hypocapnea)
- Oxygen saturation of Hgb
  - ■ Percent of oxygen in the blood transported as oxyhemoglobin
  - ■ Measures may be taken for arterial or venous blood to determine oxygen levels
  - ■ SaO_2
    - ▸ Invasive
      - ○ Normal values: Typically 98%
      - ○ Therapy is contraindicated when values fall below 90% in most clinics
    - ▸ Noninvasive via a sensor and converted by a transducer to a pulse oximeter (SpO_2), values are the same
  - ■ Oxygen saturation of venous blood (SvO_2)
    - ▸ Invasive
      - ○ Normal values: 75%
      - ○ Therapy is contraindicated when values fall below 58%

PHARMACOLOGY

The following medications are used primarily to manage HTN, angina, arrhythmias, heart failure, and coagulation disorders arising from cardiovascular pump dysfunction or failure. A summary of the common medications, the conditions affecting the cardiovascular pump function, any side effects (precautions), and the impact of the medication on physiologic responses at rest and during exercise is available in Table 4-4. Full descriptions of the mechanisms for each medication and the advantages and disadvantages with regard to the interaction of exercise are described in detail in the References.[12,47-50]

- ◆ ACE inhibitors
  - Examples: Captopril (Capoten) and enalapril (Vasotec)
  - Actions: Limit production of angiotensin II to decrease BP and proliferation of vascular smooth muscle and myocardial cell growth
  - Side effects: Dizziness, hyperkalemia, skin rash, weight loss/altered taste
- ◆ Antiarrhythmic
  - Examples: Digoxin (Lanoxin), adenosine, lidocaine, amiodarone (Betapace), and magnesium chloride (Slow-Mag)

Table 4-4

Common Medications: Conditions, Precautions, and Impact on Activity Tolerance

Medications	Conditions	Precautions	HR Rest	HR Exercise	BP Rest	BP Exercise	Exercise Capacity
Diuretics • Thiazides • Loop • Potassium Sparing	HTN CHF	Dehydration/orthostasis Electrolyte imbalance (K+, Na+): ↑ risk for arrhythmias Impairs glycemic control	↔	↔	↔ or ↓	↔ or ↓	↑ in patients with CHF Primary effect is ↓ intravascular fluid

Beta Blockers
• Cardio Selective
  Atenolol
  Metoprolol
• Nonselective
  Propranolol
  Timolol
  Nadolol
	HTN
	Angina/CAD
	Arrhythmias
	MI
	CHF
		Orthostatic hypotension
		Bradycardia
		Exercise hypotension/dizziness
		  (may mask hypoglycemia)
		GI distress
		Bronchoconstriction
		  (may worsen asthma)
		Impairs heat dissipation
		Depression
			↓	↓	↓	↓	↑ in patients with angina
							
							Primary effect is to ↓ cardiac work by blocking catecholamines to ↓ HR and contractility
							Lower HR=↑ diastolic time improving myocardial O_2 supply

Ca+Channel Blockers • Verapamil • Diltiazem • Nifedipine	HTN Variant Angina Arrhythmias	Verapamil for supraventricular tachycardia Orthostatic hypotension Dizziness Headache ↑ risk of CHF	↓ or ↑ with Nifedipine	↓ or ↑ with Nifedipine	↓	↓	↑ in patients with angina Primary effect is to ↓ afterload via vascular smooth muscle relaxation. Less ischemia on ECG
Nitrates • Nitroglycerin • Isorbide dinitrate • Amyl nitrite	Angina Postsurgically to ↓ BP	Headaches Dizziness Orthostatic hypotension	↑	↑ or ↔	↓	↓ or ↔	↑ in patients with angina Primary effect is to inhibit vasoconstriction of smooth muscle in coronary artery and reduce preload and afterload in systemic vasculature Note: Patients with severe CAD may not see coronary vascular relaxation.

continued

↑=increased, ↓=decreased, ↔=unchanged. HTN=hypertension, CHF=congestive heart failure, K+=potassium, Na+=sodium, CAD=coronary artery disease, MI=myocardial infarction, GI=gastrointestinal, HR=heart rate, Ca+=calcium, ECG=electrocardiogram, BP=blood pressure, ACE=angiotensin converting enzyme, 2°=secondary, Angio=angiotensin, A-fib=atrial fibrillation, CNS=central nervous system, ST=refers to the S wave and T wave on electrocardiogram, SV=stroke volume, LDL=low-density lipoprotein

Table 4-4 (continued)

COMMON MEDICATIONS: CONDITIONS, PRECAUTIONS, AND IMPACT ON ACTIVITY TOLERANCE

Medications	Conditions	Precautions	HR Rest	HR Exercise	BP Rest	BP Exercise	Exercise Capacity

Vasodilators
• Antiadrenergic
  Clonidine
  Methyldopa
  Reserpine
	HTN	Tachycardia
		Postural hypotension
		Dizziness
		Headaches
			↓ or ↔	↓ or ↔	↓	↓	↑ or ↔ in exercise capacity in CHF

• Nonadrenergic
  Hydralazine
  Minoxidil
			↑ or ↔	↑ or ↔	↓	↓	Primary effect is dilation of peripheral vessels

ACE Inhibitors • Captopril • Enalapril	HTN CHF	Exercise induced asthma ↑ risk (2° dehydration) Hypotension—if combined with diuretics	↔	↔	↓	↓	↑ in patients with CHF Primary effect is to lower BP by preventing conversion of Angiotensin I → Angio II
Cardiac Glycosides • Digitoxin • Digoxin	CHF, A-fib Arrhythmias	CNS disturbance (confusion) GI distress Arrhythmias Note: ECG review of ST-segment depression is not reliable indicator of ischemia when patient is on these medications.	↓	↓	↔	↔	↑ in patients with CHF ↑ in patients with a-fib Primary effect is to ↑ force and velocity of cardiac contraction. Also ↓'s conduction velocity through atrioventricular node.

Positive Inotropics
• Phosphodiesterase inhibitors (PDE)
  Amrinone
  Milrinone
  Dobutamine
  Dopamine
	CHF	↑ risk arrhythmias	↓	↓	↔	↔	Variable effects on activity tolerance-dose dependent differences in periphery.
							Primary effect is to ↑ force and velocity of cardiac contraction by stimulating the beta₁ adrenergic receptors to ↑ SV and vasodilate peripherally

continued

Table 4-4 (continued)

COMMON MEDICATIONS: CONDITIONS, PRECAUTIONS, AND IMPACT ON ACTIVITY TOLERANCE

Medications	Conditions	Precautions	HR Rest	HR Exercise	BP Rest	BP Exercise	Exercise Capacity

Antiarrhythmic
• Class I
  Quinidine
  Procanimide
  Lidocaine
• Class II-β-blockers
• Class III-
  Amidarone
• Class IV—Ca+ Blockers
	Arrhythmias	Observe impact of any change in medication on exercise for proarrhythmic effect. Arrhythmias may worsen with exercise.	↓ Classes II-IV	↓ Classes II-IV	↔	↔	↔ on exercise capacity

Anticoagulants • Heparin • Warfarin • Dipyridamole	Venous thrombosis	Propensity to ↑ bleeding, especially in patients with thrombocytopenia and those with indwelling catheters	↔	↔	↔	↔	↔ on exercise capacity Primary effect is to ↑ circulating protein, anti-thrombin III (heparin) or ↓ synthesis of clotting factors (warfarin)
Antithrombolytics • Aspirin	Prevention of vascular thrombosis or emboli	Avoid prior to surgeries 2° ↑ risk of bleeding	↔	↔	↔	↔	↔ Primary effect is inhibition of platelet activity
Thrombolytics • Streptokinase • Urokinase • Tissue plasminogen activator	Acute extensive thromboembolis to coronary artery or Post-MI	↑ risk of bleeding	↔	↔	↔	↔	↔ Primary effect is clot breakdown
Anti-inflammatory • Corticosteroids	CHF Transplant	Type II atrophy Osteoporosis Skin breakdown	↔	↔	↔	↔	↔
Antihyperlipidemic • Lovastatin • Pravastatin • Simvastatin	↑ cholesterol, at risk for CAD	Rhabdomyolysis Liver damage	↔	↔	↔	↔	↔ Primary effect is to inhibit cholesterol biosynthesis and ↓ serum LDL

Adapted from: American College of Sports Medicine. Appendix A. *Guidelines for Exercise Testing and Prescription.* 7th ed. Philadelphia, Pa: Lippincott Williams & Wilkins; 2006. Interpretations from Ciccone CD. *Pharmacology in Rehabilitation.* 2nd ed. Philadelphia, Pa: FA Davis Co; 1996. Shannon MT, Wilson BA, Stang CL, eds. *Prentice Hall Health Professionals Drug Guide 2003.* Upper Saddle River, NJ: Pearson Education Inc; 2003.

↑=increased, ↓=decreased, ↔=unchanged. HTN=hypertension, CHF=congestive heart failure, K+=potassium, Na+=sodium, CAD=coronary artery disease, MI=myocardial infarction, GI=gastrointestinal, HR=heart rate, Ca+=calcium, ECG=electrocardiogram, BP=blood pressure, ACE=angiotensin converting enzyme, 2°=secondary, Angio=angiotensin, A-fib=atrial fibrillation, CNS=central nervous system, ST=refers to the S wave and T wave on electrocardiogram, SV=stroke volume, LDL=low-density lipoprotein

- Actions:
  - Digoxin controls atrial fibrillation (A-fib), atrial flutter (A-flutter), and paroxysmal atrial tachycardia (PAT) by slowing conduction in AV node
  - Adenosine/Lidocaine slows conduction in SA and AV nodes
  - Amiodorone slows conduction and increases blood flow by acting to relax arterial smooth muscle, thereby decreasing risk for arrhythmia
- Side effects: Confusion, fatigue, headache, hypotension (via bradycardia), muscle weakness, and nausea

♦ Anticoagulants
  - Examples: Heparin, warfarin (Coumadin), and enoxaparin (Lovenox)
  - Actions: Increase antithrombin III and lower clotting risk
  - Side effects: Increases risk of bleeding

♦ Anti-inflammatory drugs
  - Examples: Corticosteroids (Medrol, Prednisone)
  - Actions: Decrease inflammation
  - Side effects: Cushingoid features, delayed wound healing, hyperglycemia. hypokalemia, insomnia, muscle weakness, nausea, osteoporosis, and psychosis

♦ Beta-adrenergic blockers
  - Cardio selective
    - Examples: Atenolol (Tenormin) and metoprolol (Lopressor, Toprol XL)
    - Actions: Lower HR and vasodilate to lower BP
    - Side effects: Dizziness, drowsiness, fatigue, hypotension, insomnia, and syncope and may mask hypoglycemia
  - Nonselective
    - Examples: Propranolol (Inderal), penbutolol (Levatol), and carteolol (Cartrol)
    - Actions: Lower HR and BP, decrease myocardial irritability, decrease AV and intraventricular conduction velocity
    - Side effects: Fatigue, dizziness, syncope, and large dose may cause bronchospasm in patients with lung disease

♦ Calcium channel blockers
  - Examples: Verapamil (Verelan, Calan, Isoptin), diltiazem (Cardizem, Dilacor), and nifedipine (Adalat, Procardia)
  - Actions: Inhibit vascular smooth muscle cell proliferation to decrease vascular resistance and vasodilate
  - Side effects: Headache, orthostatic hypotension, nausea, swelling in ankles

♦ Digitalis glycoside and inotropic agents
  - Examples: Digitoxin (Digitaline), digoxin (Lanoxin), dopamine (Dopastat), and dobutamine (Dobutrex)
  - Actions: Increase force of contractility and therefore increase SV and CO; Digoxin decreases conduction through AV node
  - Side effects
    - Digoxin increases risk of arrhythmia; toxicity prone effects also include confusion, fatigue, and gastrointestinal problems; toxic if >2 u/mL
    - Side effects: Dopamine increases risk of arrhythmia; contraindicated in patients with history of occlusive vascular disease

♦ Diuretics
  - Loop
    - Examples: Furosemide (Lasix)
    - Actions: Act on the ascending loop of Henle in the kidney to decrease fluid volume
    - Side effects: Arrhythmias, dehydration, electrolyte imbalance, impairment of glycemic control
  - Potassium sparing
    - Examples: Amiloride (Midamor) and spironolactone (Aldactone), and triamterene (Dyrenium)
    - Actions: Decrease fluid volume, spares potassium, and decreases risk of arrhythmias
    - Side effects: Dehydration and impaired glycemic control
  - Thiazides
    - Examples: Chlorthalidone (Clorpres, Tenoretic, Thalitone) and hydrochlorothiazide (Aldactazide, Capozide, Dyazide, HydroDIURIL, Lopressor HCT, Maxzide, Vaseretic)
    - Actions: Block reabsoprtion of sodium in distal tubules of the kidneys and thus decrease fluid volume in vascular system to lower BP
    - Side effects: Dehydration, electrolyte imbalance, glucose intolerance, and increase triglyceride and cholesterol levels

♦ Lipid-lowering
  - Examples: Simvastatin (Zocor) and atorvastatin calcium (Lipitor)
  - Actions: Inhibit cholesterol production
  - Side effects: May cause liver damage and rhabdomyolysis

♦ Nitrates
  - Examples
    - Nitroglycerin
      - Sublinguinal/chewable/buccal: Isordil, nitrogard, Nitrostat
      - Systemic oral: Dilatrate, IMDUR, Nitrocot

> ▸ Skin patch: Deponit, Minitran, Nitrek, Nitro-Dur
>
> ▸ Transdermal patch: Minitran, Nitro-Bid, Nitro-Dur
- ■ Isosorbide dinitrate
  > ▸ Sublinguinal/chewable/buccal: Isordil, Nitrogard, Nitrostat, Sorbitrate
  >
  > ▸ Systemic: Dilatrate-SR, IMDUR, ISMO, Monoket, Nitrocot, Nitro-par, Sorbitrate
- ■ Amyl nitrite
- • Actions: Vasodilate peripheral vessels to decrease preload and after load
- • Side effects: May cause dizziness and orthostasis
♦ Thrombolytics
- • Examples: Streptokinase (Abbokinase, Activase, Retavase, Streptase)
- • Actions: Promote thrombolysis for reperfusion of coronary arteries
- • Side effects: Increases risk of bleeding
♦ Vasodilators
- • Examples:
  - ■ Antiadrenergic: Propranolol (Inderal), metoprolol (Lopressor, Toprol XL)
  - ■ Nonadrenergic: Isoxsuprine hydrochloride (Vasodilan), hydralazine hydrochloride (Apresoline)
- • Actions: Decrease BP
- • Side effects: Decreased mental acuity, dizziness, fluid retention, nausea, syncope, and weight gain

---

Case Study #1: Complicated Myocardial Infarction, Congestive Heart Failure, High Risk

Mr. George Hartman is a 76-year-old male who was admitted through the emergency department with onset of diffuse chest pressure, weakness, shortness of breath, and diaphoresis.

PHYSICAL THERAPIST EXAMINATION

HISTORY

♦ General demographics: Mr. Hartman is a 76-year-old, black, English-speaking male. He is a high school graduate and attended some college before deciding to become a carpenter's apprentice.

♦ Social history: Mr. Hartman is a widower. He is independent in ADL; however, his daughter performs most household tasks. His wife died 6 years ago.

♦ Employment/work: Mr. Hartman is a retired carpenter.

♦ Living environment: He lives on the first floor of his daughter's 2-level home.

♦ General health status
- • General health perception: Mr. Hartman realizes smoking contributed to his lung problems, and he quit right after his wife died 6 years ago. He has tried to diet and stay away from salt but finds it difficult. He understands the hereditary nature of his HTN, diabetes, and CAD. He denies previous chest pain.
- • Physical function: Mr. Hartman reports that his body is falling apart but he only needs help when he leaves home. He is accepting of some help and equipment for community function. He does not want to use a walker for community mobility. He seems unaware of his risk for falling. His goal is to return home without a rehab stay.
- • Psychological function: Normal.
- • Role function: Father, grandfather, friend to many in church and community.
- • Social function: He plays board games with his grandchildren and bingo with his friends at church, and he is a long-time resident of his community.

♦ Social/health habits: Mr. Hartman was a former two-packs-per-day smoker and quit when his wife died of COPD 6 years ago. He occasionally uses alcohol socially.

♦ Family history: His father died of heart disease. His mother died of the sequelae of diabetes mellitus.

♦ Medical/surgical history: He has a history of HTN (25 years), COPD (10 years), and Type 2 diabetes mellitus (18 years). Mr. Hartman had an outpatient GXT 10 years ago, and the results were positive for ischemia. CAD was confirmed on a follow-up catheterization that documented three-vessel disease with 75% blockage of the middle 1/3 of the circumflex artery. Diffuse 50% to 60% blockages were found in many portions of the left anterior descending (LAD) and right coronary artery (RCA) vessels. PTCA was performed in multiple sites and reduced the lesion in the circumflex to 30%. Mr. Hartman had an EF of 55% at that time. He had 2 prior admissions for asthma attacks related to his COPD. His last recorded (3 weeks ago) PFTs revealed the following: FVC=60% predicted; and FEV_1=65% predicted. Mr. Hartman has signs of circulatory damage; PVD (ABI=0.88), visual impairments, and macular degeneration versus retinopathy. He had a small inferior MI, but there is no record of admission.

♦ Current condition(s)/chief complaint(s)

Table 4-5

CASE STUDY #1: SUMMARY OF HOSPITAL EVENTS SINCE ADMISSION

Day	Event
1	Admitted to ICU ECG: ST elevation V_1-V_4 Started on heparin, SL NTG, IV streptokinase, furosemide Placed on 40% face mask
2	Diffuse chest discomfort, increased shortness of breath, some dizziness ABGs: pH=7.48, PaO_2=60; PCO_2=50; HCO_3=20 Placed on rebreather mask, 80% ECHO: Markedly dilated left ventricle, moderately dilated right ventricle LVEF: 35% CK 60*, CK-MB index 3% Meds: Insulin, IV nitroglycerin added to furosemide
3	Increasing somnolence ABGs: pH=7.50, PaO_2=50; PCO_2=60; HCO_3=15 ECG: A-fib with runs of PVCs, some couplets Placed on mechanical ventilation, SIMV mode Central line, a-line placed HR: 120 bpm CVP: 10 mmHg PAWP: 20 mmHg AP: 96/70 mmHg MAP: 78 mmHg
4-7	Patient remains somnolent, on mechanical ventilation CT of head remarkable for age-related changes ECG: A fib with few PVCs, ST-segment elevation resolving, Q waves Medications: Digitalis added, IV nitro DC'd, SL NTG available, furosemide switched to spironolactone.
8-10	Ventilator weaning begins
11	Patient awake and alert Placed on 40% facemask TEE: Markedly dilated left ventricle with anterior wall hypokinesis, moderately dilated right ventricle LVEF: 40% Mild mitral and aortic regurgitation
12	PT consulted Labs: Hgb=13.8; Hct=42.0; Na=140; K=4.0; INR=2.5*; Glucose=180* pH=7.42; PaO_2=75; PCO_2=35; HCO_3=35 ECG: Sinus tachycardia, pathologic Q wave in V_2-V_4 HR: 110 bpm CVP: 8 mmHg PAP: 18 mmHg BP: 100/80 mmHg, MAP 88 No reports of angina, mild shortness of breath at rest in bed at 60 degrees upright, two to three episodes of dizziness with changes in position in bed with nursing

*Abnormal values

- Mr. Hartman was hospitalized for 12 days after an anterior MI that was complicated by CHF and pulmonary edema. Table 4-5 details the hospital admission events.
- He was managed in ICU with mechanical ventilation and hemodynamic monitoring.
- He was slow to wean from the ventilator.
- Mr. Hartman is scheduled for transfer to the step down unit and still on hemodynamic monitoring with telemetry.
- He requires 40% of supplemental oxygen via facemask.
- He complains of general fatigue, dizziness upon sitting or standing, and has shortness of breath with minimal activity.

♦ Functional status and activity level: Mr. Hartman had been ambulating independently without a device at home, but he used a cane and portable oxygen when he went out. His family drove him to church and bingo weekly.

♦ Medications: Prior to admission he was taking simvastatin (cholesterol lowering), atenolol (beta-blocker), spironolactone (potassium-sparing diuretic), albuterol neubilizer Q 4 hrs/PRN (bronchodilator for COPD), and chlorpropamide (oral hypoglycemic agent for diabetes). Currently (day 12) he is on digitalis, heparin spironolactone, albuterol neubilizer, simvastatin, and insulin.

♦ Other clinical tests: Noted in the chart, not documented directly in the physical therapy note; lab values indicated by * are abnormal
  - Hgb=14.4 gm/dL
  - Hct=43.2%
  - WBC=12,000/mm³
  - PT=14.4 sec
  - International Normalized Ratio (INR): 1.12 (normal =0.8 to 1.2)
  - Na=147* mEq/L (135 to 146 mEq/L)
  - K=3.4* mEq/L (3.5 to 5.0 mEq/L)
  - Cl=110 mEq/L
  - CK=60 u/L (60 to 400 u/L males)
  - CK-MB=2.4 u/L (<12 u/L if total CK is <400 u/L)
  - CK-MB index=3% (0 to 3% relative index)
  - Myoglobin=80 ng/mL (<100 ng/mL)
  - BPN=160 pg/dL
  - Chol=250* mg/dL (desirable is <200 mg/dL)
  - Glucose=350* mg/dL (normal fasting is 80 to 100 mg/dL and post prandial is <200 mg/dL)
  - Chest x-ray: Enlarged cardiac shadow, right lower lobe atelectasis
  - ECG: A fib/flutter, 1 mm ST-segment change, wide variation in HR

SYSTEMS REVIEW

♦ Cardiovascular/pulmonary
  - BP: 110/80 mmHg
  - Edema: 1+ bilateral lower extremity (BLE) pitting edema
  - HR: 110 bpm
  - RR: 20 bpm

♦ Integumentary
  - Skin color: Dusky dark brown/purple
  - Skin integrity
    - BLE skin dry and flaking
    - Grade 2 pressure ulcer sacrum
    - No hair on lower legs or toes

♦ Musculoskeletal
  - Gross range of motion: Decreased in most peripheral and spinal joints, but age appropriate
  - Gross strength
    - Decreased in feet/ankles, remainder WFL
    - Atrophy in calves bilaterally
  - Gross symmetry: Age appropriate with mild kyphosis and an elevated right shoulder
  - Height: 5'7" (1.7 m)
  - Weight: 200 lbs (90.7 kg)

♦ Neuromuscular
  - Balance: Decreased, two falls in past month
  - Locomotion, transfers, and transitions: WFL

♦ Communication, affect, cognition, language, and learning style
  - Communication, affect, cognition, and language: Alert, oriented x2
  - Appears anxious
  - Learning preferences: Concrete experiential

TESTS AND MEASURES[44,50-57]

♦ Aerobic capacity/endurance: The first evaluation of activity in an acute care setting for this patient with extremely marginal condition requires progressing the patient within the ACSM Class I Activity Status[51] using a self care monitor.[52-53] Progressing the patient on the initial visit does not go beyond building sitting tolerance. Activity is guided by vital signs and ECG using approved guidelines.[12,14] The patient is progressed at relatively low levels to prevent adverse pressure load to the heart. The HR of 120 [or resting HR +20] is not to be exceeded and BP must be adaptive. Falling BP and excessive HR are reasons for terminating the initial session (see Table 4-6).
  - Activities: Rest-supine 45 degrees; raising head of bed 75 degrees; slow deep breathing; sitting with some UE support; supine 45 degrees; ankle pumps; 2-minute recovery (see Table 4-6 for results)

Table 4-6 CASE STUDY #1: SELF-CARE MONITOR						
Activity/Workload	*HR*	*BP*	*RR*	*O_2 Sat*	*ECG*	*Symptoms*
Rest–Supine 45 degrees	110	100/80	20	90%	Q waves (V2-4)	Upper chest breathing
Raising head of bed 75 degrees	112	102/78	24	92%	Q waves	Upper chest breathing
Slow deep breathing	100	105/80	18	94%	Q waves	Normalized breathing
Sitting (some UE support)	130*	90/70*	22	90%	1 mm ST dep -V_5	Lightheaded
Supine 45 degrees	125	100/70	22	90%	Occasional PVC's	
Ankle pumps	115	102/76	20	92%	Q waves	Normalized breathing
2-minute recovery	112	100/76	22	90%	Q waves	

*LE dressing/transfer/sitting in chair deferred due to HR endpoint and falling systolic BP with LE dependent.

- ACSM Activity Class I: Inpatient Cardiac Rehab[51]
  - Functional ADL/self-care monitor[52-54]
- Anthropometric characteristics
  - BMI (kg/m[2]: weight/height)=31.39; Class I Obesity[12]
  - 1+ pitting edema BLE
- Arousal, attention, and cognition
  - Alert, oriented x2 ("hospital")
- Circulation
  - HR
    - Tachycardia 110 bpm at rest
    - Increases to endpoint 130 bpm in sitting/legs dependent
  - BP
    - Falling from 100/80 mmHg at rest-supine head of bed (HOB) 45 degrees to 90/70 mmHg with sitting/legs dependent
  - Auscultation
    - S_4 pre- and posttreatment
    - Unremarkable for S_3
  - Pulse quality
    - Varies from regular to irregular-irregular (premature ventricular contractions [PVCs])
    - Bilateral dorsalis pedis pulse weak: Grade 1
  - JVD: Present bilaterally
  - ECG
    - Occasional PVCs 10 to 12 per minute
    - Isolated unifocal
  - Extremities
    - Cool to touch
    - Mild cyanosis
  - Occasional dizziness reported with position changes
- Integumentary integrity[37]
  - Impaired in stocking pattern; protective sensation (>5.09 monofilament)
- Muscle performance
  - Modified tests performed in bed
  - All muscle groups intact (at least 3+) except:
    - Ankle plantarflexion bilaterally=3/5 (manual test)
    - Toe flexion and extension bilaterally=3/5
  - Exhales with effort
- Pain
  - No trigger points on chest wall exam
  - No reports of pain with activity during this session
- Posture
  - Sitting in semi-fowler's on exam
  - Forward head with severe thoracic kyphosis
  - Attempts to supports self with UEs
- Range of motion
  - WNL for age except
    - Decreased chest wall expansion (CWE)[57] (Table 4-7)
      - Axilla=2.0 cm
      - Xiphoid=2.5 cm
    - CWE: L>R on palpation
- Self-care and home management
  - Rolls with minimal assistance of one
  - Moves to sitting at edge of bed with minimal assistance of one

Age	Axilla (cm)		Xiphoid (cm)	
	SUPINE	STAND	SUPINE	STAND
20-29	5.1	5.3	5.9	6.2
30-39	5.1	5.6	5.3	5.7
40-49	4.1	4.5	4.3	4.5
50-59	2.7	3.1	3.0	4.1
60-69	3.2	3.3	3.3	4.1
70+	2.7	2.8	2.5	2.9

Table 4-7
NORMATIVE DATA FOR CHEST WIDTH EXPANSION USING VITAL CAPACITY MANEUVER[57]

- Testing limited by physiological responses (light-headed, unsafe systolic BP)
- ◆ Ventilation and respiration/gas exchange
  - Auscultation
    - Coarse crackles bilateral lower lobes, do not clear with cough
    - No change preexercise to postexercise
  - Breathing pattern
    - Upper chest breather
    - Recruits diaphragm with cues
  - Respiratory pattern
    - Occasional Cheyne Stokes
    - Increased rate (breaths per min)=20 bpm rest; 22 to 24 bpm with sitting upright
  - Dyspnea rated 1/4 at rest and increased to 2/4 (Ventilatory Response Index) with sitting at 75 to 90 degrees[58]
  - RPE increased from 6/20 at rest to 11/20 sitting (Borg Scale)[59,60] indicating difficulty with even the most basic activity
  - SaO_2
    - 90% at rest while on 40% O_2 increasing to 94% with deep breathing while sitting >75 degrees
- ◆ Work, community, and leisure integration or reintegration
  - Previously, Mr. Hartman was minimally assisted in the community, demonstrating activities of approximately 4 MET capacity that were limited by general fatigue

EVALUATION

The history and findings are consistent with Mr. Hartman's diagnosis of MI, CHF, and COPD. He is a patient who complains of dizziness limiting upright tolerance for function. Dizziness corresponds to a 15 mmHg fall in systolic BP, 1 mm ST-depression in V_5, and isolated unifocal PVCs (6 to 10 per minute) upon sitting upright. Orthostatic intolerance is due to cardiovascular pump failure resulting from a com-

plicated anterior wall MI and may be related to medications (excess diuretics, nitrates), effects of bed rest, and decreased venous return in sitting. The patient is stratified into the high-risk category[12,14] (Table 4-8) and requires close physiological monitoring.

He is at risk for chronic decompensating CHF as his EF is marginal, resulting in activity limiting (<5 METs) dizziness and falling BP. Mr. Hartman is also experiencing shortness of breath and impaired gas exchange secondary to CHF-related pulmonary edema superimposed on obstructive lung disease in an anxious patient. His breathing strategy also is impaired. Prior to admission, Mr. Hartman was minimally assisted in the community and performing activities at about a 4 MET capacity that were limited by general fatigue.

DIAGNOSIS

Mr. Hartman is a patient who has had an MI and has CHF and COPD. In addition, he has impaired: aerobic capacity/endurance; anthropometric characteristics; circulation; integumentary integrity; muscle performance; posture; range of motion; and ventilation and respiration/gas exchange. He is functionally limited in self-care and home management and in community and leisure actions, tasks, and activities. These findings are consistent with placement in Pattern D: Impaired Aerobic Capacity/Endurance Associated With Cardiovascular Pump Dysfunction or Failure.[11] Because of the multiplicity of findings, Mr. Hartman may also be classified in additional patterns (eg, Pattern E).[11] The identified impairments and functional limitations will be addressed in determining the prognosis and the plan of care.

PROGNOSIS AND PLAN OF CARE

The objective for Mr. Hartman at this time is to achieve adequate stability in acute physiological responses to allow safety in the upright position for ADL and then transfer to either a long-term acute care or rehabilitation unit.[14] A long and carefully supervised rehabilitation period will be required (16 weeks) during cardiovascular pump healing to avoid

Table 4-8
STRATIFICATION OF RISK FOR EXERCISE EVENTS

Characteristics of patients at lowest risk for exercise participation (all characteristics listed must be present for patient to be at lowest risk)

- Absence of complex ventricular arrhythmias during exercise testing and recovery
- Absence of angina or other significant symptoms (eg, unusual shortness of breath, light-headedness, or dizziness during exercise testing and recovery)
- Presence of normal hemodynamics during exercise testing and recovery (ie, appropriate increases and decreases in HR and systolic BP with increasing workloads and recovery)
- Functional capacity ≥7 METs

Non-exercise testing findings:
- Rest EF ≥50%
- Uncomplicated MI or revascularization procedure
- Absence of complicated ventricular arrhythmias at rest
- Absence of CHF
- Absence of signs or symptoms or postevent/postprocedure ischemia
- Absence of clinical depression

Characteristics of patients at moderate risk for exercise participation (any one or combination of these findings places a patient at moderate risk)

- Presence of angina or other significant symptoms (eg, unusual shortness of breath, light-headedness, or dizziness occurring only at high levels of exertion [≥7 METs])
- Mild to moderate level of silent ischemia during exercise testing or recovery (ST-segment depression <2 mm from baseline)
- Functional capacity <5 METs

Non-exercise testing findings:
- Rest EF=40% to 49%

Characteristics of patients at high risk for exercise participation (any one or combination of these findings places a patient at high risk)

- Presence of complex ventricular arrhythmias during exercise testing or recovery
- Presence of angina or other significant symptoms (eg, unusual shortness of breath, light-headedness, or dizziness at low levels of exertion [<5 METs] or during recovery)
- High level of silent ischemia (ST-segment depression ≥2 mm from baseline) during exercise testing or recovery
- Presence of abnormal hemodynamics with exercise testing (ie, chronotropic incompetence or flat or decreasing systolic BP with increasing workloads) or recovery (ie, severe postexercise hypotension)

Non-exercise testing findings:
- Rest EF <40%
- History of cardiac arrest or sudden death
- Complex dysrhythmias at rest
- Complicated MI or revascularization procedure
- Presence of CHF
- Presence of signs or symptoms of postevent/postprocedure ischemia
- Presence of clinical depression

Reprinted with permission from American Association of Cardiovascular and Pulmonary Rehabilitation. *Guidelines for Cardiac Rehabilitation and Secondary Prevention.* 4th ed. Champaign, Ill: Human Kinetics Books; 2004:63.

overstretching the LV with high activity demands.[2,4] Over the course of visits, the following mutually established acute care outcomes have been determined:

- A safe environment during therapeutic sessions through daily chart review, physiological monitoring with activity, and consultation with medical staff is achieved
- Breathing during activity is controlled
- Cardiovascular risk is avoided with cueing
- Functional work capacity (FWC) is increased
  - This is defined as the highest level of submaximal work performed without unwanted signs or symptoms. It is the level of safely sustainable work: in this case, without falling SBP, ST depression >2 mm, serious arrhythmias, without symptoms of SOB, diaphoresis, or dizziness. No pulmonary rales or S_3 heart sounds noted postexercise on auscultation.
- Independence in bed mobility is achieved
- Risk of skin breakdown is reduced
- Secondary effects of bed rest are prevented[61-63]
- Sitting tolerance is increased
- Tolerance is improved for supervised standing with walker

Based on the diagnosis and prognosis, Mr. Hartman is expected to require twice daily visits (12 to 16 visits) during approximately 2 weeks of physical therapy acute care services.

To achieve these outcomes, the appropriate interventions for this patient are determined. These will include: coordination, communication, and documentation; patient/client-related instruction; therapeutic exercise; functional training in self-care and home management; and airway clearance techniques.

Mr. Hartman will need a transfer after the acute care phase to an inpatient acute rehabilitation service to improve aerobic capacity and endurance and return to supervised community level status. Mr. Hartman would benefit from further assessment of his neuromusculoskeletal status, a differential diagnosis of his dizziness, a fall prevention program, an ambulation program, and patient/family education for safety and home management. Over the course of the visits, the following mutually established rehabilitation/subacute outcomes have been determined:

- Aerobic capacity/endurance and physical work capacity (PWC) are increased
  - This is defined as the maximal amount of work that can be performed during a maximal effort during a GXT. It indicates the cardiac reserve or VO_2 max and offers myocardial protection during activity. As PWC increases, the submaximal HR lowers, and the onset of symptoms that limit activity occur at higher MET levels.

- FWC and activity tolerance for independence in household ADL are increased
- Gait, locomotion, and balance are increased
- Patient will demonstrate decreased risk for falling[64,65] (Functional Reach,[66] Tinetti,[67] and Berg[68])
- Sitting tolerance is increased
- UE cardiac precautions prior to discharge (week 3) are obtained from the physician

To achieve these outcomes, the appropriate interventions for this patient are determined. These will include: coordination, communication, and documentation; patient/client-related instruction; therapeutic exercise; functional training in self-care and home management; functional training in work, community, and leisure integration or reintegration; and airway clearance techniques.

Based on the diagnosis and prognosis, Mr. Hartman is expected to now require twice daily visits (14 to 44 visits) over the course of 3 weeks during this rehabilitation phase.

INTERVENTIONS

RATIONALE FOR SELECTED INTERVENTIONS

Therapeutic Exercise

The patient has cardiovascular pump failure due to having had a complicated MI[24] and is considered high risk.[12,14] The physical therapist should consider the patient as classified in Activity Class I for inpatient cardiac rehabilitation[60] and observe limits for HR, BP, and SaO_2.[12] Cardiac precautions will be followed during all therapeutic sessions. Activity sessions will be guided by the following: facility-approved guidelines using the ACSM contraindications for inpatient cardiac rehabilitation (Table 4-9), the AACVPR criteria for inpatient exercise discontinuation criteria (Table 4-10), and by physician prescribed limits.[12,14] Systolic BP must also be >90 mmHg to begin activity.[24] During activity, the session may be guided by RPE <13 on the Borg Scale (6 to 20 scale)[12,59]; HR <120 or HR_{rest} +20 bpm[12]; oxygen saturation >90%; as well as applying and observing AACVPR criteria for discontinuation of inpatient exercise. Upright activities require monitoring and minimal assistance of one for safety.

Using the ACSM activity classification during phase I offers a stepwise approach to progressing activity that assists in facilitation of communication with physicians and documenting patient progress.[51] However, clinical decision making for progression of activity is based on achieving symptom-limited tolerance and patient safety within the agreed upon physiologic guidelines to provide the most cost-effective use of hospital resources.[69]

Table 4-9

CLINICAL INDICATIONS AND CONTRAINDICATIONS FOR INPATIENT AND OUTPATIENT CARDIAC REHABILITATION

Indications

- Medically stable post MI
- Stable angina
- Coronary artery bypass graft surgery
- PTCA or other transcatheter procedure
- Compensated CHF
- Cardiomyopathy
- Heart or other organ transplantation
- Other cardiac surgery including valvular and pacemaker insertion (including implantable cardioverter defibrillator)
- PAD
- High-risk cardiovascular disease ineligible for surgical intervention
- Sudden cardiac death syndrome
- End-stage renal disease
- At risk for CAD, with diagnoses of diabetes mellitus, dyslipidemia, HTN, etc
- Other patients who may benefit from structured exercise and/or patient education (based on physician referral and consensus of the rehabilitation team)

Contraindications

- Unstable angina
- Resting systolic BP of >200 mmHg or resting diastolic BP of >110 mmHg should be evaluated on a case-by-case basis
- Orthostatic BP drop of >20 mmHg with symptoms
- Critical aortic stenosis (peak systolic pressure gradient of >50 mmHg with an aortic valve orifice area of <0.75 cm^2 in an average size adult)
- Acute system illness or fever
- Uncontrolled atrial or ventricular dysrhythmias
- Uncontrolled sinus tachycardia (>120 bpm)
- Uncompensated congestive heart failure
- 3-degree AV block (without pacemaker)
- Active pericarditis or myocarditis
- Recent embolism
- Thrombophlebitis
- Resting ST segment displacement (>2 mm)
- Uncontrolled diabetes (resting blood glucose of >300 mg·dL^{-1}) or >250 mg·dL^{-1} with ketones present
- Severe orthopedic conditions that would prohibit exercise
- Other metabolic conditions, such as acute thyroiditis, hypokalemia or hyperkalemia, hypovolemia, etc

Reprinted with permission from American College of Sports Medicine: *Guidelines for Exercise Testing and Prescription.* 7th ed. Philadelphia, Pa: Lippincott Williams & Wilkins; 2006:176.

Early mobilization decreases the risk of clot development by preventing blood pooling and stasis.[70,71] Upright posturing will decrease atelectasis and improve tidal volume breathing and oxygenation.[61] However, fluid shifts in upright decrease venous return drastically in this case. LE weightbearing in sitting will enhance sympathetic input to vasoconstriction and encourage muscle activation to support venous return and avoid orthostasis. Gravitation stimulus will encourage resetting of the baroreceptor signal.[61] Weightbearing tasks increase osteoblastic activity preventing osteoporosis and reducing hypercalcemia that may cause urinary tract infections.[61-63]

Mr. Hartman will take longer to accommodate to positional changes due to age-related changes and to the severity of his cardiovascular pump dysfunction and co-morbidities.[72-75] Therefore, frequent intermittent work bouts emphasizing breathing maneuvers to improve oxygenation are utilized. Mobilization using large muscle groups reduces hemodynamic stress that is caused when stabilizing muscles are activated.[76] Isometric and resistive exercises are initially contraindicated

Table 4-10

ADVERSE RESPONSES TO INPATIENT EXERCISE LEADING TO EXERCISE DISCONTINUATION

- Diastolic BP ≥110 mmHg
- Decrease in systolic BP >10 mmHg
- Significant ventricular or atrial arrhythmias
- Second- or third-degree heart block
- Signs/symptoms of exercise intolerance, including angina pectoris, marked dyspnea, and ECG changes suggestive of ischemia

Reprinted with permission from American Association of Cardiovascular and Pulmonary Rehabilitation. *Guidelines for Cardiac Rehabilitation and Secondary Prevention.* 4th ed. Champaign, Ill: Human Kinetics Books; 2004:36.

because HR, systolic BP, and total peripheral resistance increase, while SV decreases when muscle contractions exceed 50% of the maximal voluntary contraction.[77,78] Progression by increasing duration first is recommended for safety reasons, to enhance compliance[4] and to provide time for this older individual to adapt to cardiovascular stress.[72-75] Increasing ambulation distance will improve overall endurance and aerobic capacity while decreasing the risk for mortality.[79]

Management considerations for therapeutic exercise include:

1. Monitoring for signs of medical instability (history of inconsistent mental status, review chart daily for complex arrhythmias, and use ECG/telemetry during physical therapy interventions [check V_5 ischemia])

2. Monitoring lab values and documenting vital signs (check electrolytes especially K^+ for increased risk of arrhythmia, check glucose medications as orthostasis may mask hypoglycemia, regulate breathing strategy impacting on SaO_2 and preload, as well as checking BP adaptations with new activities)

3. Monitoring asthma[80] (check PEFR when expiratory effort permitted and watch bronchodilator use that impacts on HR)

4. Check for signs and symptoms of decompensation (auscultate lung fields pre- and postexercise and record S3 or increased rales post-exercise; check preexercise to determine if patient gained 2 to 3 lbs overnight, had increased coarse rales, has dyspnea at rest, or had sleep disturbed due to orthopnea; ascertain whether systolic BP is falling with increased workload and whether the pulse pressure is <10 mmHg)[2,12,14]

5. Observing for autonomic neuropathy (observe and record for angina equivalents—diaphoresis, pallor, sudden shortness of breath, overwhelming fatigue—and use ECG when possible to detect ischemia, using RPP to document angina or angina equivalent onset where indicated)

6. Ascertaining the history of retinopathy and peripheral neuropathy[37] (observing appropriate BP management

with systolic BP >90 mmHg or <170 mmHg [per ADA recommendations] to start exercise, differentiating dizziness due to balance difficulties versus orthostasis/cardiovascular dysfunction, and avoiding jarring activities).

Patient/family/hospital personnel must keep an activity log of time for all activities. New or unusual symptoms and vital signs (dyspnea level or RPE and HR) are recorded.

Breathing strategies will enhance alveolar ventilation, improve ventilation perfusion matching, and augment venous return.[81-86] Gentle pursed lip breathing will increase intrathoracic pressure slightly slowing the blood flow through the pulmonary circulation.[44,86] This will increase time for oxygen to reach the red blood cells and enhance oxygen saturation on hemoglobin.[87] Airway stability is improved minimizing obstruction to airflow and providing better elimination of carbon dioxide.[88] Mild increases (5 to 10 mmHg) in intrathoracic pressure induced mechanically by ventilators have resulted in reduced preload and lower afterload with improved EF.[87,89-91] Therefore, gentle pursed lip breathing may assist in providing mild elevation of intrathoracic pressure, thus reducing preload and optimizing CO after this patient is removed from mechanical ventilation.[44,86] Cardiac pump function is optimized and systolic BP should improve and may be used as a guiding parameter during execution of pursed lip breathing.[44,86] Because breathing activities impose a change in intrathoracic pressure, these should be evaluated independently prior to incorporation into the activity program.[44,52] Changes in abdominal pressure will have an impact on left ventricular performance and regional blood flow.[92] The therapist should discriminate physiological changes related to activity (increased O_2 demand) and changes related to the impact of breathing on intrathoracic pressure and vascular compartment.[38]

Prescription, Application, and, as Appropriate, Fabrication of Devices and Equipment

♦ Certain compression stockings or devices may be contraindicated at this time as they may increase preload to the heart[93]

♦ Light-weight hose provides enough support to reduce blood pooling and risk for clot without over accentuating venous return while Mr. Hartman is confined to bed

Airway Clearance Techniques

Airway clearance techniques will be taught to Mr. Hartman during his hospital stay to provide optimal oxygenation of blood traveling to the coronary and peripheral arteries. Some strategies may also improve cardiovascular pump function via alterations in preload (pursed lip breathing),[86] while other strategies are important for reducing energy demands associated with inefficient breathing (paced breathing, coordinated breathing).[94,95] Learning forced expiratory techniques for coughing/sneezing is critical to avoid extremely high intrathoracic pressures associated with the onset of Valsalva, where high abdominal muscle contraction may increase left ventricular wall tension.[92,94] Forced expiratory techniques will also promote airway clearance, improve oxygen saturation, and reduce the risk of pneumonia.[96]

COORDINATION, COMMUNICATION, AND DOCUMENTATION

Communication will occur with Mr. Hartman, with all members of the medical team, and with family members to support him in following through with the medical and therapeutic plans. During the acute care stay, the priority is directed toward communicating signs and symptoms at rest and during activity to all members of the medical team so medications can be adjusted and stability achieved.[97,98] The team will have clearly defined physiologic guidelines for activity sessions (activity HR=resting HR level + 20; RPE <13; systolic BP >90 mmHg prior to a therapeutic session; and falling BP <10 mmHg with activity will lead to termination of a therapeutic session).[12,14] The physical therapist will communicate verbally with the critical care nurse in charge by requesting any changes in status prior to each session. Any new therapeutic plans are verbally presented to the nurse, and sessions are scheduled around medical interventions (eg, PCWP readings, x-rays, etc).

Communication and coordination of care occurs through daily rounds, patient/family conferences, and individual meetings between various members of the team. Daily reexamination is implemented by physical therapy, including chart review of pertinent lab results and hemodynamic measures. Activity responses of each session are documented so the patient may receive help from the medical team. Examples of reexamination activity tolerance reports during the acute care stay are listed in Table 4-11. Written guidelines defining "cardiac precautions" will be provided to the family and hospital caregivers. All elements of the patient's management will be documented.

PATIENT/CLIENT-RELATED INSTRUCTION

The focus in acute care is on teaching the patient and family contraindications and precautions.[94,97,98] The patient will be taught basic self-monitoring tools, but he is not expected to be independent. Reeducation for risk-factor reduction and lifestyle modification will be reinforced with the patient and family. New information on secondary disease prevention will be deferred until the rehabilitation stage so the family can attend to and comply with reducing life-threatening behaviors. Instruction should address the following:

♦ Understanding of current pathophysiology responsible for producing symptoms limiting function

♦ Need for compliance with cardiac precautions for activity to enhance safety (no breath holding, no weightbearing on arms, no lifting or straining, keep head of bed upright to at least 30 degrees or as prescribed, etc)

♦ Recognition of signs and symptoms associated with cardiopulmonary compromise and emergency response, cardiopulmonary resuscitation (CPR)[99]

♦ Ways to access emergency response systems

♦ Importance of compliance with nutritional plan (no salt, insulin/glucose intake) and impact on activity program

♦ Identification of signs and symptoms of decompensation of CHF[2,4,38]

♦ Identification of signs and symptoms of activity-related distress and techniques for managing symptoms.

♦ Careful observation during the postexercise period

♦ Skin inspection and identification of vascular incompetence

♦ Benefits of exercise training program and activity guidelines

♦ Recognition of functional limitation with regard to risk for falling and prevention strategies (orthostasis, hypoglycemia, cardiovascular pump incompetence)

♦ Proper use of inhaler and timing prior to activity[80]

THERAPEUTIC EXERCISE

♦ Acute Care Phase
  • Aerobic capacity/endurance conditioning
    ▪ Parameters for endurance conditioning[12,14]
      ► Mode
        ○ Use of large muscles and natural movements
        ○ Variable modes using tasks related to ADL to apply specificity and motor learning principles
          ♦ Sitting for increasing periods of time
          ♦ Transfers
          ♦ Standing for increasing periods of time
          ♦ Ambulation

Table 4-11

CASE STUDY #1: EXAMPLES OF ACTIVITY TOLERANCE REPORTS: DAILY REEXAMINATION DOCUMENTED BY PHYSICAL THERAPIST

PT Day 2

Medical Chart Review:
- RN report: Uneventful night
- Labs: Hgb=13.8; Hct=42.0; Na=140; K=4.0; INR=2.5*; Glucose=140*; pH=7.42; PaO_2=75; PCO_2=35; HCO_3=35
- ECG: Sinus tachycardia, 1 mm ST-segment depression V_5, pathologic Q wave, occasional PVCs
- HR=100 to 110 bpm; BP=100/80 mmHg; MAP=88; CVP=8 mmHg; PAP 18=mmHg
- One report of shortness of breath (SOB), L1 angina with diaphoresis, relieved by sublingual nitroglycerin (SL NTG)

Activity:
- 10 repetitions AROM in supine
- Sat at bedside 4 minutes, transferred to chair with min assist, sat up for 30 minutes

Activity Tolerance:

Activity/Workload	HR	BP	RR/SOB	O_2 SAT	ECG	Symptoms
Rest–Supine	90	100/80	20/1	90%	Q waves (V1-4)	Not remarkable
Supine AROM (post)	100	100/80	22/1+	90%	Occasional PVCs	Palpitations
Sitting 4 minutes	105	96/75	22/1+	90%		
Transfer	138	110/78	22/2+	89%	1 mm ST depress V_5	L1 Angina/shortness of breath RPP=15180
Posttransfer	130	110/70	22/1+	90%	Occasional PVCs couplet	Palpitations

Ausculation:
Clear pre-/postexercise, $+S_4$

PT Day 5—Monitored Floor

Medical Chart Review:
- RN report: Uneventful night
- Hgb=14; Hct=42.0; Na=139; K=4.0; INR=2.5*; Glucose=90*
- ECG: Sinus tachycardia, elevated ST-segment, pathologic Q wave, occasional PVCs
- HR=100 to 110 bpm; BP=100/80 mmHg
- No report of angina

Activity:
- 20 repetitions AROM in supine
- Ambulated 50 feet with rolling walker

Activity Tolerance:

Activity/Workload	HR	BP	RR/SOB	O_2 SAT	ECG	Symptoms
Rest–Supine	90	100/80	18/1	90%	Q waves (V1-4)	Not remarkable
Supine AROM (post)	90	100/80	22/1+	90%	Occasional PVCs	Palpitations
Sitting 30 seconds	108	98/76	22/1+	92%	Q waves	
Standing 1 minute	105	100/84	22/1+	92%	Q waves	No shortness of breath/angina
Ambulating 50 Feet	125	110/70	24/2	90%	Q waves, flip T	Increased diaphragmatic breathing
Post Ambulation— Standing	120	100/70	22/1+	90%	Occassional PVCs, couplet	Palpitations

*Abnormal value

continued

Ausculation:
- Lungs: Clear pre-/postexercise
- Heart: No S_3, +S_4

PT Day 7—Medical/Surgical Floor

Medical Chart Review:
- RN report: Uneventful night
- Hgb=13.6; Hct=41.8; Na=141; K=3.9; INR=2.5*; Glucose=220*
- HR=100 to 110 bpm; BP=100/80 mmHg
- One report of L1 angina/diaphoresis and shortness of breath, relieved by SL NTG

Activity:
- 20 repetitions AROM in sitting
- Ambulated 50 feet with rolling walker
- 3 minutes sitting step-ups

*Abnormal value

- ▶ Duration
  - ○ Intermittent bouts lasting 3 to 5 minutes
  - ○ Rest periods at patient's request, lasting 1 to 2 minutes, decreasing over time
  - ○ Total duration of up to 20 minutes
- ▶ Intensity
  - ○ Use any physician-prescribed endpoints
  - ○ RPE less than 13 (6 to 20 scale)
  - ○ Oxygen saturation >90%
  - ○ Observe for signs of contraindications; systolic BP and ECG are critical
  - ○ To tolerance if shortness of breath, dizziness, or angina/angina equivalents appear
- ▶ Frequency
  - ○ Three to four times daily (PT treatment days 1 through 3)
  - ○ Twice daily (PT treatment day 4)
- ▶ Progression
  - ○ Emphasis on increasing duration first before intensity is increased
  - ○ Continue to consult medical staff; physiologic endpoints for activity
- ● Flexibility exercises
  - ■ AROM: LE exercise into full flexion and extension in semi fowler position or modified sidelying in bed
  - ■ Active open-chain UE tasks that challenge mobility
    - ▶ Moving arms into shoulder and elbow flexion and then reaching into extension to put on button-down shirt
    - ▶ Keeping arms below 90 degrees shoulder flexion and abduction

- ▶ Later (if physiologic measures are adaptive) adding shoulder external rotation and abduction above 90 degrees while combing hair
- ■ Body positioning lying on left in modified position of 30 to 45 degrees incline[61]
  - ▶ Manual mobilization of chest wall on right combined with deep breathing to decrease atelectasis
  - ▶ Therapist stabilizes lower ribs where indicated
  - ▶ Repeat while lying on right if tolerated to increase chest wall mobility on left
  - ▶ Repeat in sitting when tolerated
  - ▶ Exhalation encouraged during effort, no isometric holding
- ● Gait and locomotion training
  - ■ Ambulation 50 to 100 feet as tolerated up to three times per day (Activity Class III)[51]
  - ■ Proper use of rolling walker; eliminate patient excessive gripping and UE weightbearing through the walker, utilization of exhalation during effort
    - ▶ Gripping may introduce isometrics in UE or elicit a pressor response.
    - ▶ Therefore, patient is considered minimally assisted in many upright activities to discourage excessive contraction in muscles of the UEs.
- ● Relaxation
  - ■ Breathing relaxation strategies to decrease anxiety[95]
  - ■ Deep breathing with emphasis on prolonged exhalation (two times exhalation to one time inhalation)[95,100]
  - ■ Gentle pursed lipped breathing during activity[86]

- Strength, power, and endurance training
  - Scapular retractions, back extension, ankle pumps, heel slides, heel and toe raises in sitting
  - Standing toe raises (three sets, 10 reps, two to three times daily)
    - ► Performed if cleared medically, prior to transfer to rehabilitation
    - ► Exhalation during effort
  - Sit to semi-stand activity with exhalation (15 reps, two to three times daily)
  - LE endurance exercises using a restorator (10 to 20 minutes total time performed in intermittent bouts to patient tolerance working toward 2 to 3 times daily)
  - Step-ups in sitting (patient will alternate LEs and step up on 2-inch block repetitively for 10 to 20 minutes total time performed in intermittent bouts to patient tolerance working toward 2 to 3 times daily). Increase step-up height to progress.
  - Active open-chain UE tasks that challenge muscle endurance
    - ► Playing Bingo with ink blotter (dabber) for 10 minutes
    - ► Participate in hygiene tasks of washing face with washcloth, brushing teeth, combing hair, and shaving for 10 minutes
- ◆ Rehabilitation/Subacute Phase
  - Aerobic capacity/endurance conditioning
    - Parameters for endurance conditioning[12,14]
      - ► Mode
        - ○ Continue use of large muscles and natural movements
        - ○ Progressive ambulation
        - ○ Begin LE recumbent bicycle
      - ► Duration
        - ○ Bouts of ambulation lasting 20 minutes
        - ○ Begin recumbent bicycle with 3 to 5 minutes and progress to 20 minutes
        - ○ Rest periods as needed
        - ○ Total duration 60 minutes over 3 therapy sessions
      - ► Intensity
        - ○ Use any physician-prescribed endpoints and ACSM/AACVPR guidelines[12,14]
        - ○ RPE less than 13 (6 to 20 scale)
        - ○ Oxygen saturation >90%
        - ○ Observe for signs of contraindications; systolic BP and ECG are critical
        - ○ To tolerance if shortness of breath, dizziness, or angina/angina equivalents appear

- ○ Document RPP for onset of unusual signs or symptoms and for peak work, quantify work in METs
  - ► Frequency
    - ○ 3 times daily: 2 ambulation, 1 recumbent bicycle
  - ► Progression
    - ○ Emphasis on increasing intensity (RPE up to 12/20) after duration has been increased
    - ○ Continue to consult medical staff; physiologic endpoints for activity
    - ○ Increase ambulation distance to 500 feet (Activity Class V)[51]
- Flexibility exercises
  - AROM: UE and LE exercises
  - Active open-chain UE tasks that challenge mobility
    - ► Shoulder flexion and abduction overhead (beyond 90 degrees)
    - ► Placing arms through a T-shirt
  - Continue chest mobilization as needed in sitting combined with UE AROM
  - Trunk flexion, trunk extension, trunk lateral flexion, trunk rotation in sitting
    - ► Exhalation encouraged during effort, no isometric holding
- Gait, locomotion, and balance training
  - Continue proper use of rolling walker and increase distance
    - ► Increase distance to 200 feet (Activity Classes IV) and progress to 500 feet (Activity Class VI)[51]
    - ► Walking speed increases from 40 m/min to 70 m/min
    - ► Progress from minimal assist to supervised with ambulation using rolling walker
  - Balance activities (Minimal handheld assist provided)
    - ► Weight shift
    - ► Bilateral toe raises; alternating weight to either side
    - ► One leg stand, tandem standing
    - ► Side step using hallway patient railing
    - ► Obstacle negotiation; stepping over and around lines and cones placed on floor
    - ► Progress from minimum handheld assist to supervised
- Relaxation
  - Continue breathing relaxation strategies
  - Continue pacing activities, but taking less frequent rest breaks

- Strength, power, and endurance training
  - Coordinated breathing strategies[95,100]
    - Emphasis on inhalation through the nose with motions that open the chest and exhalation on reverse motions as in the following examples:
      - Inhale as patient performs shoulder flexion or abduction and exhale through gentle pursed lips when returning back to starting position[100]
      - Inhale as patient performs trunk extension and exhale as patient moves into trunk flexion
      - Inhale as patient moves knee to chest in sitting and exhale as the leg is lowered down
  - LE strengthening in sitting and standing
    - Hip flexion, hip abduction, knee extension, knee flexion, ankle plantarflexion, ankle dorsiflexion
    - May begin light cuff and hand weights (1 to 5 lbs) 3 weeks post MI provided there are no unwanted physiologic events or contraindications
    - The patient should exhale with lifting[12]
  - UE strengthening and endurance
    - Scapular retractions
    - Active open-chain UE exercises
  - Step-ups in standing progressing to standard height step; minimally assisted with handheld assist in preparation for stair climbing with railing
  - Stair climbing 12 steps with railing at 60% normal velocity

FUNCTIONAL TRAINING IN SELF-CARE AND HOME MANAGEMENT

- Acute Care Phase
  - Self-care and home management
    - Review all activities and postural alignment for self-care and home management
    - Energy conservations strategies for ADL level functioning[93]
    - Bed mobility and transfer training
    - Increase sitting tolerance to 3 hours in chair with back support
    - Dressing and grooming activities in sitting (rest periods are encouraged)
    - Toileting
    - Incorporate breathing with ADL[100]
    - Exhale reaching down to put on pants and inhale when coming up
    - Patient will be instructed in pacing activities, taking frequent rest breaks, and paying attention to symptoms[94,95]

- Injury prevention education during self-care
- Injury prevention with use of walker
- Safety awareness training during self-care
- Organize the work area prior to performing ADL
- Have height of objects adjusted to avoid lifting, straining, pushing, pulling, or breath holding
- Rehabilitation/Subacute Phase
  - Self-care and home management
    - Review all activities and postural alignment for self-care and home management stressing energy conservation techniques and appropriate breathing strategies with self-care and home management activities
    - Progress to standing at bedside table/bathroom sink for ADL (sitting as necessary or for selected tasks)
    - Simulated home management tasks and task adaptation
    - Injury prevention education during home management
    - Safety awareness training during home management
    - Have height of objects adjusted at home to avoid lifting, straining, pushing, pulling, or breath holding when he is discharged

FUNCTIONAL TRAINING IN WORK, COMMUNITY, AND LEISURE INTEGRATION OR REINTEGRATION

- Community
  - Review all activities, postural alignment, and breathing for community activities
  - Safety awareness training during community activities
- Leisure
  - Playing Bingo while seated
  - Safety awareness training during leisure activities

PRESCRIPTION, APPLICATION, AND, AS APPROPRIATE, FABRICATION OF DEVICES AND EQUIPMENT

- Acute Care Phase
  - Assistive devices
    - Rolling walker
  - Supportive devices
    - Lightweight knee-length hose[93]
- Rehabilitation/Subacute Phase
  - Assistive devices
    - Rolling walker

- Supportive devices
  - Over-the-counter midcalf-length socks with light support

AIRWAY CLEARANCE TECHNIQUES

- Acute Care Phase
  - Breathing strategies
    - Active chest expansion exercises: Directed at increasing lateral costal expansion and activating diaphragm[95,98]
    - Segmental breathing to right lower lobe: Manual cues on chest wall and directed expansion of right lower lobe[95]
    - Modified cough: Forced expiratory technique at low to mid lung volumes[96,101]
    - Use of huff coughing/sneeze techniques to avoid high intrathoracic pressures
    - Paced breathing: Prolonged exhalation
    - Coordinated breathing: Inhalation on arm elevation, back extension; exhalation with reaching to the floor, trunk and hip flexion[95,100]
    - Gentle pursed lip breathing: Prolongs exhalation and decreases respiratory rate[88]
    - Ventilation strategies to encourage relaxation and optimize oxygenation
- Rehabilitation/Subacute Phase
  - Breathing strategies
    - Continue modified cough and huff coughing/sneeze techniques
    - Continue paced breathing, coordinated breathing with activities, and gentle pursed lip breathing
    - Continue ventilation strategies to encourage relaxation and optimize oxygenation

ANTICIPATED GOALS AND EXPECTED OUTCOMES

Acute Care Phase

- Impact on pathology/pathophysiology
  - Atelectasis is decreased.
  - Oxygenation is improved to support metabolic demands.
  - Physiological response to increased metabolic demand is improved.
  - Symptoms associated with increased oxygen demand are decreased.
- Impact on impairments
  - Aerobic capacity/endurance for activity in upright is increased.
  - Airway clearance is improved.

- Energy expenditure per unit of work is decreased as work of breathing decreases and alveolar/arterial oxygenation and tissue perfusion increases.
- Level of alertness is improved.
- Locomotion is improved such that minimally assisted ambulation 50 feet at 40 m/min with wheeled walker (ACSM Activity Class III)[51] is achieved (2.5 METs).[14]
- Motor performance is improved and strength is 3+/5 to 4-/5.
- Ventilation and respiration/gas exchange is improved through breathing control during activity:
  - Medical clearance for physiological examination of hyperventilation and breath holding prior to transfer from intensive care[52] is obtained.
  - Medical clearance for physiological examination of gentle pursed lip breathing and effect on systolic BP, SaO_2, and ECG is obtained prior to implementation in activity program.[44,86]
- Impact on functional limitations
  - Ability to perform physical actions, tasks, and activities related to self-care and home management is increased:
    - FWC is increased to 2.5 METs for:
      - Minimally assisted transfers.
      - Dressing and self-care activities.
    - Independence in bed mobility is achieved.
    - Sitting tolerance is increased to 3 hours in a chair with back support.
    - Tolerance for supervised standing with rolling walker for functional activities is increased.
    - Level of supervision required for task performance is decreased.
    - Patient organizes environment, selects, and utilizes equipment (stools, bed tables, reachers) to modify daily routine.
    - Tolerance of positional changes is improved to allow upright functioning.
- Risk reduction/prevention
  - A safe environment during therapeutic sessions through daily chart review, physiological monitoring with activity, and consultation with medical staff is achieved.
  - Behaviors support medical management plan so risk and therefore disability associated with acute illness is reduced.
  - Cardiovascular risk is avoided with cueing for the following:
    - Exhalation during effort related tasks is achieved.
    - Self-monitoring of HR, RPE,[59,60] and dyspnea[58] is achieved.
    - UE support/tasks are decreased until cleared.

- Symptoms of decompensating CHF (overnight weight gain of 2 to 3 lbs, greater than usual dyspnea, unusual sleep requiring increased number of pillows, and severe peripheral edema)[4] are recognized by patient and family.
  - Patient and family are compliant with dietary recommendations (coordinate meals with activity, monitor glucose/insulin per activity, and support recommendations from nutritional consult).[37]
- Risk of stroke or recurrent myocardial event is reduced.
- Safety of patient is improved as risk of recurrence of condition is reduced.
- Secondary effects of bed rest (DVT or emboli, decreased strength and ROM, skin problems)[61-63] are prevented.
- Self-management of symptoms is improved.

◆ Impact on health, wellness, and fitness
  - Health status is improved as risk of pneumonia is minimized.
  - Patient is able to progress toward greater medical stability.
  - Physical function is improved.

◆ Impact on societal resources
  - Baseline physiological responses are clarified and decision making enhanced to allow effective utilization of resources.
  - Documentation occurs throughout patient management and across settings and follows APTA's *Guidelines for Physical Therapy Documentation*.[11]
  - Interdisciplinary collaboration occurs through case conferences, patient care rounds, and patient family meetings.
  - Referrals or communication regarding changes in patient status are provided where indicated.
  - Utilization of physical therapy services is optimized.

◆ Patient/client satisfaction
  - Intensity of care is decreased.
  - Patient and family knowledge and awareness of diagnosis, prognosis, interventions, and anticipated goals and expected outcomes is increased.
  - Sense of well-being is improved.
  - Stressors are decreased, and less anxiety impacts positively on HR.
  - Stressors related to possible cardiac event are decreased.

Rehabilitation/Subacute Phase

◆ Impact on pathology/pathophysiology
  - Physiological response to increased metabolic demand is improved.

- Symptoms associated with increased oxygen demand are decreased.

◆ Impact on impairments
  - Aerobic capacity/endurance and PWC is increased to tolerance (>5 METs) so that:
    - Independence is achieved in consistently self-monitoring exercise intensity during exercise training (HR, RPE, or dyspnea).
    - Cardiac precautions are applied independently.
    - LE recumbent bicycling is increased with dyspnea at 12/20 Borg to build aerobic capacity exercise training.
  - Balance recovery strategies are improved.
  - Locomotion is improved so that:
    - Independent household ambulation is increased to 50 feet without loss of balance using a cane.
    - Supervised community ambulation is achieved to 500 feet at 70 m/min with rolling walker (ACSM Activity Class VI).[51]
    - Self-paced stair ambulation is achieved at >60% normal rate/speed.
  - Muscle performance is increased so that:
    - Bilateral LE plantarflexor and toe flexion and extension strength are increased to 4/5.
    - Biomechanical efficiency of the LEs is increased through resistance training.
    - Gentle pursed lip breathing during activity is increased, and differentiation is achieved between diaphragm activation and accessory muscle use.
  - ROM of chest wall mobility is increased to decrease work of breathing (expansion at level of axilla is from 3.0 to 3.5 cm and expansion at level of xiphoid is from 2.5 to 3.0 cm).
  - Ventilation and respiration/gas exchange is improved.

◆ Impact on functional limitations
  - Ability to perform physical actions, tasks, and activities related to self-care and home management is increased so that:
    - FWC is increased to 4 METs so that:
      ▶ Independence in transfers is achieved with appropriate device (cane versus walker).
      ▶ Independence in all self-care activities and bathing is achieved.
    - Level of supervision required for task performance is decreased.

◆ Risk reduction/prevention
  - Activities where patient may need close supervision or assistance are known by patient and family.
  - Home evaluation and assessment for safety are performed.

- Patient will demonstrate decreased risk for falling[64,65] (Functional Reach,[66] Tinetti,[67] and Berg[68]).
- Safety of patient is improved as risk of recurrence of condition is reduced.
- Self-management of symptoms is improved.

◆ Impact on health, wellness, and fitness
- Physical function and PWC is improved.
- Risk for morbidity and mortality are decreased.[12]

◆ Impact on societal resources
- Documentation occurs reporting dizziness events related to cardiovascular problems (ie, irregular pulse), hypoglycemia, and unsteadiness due to musculoskeletal problems.
- Documentation occurs throughout patient management and across settings and follows APTA's *Guidelines for Physical Therapy Documentation*.[11]
- Interdisciplinary collaboration occurs through case conferences, patient care rounds, and patient family meetings.
- Utilization of physical therapy services is optimized.

◆ Patient/client satisfaction
- Coordination of care is acceptable to patient.
- Discharge planning is coordinated, and discharge disposition is acceptable to the patient and family.
- Patient and family knowledge and awareness of diagnosis, prognosis, interventions, and anticipated goals and expected outcomes are increased.
- Sense of well-being is improved.
- Stressors are decreased and less anxiety impacts positively on HR.
- Stressors related to possible cardiac event are decreased.
- UE cardiac precautions prior to discharge (week 3) are obtained from the physician.
- Physiological monitoring report of UE tasks is submitted to medical team.
- Guidelines for UE tasks/functions are developed.
- Clearance/consultation regarding ventilatory muscle training is obtained.[4,38]

REEXAMINATION

Reexamination is performed throughout the episode of care. It is anticipated that patients placed in this pattern will require multiple episodes of care over the lifetime. Periodic reexamination and initiation of new episodes of care should occur as the patient's functional limitations or disability changes. This will allow the patient to continue to be safe and effectively adapt as a result of changes in multiple factors including his own physical status, caregivers, environment, or task demands.

DISCHARGE

Mr. Hartman is discharged from his in-hospital stay after a total of 12 to 16 physical therapy sessions over a period of 2 weeks. The acute care stay is followed by a transfer to subacute rehabilitation for 3 weeks prior to discharge to outpatient home health services. A long and carefully supervised rehabilitation period will be required (16 weeks) after this episode during cardiovascular pump healing to increase his aerobic capacity, his strength and endurance, and his functional activities.

PSYCHOLOGICAL ASPECTS

Mr. Hartman is anxious about his cardiac status and risk for another cardiac event. It is important to reassure him and calmly explain a few precautions for him to follow. Providing written instructions to the family and patient will help him review this important information as he may be preoccupied with symptoms and less focused due to changes in mental status. Reinforcement in the therapeutic routine will be helpful.

Mr. Hartman has a supportive daughter, who has been assisting him with household tasks and providing transportation to community outings. Although Mr. Hartman hates hospitals, it would be unsafe to discharge him to home directly from the acute care setting. Enhancing aerobic capacity through endurance training in a rehabilitation/subacute setting will decrease the likelihood that he will decompensate with activity at home. Additionally, Mr. Hartman is at risk for falling. The team must prioritize Mr. Hartman's safety over personal preference. Patients who are post-MI often have denial of the event. Mr. Hartman does not experience typical chest pain, which may make it easier for him to deny the seriousness of his condition. It is important that the family support his transfer to the rehabilitation/subacute facility prior to his discharge to home by reassuring him, bringing in items from home, visiting regularly, and encouraging friends to stop by.

Lifestyle modification will begin more intensively in the rehabilitation phases and will present further psychological challenges. At this stage, it is important to have the family and the patient verbally describe the plan for lifestyle modification as it relates to prevention of decompensating heart failure. Although the family may verbally describe important lifestyle changes (no salt, low cholesterol diet, regular medication schedule), they should also be expected to comply with the plan. Any inconsistencies are to be identified to the patient and family.

Case Study #2: Adult Atrial Septal Defect, Moderate to Severe Tricuspid Valve Regurgitation, Dilated Right Atrium and Ventricle

Ms. Beth Lynch is a 63-year-old female who was admitted through the emergency department with a 5-day history of shortness of breath and dizziness, and a 1-day history of "tightness" across her chest.[102]

PHYSICAL THERAPIST EXAMINATION

HISTORY

♦ General demographics: Ms. Lynch is a 63-year-old, white, English-speaking female. She graduated from a 4-year college with a degree in communications and a minor in business marketing.

♦ Social history: Ms. Lynch is divorced and lives alone in a two-story family home with three steps to enter and 10 steps to the second floor. She has two grown children. Her daughter, son-in-law, and two grandchildren live nearby. Her son and his family are 3 hours away from her.

♦ Employment/work: Ms. Lynch works as an administrative assistant for a chief executive officer in a large corporation. She participates in regular exercise at the local health club where she meets friends for regular workouts 3 to 5 times a week.

♦ General health status
  • General health perception: Ms. Lynch does not know why she was having such severe shortness of breath. She eats right and is active at the health club 3 to 5 days per week, following the recommendations of her physician. Ms. Lynch recognizes that regular exercise and a healthy diet will help control her HTN.
  • Physical function: Ms. Lynch reports she is independent in all ADL without equipment. Her exercise regime consists of walking, stationary bike, and rower for 30 to 45 minutes 3 to 5 times per week. Lately the workouts have caused overwhelming fatigue and unusual shortness of breath.
  • Psychological function: Normal. Ms. Lynch has been divorced for 12 years and is well adjusted to a single lifestyle.
  • Role function: Mother, grandmother, administrative assistant, friend to coworkers and health club exercise group.

  • Social function: She lunches with coworkers and dines with friends from the health club after workouts. She visits her grandchildren on holidays and helps her daughter with errands related to her grandchildren's school activities and soccer team events.

♦ Social/health habits: Ms. Lynch is very outgoing and drinks socially with friends when eating out. She selects heart healthy meals. Her risk factor profile is good. She denies smoking and has no family history of CAD, MI, or diabetes.

♦ Family history: Negative for CAD, diabetes, and obesity. Her mother died of cancer, and her father died in motor vehicle accident.

♦ Medical/surgical history: Ms. Lynch has a history of HTN (7 years) managed with exercise, diet, and Verlan 240 mg QID. She has had surgeries, including a tonsillectomy (age 6) and hysterectomy (age 53). She has mild degenerative joint disease (DJD) in her LEs characterized by early morning stiffness. She requires anti-inflammatory medications on days when she exercises. Four days prior to this admission Ms. Lynch was seen by her primary care physician, who sent her to the emergency department (ED) after office ECG revealed sinus tachycardia and episodes of supraventricular tachycardia (SVT) with HRs of 200 bpm. The ED physician gave her Adenosine and sent her home on Verapamil, 80 mg QID. She returned to her primary care physician 2 days later with persistent shortness of breath. Verapamil was adjusted to 80 mg TID, and she was referred for cardiology consult. The cardiologist saw Ms. Lynch the next day and changed medications to Betapace, Coumadin, and Lanoxin.

♦ Current condition(s)/chief complaint(s)
  • Ms. Lynch experienced increased shortness of breath and chest tightness that precipitated her seeking medical advice, leading eventually to admission to the ED.
  • After ED admission and 5 days of acute care hospitalization and full cardiac work-up, surgical repairs of an atrial septal defect (ASD) and tricuspid valve were performed.
  • She had minimal time on the cardiopulmonary bypass and was weaned quickly from the ventilator. She is presently on 2 L of oxygen via nasal cannula.
  • She is being seen 1 day postsurgery in the ICU by the physical therapist for initial examination. A temporary pacemaker, CVP line, and arterial line are in place. The chest tubes were removed at 2 pm.
  • She is scheduled for discontinuation of the pacemaker and transfer to the Medical/Surgical Floor with portable telemetry.
  • The patient is complaining of nausea.

♦ Functional status and activity level: Preoperatively, Ms. Lynch was independent in ambulation and all ADL without devices, working full time, and participating in regular aerobic exercise.

♦ Medications: Prior to the onset of chest discomfort, the patient was taking Verlan 240 mg QID for HTN and Advil 20 mg PRN for LE pain and inflammation due to DJD. Upon admission to the ED, medications included Lasix 40 mg IV, Coumadin 2.5 mg QID, Digoxin 0.25 QID, Verapamil 80 mg TID, Betapace 80 mg BID. Postoperative medications now include: Tylenol, Darvocet (prn for musculoskeletal pain), Riopan (antacid), Reglan (prevents nausea), acetylsalicylic acid, Benadryl (for sleep), Colace (stool softener), and Slow Magnesium 64 mg. Table 4-12 details the timeline of hospital events.[102]

♦ Other clinical tests: Noted in the chart, not documented directly in the physical therapy note.
  • Cardiac catheterization: Mild pulmonary HTN, pulmonary to systemic shunt ratio of 0.64, coronary arteries without significant disease.
  • Transesophageal echocardiogram (TEE): 2 cm ASD with significant left to right shunting, moderate to severe tricuspid regurgitation and markedly dilated right atrium and ventricle. Right ventricular ejection fraction (RVEF): 30%, LVEF: 65%.
  • Lab values (preop and postop): An * indicates an abnormal value
    ▪ Hgb: 14.4 and 12.8 g/dL
    ▪ Hct: 42.2% and 40.4%
    ▪ WBC: 7,000 and 8,500 mm³
    ▪ CK: 56 and 156* µ/L (normal for females=40 to 150 µ/L)
    ▪ Chol: 216* and 240* mg/dL (desirable <200 mg/dL)
    ▪ PT: 14.4* and 15.6* sec (normal=11.0 to 12.5 sec)
    ▪ PTT: 27.6 and 34 sec
    ▪ INR: 1.37 and 2.5* (normal=0.8 to 1.2)
  • Chest x-ray: Preop showed mild cardiomegaly, right perihilar plate atelectasis, dextrocardia versus right atrial hypertrophy (RAH). Postop chest x-ray shows slight reduction in atelectasis, mild cardiomegaly persists.
  • 12-lead ECG: Preop showed A-fib/A-flutter, right axis deviation, intraventricular conduction delays, RAH, ST-T abnormalities V1-2 with HR variable to 200 bpm. Postop ECG showed paced rhythm during physical therapist examination in ICU with HR of 70 bpm.
  • PFT: Preop revealed FVC=2950 ml (103% predicted); FEV$_1$/ FVC=2428 ml/2950 ml (ratio 82%); FEF^{50}=71% predicted (due to right perihilar plate atelectasis). Postop testing has been deferred.

SYSTEMS REVIEW

♦ Cardiovascular/pulmonary
  • BP: 127/70 mmHg
  • Edema: None
  • HR: 70 paced, consistent spikes on ECG
  • RR: 18 bpm
♦ Integumentary
  • Presence of scar formation: 6-inch incision over the sternum
  • Skin color: Redness and inflammation around the incision
  • Skin integrity: Clean wound, no exudate
♦ Musculoskeletal
  • Gross range of motion: Limited bilateral upper extremity (BUE) movement beyond 60 degrees shoulder flexion and abduction 2° pain and post surgical wound healing precautions[103,104]
  • Gross strength
    ▪ Limited UE strength examination to observable motion only due to sternal precautions/pain
    ▪ LE strength intact and WFL
  • Gross symmetry: Right knee with mild valgus deformity secondary to DJD
  • Height: 5'3" (1.6 m)
  • Weight: 126 lbs (57.3 kg)
♦ Neuromuscular
  • Gross coordinated movements (eg, balance, locomotion, transfers, transitions): Unimpaired
♦ Communication, affect, cognition, language, and learning style
  • Alert and oriented, responding to questions, voice muffled and hoarse
  • Learning preferences: Inquisitive, active participatory

TESTS AND MEASURES

The physical therapist will be offering information to the medical staff to assist management of the cardiovascular status. The process occurs over several visits to see the patient in the ICU and Medical/Surgical Floor, while medical interventions are modified according to the physiological responses observed during functional activity sessions.[52,53,69] The physical therapist will begin with examination of positional changes and sitting tolerance and progress to functional activities in subsequent reexamination sessions.[33,61] This case demonstrates how the physical therapist's examination and documentation of physiological responses may be used to optimize the medical outcomes and progress the patient safely toward recovery. Table 4-12 details the timeline of events.[102]

The following tests and measures were selected for this patient while in the ICU on day 11. The results are indicated below:

Table 4-12

CASE STUDY #2: TIMELINE OF EVENTS LEADING TO HOSPITALIZATION AND INITIAL ACTIVITY TOLERANCE REPORTS DOCUMENTED BY PHYSICAL THERAPIST

Day	Event
1	• Seen by primary care physician with chief complaint of shortness of breath, dizziness • ECG: Sinus tach/supraventricular tachycardia with rates to 200 • Sent to ED, where she was given Adenosine, home with Verapamil, 80 mg QD
2	• Back to physician with persistent shortness of breath • Adjusted Verapamil to 80 mg TID • Scheduled for cardiology consult
3	• Saw cardiologist • Medications changed to: Betapace, Coumadin, Lanoxin
4-5	• Increased shortness of breath, admitted to acute hospital via ED with complaints of chest tightness, shortness of breath • Medications on admission: Lasix 40 IV, Coumadin 2.5 mg QID, Dig 0.25 QD, Verapamil 80 mg RID, Betapace 80 mg BID • Cardiac catheterization: Mild pulmonary HTN, shunt ratio of 0.64, coronary arteries without significant disease • TEE: 2 cm ASD with significant left to right shunting, moderate to severe tricuspid regurgitation and a markedly dilated right atrium and ventricle. RVEF: 30%, LVEF: 65% • Chest x-ray: Mild cardiomegaly; right perihilar plate atelectasis, dextrocardia vs RAH • ECG: A fib/A flutter, right axis deviation, intraventricular conduction delays, RAH, ST-T abnormalities
6-9	• Started on Heparin drip due to continued arrhythmias • Treated with aerosolized medications and deep breathing to reverse atelectasis
10	• Surgical repair of ASD and tricuspid valve • Medications: Tylenol, Morphine Sulfate for pain/temp, Darvocet prn, Riopan, Reglan, acetylsalicylic acid, Benadryl for sleep, Colace, Slow Magnesium 64 mg
11	• Initial PT examination in ICU • Pacemaker (overdrive), central line, A-line, chest tubes removed at 2 pm • CVP=12 mmHg, MAP=90 mmHg, PaO_2=85 (2 LPM O_2 via nasal cannula) • Activity: Sat at bedside x 8 minutes, then returned to supine due to nausea

Activity	HR	BP	O₂ Sat	ECG	Symptoms
Rest	*70*	*127/70*	*94%*	*PACED*	*Nausea*
Sitting	*72*	*104/60*	*93%*	*PACED*	*Nausea*
Supine	*70*	*114/57*	*94%*	*PACED*	*Nausea*

	• Pacemaker removed 60 minutes after PT session • ECG (after pacer removed): Sinus tachycardia, HR=139, right axis deviation, RVH
12	• On Medical/Surgical Floor with portable telemetry • Physical therapy reexamination in am. Patient ambulating 200 feet with rolling walker for safety without complaint. Resting O_2 Sat=96%. • ECG: Normal sinus rhythm (NSR) with occasional premature atrial contractions (PACs)

Activity	HR	BP	ECG	Symptoms
Rest	*91*	*134/59*	*NSR c̄ Rare PACs*	*No c/o*
*Amb. *=BP sitting*	*101*	*130/59 **	*NSR c̄ Rare PACs*	*No c/o*
Supine	*87*	*122/55*	*NSR c̄ Rare PACs*	*No c/o*

	• Converted to A-fib in afternoon; medication adjustment to: Coumadin 5 mg and Dig 0.125 mg in attempt to convert to NSR; no pm PT session • Chest x-ray: Cardiomegaly with mild pulmonary vasculature congestion • Right/left perihilar plate atelectasis slightly improved

continued

Table 4-12 continued
CASE STUDY #2: TIMELINE OF EVENTS LEADING TO HOSPITALIZATION AND INITIAL ACTIVITY TOLERANCE REPORTS DOCUMENTED BY PHYSICAL THERAPIST

Day	Event				
13	*PT defers treatment when A-flutter ratio deteriorates from 2:1 to 3:1.*				
14	**Activity**	**HR**	**BP**	**ECG**	**Symptoms**
	Rest 45° Supine	100	123/69	A fib/ A flutter	No c/o
	Sitting edge of bed (EOB)	116	138/70	A flutter	Fatigue
	Stand/Transfer	130	98/64*	A flutter	Fatigue
	Supine 30°	88	108/80	A fib/ A flutter	Fatigue

- Blood pressure responses are hypoadaptive. Activity session is terminated per AACVPR criteria. Medications are adjusted so Digoxin is increased to 0.5 mg.

15-21	• The patient continued to be refractory to pharmacological management and eventually receives a surgical ablation of aberrant pathways along with implantation of an antitachycardia dual chambered programmable pacemaker with IAD (implanted atrial defibrillator) capability.

*= BP sitting post
Adapted from Carrothers L, Bailey M, Irwin S, Zadai C. A patient with a complicated recovery following open heart surgery. A presentation handout from the Annual Conference and Exposition of the American Physical Therapy Association compendium of handouts. *Physical Therapy '99 Course Materials: Part 2.* Orlando, Fla; June 7, 1999:351-355.

- ◆ Aerobic capacity/endurance
  - Tolerance to sitting bedside for 8 minutes limited by symptoms of nausea
- ◆ Anthropometric characteristics
  - BMI (kg/m^2: weight/height)=22.38 indicating that she is average[12]
- ◆ Arousal, attention, and cognition
  - Oriented x3
  - Limited attention, distracted by pain/nausea
- ◆ Circulation
  - HR
    - Determination of type of pacing (overdrive pacing)[105-108]
    - 70 bpm while lying supine
    - Increased to 72 bpm with sitting
    - Recovery in supine back to 70 bpm within 30 seconds
  - BP
    - 127/70 mmHg in supine at rest
    - 104/60 mmHg in sitting
    - 114/57 mmHg during recovery in supine (1-minute post)
  - Auscultation
    - S$_4$ heart sound, wide splitting of S$_2$

- No carotid bruits
- ◆ Pulse quality
  - Immediate–postactivity pulse quality–faint
- ◆ JVD
  - None detected
- ◆ ECG
  - Atrial overdrive pacing, spikes observed on monitor
  - Pacemaker set in overdrive burst mode to control aberrant tachycardia[108]
- ◆ Integumentary integrity
  - Warm, dry extremities
  - Sternal incision warm, red, and tender to touch
- ◆ Muscle performance
  - Modified tests in bed
  - Intact muscle groups (tested to 3+)
    - LE hip flexors, quadriceps, hamstrings, dorsiflexors, and plantarflexors
    - Palpable contractions for gluteals (2/5 since testing limited by physiological responses)
    - UE shoulder flexion and abduction to 60 degrees limited by incisional pain
    - UE elbow and wrist flexion and extension and grip intact (at least 3+/5)

- Accessory muscle use for inspiration
♦ Neuromotor development and sensory integration
  - Poor speech quality postextubation
♦ Pain
  - Tender over incision
  - Shoulder flexion and abduction (beyond 60 degrees) pain is 7/10 (0=no pain, 10=worst ever)
  - No trigger points over right mid clavicular line in 4th intercostals space, adjacent V_1 electrode
  - Point tenderness (4/10) near right lateral sternum consistent with postsurgical inflammation
  - Anterior sternal pain on deep inspiration (5/10)
  - No reports of increased pain with eating or changes in position during activity to sitting upright
♦ Posture
  - Scapula protracted, shoulders internally rotated
  - Intentional forward head posture
♦ Range of motion
  - WNL for age except
    - Decreased CWE—limited by pain
      - Axilla=2.5 cm
      - Xiphoid=1.0 cm
    - Poor bilateral lateral costal expansion on palpation
    - UE shoulder flexion, abduction AROM limited to 60 degrees 2° pain
    - Pain limits UE shoulder external rotation passive range of motion (PROM) to 30 degrees past neutral (tested with 30 degrees of shoulder abduction, patient inclined 45 degrees supine)
♦ Self-care and home management
  - Positioned in 45 degrees supine, rolls to sidelying on right with minimal assistance of one
  - Sitting at edge of bed with moderate assist of one, limited by nausea and pain
  - Physiologic response and nausea limit full testing this session
♦ Ventilation and respiration/gas exchange
  - Auscultation revealed decreased breath sounds bilateral posterior and lateral basal segments of lower lobes
  - Breathing with an upper chest pattern using clavicular elevation
  - Limited pump handle motion and poor costal expansion
  - Respiratory pattern=Tachypnic
  - Oximetry on 2 L of oxygen via nasal cannula revealed an O_2 saturation of 94% in supine
  - Review of pulmonary function found:
    - FVC=2200 ml (76% predicted)
    - FEV_1/FVC=2000 ml/2200 ml (ratio=91%; test limited by postop pain and precautions)

♦ Work, community and leisure integration or reintegration
  - Ms. Lynch's return to work is contingent upon physiological response to exercise as she recovers
  - Her return to prior leisure activity is unlikely due to permanent right ventricular damage and poor CO.
  - Lifestyle modification and guidance toward resuming some former activities will require several months of cardiac rehabilitation and close physiologic monitoring

EVALUATION

Her history and findings are consistent with a diagnosis of postoperative repair of adult ASD that manifested itself in excessive blood flow from the left heart into the right atria and ventricle. The pressure loads imposed on the right myocardium became excessive, damaging the tricuspid valve, imposing electrical remodeling to the conduction system, and leading to high pressure in the pulmonary system.[109] The ASD and tricuspid values were repaired surgically. Such surgical repairs are complicated by sustained atrial fibrillation or flutter prior to surgery in about 1/5 of patients with ASD.[110] Patients with ASD who have preoperative arrhythmias are typically older and have higher pulmonary artery pressures than patients without preoperative arrhythmias. Ms. Lynch fits the profile.

Postsurgically, the physical therapist must consider that Ms. Lynch will continue to be at risk for persistent atrial arrhythmias that will increase her risk for stroke and emboli.[111] Although the pressure load is reduced by surgical repair, the damage to the right heart is not reversible and continues to contribute to ongoing risks.[102,109,110] The myocardium has stretched, and the patient has poor CO as right heart failure impacts on left heart function (see Figure 4-2)[29] causing drops in systolic BP and poor activity tolerance. At this time, shortness of breath is no longer the factor limiting functional training. Nausea and pain now limit activity in addition to a physiologically inadequate CO that prohibits safe participation in the physical therapy program.

Aberrant arrhythmias persist. A falling systolic BP with positional change and inability to adapt with an appropriate compensatory rise in ventricular rate cause the physical therapist to consider this patient to be high risk.[12,14] Thus, a process of continual reexamination is required by physical therapy along with detailed communication with the medical staff. The physical therapist plays a critical role in providing a complete report of the patient's physiological responses to positional changes and activity for each session. The medical staff will adjust medications and interventions according to these reports. A complete review of the physical therapy reexamination session and adjustments in medical management is summarized in Table 4-11.[102]

DIAGNOSIS

Ms. Lynch is a patient who now has a postsurgical repair of an ASD and tricuspid valve complicated by right ventricular heart failure (RVHF) and aberrant atrial fibrillation placing her at risk for stroke.[102,111] She has pain over and around the incision area. She has impaired: aerobic capacity/endurance; circulation; muscle performance; posture; range of motion; and ventilation and respiration/gas exchange. She is functionally limited in self-care and home management and in work, community, and leisure actions, tasks, and activities. These findings are consistent with placement in Pattern D: Impaired Aerobic Capacity/Endurance Associated With Cardiovascular Pump Dysfunction and Failure.[11] During the early postoperative period, pain and poor ventilation mechanics increases the risk for pneumonia.[112-115] Therefore, Ms. Lynch may also be classified in additional patterns (Cardiovascular/Pulmonary Pattern E).[11] The identified impairments will be addressed in determining the prognosis and the plan of care.

PROGNOSIS AND PLAN OF CARE

The primary objective for Ms. Lynch at this time is to achieve stability in physiological responses to allow safety in upright for ADL and transfer to the Medical/Surgical Floor and then home with outpatient physical therapy. Pain management and restoration of alveolar ventilation to the lower lobes of the lung will be an important part of the physical therapy plan to prevent onset of pneumonia.[94,95,98] Ms. Lynch's surgical incision will be monitored for healing and signs of infection.

Since her right ventricular dysfunction is long standing and chronic, a plan of modifying her lifestyle will be necessary. Ms. Lynch will be instructed in the limitations of permanent cardiac muscle (central) impairment. Increasing aerobic capacity will offer a modest peripheral conditioning benefit that will improve her function, but it is unlikely that Ms. Lynch can expect full normalization of her CO.[102] Additionally, Ms. Lynch will need to be educated in sternal and cardiac precautions[104] and the importance of following the medical plan to minimize the risk of emboli associated with atrial fibrillation and decrease the potential for stroke, pulmonary emboli, and DVT. Over the course of the next week, 8 to 12 visits at least twice a day will be required, and the following mutually established acute care outcomes have been determined:

♦ A safe environment during therapeutic sessions through daily chart review, physiological monitoring with activity, and consultation with medical staff is achieved[52,53]

♦ Independence in bed mobility is achieved

♦ Secondary effects of bed rest are prevented

♦ Supervised standing and ambulation is achieved

♦ Tolerance to sitting is achieved

Upon transfer to the Medical/Surgical Floor, the following mutually established outcomes prior to discharge from acute care have been determined:

♦ Aerobic capacity is increased

♦ Breathing pattern is normalized at rest and during activity

♦ Cardiovascular risk is minimized and sternal precautions are followed

♦ Functional work capacity is increased

♦ Pain over sternal incision is decreased

♦ Posture is improved

♦ ROM is increased for participation of UE in functional tasks

To achieve these outcomes, the appropriate interventions for this patient are determined. These will include: coordination, communication, and documentation; patient/client-related instruction; therapeutic exercise; functional training in self-care and home management; and airway clearance techniques.

Ms. Lynch will be discharged to home with a recommendation for supervision by a family member along with a plan for emergency management at home. Due to the risk of arrhythmias, compliance with lifestyle modification recommendations will need further evaluation through home health medical services. Ms. Lynch will be scheduled for six visits of physical therapy in the home to perform physiological monitoring during usual ADL. Additionally, the physical therapist will design an exercise prescription to build aerobic capacity within safe physiologic limits. After 2 weeks of home physical therapy, Ms. Lynch will attend a monitored, phase 2, outpatient cardiac rehabilitation program. Over the course of 12 weeks, 14 to 36 visits 3 times per week will be needed to enhance aerobic capacity and allow Ms. Lynch to return to full-time employment in a modified capacity and safe participation in modified leisure activities.

INTERVENTIONS

RATIONALE FOR SELECTED INTERVENTIONS

Therapeutic Exercise

All therapeutic exercise sessions will be guided by facility approved ACSM criteria for contraindications (see Table 4-9) and AACVPR criteria to terminate activity for inpatients (see Table 4-10).[12,14] Additionally, physiologic limits will be determined through collaborative discussions with the medical team. For Ms. Lynch it will be especially important to have ECG and BP monitored sessions. Patient participation in the initial ICU session is limited by nausea secondary to postop anesthesia, poor HR response secondary to overdrive pacing (now 70 to 72 bpm), and falling BP with positional changes (127/70 mmHg to 104/60 mmHg). Atrial overdrive pacing interrupts the aberrant rhythms (SVT and uncontrolled atrial fibrillation) providing a safe ventricular rate but does not allow for a baroreceptor mediated compensatory HR response.[105-108] The HR returned to 139 bpm after removal of the pacemaker so digitalis was used to slow the conduction through the heart. This resulted in an acceptable rhythm (normal sinus rhythm [NSR] with multiple premature atrial contractions [PACs]) that does not contraindicate activity. Yet later, after physical therapy on day 12, the patient does not maintain the rhythm and converts back to atrial fibrillation.

Temporary overdrive pacing is intended to correct the atrial rhythm and decrease the ventricular rate. Theoretically, this should improve atrial contraction and provide more complete filling of a weakened right ventricle during diastole.[116] In a mildly compromised heart, the increased ventricular filling would offer improved CO by optimizing the length tension effect in the heart. However, in this case, the BP measures revealed myocardial incompetence suggesting extra filling compromises the length tension of the right ventricle, further contributing to overstretching the right ventricular myocardium. Although the risk of stroke and tachycardia may decrease with pacing,[116,117] in this case pacing compromises CO, so a drop in BP is observed. This patient has a fragile CO response to medical interventions that slow the atrial conduction, yet faster atrial rates also compromise safety.

The physical therapist continually reviews the medical management plan when determining treatment options for each therapeutic session. Although the patient achieves a period of acceptable cardiac rhythms that permit functional training, the rhythm later deteriorates. The initial pharmacological management with digitalis occurs with a dose that is insufficient. The therapist recognizes uncontrolled atrial fibrillation and flutter as a contraindication to activity and postpones the treatment session on day 13.[12,14] The therapist learns that the medical management options for this patient are: 1) further pharmacological management, 2) mapping of the conduction system and surgical ablation of aberrant conduction pathways, or 3) permanent implantable atrial defibrillator (IAD) combined with a dual chamber pacemaker.[116-119] The medical team agrees that further pharmacological management will be the first strategy attempted.

Atrial fibrillation interferes with cardiac function in two ways. First, there is incomplete filling of the ventricles to assist in augmenting preload to optimizing length tension for SV (contributing to a decrease in systolic BP). Second, it may be an indication that there is electrical remodeling due to long-standing right atrial enlargement,[109] which then contributes to the potential for uncontrolled ventricular con-

duction (disturbing the HR component of CO). Therefore, the physical therapist not only examines BP but also reviews the ECG and considers the ventricular rate and the number of atrial beats between ventricular contractions. The AV ratio of conduction is critical to determining whether CO will be able to increase adequately during activity.[102] Further adjustments in the pharmacological management appear to be necessary as the benefits of some medications designed to control for SVT and atrial fibrillation may be reversed when small amounts of catecholamine are introduced, as occurs with exercise.[117,120] When working with Ms. Lynch, if the BP does not adapt to activity or atrial flutter results in an A-V conduction ratio that increases from 2:1 to 3:1 to 4:1, activity sessions are deferred (see Table 4-12, day 13). The physical therapist speaks to the physician about the possibility of increasing Digoxin dosage and minimizing any vasodilating medications that may result in hypotensive BP responses.[102] Because the patient's rhythm deteriorated after exercise, the medical team recognizes that catecholamine may have diminished the effectiveness of the initial pharmacological management, and the Digoxin dosage is increased to 0.5 mg.

Throughout the inpatient acute care stay, Ms. Lynch has episodes of uncontrolled atrial fibrillation with ventricular rates at rest that exceed 120 bpm. Ms. Lynch is classified as having cardiovascular pump failure due to the arrhythmia and falling BP with changes in position.[12,14,38] Selection of activities during each therapeutic session is dependent on careful observation for signs of medical instability and cardiac decompensation. The physical therapist must judge changes in medications for their potential to assist in improving CO to meet activity demands. Over demanding exercise could result in excessive increases in preload to the RV and push the patient into acute failure. Additionally, catecholamine input during exercise will have an impact on conduction and may interact with pharmacological agents, reversing their beneficial effects.[117,120]

When the patient is stable, the physical therapist considers the ACSM recommendations for HR limits during activity for postsurgical inpatients and uses HR_{rest}+ 30 beats/min^{-1} limits as a guide during activity in addition to preactivity screening for contraindications to exercise (see Table 4-9).[12] Activity is discontinued whenever the patient demonstrates atrial fibrillation or SVT as the physical therapist observes AACVPR criteria (see Table 4-10).[14] However, the physical therapist is also cognizant of the evidence in the literature that suggests physical conditioning in patients with compensated heart failure results in reduced symptoms improving quality of life and functional capacity.[121] Therefore, the patient is encouraged to increase ambulation time. Mobilization will minimize the risk of clot formation[70,71] while also improving ventilation/perfusion matching and lowering the risk of pneumonia.[61] The physical therapist also considers the effect of anticoagulants on increased soft tissue bruising when selecting activities and monitors INR values, which should remain purposely elevated.[76] The physical therapist observes for signs of bleeding.

Therapeutic exercises will also focus on gradual restoration of UE ROM and maintenance of LE strength and mobility. Postoperative pain will diminish within 4 to 5 days. As pain decreases, the physical therapist will need to emphasize the importance of maintaining sternal precautions while encouraging UE AROM. The physical therapist will be vigilant in examining the wound for signs of infection (foul smell or excessive discolored drainage) as the patient increases UE function. Additionally, progression of UE ROM activities will be guided by the type of surgical and sternal stabilization procedures employed.[122] The physical therapist will examine the chest wall for sternal stability (observing for even rise and fall of the chest on both sides of the wound during deep inspiration and confirming by auscultation that there is no click or rubbing noise) before implementing more aggressive UE motions.[104] Ms. Lynch is instructed to avoid bilateral UE movements overhead, horizontal adduction across midline, and horizontal adduction past the coronal plane.[104] UE weightlifting will be limited to 10 to 15 repetitions with light weights (1 to 3 lbs) to prevent complications associated with inactivity.

As Ms. Lynch progresses through the episode of care, therapeutic sessions will also be guided by ACSM and AACVPR recommendations.[12,14] UE AROM with light weights (1 to 3 lbs) will be important initially to prevent muscle atrophy and postsurgical scarring. However, formal resisted exercise progression will not be appropriate for the UE for 3 months, in order to ensure complete healing.[12,123] LE weight training will be guided by BP and HR responses and limited to less than 50% 1 RM with proper breathing to avoid excessive sympathetic outflow.[14]

Airway Clearance Techniques

Postsurgical management of musculoskeletal and integumentary systems must also be addressed by physical therapy. Pain management is critical for achieving increased chest expansion and good inspiratory volume prior to gentle huff coughing for airway clearance.[123] Therefore, breathing and coughing activities are planned after pain medications. Postsurgical patients are at increased risk of pneumonia.[112-115] Diaphragmatic and deep breathing exercises are important for increasing inspiratory volume as phrenic nerve inhibition may lower diaphragmatic tone after a period of anesthesia.[114,124] Splinting with a pillow or towel over the sternal incision encourages deep breathing while controlling pain and preventing wound dehiscence.[95]

COORDINATION, COMMUNICATION, AND DOCUMENTATION

Communication will occur daily with the medical team during acute care to obtain the optimal medical manage-

ment for Ms. Lynch.[98] The physical therapist will review the medical chart and communicate with the medical team to determine the appropriate therapeutic strategy for treatment prior to every session. The medical team will have clearly defined and agreed upon limits for lab values (INR and/or PT/PTT)[41,42,49] and physiologic guidelines (ECG and systolic BP) for initiation of activity sessions.[12,14] The physical therapist is familiar with established hospital unit protocols for session to session judgments by the critical care nurse or physician on site. The physical therapist communicates verbally with the appropriate person requesting any changes in status prior to each session. The physical therapist meets with family members to discuss activities that support the medical and therapeutic plans for Ms. Lynch.

The physical therapist will discuss with the medical staff plans for managing poor BP and ECG findings that contraindicate activity or cause a therapeutic exercise session to be discontinued. Specifically for Ms Lynch, it may be important to confirm that the physician sees and believes the report of physiologic responses (specifically falling systolic BPs) obtained during activity. Clear documentation of the patient's physiologic responses by physical therapy assists the medical team in optimal management. The physical therapist seeks to understand the physiologic rationale behind the patient's physiologic responses and symptoms and the adequacy of the medical management plan in improving outcome for activity. The physical therapist discusses options with the medical team in order to seek medical management that will improve the patient's CO during activity. Activity tolerance reports with complete notation of all physiologic variables are used during discussions with the physician to learn whether there will be further modifications of medications to improve CO[102] and to learn whether there is a possibility of surgical ablation of aberrant conduction pathways and/or a permanent anti-tachycardia pacemaker with defibrillation capability. Long-term cardiac stability during ambulation and ADL is essential for participation in cardiac rehabilitation and safe discharge to home.

Communication and coordination of care occurs through case conferences, patient/family meetings, daily rounds, timely data collection, analysis, and reporting in the medical record. Daily reexamination by the physical therapist includes chart review of pertinent lab results, vital signs, and ECG. Interdisciplinary team member comments will also be sought. Activity responses will be recorded in the medical chart to assist the medical team in adjusting medications and assessing overall progress toward achieving cardiac stability. Examples of reexamination activity tolerance reports during the acute care stay are listed in Table 4-12.[102] Written guidelines defining "cardiac and surgical precautions" will be provided to the family and hospital caregivers. Signs will be placed over the patient bed to remind caregivers not to pull on the UEs when assisting the patient with bed mobility. Mini training sessions will be provided to ensure understanding of possible complications pertaining to safety and healing of the sternum for Ms. Lynch.

PATIENT/CLIENT-RELATED INSTRUCTION

In acute care, the focus is on teaching the patient and family postsurgical and cardiac precautions.[97,104] Family members may see Ms. Lynch as having full function with some postsurgical pain. The family may want to encourage her to get up and move despite the risk of arrhythmia and clotting disorder. The seriousness of the disorder will be communicated and will include education about important signs and symptoms to observe and report to nursing. The medical plan for pain reduction and wound healing as well as limb protection to avoid bruising will be explained to the family. Instruction should address the following:

♦ Recognition of signs and symptoms associated with cardiopulmonary compromise and emergency response, CPR[98]

♦ Ways to access emergency response system

♦ Understanding of current pathophysiology responsible for inconsistent ECG and what medically is being done to manage the disorder

♦ Need for compliance with cardiac and sternal precautions to enhance safety (no breath holding, no weight-bearing on arms, no lifting or straining, no raising of arms beyond 60 degrees initially, no extreme horizontal abduction or adduction)[104]

♦ Use of pillow splinting over sternum and huff cough/sneezing techniques[95,98]

♦ Identification of signs of decompensation of right heart (abdominal pain, bloating, overwhelming fatigue, and ankle swelling) as well as secondary impact of decompensation of left heart (shortness of breath out of proportion and increased incline required in bed)[2,4]

♦ Importance of regular medication and blood clotting management

♦ Skin protection strategies during mobility

THERAPEUTIC EXERCISE

In the early acute stage on the Medical/Surgical Floor, ECG telemetry monitoring is in use; however, all central lines were removed so BP monitoring by the physical therapist occurs with each change in position or task. Cardiac and sternal precautions will be followed during each therapeutic session. Therapeutic sessions are scheduled 30 minutes after pain medications at this time. Activity sessions will be guided by facility approved ACSM criteria for contraindications and AACVPR criteria to terminate activity (see Tables 4-9 and 4-10). Therefore, the activity prescription for intensity will be: HR=HR$_{rest}$ +30; RPE <13; and systolic BP >90 mmHg for activity.[12,14,24] Although Ms. Lynch is very functional, she is supervised in all tasks due to her risk for arrhythmia and potential for sudden fainting. Management considerations for therapeutic exercise include:

1. Monitoring for signs of medical instability (ECG review for SVT, A-fib/flutter with uncontrolled rate, low BP)

2. Screening for signs and symptoms of decompensation and worsening heart failure (JVD, abdominal pain, extreme swelling in LE, RR >30 bpm or significant shortness of breath at rest, coarse pulmonary rales in greater than half the lung fields, overwhelming fatigue at rest)[2,4] that would contraindicate activity

3. Monitoring lab values and observing for signs of clotting or bleeding (checking INR and PTT prior to therapeutic sessions and observing for signs of DVT, pulmonary embolism, or impending stroke)

4. Attending to new signs of respiratory distress that may signal infection or pneumonias through auscultation

5. Modifying treatment according to level of pain

6. Applying therapeutic interventions while respecting wound healing status.

♦ Aerobic capacity/endurance conditioning
  • Parameters for endurance[12]
    ■ Mode
      ► Marching while seated at bedside progressing to hallway walking so that large muscles and natural movements of the LEs are used
      ► No UE demands for aerobic training
    ■ Duration
      ► Intermittent bouts lasting 3 to 5 minutes
      ► Rest period should be half the exercise period
    ■ Intensity
      ► Use any team prescribed endpoints (BP lower limit, HR upper limit)
      ► Observe for signs of contraindications
      ► HR is <120 mmHg at rest and rhythm is consistent[12]
      ► ECG demonstrates adequate ventricular conduction ratios <3:1 atrial to ventricular rates
      ► Exercise HR and BP is adaptive and amount of rise is appropriate to medication regime[29,52]
      ► Note MET level of activity that precipitates any aberrant rhythm and keep functional and aerobic training below that level[38]
    ■ Frequency
      ► 2 to 3 times daily
    ■ Progression
      ► To tolerance and appropriate physiologic responses
      ► According to agreed upon criteria for continuation of activity
      ► Working toward continuous exercise of 10 to 15 minutes each session during the inpatient phase

- ◆ Body mechanics and postural stabilization
  - Encourage movement in bed and posturing in upright using core trunk muscles and not UEs
  - Exhalation during changes in position to avoid strain and high intrathoracic pressure
  - Discourage forward head, rounded shoulders, and kyphosis resulting from splinting the painful sternal incision
  - Encourage axial extension of head, easy correct alignment of shoulders, gentle retraction of scapula in all positions
- ◆ Flexibility exercises (as wound healing allows)
  - Towel rolls (less than 2 inches in diameter) will be placed vertically under the spine while lying supine at a 30-degree incline to promote anterior chest expansion with gentle stretch to pectorals[100]
  - Towel rolls (less than 2 inches in diameter) will be placed horizontally under the upper thoracic spine at the level of the axilla while lying supine in bed at a 30-degree incline to decrease thoracic kyphosis and improve upper chest mobility[100]
  - AROM for UE to 60 degrees of shoulder flexion and abduction until wound healing allows for progression to 90 degrees during acute care
  - Scapular retraction performed in sitting as physiologic tolerance to upright improves
  - Add inspiration during scapular retraction and expiration as patient relaxes to improve chest mobility
  - Any breath holding will be discouraged
  - Progress to AROM shoulder flexion and abduction with inspiration while seated upright as wound healing occurs[100]
- ◆ Gait and locomotion training
  - Ambulation 200 to 500 feet progressing to 3 times daily (Activity Class V)[51]
  - Stair climbing on 2-inch high therapy stairs for 2 steps up/down with therapist supervision for balance
- ◆ Strength, power, and endurance training
  - Breathing exercises
    - Active deep breathing emphasizing lateral costal expansion will be added as wound healing allows
    - Emphasis on exhalation with effort and close BP monitoring
    - Ventilatory muscle strengthening using deep breathing with tactile cures for lateral costal breathing emphasizing ventilation to lower lobes[95,98]
  - Ankle circles 10 repetitions hourly until medically stable and ambulatory
  - No isometric exercises
  - Once medically stable, add LE resistance training with weights for major muscle groups (hip extensors, quadriceps, hip and knee flexors) up to 5 lbs.

- Light elastic bands for ankles motions.[12]
- Seek medical clearance for increasing LE resistance and progress to 50% of 1 RM load for 12 to 15 repetitions to large muscles as this is critical for ambulation and function[12]
- Progress according to patient comfort
- Once medically stable, UE resistance training with weights may be added, but is limited to 1 to 3 lbs for 12 to 15 reps according to patient comfort[12]
- Tight gripping of weights is discouraged
- No heaving lifting for 3 months post surgery[12]

FUNCTIONAL TRAINING IN SELF-CARE AND HOME MANAGEMENT

- ◆ Safety awareness training prior to and during self-care and home management
  - Devices and equipment use and training
    - Use of hospital bed with mechanical elevation features to assist in moving into sitting without UE support
  - Attending to symptoms that may require patient to sit down
  - Avoiding activities that are beyond the margin of safety and may precipitate aberrant rhythms
- ◆ Functional training programs
  - Use of simulated environments emphasizing identification of MET level for various functional tasks
  - Practice getting up out of chair or sofa, reaching for kitchen items and clothing in modular home station within the hospital
  - Providing ECG monitoring to demonstrate activities that may precipitate aberrant rhythms
  - Organizing the work area prior to performing ADL and self-care
  - Procedures for modifying ADL to avoid UE support when:
    - Getting out of bed at home
    - Getting into and out of the bathtub
    - Getting up from a low chair

AIRWAY CLEARANCE TECHNIQUES

- ◆ Breathing strategies
  - Active deep breathing using tactile cueing to lateral lower intercostals prior to breath stacking attempts (no glottis closure or breath holding) to increase inspiratory volume[100]
  - Forced expiratory technique for coughing using low to mid lung volumes and pillow splinting to sternum
  - Progression to high volume huffing[95,96,98]

- Coordinated breathing activities; coordinating inhalation with thoracic extension and exhalation with trunk and hip flexion[100]
- Positioning
  - Encourage patient to be upright and out of bed during periods of medical stability to prevent pneumonia and improve ventilation and perfusion[61]

ANTICIPATED GOALS AND EXPECTED OUTCOMES

- Impact on pathology/pathophysiology
  - Atelectasis is decreased as airway clearance improves.
  - Edema of distal extremities is reduced.
  - Pain over sternal incision is decreased to 0/10 at rest and ≤3/10 with UE movement to 70 degrees of shoulder abduction or flexion.
  - Physiologic response to increased activity is improved.
  - Symptoms limiting participation in activity are reduced.
  - Tissue perfusion and oxygenation are enhanced.
- Impact on impairments
  - Aerobic capacity is increased to permit supervised ambulation on the unit >500 feet at 60 m/min at least three times a day (Activity Class V ACSM).[51]
  - Airway clearance and cough are improved.
  - Breathing pattern is normalized at rest and during activity so that:
    - Lateral costal expansion is achieved bilaterally with ≤2/10 pain during deep inspiration.
    - RR is decreased to 12 to 14 bpm.
    - Accessory muscle use is decreased.
    - FVC of 2800 ml or >90% predicted is achieved.
    - Improved inspiration and pillow splint coughing provides enhanced airway clearance decreasing the risk of pneumonia.
  - Energy expenditure for mobility is decreased.
  - Energy expenditure for sitting balance and transfers is reduced.
  - Locomotion is improved so that:
    - Independence in household ambulation on level surfaces is achieved.
    - Stair climbing for 10 stairs with railing for balance is achieved.
  - Muscle performance is increased.
  - Optimal spinal alignment is achieved.
  - Postural control is increased so that:
    - Head is aligned over cervical spine.
    - Humeral head sits naturally in the glenoid fossa without excessive anterior placement or internal rotation.
    - Scapulae are symmetrical and thoracic alignment is normal.
  - ROM is increased for participation of UEs in functional tasks and optimal pulmonary ventilation. The following are achieved:
    - CWE is increased to 2.5 cm at the xiphoid level.
    - Shoulder flexion/abduction AROM is increased to at least 70 degrees with minimal (≤3/10) pain.
    - Shoulder flexion/abduction PROM is increased to 90 degrees per sternal precautions, pending no wound healing problems, for dressing and self-care activity.
  - Ventilation and respiration/gas exchange are improved.
  - Work of breathing is decreased.
- Impact on functional limitations
  - Ability to participate in physical actions, tasks, and activities related to self-care and home management is improved.
  - Functional capacity is increased to 5 METs to allow:
    - Independent dressing and self-care activities.
    - Independent bed mobility and basic transfers.
    - Transfers with modifications to manage sternal precautions and optimize wound healing.
    - Supervised community ambulation.
  - Functional performance of ADL improves as follows:
    - Level of assistance required for physical actions, tasks, and activities related to self-care is decreased.
    - Level of supervision required for task performance is decreased.
  - Participation in physical actions, tasks, and activities related to self-care and role in family activities is increased.
- Risk reduction/prevention
  - Activity demands are safe within physiologic tolerance and limits of CO.
  - Behaviors that promote healing and reduce risk of stroke or cardiac events are acquired.
  - Cardiovascular risk is minimized and sternal precautions are followed with cueing so that:
    - AROM to bilateral ankles hourly and out of bed (OOB) to tolerance to reduce risk of emboli.
    - Episodes of heart palpitations (a-fib) and dizziness are reported to the medical staff.
    - Exhalation during effort-related tasks is achieved.
    - Huff coughing and pillow splinting techniques are employed.[96,98,101]
    - Patient and family are compliant with medical staff recommendations for timely intake of medications.

- Self-monitoring of HR, RPE, and dyspnea is achieved.
- UE support/tasks are decreased until cleared.
- Wound inspection before and after all therapy sessions confirms no activity related stress to healing of surgical site.

- Established emergency management plans and agreed upon guidelines allow for safe participation in the therapeutic program.
- Patient safety is enhanced.
- Protection of body parts is increased and bruising reduced.
- Risks of acquiring a DVT, pulmonary embolism, pneumonia, wound dehiscense, and occurrence of cardiac event or stroke are reduced.
- Safety is improved.
- Self-management of symptoms is improved.

♦ Impact on health, wellness, and fitness
  - Physical function is improved.

♦ Impact on societal resources
  - Accountability for services is increased.
  - Advanced directive, individualized family service, and education plan are obtained.
  - Decision making for medical management and appropriate implementation of the therapeutic plan is enhanced through full interpretation of documented physiologic response to activity.
  - Documentation occurs throughout patient management and across settings to ensure continuity of care and to optimize patient safety while enhancing decision making.
  - Individual physical therapy session summaries are prepared according to the APTA's *Guidelines for Physical Therapy Documentation.*[11]
  - Intensity of care is decreased and disability associated with acute illness is reduced.
  - Utilization of physical therapy services is optimized, and cost of health care services is decreased.

♦ Patient/client satisfaction
  - Access, availability, and services provided are acceptable to patient.
  - Discharge disposition is acceptable.
  - Intensity of care and cost of health care services are decreased.
  - Patient, family, and caregiver knowledge and awareness of diagnosis, prognosis, interventions, and anticipated goals and expected outcomes are increased.
  - Patient sense of well-being is improved.
  - Stressors are decreased.
  - Therapeutic plan is implemented without adverse events or delays.

REEXAMINATION

Reexamination is performed throughout the episode of care. It is anticipated that patients placed in this pattern may require multiple episodes of care. Periodic reexamination and initiation of new episodes of care should occur as the patient's functional limitations or disability changes. This will allow the patient to continue to be safe and effectively adapt as a result of changes in multiple factors including her own physical status, environment, or task demands.

Initially reexamination focuses on achieving medical stability and managing patient risk of pneumonia, clotting, and decompensating heart failure. Auscultation reveals gradual clearing of atelectasis. Oxygen saturation improvement corresponds to clearing by day 12 (see Table 4-12). Auscultation of lung fields occurs daily prior to exercise and confirms that there is no pulmonary edema occurring and no left ventricular compromise from mechanic encroachment of right ventricular failure (see Figure 4-2). Each day the therapist confirms that right ventricular function is adequate by noting that there is no JVD, abdominal pain, or excessive peripheral edema and that auscultation of the heart reveals no split S_2 at rest.[44] The physical therapist also monitors the BP during activity and positional changes, which indicate whether the patient's heart failure is compensated. The therapist notes an appropriate HR and BP response prior to and during ambulation briefly after pacemaker removal on day 12. The ECG is observed on monitors in the hall as the patient ambulates. Normal sinus rhythm is present with occasional PACs, and the patient is able to ambulate 200 feet. Heart and lung sounds occurring before and after do not change. However, the rhythm converts to atrial fibrillation by afternoon on day 12 and a contraindicated rhythm is observed on day 13 so this session is postponed. The physical therapist awaits further medical management.

Patient/family/hospital personnel keep an activity log of time for all activities. ECG and BP responses are documented and follow the patient from one setting or hospital unit to another. The role of the physical therapist shifts depending upon patient medical status. During the initial period of medical instability the role of the physical therapist is careful physiologic monitoring with documentation and communication that facilitate decision making for the medical team. The physical therapist is also responsible for prevention of adverse affects of bed rest and immobility (contractures, muscle atrophy, pneumonia, DVT, etc) at this time.[61-63] Prevention may be achieved through frequent monitored postural perturbations during therapeutic sessions.[61,76]

Over time, the medical team determines the patient's heart is refractory to pharmacological management, a second surgery will need to be performed. Eventually, the patient receives surgical ablation of aberrant conduction pathways and implantable defibrillator with dual chamber pacemaker functions. The physical therapist learns how the pacemaker is programmed and how it may affect the CO during activity. During the subacute phase, interventions are directed toward safe recovery of function and discharge to her daughter's home. The physical therapist in the acute care setting recommends discharge to her daughter's home with home physical therapy.

The home physical therapist will provide further examination of the physiologic responses during ADL and document the workload imposed. Ms. Lynch will be educated about which tasks may precipitate decompensation or pacemaker activation. The home physical therapist will communicate physiologic reports to the physician to facilitate appropriate programming of the pacemaker. The home physical therapist will assist in identifying safe participation in self-care and home management tasks. Auscultation of heart and lung sounds occurs before and after each session, as well as screening for signs of decompensation or inappropriate pacemaker response (pulse palpation, BP responses, shortness of breath out of proportion, sudden overnight weight gain, etc) during every visit by the home physical therapist. Ms. Lynch will then be cleared for safe participation in outpatient cardiac rehabilitation.

DISCHARGE

Ms. Lynch is discharged from her acute care stay after a total of 15 to 20 physical therapy sessions over a period of 3 weeks. These sessions have been a continuation of an episode of care that began in the ICU, progressed to a Medical/Surgical Floor, and continued on a monitored floor. Reexamination procedures performed in physical therapy assist the medical team in selection of the optimal medical and surgical management. The patient recovers after a second surgical procedure. The long-term outcomes at home will continue to build endurance for home management. Increasing endurance will increase cardiac reserve that will offer protection against cardiac decompensation and development of comorbidities (pneumonia, respiratory tract infections, etc).

REFERENCES

1. Ellestad M. Cardiovascular and pulmonary responses to exercise. In: Ellestad M, ed. *Stress Testing. Principles and Practice.* 3rd ed. Philadelphia, Pa: FA Davis; 1986:9-37.
2. Cahalin L. Cardiac muscle dysfunction. In: Hillegass EA, Sadowsky HS, eds. *Essentials of Cardiopulmonary Physical Therapy.* 2nd ed. Philadelphia, Pa: WB Saunders Co; 2001:106-181.
3. Skloven ZD. Hemodynamics. In: Irwin S, Tecklin JS, eds. *Cardiopulmonary Physical Therapy.* 3rd ed. St. Louis, Mo: Mosby; 1995:22-33.
4. Cahalin LP. Heart failure. *Phys Ther.* 1996;76(5):516-534.
5. Certo C. Guidelines for exercise prescription in congestive heart failure. *Cardiopulm Phys Ther.* 2001;12(2):39-45.
6. Watchie J. Cardiopulmonary pathology. In: Watchie J, ed. *Cardiopulmonary Physical Therapy. A Clinical Manual.* Philadelphia, Pa: WB Saunders Co; 1995:67-84.
7. Wilmore JH, Costill DL. Cardiovascular and respiratory adaptations to training. In: *Physiology of Sport and Exercise.* 3rd ed. Champagne, Ill: Human Kinetics; 2004:271-301.
8. Morey MC, Pieper CF, Cornoni-Huntley J. Physical fitness and functional limitations in community-dwelling older adults. *Med Sci Sports Exerc.* 1998;30:715-723.
9. Morey MC, Pieper CF, Cornoni-Huntley J. Is there a threshold between peak oxygen uptake and self-reported physical functioning in older adults? *Med Sci Sports Exerc.* 1998;30:1223-1229.
10. Tepper, S. Examination and treatment for patients with endurance impairments: an intermediate level course for practicing therapists. A presentation handout from APTA Combined Sections Meeting Pre-conference Course. San Antonio, Texas; February 14, 2001:4.
11. American Physical Therapy Association. *Guide to Physical Therapist Practice.* Rev 2nd ed. Alexandria, Va: American Physical Therapy Association; 2003.
12. American College of Sports Medicine. *Guidelines for Exercise Testing and Prescription.* 7th ed. Philadelphia, Pa: Lippincott Williams & Wilkins; 2006.
13. The Criteria Committee of the New York Heart Association. *Nomenclature and Criteria for Diagnosis of Diseases of the Heart and Great Vessels.* 9th ed. Boston, Mass: Little, Brown & Co; 1994:253-256.
14. American Association of Cardiovascular and Pulmonary Rehabilitation. *Guidelines for Cardiac Rehabilitation and Secondary Prevention.* 4th ed. Champaign, Ill: Human Kinetics Books; 2004.
15. Agency for Health Care Policy and Research. Clinical Practice Guideline (No. 17). *Cardiac Rehabilitation.* US Department of Health and Human Services. AHCPR publication no. 96-0672, October 1995.
16. Cohen M, Michel TH. *Cardiopulmonary Symptoms in Physical Therapy Practice.* New York, NY: Churchill Livingstone; 1988.
17. Grimes K. Heart disease. In: O'Sullivan SB, Schmitz TJ, eds. *Physical Rehabilitation: Assessment and Treatment.* 4th ed. Philadelphia, Pa: FA Davis Co; 2001:471-518.
18. Watchie J. Cardiopulmonary implications of specific diseases. In: Hillegass EA, Sadowsky HS, eds. *Essentials of Cardiopulmonary Physical Therapy.* 2nd ed. Philadelphia, Pa: WB Saunders Co; 2001:285-292.
19. Irwin S. Normal and abnormal cardiopulmonary responses to exercise. In: Irwin S, Tecklin JS, eds. *Cardiopulmonary Physical Therapy. A Guide to Practice.* 4th ed. St. Louis, Mo: Mosby; 2004:82-101.
20. Sheps DS, Ernst JC, Briese FW, Myerburg RJ. Exercise-induced increase in diastolic pressure: indicator of severe coronary artery disease. *Am J Cardiol.* 1979;43:708-712.

21. Go BM, Sheffield D, Krittayaphong R, et al. Association of systolic BP at time of myocardial ischemia with angina pectoris during exercise testing. *Am J Cardiol.* 1997;79:954-956.

22. Ellestad M. Physiology of cardiac ischemia. In: Ellestad M, ed. *Stress Testing. Principles and Practice.* 3rd ed. Philadelphia, Pa: FA Davis Co; 1986:71-104.

23. Irwin S. Cardiac disease and pathophysiology. In: Irwin S, Tecklin JS, eds. *Cardiopulmonary Physical Therapy. A Guide to Practice.* 4th ed. St. Louis, Mo: Mosby; 2004:123-144.

24. McNeer JF, Wallance AG, Wagner GS, et al. The course of acute myocardial infarction. Feasibility of early discharge of the uncomplicated patient. *Circulation.* 1975;51(3):410-413.

25. Watchie J. Cardiology. In: Watchie J, ed. *Cardiopulmonary Physical Therapy. A Clinical Manual.* Philadelphia, Pa: WB Saunders Co; 1995:22-23.

26. Ceisla ND, Murdock KR. Lines, tubes, catheters, and physiological monitoring in the ICU. *Cardiopul Phys Ther.* 2000;11(1):16-25.

27. Hillegass EA. Cardiovasculascular diagnostic tests and procedures. In: Hillegass EA, Sadowsky HS, eds. *Essentials of Cardiopulmonary Physical Therapy.* 2nd ed. Philadelphia, Pa: WB Saunders Co; 2001:336-377.

28. Sadowsky HS. Monitoring and life-support equipment. In: Hillegass EA, Sadowsky HS, eds. *Essentials of Cardiopulmonary Physical Therapy.* 2nd ed. Philadelphia, Pa: WB Saunders Co; 2001:509-534.

29. Marino PL. *The ICU Book.* Malvern, Pa: Lea and Febiger; 1991.

30. Austin GL, Greenfield LJ. Respiratory care in cardiac failure and pulmonary edema. *Surg Clin N Am.* 1980; 60:1565-1575.

31. Matthay MA. Pathophysiology of pulmonary edema. *Clinics in Chest Medicine.* 1985;6:301-314.

32. Cahalin L. Pulmonary hypertension and exercise. *Cardiopulm Phys Ther.* 1995;6:3-12.

33. Gibbs JSR, Keegan J, Wright C, et al. Pulmonary artery pressure changes during exercise and daily activities in chronic heart failure. *J Am Coll Cardiol.* 1990;15:52.

34. Widmaier EP, Raff H, Strang KT. Cardiovascular physiology. In: Widmaier EP, Raff H, Strang KT, eds. *Vander's Human Physiology. The Mechanisms of Body Function.* 10th ed. Boston, Mass: The McGraw Hill Co; 2006:387-458.

35. Drexler H, Riede U, Munzel T, et al. Alterations of skeletal muscle in chronic heart failure. *Circulation.* 1992;85:1751-1759.

36. Cicoira M, Zanolla L, Franceschini L, et al. Skeletal muscle mass independently predicts peak oxygen consumption and ventilatory response during exercise in noncachectic patients with chronic heart failure. *J Am Coll Cardiol.* 2001;37:2080-2085.

37. American Diabetes Association Position Statements. 2004;27: S1-137. Available at: http://care.diabetesjournals.org/cgi/content/full/27/suppl_1/s58. Accessed January 13, 2004.

38. Cahalin LP, Buck LA. Physical therapy associated with cardiovascular pump dysfunction and failure. In: DeTurk WE, Cahalin LP, eds. *Cardiovascular and Pulmonary Physical Therapy: An Evidence-Based Approach.* New York, NY: McGraw-Hill Co; 2004.

39. Seventh Report of the Joint National Committee on Prevention, Detection, Evaluation, and Treatment of High BP

(JNC 7). NIH Publication No. 03-5231, May 2003. Available at: http//www.nhlbi.nih.gov. Accessed October 10, 2003.

40. Lown B, Wolf M. Approaches to sudden death from coronary heart disease. *Circulation.* 1971;44:130-142.

41. Polich S, Faynor SM. Interpreting lab test values. *PT Magazine.* 1996;4:76-88.

42. Irion GL. Lab values update. *Acute Care Perspectives.* 2004; 13(1):1-5.

43. Knudsen CW, Omland T, Clopton P, et al. Diagnostic value of B-type naturetic peptide and chest radiographic findings in patients with acute dyspnea. *Am J Med.* 2004;116:363-368.

44. Cahalin LP. Cardiovascular evaluation. In: DeTurk WE, Cahalin LP, eds. *Cardiovascular and Pulmonary Physical Therapy: An Evidence-Based Approach.* New York, NY: McGraw-Hill Co; 2004.

45. Widmaier EP, Raff H, Strang KT. Respiratory physiology. In: Widmaier EP, Raff H, Strang KT, eds. *Vander's Human Physiology. The Mechanisms of Body Function.* 10th ed. Boston, Mass: McGraw Hill Co; 2006:477-500.

46. Beckman Coulter, Inc. Array® Protein System. Available at: http://www.beckmancoulter.com/literature/ClinDiag/array.pdf. Accessed September 12, 2006.

47. Bank AJ, Kubo SH. Congestive heart failure: inotropic agents. In: Parillo JE, Herrick JB, eds. *Current Therapy in Critical Care Medicine.* 2nd ed. Philadelphia, Pa: BC Decker; 1991:92-96.

48. Ciccone CD. Current trends in cardiovascular pharmacology. *Phys Ther.* 1996;76(5):481-497.

49. Ciccone CD. *Pharmacology in Rehabilitation.* 2nd ed. Philadelphia, Pa: FA Davis Co; 1996.

50. Shannon MT, Wilson BA, Stang CL, eds. *Prentice Hall Health Professionals Drug Guide 2003.* Upper Saddle River, NJ: Pearson Education Inc; 2003.

51. American College of Sports Medicine. *Guidelines for Exercise Testing and Prescription.* 6th ed. Philadelphia, Pa: Lippincott Williams & Wilkins; 2000.

52. Irwin S, Blessey RL. Patient evaluation. In: Irwin S, Tecklin JS, eds. *Cardiopulmonary Physical Therapy.* 3rd ed. St. Louis, Mo: Mosby; 1995:106-141.

53. Butler SM. Phase one cardiac rehabilitation: the role of functional evaluation in patient progression. Master's thesis. Atlanta, Ga: Emory University; 1983.

54. Comoss PM. The new infrastructure for cardiac rehabilitation practice. In: Wenger NK, Smith LK, Froelicher ES, Comoss PM, eds. *Cardiac Rehabilitation: A Guide to Practice in the 21st Century.* New York, NY: Marcel Dekker; 1999:315-326.

55. LaPier TK. Assessment and intervention during phase I cardiac rehabilitation. *Acute Care Perspectives.* 2000;8(3):6-14.

56. Eason JM. Cardiopulmonary assessment. *Cardiopulm Phys Ther.* 1999;10(4):135-142.

57. Kinney LaPier T, Jones C, Kreizenbeck H, McDowell R. Normal rib mobility: chest wall excursion values in supine and standing (Abstract). *Cardiopulm Phys Ther.* 2000;11(4):161.

58. Frownfelter D, Ryan J. Dyspnea: measurement and evaluation. *Cardiopulm Phys Ther.* 2000;11(1):7-15.

59. Borg G. Psychophysiological bases of perceived exertion. *Med Sci Sports Exerc.* 1982;14:77-381.

60. Scherer S, Cassady SL. Rating of perceived exertion: development and clinical applications for physical therapy exercise testing and prescription. *Cardiopulm Phys Ther.* 1999; 10(4):143-147.

61. Dean E. Body positioning. In: Frownfelter D, Dean E, eds. *Cardiovascular and Pulmonary Physical Therapy. Evidence for Practice.* 4th ed. St. Louis, Mo: Mosby; 2006:307-324.

62. Convertino VA, Bloomfield SA, Greenleaf JE. An overview of the issues: physiological effects of bed rest and restricted physical activity. *Med Sci Sports Exerc.* 1997;29(2):187-190.

63. Convertino VA. Cardiovascular consequences of bed rest: effect on maximal oxygen uptake. *Med Sci Sports Exerc.* 1997; 29(2):191-196.

64. Shumway-Cook A, Baldwin M, Pollisar N, Gruber W. Predicting the probability of falls in community dwelling older adults. *Phys Ther.* 1997;77:812-819.

65. Shumway-Cook A, Gruber W, Baldwin M, Liao S. The effect of multidimensional exercises on balance, mobility and fall risk in community dwelling older adults. *Phys Ther.* 1997;77:46-57.

66. Duncan P, Studenski S, Chandler J, Prescott B. Functional reach: a new clinical measure of balance. *J Gerontol.* 1990;45: M192-M197.

67. Tinetti ME. Performance oriented assessment of mobility problems in elderly patients. *J Am Geriatr Soc.* 1986;34:119-126.

68. Berg K, Wood-Dauphinee S, Williams J, Gayton D. Measuring balance in the elderly: preliminary development of an instrument. *Physiother Canada.* 1989;41:304-308.

69. Cronqvist A, Faager G, Larsen FF, Schenck-Gustafsson K. Stepwise versus symptom-limited in-hospital mobilization after acute myocardial infarction. *Physiother Theory Pract.* 1996;12:67-75.

70. Weill-Engerer S, Meaume S, Lahlou A, et al. Risk factors for deep vein thrombosis in inpatients aged 65 and older: a case-control multicenter study. *J Am Geriatr Soc.* 2004;52(8):1299-1304.

71. Partsch H, Blattler W. Compression and walking versus bed rest in the treatment of proximal deep venous thrombosis with low molecular weight heparin. *J Vasc Surg.* 2000; 32:861-869.

72. Protas E. The aging patient. In: Frownfelter D, Dean E, eds. *Cardiovascular and Pulmonary Physical Therapy. Evidence for Practice.* 4th ed. St. Louis, Mo: Mosby; 2006:685-693.

73. Chandler JM, Hadley EC. Exercise to improve physiologic and functional performance in old age. *Clin Geriatr Med.* 1996;12(4):761-784.

74. Polich S, Wetzel J. Declining functional status in a deconditioned geriatric patient. *Phys Ther Case Reports.* 2000; 3(4): 171-180.

75. Smith EL, Gilligan C. Physical activity prescription for the older adult. *Phys and Sports Med.* 1983;11(8):91-101.

76. Dean E. Intensive care management of individuals with primary cardiopulmonary dysfunction. In: Frownfelter D, Dean E, eds. *Cardiovascular and Pulmonary Physical Therapy. Evidence for Practice.* 4th ed. St. Louis, Mo: Mosby; 2006:625-638.

77. Pollock ML, Franklin BA, Balady GJ, et al. Resistance exercise in individuals with and without cardiovascular disease: benefits, rationale, safety and prescription. An advisory from the Committee on Exercise, Rehabilitation, and Prevention, Council on Clinical Cardiology, American Heart Association. Position paper endorsed by the American College of Sports Medicine. *Circulation.* 2000;101(7):828-833.

78. Hanson P, Nagle F. Isometric exercise: cardiovascular responses in normal and cardiac populations. In: Hanson P, ed. *Exercise and the Heart.* Philadelphia, Pa: WB Saunders Co; 1987.

79. Cahalin LP, Mathier MA, Semigran MJ, et al. The six-minute walk test predicts peak oxygen uptake and survival in patients with advanced heart failure. *Chest.* 1996;110:325-332.

80. Chesnutt MS. Management of asthma exacerbations. Clin Cornerstone. Posted 9/05/2002;4(6):1-17. Available at: http://www.medscape.com/viewarticle/439359. Accessed November 12, 2002.

81. Takata M, Robotham JL. Effects of inspiratory diaphragmatic descent on inferior vena caval venous return. *J Appl Phys.* 1992;72(2):597-607.

82. Takata M, Wise RA, Robotham JL. Effects of abdominal pressure on venous return: abdominal vascular zone conditions. *J Appl Phys.* 1990;69(6):1961-1972.

83. Ferguson JJ 3rd, Miller MJ, Sahagian P, et al. Effects of respiration and vasodilation on venous volume in animals and man, as measured with an impedance catheter. *Catheterization Cardiovasc Diag.* 1989;16(1):25-34.

84. Willeput R, Rondeux C, De Troyer A. Breathing affects venous return from legs in humans. *J Appl Phys.* 1984; 57(4):971-976.

85. Lloyd TC Jr. Effect on breathing of acute pressure rise in pulmonary artery and right ventricle. *J Appl Phys.* 1984; 57(1):110-116.

86. Cahalin LP. Cardiopulmonary dysfunction: practical application of physiologic principles. In: *Physical Therapy '98 Course Materials: A Compendium of Conference Handouts.* Part 2. Washington, DC: American Physical Therapy Association; 1998:281-285.

87. Genovese J, Moskowitz M, Tarasiuk A, et al. Effects of continuous positive airway pressure on cardiac output in normal and hypovolemic unanesthetized pigs. *Am J Respir Crit Care Med.* 1994;150:752-758.

88. Dechman G, Wilson CR. Evidence underlying breathing retraining in people with stable chronic obstructive pulmonary disease. *Phys Ther.* 2004;84:1189-1197.

89. Acosta B, DiBenedetto R, Rahimi A, et al. Hemodynamic effects of noninvasive bi-level positive airway pressure on patients with chronic congestive heart failure with systolic dysfunction. *Chest.* 2000;118(4):1004-1009.

90. Naughton MT, Rahman A, Hara K, et al. Effect of continuous positive airway pressure on intrathoracic and left ventricular transmural pressures in patients with congestive heart failure. *Circulation.* 1995;91:1725-1731.

91. O'Donnell DE, D'Arsigny C, Raj S, et al. Ventilatory assistance improves exercise endurance in stable congestive heart failure. *Am J Resp Crit Care Med.* 1999;160:1804-1811.

92. Robotham JL, Wise RA, Bromberger-Barnea B. Effects of changes in abdominal pressure on left ventricular performance and regional blood flow. *Critical Care Medicine.* 1985; 13(10):803-809.

93. Reid T. Congestive heart failure. Dr. Reid's Corner. Peninsula Medical, Inc. Available at: http://www.lymphedema.com/heart.htm. Accessed August 22, 2005.

94. Watchie J. Cardiopulmonary physical therapy treatment. In: Watchie J, ed. *Cardiopulmonary Physical Therapy. A Clinical Manual.* Philadelphia, Pa: WB Saunders Co: 1995:197-225.

95. Kisner C, Colby LA. Management of pulmonary conditions. In: Kisner C, Colby LA, eds. *Therapeutic Exercise Foundations and Techniques.* 4th ed. Philadelphia, Pa: FA Davis Co; 2002:758-760.

96. Downs AM. Clinical application of airway clearance techniques. In: Frownfelter D, Dean E, eds. *Cardiovascular and Pulmonary Physical Therapy. Evidence for Practice.* 4th ed. St. Louis, Mo: Mosby; 2006:341-362.

97. LaPier TK. Patient education during phase I cardiac rehabilitation: a case example. *Acute Care Perspectives.* 2000;8(3):1-5, 20-22.

98. Sciaky A, Stockford J, Nixon E. Treatment of acute cardiopulmonary conditions. In: Hillegass EA, Sadowsky HS, eds. *Essentials of Cardiopulmonary Physical Therapy.* 2nd ed. Philadelphia, Pa: WB Saunders Co; 2001:647-675.

99. 2005 American Heart Association Guidelines for Cardiopulmonary Resuscitation and Emergency Cardiovascular Care. Circulation. 2005;112(Suppl I):IV18-IV34. Available at http://www.circuationaha.org. Accessed January 12, 2006.

100. Frownfelter D, Massery M. Facilitating ventilation patterns and breathing strategies. In Frownfelter D, Dean E, eds. *Cardiovascular and Pulmonary Physical Therapy. Evidence for Practice.* 4th ed. St. Louis, Mo: Mosby; 2006:377-403.

101. Pryor JA. The forced expiratory technique. In: Pryor JA. ed. *Respiratory Care.* Edinburgh: Churchill Livingstone; 1991.

102. Carrothers L, Bailey M, Irwin S, Zadai C. A patient with a complicated recovery following open heart surgery. A presentation handout from the Annual Conference and Exposition of the American Physical Therapy Association compendium of handouts. Physical Therapy '99 Course Materials: Part 2. Orlando, Fla; June 7, 1999:351-355.

103. Robicsek F, Daugherty HK, Cook JW. The prevention and treatment of sternum separation following open-heart surgery. *J Thorac Cardiovasc Surg.* 1977;73:267-268.

104. Malone D. Cardiovascular disease and disorders. In: Malone D, ed. *Physical Therapy in Acute Care: A Clinician's Guide.* Thorofare, NJ: SLACK Incorporated; 2006.

105. Israel CW, Gronefeld G, Ehrlich JR, Hohnloser SH. Suppression of atrial tachyarrhythmias by pacing. *Journal of Cardiovascular Electrophysiology.* 2002;13(1 Suppl):S31-S39.

106. Maisel WH, Rawn JD, Stevenson WG. Atrial fibrillation after cardiac surgery. *Annals of Internal Medicine.* 2001;135(12):1061-1073.

107. Knight BP, Gersh BJ, Carlson MD, et al. American Heart Association Council on Clinical Cardiology (Subcommittee on Electrocardiography and Arrhythmias). Quality of Care and Outcomes Research Interdisciplinary Working Group. Heart Rhythm Society. AHA Writing Group. Role of permanent pacing to prevent atrial fibrillation: science advisory from the American Heart Association Council on Clinical Cardiology (Subcommittee on Electrocardiography and Arrhythmias) and the Quality of Care and Outcomes Research Interdisciplinary Working Group, in collaboration with the Heart Rhythm Society. *Circulation.* 2005;111(2):240-243.

108. Lau CP. Pacing for atrial fibrillation. *Heart.* 2003;89(1):106-112.

109. Morton JB, Sanders P, Vohra JK, et al. Effect of chronic right atrial stretch on atrial electrical remodeling in patients with an atrial septal defect. *Circulation.* 2003;107(13):1775-1782.

110. Gatzoulis MA, Freeman MS, Siu SC, et al. Atrial arrhythmia after surgical closure of atrial septal defects in adults. *N Engl J Med.* 1999;340:839-846.

111. American Heart Association. *2001 Heart and stroke statistical update.* Dallas, Texas: American Heart Association; 2000.

112. Brooks-Brunn JA. Postoperative atelectasis and pneumonia: risk factors. *Am J Critical Care.* 1995;4(5):340-349.

113. Leroy O, Soubrier S. Hospital-acquired pneumonia: risk factors, clinical features, management, and antibiotic resistance. *Current Opinions in Pulm Med.* 2004;10(3):171-175.

114. Dean E. Individuals with acute surgical conditions. In: Frownfelter D, Dean E, eds. *Cardiovascular and Pulmonary Physical Therapy. Evidence for Practice.* 4th ed. St. Louis, Mo: Mosby; 2006:529-542.

115. Avery RK, Longworth DL. Viral pulmonary infections in thoracic and cardiovascular surgery. *Semin Thorac Cardiovasc Surg.* 1995;7(2):88-94.

116. Cooper JM, Katcher MS, Orlov MV. Implantable devices for the treatment of atrial fibrillation. *N Engl J Med.* 2002; 346(26):2062-2068.

117. Edmunds LH. Therapeutic choices for cardiac arrhythmias. Available at: http://www.ctsnet.org/edmunds/Chapter25section3.html. Accessed February 20, 2006.

118. Geller JC, Reek S, Timmermans C, et al. Treatment of atrial fibrillation with an implantable atrial defibrillator. *Eur Heart J.* 2003;24(23):2083-2089.

119. Houghton T, Kaye GC. ABC of interventional cardiology. Implantable devices for treating tachyarrhythmias. *BJM.* 2003;327:333-336.

120. Calkins H, Sousa J, EI AR, et al: Reversal of antiarrhythmic drug effects by epinephrine: quinidine versus amiodarone. *J Am Coll Cardiol.* 1992;19:137.

121. Belardinelli R, Georgiou D, Cianci G, Purcaro A. Randomized, controlled trial of long-term moderate exercise training in chronic heart failure: effects on functional capacity, quality of life, and clinical outcome. *Circulation.* 1999;99:1173-1182.

122. Mcgregor W, Trumble D, Magovern J. Mechanical analysis of midline sternotomy wound closure. *J Thoracic Cardovasc Surg.* 1999;117:1144-1150.

123. Pollock ML, Franklin BA, Balady GJ. Resistance exercise in individuals with and without cardiovascular disease: benefits, rationale, safety and prescription. *Circulation.* 2000;101:828-833.

124. Ford GT, Guenter CA. Toward prevention of postoperative complications. *Am Rev Resp Dis.* 1984;130:4-5.

RECOMMENDED READINGS

ECG

Huff J. *The ECG Workout: Exercises in Arrhythmia Interpretation.* 4th ed. Philadelphia, Pa: Lippincott Williams & Wilkins; 2006.

Thaler MS. *The Only ECG Book You'll Ever Need.* 3rd ed. Philadelphia, Pa: Lippincott Williams & Wilkins; 1999.

AUSCULTATION

Erickson B. *Heart Sounds and Murmurs: A Practical Guide.* 2nd ed. St. Louis, Mo: Mosby Co; 1991.

Wilks RL, Hodgkin JE, Lopez B. *Lung Sounds: A Practical Guide.* St. Louis, Mo: Mosby Co; 1988

Impaired Ventilation and Respiration/Gas Exchange Associated With Ventilatory Pump Dysfunction or Failure (Pattern E)

Alexandra Sciaky, PT, MS, CCS

ANATOMY

The pulmonary and cardiovascular systems provide the delivery of oxygenated blood to the body's tissues and the return of partially desaturated blood to the lungs. The function of the ventilatory pump, consisting of the lungs, airways, bony thorax, nerve, muscle, and connective tissues of the chest and abdomen, is the focus of this practice pattern. This neuromusculoskeletal pump creates the pressure changes within the chest cavity that result in the gas volume flow and pressure changes required for breathing and coughing. The anatomy of the lungs and airways has been described in detail in Pattern A.

The bony thorax consists of the 12 thoracic vertebrae, 12 pairs of ribs, sternum, and costal cartilages. These structures form a conically shaped cage, with a greater lateral diameter as compared to its anterior-posterior diameter. Its function is to provide a protective housing for the lungs and mediastinal structures and form a flexible frame to which the respiratory muscles attach. Each rib has a costal groove that extends along the inferior border dorsally and to the internal surface at the angle of the rib. This groove houses the intercostals vessels and nerves.[1]

The sternum has three parts—the manubrium, body, and xyphoid process. The manubrium and the body are on slightly different planes, creating the sternal angle. The superior border of the manubrium is concave, forming the sternal notch, which is the bony landmark used to locate the approximate level of the carina. The clavicles, first rib, and second rib articulate with the manubrium. The 2nd through 7th ribs articulate with the body. The costal cartilages of the 8th through the 10th ribs are attached to the rib above, without a direct connection to the sternum. The ventral ends of the 11th and 12th ribs (floating ribs) have no skeletal attachment.[1,2]

The respiratory muscles may be categorized according to their function: for inspiration, for expiration, and for accessory use. Inspiration is primarily the result of the contraction of the diaphragm. It is responsible for approximately 60% to 70% of quiet ventilation when upright and approximately 75% when supine. Other muscles that are involved in quiet inspiration are the external intercostals, internal intercostals, and scalene muscles. The diaphragm is a large, dome-shaped muscle that forms the base of the chest cavity, separating it from the abdominal cavity and supporting the mediastinum and lungs. The portions of the diaphragm on each side of the central tendon are often referred to as the right and left hemidiaphragms. Its position varies with inspiration, expiration, postural position, postural deformity, and size of the abdominal organs. The external intercostal muscles are located in the spaces between the ribs. These short muscle fibers extend from the lower border of the rib above to the upper border of the rib below at a posterior-superior angle. Contraction of these muscles draws the ribs below superiorly and laterally, increasing the volume of the chest cavity. The scalene muscles have been observed to be active during quiet inspiration, and they help to expand the upper rib cage in an anteroposterior dimension.

Normal expiration is a passive process that is a function of inspiratory muscle relaxation. However, forced expiration, as occurs in huffing or coughing, compresses the lungs and increases intrathoracic and intra-abdominal pressures, thereby creating high velocity air flow out of the lungs. The primary muscles of forced expiration are the internal intercostals, rectus abdominus, external oblique abdominis, internal oblique abdominis, and transversus abdominis muscles.

Accessory muscle use occurs when deep inspiration is necessary (as in a cough) and when patients are dyspneic. The accessory muscles can serve to elevate the chest and increase its anterior-posterior diameter or extend the spine. The muscles in this category include the sternocleidomastoid; anterior, middle, and posterior scalenes; serratus anterior; pectoralis major; pectoralis minor; levatores costarum; rhomboids; trapezius; latissimus dorsi; quadratus lumborum; and erector spinae.[1,2]

Other accessory muscles may assist forced expiration by compressing the chest and decreasing its anteroposterior diameter. These muscles include the iliocostalis lumborum, transverses thoracis, latissimus dorsi, quadratus lumborum, and serratus posterior inferior.

All of the respiratory muscles are composed of striated-type muscle fibers. These fibers are made up of long, multinucleated cells. Each cell is covered with a thin membrane called the sarcolemma. The contractile apparatus of each muscle fiber is divided into myofibrils that are bundles of thick and thin filaments. Z bands are located at regular intervals along the length of the myofibrils. The portion of the myofibrils between the Z bands is called the sarcomere and is considered the contractile unit. The thin filaments and thick filaments are linked together by the cross bridges. The cross bridges contain the head groups of myosin molecules, located in the thick filaments. Cytoskeletal proteins located beneath the sarcolemma play an important role in successful muscle contractions.[3] For further information on the anatomy and physiology of skeletal muscle, see Musculoskeletal Pattern C: Impaired Muscle Performance.

PHYSIOLOGY

The pertinent physiology for this pattern is related to the function of the ventilatory pump muscles during breathing and coughing and to the exchange of oxygen and carbon dioxide between the blood and the atmosphere. Effective contraction and relaxation of the respiratory muscles drive the ventilatory pump that moves gases in and out of the lungs. The length-tension and force-velocity relationships of the musculoskeletal structures in the ventilatory pump translate into measurements of gas pressure (tension), gas

volume (length), and gas flow (velocity). These measurements are a reflection of ventilatory pump performance. Further information on the physiology of gas exchange is found in Pattern A.

The tension developed by a muscle is dependent on the final length of the muscle fibers. If muscle contraction occurs at the normal resting length of the muscle fiber, maximum tension is exerted, and all the cross bridges between the thick and thin filaments are activated. If the muscle is elongated when it begins to contract, fewer cross bridges are formed and the thin filaments do not have access to all of the available myosin head groups. Therefore, less tension develops with the muscle contraction. If the muscle is shortened or contracted, the thin filaments overlap, interfering with their interaction with the thick filaments and reducing the amount of tension the muscle can develop. The function of the muscles that drive the ventilatory pump is determined by these length tension relationships. However, since these muscles are moving gas instead of limbs, their performance is expressed in measurement of gas pressure (cm H_2O or mmHg), gas volume (cc or mL), and gas flow (L/sec).

Normal breathing consists of inspiration and expiration of varying tidal volumes (TVs) (ie, the amound of air inhaled and exhaled during normal quiet ventilation) with intermittent breaths above TV (sigh breaths). Periodic deep breaths are necessary to stimulate the production of surfactant and prevent collapse of alveoli. These deep breaths also serve to maintain the elastic properties of the lung tissues and ventilatory pump structures.

Inspiration begins with contraction of the diaphragm and inspiratory muscles. A subatmospheric pressure is generated in the chest. The chest expands symmetrically in anterior-posterior and lateral directions. Atmospheric air takes the path of least resistance through the nose or mouth, to the larynx, trachea, mainstem and segmental bronchi, and finally to the bronchioles and alveoli. Once TV is reached, the diaphragm and inspiratory muscles relax. Then exhalation occurs via the elastic recoil of the lungs and ventilatory pump structures. Both inspiration and expiration are dependent on airway patency and chest wall mobility.

Effective coughing begins with a deep inspiration followed by closure of the glottis. High thoracoabdominal pressures are generated by co-contraction of the diaphragm and expiratory muscles against the closed glottis. The deep breath dilates the airways, increases lung recoil, and allows for increased force of expiratory muscle contraction. When the glottis opens, about 2.3 L (SD + 0.5 L) of air is expelled at flows of 6 to 20 L/sec.[4] This high velocity burst of air serves to mobilize material in its path (eg, mucus) and maintain the patency of the airways. In adults, peak flow rates of at least 160 L/min are the minimum required during a cough to remove debris in the airways.[5] Coughing may be assisted manually with an abdominal thrust or mechanically with a device (eg, Cough Assist In-Exsufflator). In a retrospective study of 94 patients with Duchenne's muscular dystrophy (DMD), the authors found that when routinely monitored assisted cough peak flow rates dropped below 270 L/min, they were very likely to drop below 160 L/min during pulmonary infections and the likelihood of respiratory failure increased greatly.[6]

PATHOPHYSIOLOGY

DUCHENNE'S MUSCULAR DYSTROPHY

DMD, the most common form of muscular dystrophy, is a chronic, progressive disease.[7] It is inherited as an X-linked recessive trait (predominantly affecting boys). In DMD, the gene responsible for producing dystrophin mutates, so that muscle tissue necrosis occurs and is replaced by connective tissue and fat.[7] Serum CK levels are elevated at birth and decline as the disease progresses.[8] Manifestations begin at 3 to 5 years of age and include: delayed motor milestones, progressive muscle weakness (shoulder and pelvic girdles), pseudohypertrophy of calf muscles, joint contractures, and kyphoscoliosis. Later stages (ages 12 to 25 years of age) are characterized by pulmonary impairments resulting from respiratory muscle weakness, ineffective cough, hypoventilation, hypercapnia, aspiration, hypotonia of the pharyngeal structures, pulmonary infections, and thoracic deformity (scoliosis).[9-11] Some patients have subclinical cardiac involvement. The loss of functional muscle mass appears to limit maximal oxygen consumption.[12] Up to one-third of patients with DMD have some degree of intellectual impairment.

The process of breathing depends on the coordinated function of the respiratory muscles in generating a negative pressure and the compliance of the lungs and chest wall. Normal subjects fully expand their lungs by regularly taking deep breaths or sighs. These regularly occurring breaths stretch the lung and chest wall tissues and keep them compliant. Patients with chronic respiratory muscle weakness, including those with DMD, are not able to fully expand their lungs, and over time, develop increased lung tissue and chest wall stiffness (ie, decreased compliance).[11,13,14] This inability to take periodic deep breaths may change alveolar surface tension and increase the tendency for atelectasis.[15] Serial pulmonary function tests may be used to track the rate of deterioration so that therapeutic interventions may be implemented before a respiratory crisis occurs.[16] The passive recoil of the thoracic cage is altered by gross muscle weakness that changes the neutral position at which lung and thoracic cage recoil pressures are balanced. As a result, the respiratory muscles no longer have optimal length-tension relationships, and their peak tensions are reduced.[12,17,18] Sleep disordered breathing and nocturnal desaturation are also common.[19] The long-term inability to take deep breaths may result in recurrent respiratory infections, progressive CO_2 retention, and permanent pulmonary restriction.[9,11]

Coughing, which is vital in maintaining airway patency, is also negatively affected by impaired respiratory muscle function.[20,21] The act of coughing depends on the ability of the respiratory muscles to generate a critical volume flow and positive pressure that are coordinated with the opening and closing of the glottis. These actions may be compromised by muscle weakness in the trunk and shoulder girdle and joint contractures that impact length-tension relationships. Impaired respiratory muscle function is a dominant clinical manifestation in the late stages of several primary neurological and neuromuscular diseases, including DMD.[21] The inability to inspire a volume of air greater than 1500 cc results in reduced spontaneous and assisted cough flows and greatly increases the risk of pulmonary morbidity and mortality.[9,14,22] Structural impairments of the thorax, such as scoliosis, may occur with neuromuscular disease and further compromise the length-tension relationships of the respiratory muscles. For further information about the musculoskeletal management of patients with DMD, see Musculoskeletal Pattern C.

GUILLAIN-BARRÉ SYNDROME

Guillain-Barré syndrome (GBS) is also known as Landry's paralysis or acute inflammatory demyelinating polyradiculopathy (AIDP). GBS is one of the most common life-threatening diseases of the peripheral nervous system and has a significant effect on the patient's ventilatory pump. The disease is an autoimmune disorder characterized by acute inflammation and demyelination of the peripheral nerves, including those that supply the ventilatory pump muscles. The inflammation is manifested as perivenular and endoneurial infiltration of the nerves by lymphocytes, macrophages, and a few plasma cells. The macrophages penetrate the basement membrane of the Schwann cells, especially in the vicinity of the nodes of Ranvier, and extend between the myelin lamellae, stripping away the myelin sheath from the axon.[23]

The most common clinical feature is limb weakness occurring more proximal than distal. In about two thirds of patients, symptoms are preceded by an antecedent event such as an upper respiratory infection (40% of cases).[24] The most common type of cranial nerve involvement is facial nerve palsy, noted in 53% of patients.[25] Pain, experienced by about 90% of patients, is often severe.[26] Autonomic dysfunction, manifesting as either excess or reduced sympathetic or parasympathetic nervous system activity, occurs in about two-thirds of cases.[27] The onset of symptoms can be acute or gradual. Recovery progresses gradually after a plateau phase. Ninety-eight percent of patients reach the plateau phase 4 weeks after the onset of symptoms.[28] About 25% of patients experience ventilatory pump failure and require ventilator support.[28] Three factors that are predictive of the need for intubation and mechanical ventilation are: if the time from onset of weakness to hospital admission is less than 7 days, if the patient is unable to lift his or her head, and if the patient's vital capacity is less than 60% of predicted.[29] Complete recovery of neuromuscular function is generally observed in about two-thirds of patients at 1 year after onset.[28] IV immunoglobulin is the current treatment of choice for GBS. It is thought to act through several mechanisms including anti-idiotypic suppression of autoantibodies. The side effects may include fever, chills, headache, nausea, vomiting, and feeling faint. IV plasma exchange is an alternative treatment for GBS that has been shown to be equally as effective as immunoglobulin.[28] Its side effects are very similar to IV immunoglobulin and include chills, fever, nausea, vomiting, immunosuppression, and feeling faint. For further information about the neuromuscular management of patients with DMD, see Neuromuscular Pattern G.[30]

IMAGING

DUCHENNE'S MUSCULAR DYSTROPHY

Patients with DMD are likely to develop chronic hypoventilation and recurrent pulmonary infections due to their progressive respiratory muscle weakness. Chest radiographs are used to assess anatomic abnormalities and pathological processes in the chest of the patient with DMD. For a posteroanterior study, the chest film is positioned behind the patient's back and the x-ray source is positioned 72 inches in front.[31] Areas of low density, such as air-filled parenchyma, appear darkest on the radiograph. Areas of higher density, such as bone, appear lightest or white. Pathological processes, such as pneumonia, may cause infiltrates or consolidation in the lung parenchyma, preventing full ventilation of the affected areas and thereby increasing their density. Areas that would normally appear dark on the radiograph then appear as a lighter gray or white. An infiltrate in either lower lobe would also cause blurring of the costophrenic angle on the side of the infiltrate. The level and curvature of the hemidiaphragms on the chest radiograph are indicative of lung inflation at full inspiration. Although both sides of the diaphragm usually work in synchrony, pathological processes may affect only one lung and the corresponding hemidiaphragm. The level of each hemidiaphragm corresponds to the inflation of the lung above it. Hyperinflated lungs cause the hemidiaphragms to flatten and decrease in curvature, whereas hypoinflated lungs cause the hemidiaphragms to be elevated and increase in curvature.

GUILLAIN-BARRÉ SYNDROME

Patients with GBS are likely to develop acute hypoventilation and pulmonary infections, so chest radiographs are also an important tool to assess aeration and pathological processes in the lungs. See Imaging for DMD in the previous section for more detail.

PHARMACOLOGY

DUCHENNE'S MUSCULAR DYSTROPHY

♦ Antimicrobial agents/antibiotics
  • Examples: Cephalosporins (Ancef, Keflex), aminoglycosides (Garanmycin, Janimicin), lincomycins (Lincocin, Lincorex)
  • Actions:
    ▪ Combat organisms, such as bacteria, that cause pulmonary infections
    ▪ Cephalosporins act by inhibiting cell wall synthesis and function of a broad spectrum of bacterial organisms
    ▪ Aminoglycocides and lincomycins act by inhibiting protein synthesis of a broad spectrum of bacterial organisms
  • Administered: Intravenously and/or orally
  • Side effects: Nausea, vomiting, inflammation of the colon, impaired renal function, ototoxicity

♦ Bronchodilators
  • Examples: Beta$_2$ agonists (Alupent, Bronkaid Mist, Isuprel, Maxair, Proventil, Ventolin), anticholinergics (Atrovent), phosphodiesterase inhibitors
  • Actions:
    ▪ Open airways and optimize ventilation and airway clearance
    ▪ Bronchomotor tone is mediated by cholinergic and adrenergic stimulation
    ▪ Stimulation of adrenergic beta$_2$ receptors produces an increase in cyclic adenosine monophosphate and bronchodilation
    ▪ Stimulation of cholinergic muscarinic receptors produces an increase in cyclic guanosine monophosphate and bronchoconstriction
  • Administered: Oral inhalation
  • Side effects: Tachycardia, headache, nausea, hyperactivity

♦ Mucokinetic agents
  • Examples: Acetylcysteine (Mucomyst, Mucosil), wetting agents
  • Actions:
    ▪ Promote mobilization and removal of pulmonary secretions
    ▪ Mucolytics act on the chemical bonds in mucoid secretions, reducing their viscosity and facilitating expectoration
    ▪ Wetting agents provide humidification and lubrication of the airways to enhance expectoration
  • Administered: Oral inhalation
  • Side effects: Mucosal irritation, bronchospasm, nausea

GUILLAIN-BARRÉ SYNDROME

- ♦ Analgesics
  - • Examples: Morphine sulfate (Astramorph, Duramorph, Infumorph), oxycodone (Darvon, Dilaudid, Hydrostat IR, OxyContin, Roxanol)
  - • Actions:
    - ▪ Inhibit synaptic transmission in pain pathways of the spinal cord and brain
    - ▪ Inhibitory effect is mediated by the opioid receptors in these pathways
    - ▪ Opiods used to reduce neuromuscular pain
  - • Administered: Intravenously or orally
  - • Side effects: Respiratory suppression, drowsiness, constipation
- ♦ Anticoagulants
  - • Examples: Heparin (Calciparine, HEP-LOCK, Liquaemin), warfarin (Coumadin, Miradon)
  - • Actions:
    - ▪ Function is to prevent pulmonary embolus and DVT
    - ▪ Heparin potentiates the activity of circulating protein known as antithrombin III, which renders clotting factors inactive
    - ▪ Warfarin impairs the hepatic synthesis of several clotting factors by blocking the conversion of vitamin K epoxide to vitamin K
  - • Administered: Heparin is taken by injection, warfarin is taken orally
  - • Side effects: Thrombocytopenia, bleeding
- ♦ Antimicrobial agents/antibiotics (see above)
- ♦ Bronchodilators (see above)
- ♦ Mucokinetic agents (see above)
- ♦ Pain management
  - • Examples: Carbamazepine (Atretol, Carbatrol, Tegretol) and gabapentin (Neurontin)
  - • Actions: Used as adjuncts for pain management help reduce doses of narcotics needed to achieve relief and thereby reduce narcotic side effects
  - • Administered: Orally
  - • Side effects:
    - ▪ For carbamazepine: Dizziness, drowsiness, ataxia, blurred vision, anemia, CHF
    - ▪ For gabapentin: Sedation, dizziness, fatigue, ataxia

Case Study #1: Acute Shortness of Breath and Possible Aspiration

Mr. Thomas Downs is a 21-year-old male with Duchenne's muscular dystrophy admitted to the hospital due to acute shortness of breath and possible aspiration of food.

PHYSICAL THERAPIST EXAMINATION

HISTORY

- ♦ General demographics: Thomas is a 21-year-old white male whose primary language is English. He is a high school graduate.
- ♦ Social history: He lives with his parents who are able-bodied. He is their first and only child. Both parents continue to share in caregiver responsibilities. They are strong advocates for their son, flexing their work schedules to accommodate his needs. He is covered by a special state-sponsored insurance plan for children with chronic, progressive diseases.
- ♦ Employment/work: Thomas spends several hours a day on a computer, corresponding with his friends and playing games. He goes outside in his electric wheelchair at least three to four times a week. He attends family gatherings with his parents as much as possible.
- ♦ Growth and development: Thomas was born following a full-term pregnancy. He sat up at age 22 months and walked at 2 years, 6 months. He began showing signs of progressive weakness of his shoulder and pelvic girdle muscles at the age of 6 years. He was then diagnosed with DMD. By age 13 years, the weakness had progressed to the point he could no longer walk and required a wheelchair for mobility. He appears younger than his chronological age.
- ♦ Living environment: He lives in a two-story, three-bedroom house in a suburban neighborhood. The first floor is wheelchair accessible and contains his bedroom and bathroom.
- ♦ General health status
  - • General health perception: Thomas reports that he gets depressed sometimes because he keeps getting weaker as he gets older. He stated that his main concern is his breathing: he gets short of breath, especially at night and loses sleep because of it. He also has trouble coughing and clearing his secretions.

- Physical function: He is out of bed 6 to 8 hours per day, and he uses a power wheelchair for mobility. He requires maximum assist for sliding board transfers, dressing, and lower body hygiene care. He requires minimal assist for feeding and upper body hygiene care. At baseline, he is able to breathe spontaneously on room air without supplemental oxygen.
- Psychological function: There are no apparent cognitive or memory impairments, although he does have a depressed affect.
- Role function: Son, friend.
- Social function: Thomas has a small circle of supportive friends. He enjoys visiting with friends and family, also keeping in touch with them via e-mail.

♦ Social/health habits: He reports a recent loss of appetite.

♦ Family history: His mother has a history of depression that is well controlled on Wellbutrin. She complained of low back pain that has become progressively worse as a result of assisting Thomas with his transfers in or out of his wheelchair. His father has gout.

♦ Medical/surgical history: Thomas has a history, over the past 6 months, of upper respiratory infections leading to lower respiratory infections requiring antibiotics.

♦ Prior hospitalizations: Three months ago, Thomas came to the ED with acute shortness of breath. He was diagnosed with pneumonia and admitted for 2 weeks of IV antibiotics, oxygen, and airway clearance techniques.

♦ Preexisting medical and other health-related conditions: Thomas has a bony deformity of his left humerus as a result of a fracture at 10 years of age following a fall. He also has a scoliosis with a right thoracic convexity. He has had a history of multiple upper respiratory infections, in addition to the pneumonia noted above.

♦ Current condition(s)/chief complaint(s): His current chief complaints are difficulty breathing and clearing secretions. He came to the ED 2 days ago complaining of shortness of breath and a wet cough. He reported choking on some applesauce a week earlier. His oxygen saturation on room air was 84%. His chest x-ray showed a right lower lobe opacification consistent with aspiration pneumonia. A sputum culture was obtained and was found positive for streptococci. He was placed on 2 L of oxygen per nasal cannula and started on IV Clindamycin and admitted to the hospital's pulmonary care floor.

♦ Functional status and activity level: In addition to above, his parents perform ROM and stretching exercises to all of his extremities four times per week. In the hospital, Thomas reports he has the greatest difficulty breathing in the supine position.

♦ Medications: At home, Thomas takes a stool softener and multivitamin daily.

♦ Other clinical tests
- Arterial blood gases on room air were:
  - PaO_2: 75 mmHg (normal: 80 to 100 mmHg)
  - $PaCO_2$: 48 mmHg (normal: 35 to 45 mmHg)
  - pH: 7.33 (7.35 to 7.45)
  - HCO_3^-: 24 mEq/L (normal: 22 to 26 mEq/L)
- Pulmonary function tests/spirometry results, which are based upon age, height, ethnicity, and sex and are normally expressed as a percentage, revealed:
  - TV: 400 cc (normal approximately 500 cc)
  - FVC: 50% predicted (normal for males is 7.74 x $height_{meters}$ – 0.021 x age_{years} – 7.75 x [0.51])
  - FEV_1: 60% predicted (normal for males is 5.66 x $height_{meters}$ – 0.023 x age_{years} – 4.91 x [0.41])
  - PEFR: 140 L/min (normal peak approximately 554 to 575 L/min)
  - MIP: -48 cm H_2O (normal for 20- to 54-year-old males is 129 – [0.13 x age in years])

SYSTEMS REVIEW

♦ Cardiovascular/pulmonary
- BP: 140/70 mmHg
- Edema: None
- HR: 110 bpm
- RR: 24 bpm

♦ Integumentary
- Presence of scar formation: Well-healed scar over lateral aspect of distal left humerus; slight redness over sacrum and posterior heels
- Skin color: Pale
- Skin integrity: Intact, moist, warm

♦ Musculoskeletal
- Gross range of motion: Limited in UEs, LEs, and trunk
- Gross strength: Limited in UEs, LEs, and trunk
- Gross symmetry:
  - Scoliosis with right thoracic convexity
  - Pronounced wasting of shoulder and pelvic girdle musculature
- Height: 5'3" (1.6 m)
- Weight: 115 lbs (52.16 kg)

♦ Neuromuscular
- Maximum assist for bed mobility and transfers

♦ Communication, affect, cognition, language, and learning style
- Communication, affect, and cognition: Alert and oriented to person, place and time, intermittently anxious, able to speak softly in short sentences of four to five words in length, speech has slight wet quality
- Learning preferences: No apparent preference

Table 5-1

RESULTS OF AEROBIC CAPACITY/ENDURANCE TESTS AND MEASURES

Activity	HR	BP	RR	SaO$_2$ (FiO$_2$)	RPE
Rest	110	140/70	24	92% (28%)	12
#1 Supine to sit	120	130/70	26	92% (28%)	13
#2 Supported sitting for 10 minutes	125	135/69	28	90% (28%)	14
#3 Sliding board transfers	146	142/72	30	89% (28%)	16

TESTS AND MEASURES

- ◆ Aerobic capacity and endurance
  - Bedside observation and monitoring of vital signs, RPE, and oxygen saturation during supine to sit, supported sitting at the edge of bed for 10 minutes, and sliding board transfers from bed to wheelchair and from wheelchair to bed—See Table 5-1 for results of the tests
- ◆ Anthropometric characteristics
  - BMI (kg /m^2)=20.4; normal weight[32]
- ◆ Arousal, attention, and cognition
  - Alert and oriented to person, place, self, and time
  - Easily startled
- ◆ Assistive and adaptive devices
  - Patient uses a battery-powered wheelchair with right hand control that is approximately 2 years old
  - Observation revealed that the wheelchair fit the patient properly
  - Patient is able to operate and control the chair safely
  - A gel-type cushion is used
  - A custom support seating system is in place to accommodate for the thoracic scoliosis and secure the patient into chair
- ◆ Circulation
  - Body temperature: 99.2° F orally
- ◆ Environmental, home, and work barriers
  - Home is wheelchair accessible on the first floor
  - His bathroom and bedroom are on the first floor
- ◆ Gait, locomotion, and balance
  - Locomotion is achieved by means of powered wheelchair
  - Sitting balance is poor without supports built into wheelchair
- ◆ Integumentary integrity
  - Integument intact, moist, and warm
  - Sensation intact

- No breakdown over bony prominences, but redness over sacrum and posterior heels
- ◆ Muscle performance
  - MMTs revealed
    - Shoulder flexors: 2+/5
    - Shoulder elevators: 2/5
    - Shoulder abductors: 2/5
    - Shoulder extensors: 2-/5
    - Elbow flexors: 3-/5
    - Grip: 3+/5
    - Hip flexors: 1+/5
    - Hip extensors: 1/5
    - Hip abductors: 1/5
    - Hip adductors: 1+/5
    - Knee extensors: 1/5
    - Ankle dorsiflexors: 2/5
    - Ankle plantarflexors: 1/5
    - Swallowing
      - ▸ Bedside observation of swallowing suspicious for aspiration
      - ▸ Voice had wet quality after swallowing juice
      - ▸ Diminished elevation of thyroid cartilage noted during swallow
- ◆ Orthotic, protective, and supportive devices
  - Wearing bilateral ankle heel protectors to prevent skin breakdown on heels
  - Supplemental O$_2$ at 28% used at rest and during activity with an O$_2$ sat of 92%
- ◆ Pain: 0/10 on pain scale
- ◆ Posture
  - In sitting posture, patient observed to lean to the right, left shoulder higher than right and rotated slightly anteriorly
  - Posterior rib flare noted on left
- ◆ Range of motion
  - Shoulder flexion: R=0 to 90 degrees, L=0 to 105 degrees

- Shoulder abduction: R=0 to 85 degrees, L=0 to 100 degrees
- Shoulder internal rotation: R=0 to 70 degrees, L=0 to 75 degrees
- Shoulder external rotation: R=0 to 10 degrees, L=0 to 10 degrees
- Elbow flexion: R=5 to 115 degrees, L=10 to 110 degrees
- Hip flexion: R=10 to 110 degrees, L=10 to 110 degrees
- Hip abduction: R=0 to 25 degrees, L=0 to 30 degrees
- Bilateral hip internal rotation: 0 to 10 degrees
- Bilateral hip external rotation: 0 to 15 degrees
- Knee flexion: R=20 to 100 degrees, L=10 to 105 degrees
- Ankle plantar/dorsiflexion: R=25 to 0 degrees, L=20 to 0 degrees
- CWE: 28 inches (full expiration) to 28.5 inches (full inspiration) measured at the level of the xiphoid

◆ Reflex integrity: Patella and Achilles reflexes diminished bilaterally

◆ Self-care and home management
- Observation of patient brushing his teeth revealed that he became short of breath after 30 seconds of brushing
- Wheelchair transfers of Thomas by his mother revealed poor body mechanics on her part
- Parents had no knowledge of aspiration and its risks, measures to prevent/reduce pulmonary complications of DMD, or airway clearance techniques

◆ Ventilation and respiration/gas exchange
- Auscultation of the chest revealed diminished breath sounds over right lower lobe, positive E to A changes, and coarse breath sounds in central airways
- Dyspnea index: Rated at 1/4 at rest and increased to 4/4 with activity (Ventilatory Response Index also referred to as 15-count breathlessness index)[33]
- Respiratory rate: See Table 5-1
- Pulse oximetry: See Table 5-1
- Ventilatory pattern
  - Observation revealed shallow/restricted pattern, rapid, positive accessory muscle activation, diminished diaphragmatic movement, and inspiratory to expiratory ratio of 1:1.5
- Palpation of the chest
  - Palpation revealed bony deformity consistent with scoliosis with right thoracic convexity
  - No masses or tenderness to palpation
- Cough sequence/function

- Ineffective cough (in sitting position) characterized by low inspiratory volume, incomplete glottal closure, and low expiratory volume
- Unable to clear and expectorate mucus

● Bedside pulmonary function tests/spirometry revealed:
  - TV: 450 cc
  - FVC: 50% predicted
  - FEV_1: 60% predicted
  - PEFR: 135 L/min
  - MIP: -45 cm H_2O

◆ Work, community, and leisure integration or reintegration
- Patient has difficulty tolerating sitting in wheelchair and using laptop computer for more than 20 minutes due to shortness of breath, making keeping in touch with friends and extended family problematic

EVALUATION

Thomas has an inherited, progressive myopathy that has progressed to the point that he is dependent on caregivers and assistive devices for mobility and ADL. He also has a history of scoliosis, deformity of the left humerous as a result of the fracture, multiple upper respiratory infections, and pneumonia. The physical therapy evaluation reveals he has difficulty with airway clearance, impaired gas exchange, and ventilatory pump dysfunction. He has a low-grade fever and is having difficulty coughing and maintaining his oxygen saturation above 90% on room air. The strength and endurance of his ventilatory muscles have been further compromised by a pulmonary infection in the presence of advanced DMD. He is at risk for future pulmonary infections due to the progressive nature of his myopathy. His mother is at risk for low back injury due to improper body mechanics during transfers. The patient and his parents are lacking knowledge about the risks of aspiration with DMD, preventative measures, and airway clearance techniques.

DIAGNOSIS

Thomas is a patient with advanced DMD and with acute shortness of breath and possible aspiration associated with ventilatory pump dysfunction. He has impaired: aerobic capacity/endurance; muscle performance; posture; range of motion; and ventilation and respiration/gas exchange. He is functionally limited in self-care, home management, work, community, and leisure actions, tasks, and activities. He is also in need of devices and equipment. These findings are consistent with placement in Pattern E: Impaired Ventilation and Respiration/Gas Exchange Associated With Ventilatory Pump Dysfunction or Failure. Thomas may also be classified in other patterns to address the impairments related to his DMD (eg, Musculoskeletal Pattern C: Impaired Muscle Performance and Neuromuscular Pattern B: Impaired Neuromotor Development).[30,34,35] These impairments will be addressed in determining the prognosis and the plan of care.

PROGNOSIS AND PLAN OF CARE

Over the course of the visits, the following mutually established outcomes have been determined:

♦ Airway clearance is enhanced

♦ Endurance is improved

♦ Family, significant other, and caregiver safety is improved

♦ Health status is improved

♦ Patient is able to assume or resume some self-care, community, and leisure roles

♦ Patient is able to perform physical actions, tasks, and activities related to self-care, community, and leisure

♦ Patient, family, significant other, and caregiver knowledge and awareness of the diagnosis, prognosis, interventions, and anticipated goals and expected outcomes are increased

♦ Physical function is improved

♦ Risk of recurrence of condition is reduced

♦ Risk of secondary impairment is reduced

♦ Self-management of symptoms is improved

♦ Sense of well-being is increased

♦ Stress is reduced

♦ Tissue perfusion and oxygenation is improved

♦ Work of breathing is decreased

To achieve these outcomes, the appropriate interventions for this patient are determined. These will include: coordination, communication, and documentation; patient/client-related instruction; therapeutic exercise; functional training in self-care and home management; functional training in community and leisure integration or reintegration; manual therapy techniques; prescription, application, and, as appropriate, fabrication of devices and equipment; and airway clearance techniques.

Thomas is expected to require between 15 to 18 visits over a 2- to 3-week period of time. Thomas has good social support, is somewhat depressed, and is severely impaired.

INTERVENTIONS

RATIONALE FOR SELECTED INTERVENTIONS

The rationale presented in this chapter will relate to the cardiovascular/pulmonary systems for this patient. See additional rationale for therapeutic exercise for DMD in Musculoskeletal Pattern C: Impaired Muscle Performance.[34]

Therapeutic Exercise

Respiratory muscles, and the diaphragm in particular, have been shown to be trainable in patients with DMD with respect to endurance but not strength.[12,36-38] Implementation of breathing strategies, relaxation techniques, and optimal postural positioning may minimize the work of breathing and perception of dyspnea.[39,40]

The studies on respiratory muscle training in patients with DMD vary widely in the effects that have been achieved. These findings ranged all the way from substantial improvement in the strength and endurance of the respiratory muscles to minimal or insignificant changes in respiratory muscle performance.[41-51] The patient's ability to deep breathe, cough, and mobilize secretions has been shown to be directly related to the strength of the respiratory muscles. Inspiratory muscle training in patients with DMD has been shown to improve performance in regard to endurance but not strength.[38] It may be helpful to measure inspiratory muscle strength during recovery from an acute pulmonary infection to determine when the patient has returned to his baseline muscle strength. Use of sniff nasal pressure to measure inspiratory muscle strength in patients with DMD has been shown to be particularly useful in that it represents a major determinant of vital capacity.[52]

Manual Therapy Techniques

Prolonged stretching of the chest wall and extremities may enhance joint flexibility and prevent contractures.[10] Manual chest stretching performed segmentally to the lower, middle, and upper thoracic regions at least twice per day may help increase chest wall ROM.[53-54]

Prescription, Application, and, as Appropriate, Fabrication of Devices and Equipment

His main form of communicating with his friends and extended family is via e-mail, so it is important for Thomas to be able to use the computer keyboard accurately and frequently. Providing him with a computer tray fitted to his wheelchair would allow him greater access. Thomas is also on supplemental oxygen at rest and during activity at 28% to maintain an O_2 sat of 92%.

Daytime noninvasive ventilation (glossopharyngeal breathing, mouthpiece IPPB, and intermittent abdominal pressure ventilator) may also be used for patients with DMD. Glossopharyngeal breathing may allow short periods off mechanical ventilation and is extremely useful in the event of ventilator failure.[55] The most commonly used noninvasive technique is mouthpiece intermittent positive pressure ventilation.[56-58] The intermittent abdominal pressure ventilator (also called a Pneumo-belt) consists of an inflatable bladder placed over the abdomen that is connected to a conventional portable ventilator. With the patient seated, inflation of the bladder creates a forced exhalation (pushes the abdominal contents up against the diaphragm), and inhalation occurs as the bladder deflates and thus causes the diaphragm to passively descend and the ribcage to outwardly recoil. This method may not work in patients with scoliosis or obesity.[59,60]

Noninvasive nocturnal ventilation has been used in the management of patients with DMD, who have hypoventilation at night and sleep-disordered breathing.[61,62] Using a bilevel positive airway pressure generator or a mechanical ventilator during nocturnal nasal intermittent positive pressure ventilation (NIPPV), patients with DMD had improved survival rates, daytime gas exchange, quality of sleep, well-being, and independence. When compared to non-ventilated control subjects, the patients using NIPPV also were observed to have decreased daytime sleepiness and a slower rate of decline in pulmonary function.[63-68]

The use of bilevel positive airway pressure, through nose or mouth via facemask, may be considered for patients with DMD, who have hypoxemia due to hypoventilation. The use of supportive oxygen is not recommended in these patients just because their hypoxemia is the result of hypoventilation.[66,69] Supportive oxygen during exercise may be used to maintain the patient's O_2 sat.

The use of assisted ventilation in patients with DMD has been recognized for its benefits of prolonging life.[56] In patients with DMD in chronic respiratory failure, there is consensus that noninvasive positive pressure ventilation (NPPV) should be instituted.[70,71] See Airway Clearance Techniques for additional devices and equipment.

Airway Clearance Techniques

The management of patients with DMD has dramatically evolved in both the quality of the care rendered and the duration of survival of these patients.[72-74] In spite of these advances, the still high mortality in patients with DMD is primarily the result of deterioration of their respiratory function.[75] Bach and associates found that patients with DMD had one episode of pneumonia per year with a higher incidence in advanced disease.[76] A viral infection of the upper airways has been observed to impair already weak respiratory muscles.[77] Thus, the critical importance of intense attention to effective airway clearance is apparent in these patients to prevent atelectasis and pneumonia.[78] Early interventions aimed at improving airway clearance can prevent hospitalization and reduce the incidence of pneumonia.[9]

Ineffective peak cough flow is a predominant clinical feature of patients with DMD, and several techniques may be used to overcome it.[22,79] Maximum insufflation capacity has been defined as the maximum air volume that can be held with a closed glottis. The strength of both the oropharyngeal and laryngeal musculature affect this capacity, and a training program in the technique of air stacking (taking a series of tidal breaths without exhaling between them) has been shown to improve lung and chest wall range of motion and thus maximum insufflation capacity.[14] Clearance of secretions in the airways necessitates adequate expiratory muscle function. Of note was the finding that the expiratory muscles in patients with DMD may be affected to the same degree as the inspiratory muscles and at times more severely affected, which will significantly reduce the efficiency of the patient's cough and airway clearance.[80]

The ability to clear secretions is directly related to cough peak flows,[81] and ineffective airway clearance is associated with flows below 160 L/min.[5] Peak cough flows of 270 L/min have been used to identify those patients who would benefit from assisted cough techniques.[9] Szeinberg and associates found a correlation between the ability to generate adequate flow for effective coughing and a maximum expiratory pressure (MEP) of 60 cm H_2O and above.[80]

Assisted cough techniques may include both manual and mechanical maneuvers that have the potential of avoiding adverse respiratory problems for these patients.[82] Increasing peak expiratory flow (PEF) may be achieved by enhancing the patient's vital capacity through the use of positive pressure devices, glossopharyngeal breathing (which uses oral muscles to gulp small amounts of air into the lungs, with six or more gulps producing a tidal volume breath), or air-stacking by means of a manual resusitator.[83] These techniques may be used alone or may be used in combination with techniques (ie, manual thoracoabdominal compression or mechanical insufflation/exsufflation) to enhance expiration/peak cough flow.[14,22,79,83] Manual assisted or forced exhalation is achieved by compression on the upper abdomen or chest wall in synchrony with the subject's own cough effort. Mechanical insufflation-exsufflation simulates a cough by providing a positive pressure breath (insufflation) followed by a negative pressure exsufflation.[84,85]

Mechanical insufflation/exsufflation has been shown to be not only well-tolerated by patients, but also to be superior in generating peak cough expiratory flow rates when compared to either manual cough assistance or air stacking.[83] It is particularly important for the prevention of hospitalizations or the need for a tracheostomy for those patients with DMD whose peak cough expiratory flows were around 160 L/min.[9,86] Mechanical insufflation/exsufflation has also been shown to have several advantages over the use of traditional suctioning. These advantages include that it is more comfortable for the patient, does not produce mucosal trauma, and enables clearance of secretions from the peripheral airways.[87]

Intermittent positive pressure breathing (IPPB) assisted hyperinsufflation is another technique that has been shown to improve peak cough flow and enhance airway clearance in pediatric patients with neuromuscular disorders.[88] In addition to noninvasive positive pressure ventilation, effective treatment of lower respiratory tract secretion retention in individuals with muscular dystrophy includes mechanical mucus clearing techniques, such as chest percussion and vibration.[22,89] Use of a peak flow meter has been recommended to routinely measure peak flows during assisted coughs, since it provides an objective measure of cough effectiveness.[6]

COORDINATION, COMMUNICATION, AND DOCUMENTATION

Airway clearance techniques will be coordinated with the patient's eating schedule and aerosolized medications. Functional mobility exercises, such as transfers to the wheelchair, will be coordinated with Thomas's other inpatient activities (medical/nursing care) and tests. The physical therapist will communicate the pertinent patient care information to members of Thomas's hospital care team, family caregivers, discharge planner, case manager, and any other individuals with a "need to know." His discharge plan will be coordinated with and communicated to all parties involved (eg, family caregivers, discharge planner, home health agency, equipment company). This communication will be implemented via case conferences, patient care rounds, patient family meetings, and discharge planning procedures. Referrals to inpatient psychiatry and social work will be made for evaluation and recommendations regarding his depressed affect and need to cope with a chronic, progressive illness. All elements of the patient's management will be documented in the official record, including examination and evaluation findings, diagnosis, prognosis, interventions, and outcomes.

PATIENT/CLIENT-RELATED INSTRUCTION

The overall goal of patient-related instruction is to affect a durable cognitive improvement that results in a positive change in health-related behavior.[90] Hypoventilation and accumulation of pulmonary mucus secretions inevitably lead to acute respiratory failure in the patient with DMD.[6] Emphasizing this point in the patient-related instruction is critical in illustrating the importance of pulmonary interventions.

In the hospital setting, factors that may influence an individual's ability to learn and process information include signs and symptoms of acute illness, anxiety, fear, cognitive ability, and time constraints. Based on the evaluation of learning needs in this case, Thomas and his caregivers will be given instruction in the following areas:

- CPR
- Emergency response system access
- Infection control procedures
- Optimal body mechanics for caregivers during wheelchair transfers and airway clearance procedures
- Proper use of recommended equipment, such as mechanical percussor and hospital bed
- Risk factors related to the disease and the preventative measures need to be taken to prevent aspiration and recurrent pulmonary infections
- Signs and symptoms of cardiopulmonary compromise and emergency responses

The methods used to teach the above knowledge and skills include oral presentation with written information/instructions, demonstration by the physical therapist followed by practice by the patient/caregiver, and explanation of desired procedures using pictures and charts to illustrate.

THERAPEUTIC EXERCISE

- Aerobic capacity/endurance conditioning
  - UE endurance exercises
    - Active assistive range of motion (AAROM) exercises progressing to AROM exercises
    - Increasing the number of repetitions daily as tolerated
    - Progress to upper body ergometer (UBE) as possible
- Balance, coordination, and agility training
  - Sitting balance exercises with progressively less trunk support
  - Sitting balance combined with reaching and UE tasks
- Body mechanics and postural stabilization
  - Body mechanics training
    - Appropriate sitting posture in wheelchair
    - Appropriate use of body mechanics while utilizing computer keyboard
  - Posture control training
    - Proper alignment of head, cervical and thoracic spines, and shoulders
    - Scapula retraction and depression
    - Chicken wing position (hands behind head, horizontal abduction of shoulders)
  - Postural stabilization activities
    - Axial extension starting in supine and progressing to sitting
    - Maintenance of axial extension position with bilateral arm raises
  - Postural awareness training
    - Use of mirror for visual input of appropriate alignment
    - Notes all around home
- Flexibility exercises

- Stretching exercises should be done after warming up, using a slow and steady stretch accompanied by deep breathing, and building hold up to 30 seconds
- UE stretching at end ROM exercises
- Anterior chest wall stretching
- LE stretching
♦ Relaxation
- Guided imagery techniques
- Contract-relax techniques
♦ Strength, power, and endurance training
- Ventilatory muscle endurance exercises
- Respiratory muscle training, including use of inspiratory training device to increase strength and endurance of the ventilatory muscles
- Breathing strategies

FUNCTIONAL TRAINING IN SELF-CARE AND HOME MANAGEMENT

♦ Self-care and home management
- Bed mobility and transfer training
- Eating, including positioning for safe swallowing to protect the airway
- Grooming
- Toileting
- Safety awareness training during self-care and home management

FUNCTIONAL TRAINING IN WORK, COMMUNITY, AND LEISURE INTEGRATION OR REINTEGRATION

♦ Community and leisure integration or reintegration
- Task specific (computer keyboard) performance training

MANUAL THERAPY TECHNIQUES

♦ Mobilization/manipulation
- Chest wall stretching during expiration, assisted rib elevation during inspiration

PRESCRIPTION, APPLICATION, AND, AS APPROPRIATE, FABRICATION OF DEVICES AND EQUIPMENT

In order for Thomas and his parents to perform the recommended airway clearance program at home and monitor Thomas's need for intervention, including temporary supplemental oxygen, they will need the following durable medical equipment:

♦ Hospital bed

- To assist Thomas in assuming the various postural drainage positions
- To allow his caregivers to adjust the bed to the level of his wheelchair for transfers
♦ Oscillatory airway clearance device for home use (eg, mechanical percussor, which is an electrical clearance device that mechanically percusses the chest in lieu of the hands of the caretaker, or the Vest (formerly the ThAIRapy Vest)
- To provide high frequency chest compression by vibrating the chest wall to loosen secretions and then chest wall oscillation resulting in outward airflow
- To help his caregivers conserve energy while providing airway clearance twice a day
♦ Pulse oximeter
- To monitor Thomas's oxygen saturation
- To cue his caregivers to administer oxygen via nasal cannula when his SaO_2 drops below 93%
♦ Peak flow meter
- To monitor the speed air can be exhaled in one breath
- To objectively measure cough effectiveness
♦ Supplemental oxygen
- To treat hypoxemia and support oxygenation of the tissues
- Goal is to increase arterial oxygen content and improve peripheral tissue oxygenation
- Inhaled via nasal cannula or face mask
- After prolonged use at concentrations higher than FiO_2 of 40%, side effects may include increased capillary permeability, impaired mucociliary transport, and pulmonary fibrosis
♦ Continued use of power wheelchair/seating system

AIRWAY CLEARANCE TECHNIQUES

♦ Breathing strategies
- Assisted cough techniques
  - Maximal insufflations with self-inflating bag and mouthpiece (or other volume generating device)
  - Stacked breathing: The patient takes 2 to 4 inspirations for each expiration to maximize inspiratory and expiratory volume
  - Abdominal support (manually or with a binder)
  - Rocking
    ▶ In the sitting position, the patient inspires as deeply as possible as the therapist assists the patient in leaning backward
    ▶ Then the patient forcefully expires/coughs while the therapist assists him in leaning quickly forward

- ▸ Abdominal support is applied with a pillow or the therapist's hands during the expiratory maneuver
  - ■ Positioning for best mechanical advantage of the expiratory muscles
  - Paced breathing
    - ■ Timing breaths to conserve energy and accomplish desired tasks
  - Techniques to maximize ventilation
    - ■ Inspiratory hold maneuvers in a variety of positions
      - ▸ The patient takes a deep breath and holds it for 5 seconds for 5 to 10 repetitions in each of the following positions: Sitting, right sidelying, left sidelying, supine, and prone (if tolerated)
- ◆ Manual/mechanical techniques
  - Chest wall mobilization
  - Chest percussion, vibration, and shaking in combination with pulmonary postural drainage
    - ■ Emphasis on areas of retained secretions and decreased aeration
    - Oropharyngeal suction may be used when patient has difficulty fully expectorating the secretions
- ◆ Positioning
  - Positioning to alter work of breathing
    - ■ Sitting and semi-fowler's positions provide best mechanical advantage to reduce work of breathing
    - ■ Work of breathing is increased in the supine position
  - Positioning to maximize ventilation and perfusion
- ◆ Frequency
  - During Thomas's hospital stay, airway clearance techniques will be performed up to 3 times a day and as needed to ensure clearance of excess pulmonary secretions and optimization of his breathing, coughing, and oxygenation
  - As his condition improves, the frequency will be reduced to twice a day
  - His parents and caregivers will be instructed in a simplified airway clearance routine to do at home to reduce the likelihood of future pulmonary infections and prevent respiratory failure

ANTICIPATED GOALS AND EXPECTED OUTCOMES

- ◆ Impact on pathology/pathophysiology
  - Energy expenditure per unit of work is decreased.
  - Physiological response to increased oxygen demand is improved.
  - Symptoms associated with increased oxygen demand are decreased.
  - Tissue perfusion and oxygenation are enhanced so that the patient is able to breathe spontaneously on room air continuously and maintain a SaO_2 of 93% or greater on room air.
- ◆ Impact on impairments
  - Airway clearance is improved so that the patient's chest x-ray is clear.
  - Cough function is improved so that the patient is able to effectively clear excess pulmonary secretions with minimal to moderate assistance.
  - Endurance is increased so that the patient is able to tolerate sitting in his wheelchair and using his computer independently for 3 to 4 hours per day.
  - Optimal loading on a body part is achieved.
  - Postural control is improved.
  - Ventilation and respiration/gas exchange are improved.
  - Work of breathing is decreased so the patient is able to breathe spontaneously without complaints of shortness of breath.
- ◆ Impact on functional limitations
  - Patient is able to assume or resume required self-care, home management, work, community, and leisure roles with minimal assistance.
  - Patient is able to perform physical actions, tasks, and activities related to self-care, home management, work, community, and leisure with minimal assistance.
  - Performance of and independence in ADL with or without devices and equipment are increased.
  - Tolerance of positions and activities is increased.
- ◆ Risk reduction/prevention
  - Family, significant others, and caregivers are able to safely care for the patient.
  - Mother's body mechanics during wheelchair transfers are improved.
  - Pressure on body tissues is reduced.
  - Protection of body parts is increased.
  - Risk factors are reduced.
  - Risk of recurrence of the condition is decreased.
  - Risk of secondary impairment is reduced.
  - Safety of patient, family, significant others, and caregivers is improved.
  - Self-management of symptoms is improved so that the patient's family is able to perform airway clearance techniques properly.
- ◆ Impact on health, wellness, and fitness
  - Health status is improved.
  - Physical function is improved so that the patient is able to feed himself, perform upper body hygiene care with minimal assistance, and able to propel himself in his electric wheelchair independently.

- Impact on societal resources
  - Cost of health care services is decreased.
  - Documentation occurs throughout patient management and across settings and follows APTA's *Guidelines for Physical Therapy Documentation.*[35]
  - Resources are utilized in a cost-effective way.
  - Utilization of physical therapy services results in efficient use of health care dollars, shorter length of stay, and appropriate discharge plan.
- Patient/client satisfaction
  - Access, availability, and services provided are acceptable to patient and addresses his concerns.
  - Care is coordinated with patient, family, significant others, caregivers, and other professionals.
  - Decision making is enhanced regarding patient health and the use of health care resources by patient family, significant others, and caregivers.
  - Intensity of care is decreased.
  - Interdisciplinary collaboration occurs through case conferences, patient care rounds, and patient family meetings.
  - Patient and family report a reduction in stress level by at least 50%.
  - Patient, family, significant other, and caregiver knowledge and awareness of the diagnosis, prognosis, interventions, and anticipated goals and expected outcomes are increased.
  - Patient knowledge of personal and environmental factors associated with the condition is increased.
  - Referrals are made to other professionals or resources whenever necessary and appropriate.
  - Sense of well-being is improved with respect to consistent airway clearance, airway protection, relief of pressure areas, and swallowing.
  - Stressors related to choking and injury to caregivers during transfers are decreased.

REEXAMINATION

Reexamination is performed throughout the episode of care.

DISCHARGE

Thomas is discharged from physical therapy after a total of 16 physical therapy sessions and attainment of his goals and expectations. These sessions have covered his entire episode of care related to this cardiovascular/pulmonary episode. He is discharged because he has achieved goals and expected outcomes. Since patients with muscular dystrophy require life-long management, he may return to therapy for additional episodes of care.

PSYCHOLOGICAL ASPECTS

Mental health issues such as anxiety, social inhibition, anger, passiveness, and depression are common for patients with DMD and their families.[91-92] Dysthymic (chronic depressive mood) disorder and major depressive disorder have been found to occur significantly more often among patients with DMD than matched controls.[93] As a group, parents of adolescents with DMD show marked preoccupation with their children, great stress, and reduced expression of enjoyment.[94] These realities need to be considered by the physical therapist as part of the life experience for patients with DMD and their families. Counseling and support services for families, in-service education for health care providers, and group activities for patients with DMD may provide assistance in dealing with these psychosocial concerns. The physical therapist may facilitate the implementation of these services by recognizing the signs of depression and extreme stress and making referrals to the appropriate mental health professionals (eg, social worker, psychiatrist, psychologist).

Case Study #2

Mr. Juan Martinez is a 42-year-old male with Guillain-Barré syndrome and pneumonia admitted to the hospital due to sudden progressive weakness of the muscles in all four extremities and acute shortness of breath following an upper respiratory infection.

PHYSICAL THERAPIST EXAMINATION

HISTORY

- General demographics: Mr. Martinez is a 42-year-old Hispanic male who is bilingual, speaking both Spanish and English. He is a high school graduate with 2 years of study at a community college.
- Social history: He lives with his wife and five children, ages 11 through 17 years. He is the only wage earner, and his wife's role is to care for the children and the home. His mother lives close by and visits often. He is very active in his Roman Catholic parish and considers himself a religious person. He enjoys eating, dancing, and listening to Latin music.
- Employment/work: Mr. Martinez works at an auto assembly plant, operating a riveting machine. He works long hours to meet his family's expenses. He hopes to change jobs soon. He would like to use the skills he acquired in community college and find a position in computer programming.

Table 5-2

RESULTS OF AEROBIC CAPACITY/ENDURANCE TESTS AND MEASURES

Activity	HR	BP	RR	SaO2 (FiO$_2$)	RPE
Rest	112	150/72	28	94% (35%)	10
#1 Supine to sit	140	128/70	32	92% (35%)	13
#2 Supported sitting for 10 minutes	130	138/68	30	91% (35%)	14
#3 Sliding board transfers	152	148/68	34	88% (35%)	15

♦ Living environment: He lives in a two-story, four-bedroom house in an urban neighborhood. There are four steps to enter the house with handrails on both sides, and there are 14 steps to the second floor with a handrail on one side. His bedroom and bathroom are on the second floor. There is a full bathroom on the first floor.

♦ General health status
  ● General health perception: Mr. Martinez reports that he has enjoyed good health most of his life. He has been concerned about his weight and would like to lose about 20 lbs.
  ● Physical function: His baseline status had been independent with ambulation, transfers, and all ADL. He was also able to drive a car or small truck and operate heavy machinery.
  ● Psychological function: Mr. Martinez does not have any apparent cognitive or memory impairments, although he does admit to getting angry easily.
  ● Role: Husband, father, son, laborer, parishioner.
  ● Social function: Mr. Martinez's social community is largely comprised of his immediate family and a few other Hispanic families that attend his church. Most of his social activities outside of work involve large family meals.

♦ Social/health habits: He prefers authentic Mexican food, including refried beans made with lard. He has not seen a doctor or had a check up in 4 years. He smokes one pack of cigarettes a day.

♦ Family history: His mother has a history of Type 2 diabetes. His father died of a MI at age 50.

♦ Medical/surgical history: Mr. Martinez has a history of chronic low back pain and gastric reflux. There is no surgical history.

♦ Prior hospitalizations: None.

♦ Current condition(s)/chief complaint(s): Mr. Martinez's current chief complaints are difficulty coughing and moving his limbs. He came to the ED 3 weeks ago complaining of shortness of breath and difficulty walking. In the ED, he reported having an upper respiratory infection a week earlier. His oxygen saturation on room air was 89%. His chest x-ray was clear. He was admitted to the hospital for further tests. Within the next 24 hours, he lost the ability to walk and breathe on his own, and he was diagnosed with GBS. He required intubation and has been on mechanical ventilation for 2 weeks due to respiratory muscle weakness. Currently he is to be weaned from the ventilator as his respiratory and peripheral muscle power has been gradually increasing. His chest x-ray now shows bibasilar atelectasis.

♦ Functional status and activity level: Mr. Martinez's job entails a lot of trunk twisting and bending. His only other exercise had been occasional dancing at church functions.

♦ Medications: Previously he had taken ibuprofen 800 mg for back pain as needed. In the hospital he was given IV immunoglobulin for GBS, morphine sulfate to depress respiration while on the ventilator, and heparin to prevent clot formation.

♦ Other clinical tests (on admission):
  ● Arterial blood gases on room air were:
    ▪ PaO$_2$: 80 mmHg (normal: 80 to 100 mmHg)
    ▪ PaCO$_2$: 49 mmHg (normal: 35 to 45 mmHg)
    ▪ pH: 7.32 (7.35 to 7.45)
    ▪ HCO$_3^-$: 24 (normal: 22 to 26 mEq/L)
  ● Pulmonary function tests/spirometry revealed:
    ▪ TV: 300 cc (normal approximately 500 cc)
    ▪ FVC: 55% predicted (normal for males is 7.74 x height$_{meters}$ – 0.021 x age$_{years}$ – 7.75 x [0.51])
    ▪ FEV$_1$: 50% predicted (normal for males is 5.66 x height$_{meters}$ – 0.023 x age$_{years}$ – 4.91 x [0.41])
    ▪ PEFR: 125 L/min (normal peak approximately 600 to 630 L/min)
    ▪ MIP: -39 cm H$_2$0 (normal for 20- to 54-year-old males is 129 – [0.13 x age in years])

SYSTEMS REVIEW

♦ Cardiovascular/pulmonary
  ● BP: 165/70 mmHg

- Edema: None
- HR: 112 bpm
- RR: 12 bpm as set on ventilator

♦ Integumentary

- Presence of scar formation: None
- Skin color: Pale
- Skin integrity
  - Disrupted with tracheostomy opening for tracheal tube
  - Preliminary signs of breakdown over bony prominences resolving with increased movement of extremities

♦ Musculoskeletal

- Gross range of motion: Limited in UEs, LEs, and trunk
- Gross strength: Limited in UEs, LEs, and trunk
- Gross symmetry: Symmetrical
- Height: 5'9" (1.75 m)
- Weight: 220 lbs (99.79 kg)

♦ Neuromuscular

- He needs maximum assist for all mobility and transfers

♦ Communication, affect, cognition, language, and learning style

- Alert and oriented to person, place, and time
- Affect improved as his condition has been improving
- Learning preferences: Prefers visual demonstration

TESTS AND MEASURES

♦ Aerobic conditioning/endurance

- His first attempt at mobility required maximum assist for movement from supine to sit and to supported sitting at the edge of bed for 10 minutes (see Table 5-2 for results of the tests)
- Patient was observed to fatigue easily

♦ Anthropometric characteristics

- BMI (kg/m^2)=32.5, which places him in the obese category[32]

♦ Arousal, attention, and cognition

- Alert and oriented to person, place, self, and time

♦ Assistive and adaptive devices: None

♦ Circulation

- Body temperature: 100.0° F orally
- Pulses: Normal

♦ Gait, locomotion, and balance

- Gait not evaluated at this time, as muscle strength returns will be assessed
- Sitting balance is poor at this time

♦ Integumentary integrity

- Integument intact

- Previous signs of preliminary signs of breakdown over bony prominences (eg, sacrum and heels) resolving
- Skin disrupted at tracheostomy opening tracheal tube

♦ Muscle performance: MMTs revealed the following abnormalities:

- Shoulder flexors: 2-/5
- Shoulder elevators: 2/5
- Shoulder abductors: 2-/5
- Shoulder extensors: 2/5
- Elbow flexors: 3/5
- Grip: 3-/5
- Hip flexors: 2/5
- Hip extensors: 1/5
- Hip abductors: 2-/5
- Hip adductors: 2/5
- Knee extensors: 2-/5
- Ankle dorsiflexors: 2/5
- Ankle plantarflexors: 1/5
- Trunk flexors and extensors: 2+/5

♦ Orthotic, protective, and supportive devices

- Wearing bilateral protective heel protectors to prevent skin breakdown on his heels
- Mechanical ventilator is supporting his breathing, and interventions for weaning are being instituted
  - Mechanical ventilator settings
    - ‣ Mode: Synchronized intermittent mechanical ventilation (SIMV)
    - ‣ Set TV (V_t): 600 mL
    - ‣ Set rate: 12 bpm
    - ‣ Fraction of inspired oxygen (FiO_2): 32%
    - ‣ Positive end-expiratory pressure (PEEP): +5 cm H_2O (relative to atmospheric)
    - ‣ Pressure support: +5 cm H_2O (relative to atmospheric)

♦ Pain

- NPS
- Pain of 4/10 on the NPS (0=no pain and 10=worst possible pain) in both thighs and low back
- Downie and associates[95] described a high degree of agreement between the visual analog scale (VAS), NPS, and the simple descriptive scale (SDS), although they reported that the NPS performed better
- Jensen[96] found the NPS to be the most practical tool

♦ Posture

- In sitting, patient observed to lean forward with shoulders slumped
- Pronounced lumbar lordosis
- Forward head kyphosis

- Range of motion (only abnormal findings are included)
  - Shoulder flexion: R=0 to 160 degrees, L=0 to 165 degrees
  - Shoulder abduction: R=0 to 160 degrees, L=0 to 165 degrees
  - Shoulder internal rotation: R=0 to 80 degrees, L=0 to 85 degrees
  - Shoulder external rotation: R=0 to 55 degrees, L=0 to 55 degrees
  - Elbow flexion: R=5 to 140 degrees, L=10 to 140 degrees
  - Hip flexion: R=15 to 110 degrees, L=15 to 110 degrees
  - Hip abduction: R=0 to 30 degrees, L=0 to 30 degrees
  - Bilateral hip internal rotation: 0 to 10 degrees
  - Bilateral hip external rotation: 0 to 25 degrees
  - Knee flexion: R=0 to 120 degrees, L=0 to 120 degrees
  - Ankle plantar/dorsiflexion: R=35 to 0 degrees, L=35 to 0 degrees
  - Chest wall: 48 inches (full expiration) to 48.75 inches (full inspiration) measured at the level of the xiphoid
- Self-care and home management
  - He requires maximum assist for bed mobility and transfers
  - Patient requires maximum assistance with hygiene
  - Patient's wife is willing to assist patient at home, but will need some help
- Ventilation and respiration/gas exchange
  - Auscultation of the chest revealed diminished breath sounds over both lower lobes and coarse breath sounds in the central airways
  - Dyspnea index: Rated at 1/4 at rest and increased to 4/4 with activity (Ventilatory Response Index also referred to as 15-count breathlessness index)[33]
  - Respiratory rate: See Table 5-2
  - Pulse oximetry: See Table 5-2
  - Ventilatory pattern
    - Combination of ventilator provided breaths (12/minute) and spontaneous breaths (2 to 8/minute)
  - Palpation of the chest
    - Palpation revealed obese chest, no bony deformity
    - No masses or tenderness to palpation
  - Cough sequence/function
    - Unable to clear and expectorate secretions
    - Suctioning performed to clear airway
  - Bedside pulmonary function tests/spirometry
    - TV: 425 cc
    - FVC: 55% predicted
    - FEV1: 60% predicted
    - PEFR: 135 L/min
    - MIP: -50 cm H_2O
- Work, community, and leisure integration or reintegration
  - Patient does not have definitive plans of when he will return to work
  - He is anxious about not being able to work and provide for his family

EVALUATION

Mr. Martinez's history reveals an acute onset of progressive muscle weakness and ventilatory pump failure preceded by an upper respiratory infection. The physical therapy examination reveals that he is on mechanical ventilation (SIMV) and has impaired gas exchange and ventilatory pump dysfunction. The process of weaning from the ventilator has been initiated. He has a fever. The strength and endurance of his ventilatory muscles have been further compromised by obesity in the presence of GBS. His muscle strength testing reveals that he is not able to move his extremities fully against gravity, making him at risk for skin breakdown. Mr. Martinez has lost his independence and his ability to walk, to perform self-care, and to perform his job. His wife is willing to assist the patient but lacks the knowledge and skill to do so.

DIAGNOSIS

Mr. Martinez is a patient with GBS with ventilatory pump dysfunction. He has impaired: aerobic capacity/endurance; muscle performance; posture; range of motion; and ventilation and respiration/gas exchange. He is functionally limited in self-care, home management, work, community, and leisure actions, tasks, and activities. He is also in need of devices and equipment. These findings are consistent with placement in Cardiovascular/Pulmonary Pattern E: Impaired Ventilation and Respiration/Gas Exchange Associated With Ventilatory Pump Dysfunction or Failure. Mr. Martinez may also be classified in other patterns to address the impairments related to his GBS (eg, Musculoskeletal Pattern C: Impaired Muscle Performance and Neuromuscular Pattern G: Impaired Motor Function and Sensory Integrity Associated With Acute or Chronic Polyneuropathies).[35] These impairments will be addressed in determining the prognosis and the plan of care.

PROGNOSIS AND PLAN OF CARE

Over the course of the visits, the following mutually established outcomes have been determined:

- Airway clearance is enhanced

- Endurance is improved
- Family, significant other, and caregivers are able to safely care for the patient
- Health status is improved
- Patient is eventually able to assume or resume required self-care, home management, work, community, and leisure roles
- Patient is able to perform physical actions, tasks, and activities related to self-care, home management, work, community, and leisure
- Patient, family, significant other, and caregiver demonstrate knowledge and awareness of the diagnosis, prognosis, interventions, and anticipated goals and expected outcomes
- Physical function is improved
- Risk of recurrence of condition is reduced
- Risk of secondary impairment is reduced
- Sense of well-being is increased
- Stress is reduced
- Tissue perfusion and oxygenation is improved
- Work of breathing is decreased

To achieve these outcomes, the appropriate interventions for this patient are determined. These will include: coordination, communication, and documentation; patient/client-related instruction; therapeutic exercise; functional training in self-care and home management; functional training in work, community, and leisure integration or reintegration; manual therapy techniques; prescription, application, and, as appropriate, fabrication of devices and equipment; and airway clearance techniques.

Mr. Martinez is expected to require between 14 and 16 visits over a 2- to 3-week period of time. This may increase based on the other factors in his history. Mr. Martinez has good social support, is anxious to recover, and is severely impaired.

INTERVENTIONS

RATIONALE FOR SELECTED INTERVENTIONS

The rationale presented in this chapter will relate to the cardiovascular/pulmonary systems for this patient. See additional rationale for therapeutic exercise for GBS in Musculoskeletal Pattern C: Impaired Muscle Performance and in Neuromuscular Pattern G: Impaired Motor Function and Sensory Integrity Associated With Acute or Chronic Polyneuropathies.[30]

Therapeutic Exercise

Facilitation of Ventilator Weaning

Respiratory muscle dysfunction that may result from etiologies such as Guillain Barré has been shown to limit weaning from mechanical ventilation.[97-99] In addition, prolonged, controlled mechanical ventilation might produce disuse atrophy of the respiratory muscles. Therefore, physical therapy intervention that is coordinated with the process of weaning from the ventilator is important in the management of this patient. As the patient's oxygenation, hemodynamic stability, vital capacity, and negative inspiratory force improve to the point where he can maintain his own pulmonary function, weaning from the ventilator will progress. The goal of weaning is for the patient to return to spontaneous, continuous, independent breathing. The amount of time on mechanical ventilation is proportional to the time it takes to correct the underlying pathologies and ventilatory muscle weakness. Mechanical ventilators have modes in which the breaths initiated by the patient are synchronized with the breaths initiated by the ventilator. These modes significantly reduce the patient effort required for weaning. As the patient's ability to sustain spontaneous ventilation improves, the mechanical ventilatory support can be reduced as quickly as possible.[100,101] The physical therapist can facilitate the weaning process by having the patient perform ventilatory muscle strength and endurance exercises alternating with periods of ventilatory and/or oxygen support from the ventilator.

Horst and her colleagues found that a protocol-guided weaning program (based on evaluation for readiness to wean and a standardized process for weaning) from mechanical ventilation led to more rapid extubation than physician-directed weaning.[102]

Esteban and associates studied four different methods used to wean patients who had been on mechanical ventilation for an average of 7.5 days. The four methods were: 1) intermittent mandatory ventilation with the ventilator rate initially set at 10.0 ± 2.2 bpm and then decreased at least twice a day as possible by 2 to 4 bpm; 2) pressure-support ventilation with pressure set initially at 18.0 ± 6.1 cm of water and then reduced as possible at least twice daily by 2 to 4 cm of water; 3) multiple intermittent trials of spontaneous breathing as possible two or more times a day; or 4) a once-daily trial of spontaneous breathing. They concluded that the once-daily trial and the multiple daily trials of spontaneous breathing were equally effective in weaning patients from the ventilator and were more successful than the results in extubation using intermittent mandatory ventilation (three times more effective) and pressure-support ventilation (twice as effective).[103]

Trials of spontaneous breathing in appropriate patients on mechanical ventilation have been shown to reduce the duration of mechanical ventilation, the costs associated with intensive care, and the complications.[104]

The presence of a physical therapist as part of the weaning team has been shown to reduce patient anxiety.[105] The goal of physical therapy intervention for this patient is to avoid fatigue and to recondition the respiratory muscles by gradually shifting the work done by the ventilator to the patient, thus reducing the amount of ventilatory support required.[106] Aldrich and associates studied attaching an adjustable nonlinear resistive inspiratory training device to the patient's endotracheal tube to facilitate the weaning process. They found that both maximal inspiratory pressure and vital capacity improved, and 12 of the 27 patients in this study were weaned successfully from the ventilator.[107,108]

Other Exercise

Implementation of breathing strategies, such as mechanically assisted deep breathing and coughing, has been shown to prevent pulmonary complications in patients with neuromuscular disease.[109] Gradual, monitored exercise can assist patients in recovering their functional mobility. The physical therapist must avoid exercise that involves multiple maximal muscle contractions, which can cause overwork weakness.[110] Slow, steady exercise at approximately 30% of maximum muscle contraction can help avert signs of overwork, such as prolonged fatigue, sensation of limb heaviness, and muscle cramps.

Manual Therapy Techniques

Prolonged stretching of the chest wall and extremities may prolong joint flexibility and prevent contractures.[111] Manual chest stretching and coordinated manually assisted cough techniques can increase TV and cough effectiveness.[112-114]

Prescription, Application, and, as Appropriate, Fabrication of Devices and Equipment

Mr. Martinez's current functional mobility is impaired. The following equipment is likely to be useful in supporting him through his monitored activity progression: sliding board; reclining manual wheelchair with removable armrests and removable, elevating legrests; bilateral above knee compression hose; wheeled walker with seat; and gait belt. A semi-recumbent stepper for aerobic exercise may be used once he is able to transfer from the wheelchair with minimal assistance and walk 40 feet with the walker.

Airway Clearance Techniques

Effective treatment of atelectasis and lower respiratory tract secretion retention in patients with GBS includes noninvasive positive pressure ventilation and mechanical mucus clearing techniques, such as chest percussion and vibration. Vibration may also reduce hypercarbia, a result of hypoventilation in patients with GBS. Although no human studies have demonstrated this to date, there are animal studies that support the technique.[115,116] Ineffective peak cough flow, a predominant clinical feature of patients with GBS, may be improved by manually assisting the patient and/or by mechanical insufflation/exsufflation. The patient's ability to deep breathe, cough, and mobilize secretions is directly related to the strength of the respiratory muscles. Respiratory muscle training in patients with GBS may help improve cough effectiveness.[117] It may be helpful to measure inspiratory muscle strength during recovery to determine when the patient has returned to his baseline muscle strength. Use of a peak flow meter to routinely measure peak flows during assisted coughs provides an objective measure of cough effectiveness.[6]

COORDINATION, COMMUNICATION, AND DOCUMENTATION

During weaning from the ventilator and after, airway clearance techniques will be coordinated with the patient's eating schedule and aerosolized medications. Functional mobility exercises, such as transfers to the wheelchair, will be coordinated with Mr. Martinez's other inpatient activities (medical/nursing care) and tests. The physical therapist will communicate the pertinent patient care information to members of Mr. Martinez's hospital care team, family caregivers, discharge planner, case manager, and any other individuals with a "need to know." Mr. Martinez's discharge plan will be coordinated with and communicated to all parties involved (eg, family caregivers, discharge planner, home health agency, medical equipment company). This communication will be implemented via case conferences, patient care rounds, patient family meetings, and discharge planning procedures. Referrals to inpatient psychiatry and social work will be made for evaluation and recommendations regarding Mr. Martinez's emotional stress and need to cope with a debilitating illness. All elements of the patient's management will be documented in the official record, including examination and evaluation findings, diagnosis, prognosis, interventions, and outcomes.

PATIENT/CLIENT-RELATED INSTRUCTION

The overall goal of patient-related instruction interventions is to affect a durable cognitive improvement that results in a positive change in health-related behavior.[90] Hypoventilation and accumulation of pulmonary mucus secretions inevitably lead to acute respiratory infections. Emphasizing this point in the patient-related instruction is critical in illustrating the importance of pulmonary interventions.

In the hospital setting, factors that may influence an individual's ability to learn and process information include signs and symptoms of acute illness, anxiety, fear, cognitive ability, and time constraints. Based on the evaluation of learning needs in this case, the patient and caregivers will be instructed in the following:

♦ Airway clearance techniques including percussion, vibration, and postural drainage

♦ Airway protection, including positioning for safe swallowing

- ◆ Assisted cough techniques, including stacked breathing, abdominal support, positioning, and maximal insufflations/exsufflations using Cough Assist device
- ◆ CPR
- ◆ Emergency response system access
- ◆ Infection control procedures
- ◆ Optimal body mechanics during wheelchair transfers and airway clearance procedures
- ◆ Proper use of recommended equipment, such as airway clearance devices (eg, an Acapella™ or Flutter® device), wheelchair, and ambulatory aids
- ◆ Risk factors and preventative measures related to pulmonary infections in individuals with GBS
- ◆ Signs and symptoms of cardiopulmonary compromise and emergency response

Of importance for this patient will be the need to maintain and enhance hydration to facilitate mobilization of secretions.

The methods used to teach the above knowledge and skills include oral presentation with written information/instruction, demonstration by the physical therapist followed by practice by the patient/caregiver, and explanation of desired procedures using pictures and charts to illustrate.

THERAPEUTIC EXERCISE

- ◆ Aerobic capacity/endurance conditioning
  - UE and LE endurance exercises (AAROM exercises progressing to AROM exercises, increasing the number of repetitions daily)
  - A semi-recumbent stepper for aerobic exercise may be used once he is able to transfer from the wheelchair with minimal assistance
- ◆ Balance, coordination, and agility training
  - Static sitting balance exercises with progressively less trunk support and increasing endurance
  - Dynamic sitting balance combined with head movements, reaching, and UE tasks
- ◆ Body mechanics and postural stabilization
  - Postural awareness training
  - Postural stabilization activities
- ◆ Flexibility exercises
  - Stretching exercises should be done after warming up, using a slow and steady stretch accompanied by deep breathing, and building hold up to 30 seconds
  - UE stretching at end ROM exercises
  - LE stretching
  - Chest wall stretching
- ◆ Relaxation
  - Guided imagery techniques

- Contract-relax techniques
- ◆ Strength, power, and endurance training
  - Weaning exercises
    - Maintain good postural positioning in chair with armrests when weaning
    - Be sure primary focus of activities is on weaning at this time without interference from other activities
    - Respiratory muscle training for weaning from ventilator may include:
      - ‣ Strength: 3 to 5 sec max inspiratory and expiratory maneuvers at 20% increments over vital capacity ranges
      - ‣ Endurance: Ventilation to exhaustion three to five times a day
      - ‣ Maximal inspiratory force training: Daily inspiratory resistance training
  - Ventilatory muscle endurance exercises continued after weaning
  - Respiratory muscle strength training using varied diameter orifice device
  - Breathing strategies including assisted deep breathing coordinated with exercises (eg, inspiration with exercises that open the chest and expiration with exercises that tend to compress the chest)
  - The initiation of a more formalized strength and endurance exercise program will be added as Mr. Martinez's symptoms decrease and his functional independence increases

FUNCTIONAL TRAINING IN SELF-CARE AND HOME MANAGEMENT

- ◆ Self-care and home management
  - Bed mobility and transfer training, including sliding board transfers from bed to chair and from chair to bed while monitoring vital signs, RPE, and oxygen saturation
  - Eating
  - Grooming
  - Toileting
  - Safety awareness training during self-care and home management

FUNCTIONAL TRAINING IN WORK, COMMUNITY, AND LEISURE INTEGRATION OR REINTEGRATION

- ◆ Community and leisure integration or reintegration
  - Task-specific performance training as his functional independence increases

MANUAL THERAPY TECHNIQUES

♦ Mobilization/manipulation
  • Chest wall stretching coordinated with breathing
    ▪ Sylvester maneuver: Patient supine holds arms elbow to elbow and physical therapist raises both arms of patient up overhead while stabilizing the lower rib cage to mobilize anterior chest
    ▪ Lateral trunk flexion: Patient supine and physical therapist places one arm under the patient's upper back with the hand in opposite axilla and the other hand stabilizes the lateral lower ribs on that same side; patient's upper trunk is pulled toward the therapist in a lateral flexion maneuver, applying downward and inward pressure on the ribs
    ▪ Dorsal hyperextension: Patient supine and physical therapist places one hand under each scapula with the finger tips on the transverse processes; the therapist flexes the wrists to extend the spine at each thoracic vertebral level
    ▪ Trunk torsion: Similar to lateral trunk flexion except that the patient is rolled toward the physical therapist and the pressure on the lower ribs is at an oblique angle
  • Chest wall soft tissue mobilization

PRESCRIPTION, APPLICATION, AND, AS APPROPRIATE, FABRICATION OF DEVICES AND EQUIPMENT

♦ Hospital bed
  • To assist Mr. Martinez as muscle strength is increasing in assuming the various postural drainage positions and allow his wife to adjust the bed to the level of his wheelchair for transfers until he no longer needs the wheelchair
    ▪ Cough assist device used until pulmonary function and muscle strength are effective for a cough
    ▪ Pulse oximeter
      ▶ To monitor Mr. Martinez's oxygen saturation and cue his wife to administer oxygen via nasal cannula when his SaO_2 drops below 92%
    ▪ Peak flow meter
    ▪ Supplemental oxygen delivery system
    ▪ Sliding board
    ▪ Wheelchair with removable armrests, removable, elevating legrests, and protective seat cushion
    ▪ Bilateral above knee compression hose until he begins to ambulate
    ▪ Wheeled walker with seat

AIRWAY CLEARANCE TECHNIQUES

♦ Breathing strategies during and after weaning from ventilator
  • Use of the Acapella™ device to assist airway clearance by providing positive expiratory pressure while exhaling oscillations are created in the airway
  • Assisted cough techniques
  • Maximal insufflations with self-inflating bag and mouthpiece (or other cough assist device)
  • Stacked breathing: Patient takes two to four inspirations for each expiration to maximize inspiratory and expiratory volume
♦ Abdominal support (manually or with a binder)
♦ Rocking
  • In the sitting position, the patient inspires as deeply as possible as the therapist assists the patient in leaning backward
  • Then the patient forcefully expires/coughs while the therapist assists him in leaning quickly forward
  • Abdominal support is applied with a pillow or the therapist's hands during the expiratory maneuver
♦ Positioning for best mechanical advantage of the expiratory muscles
♦ Paced breathing
♦ Timing breaths to conserve energy and accomplish desired tasks
♦ Techniques to maximize ventilation
  • Inspiratory hold maneuvers in a variety of positions: The patient takes a deep breath and holds it for 5 seconds for 5 to 10 repetitions in each of the following positions: sitting, right sidelying, left sidelying, supine, and prone (if tolerated)
♦ Manual/mechanical techniques
  • Chest wall mobilization and stretching
  • Chest percussion, vibration, and shaking in combination with pulmonary postural drainage
  • Emphasis on areas of retained secretions and decreased aeration
  • Suctioning will be performed while on ventilator via endotracheal tube and after weaning oropharengeal suctioning may be performed
  • After weaning cough assist device may also be used when patient has difficulty fully expectorating the secretions
♦ Positioning
  • Positioning to alter work of breathing
  • Sitting and semi-fowler's positions provide best mechanical advantage to reduce work of breathing
  • Work of breathing is increased in supine position
  • Positioning to maximize ventilation and perfusion

♦ Frequency during Mr. Martinez's hospital stay

  • Up to three times a day and as needed to wean from ventilator and to ensure clearance of excess pulmonary secretions and optimization of his breathing, coughing, and oxygenation

  • As condition improves, the frequency will be reduced to twice a day

  • If Mr. Martinez is still having difficulty coughing at the time of his discharge to home, his wife will be instructed in a simplified airway clearance routine to do at home to reduce the likelihood of future pulmonary infections

ANTICIPATED GOALS AND EXPECTED OUTCOMES

♦ Impact on pathology/pathophysiology

  • Energy expenditure per unit of work is decreased.

  • Physiological response to increased oxygen demand is improved.

  • Symptoms associated with increased oxygen demand are decreased.

  • Tissue perfusion and oxygenation are enhanced so that the patient is able to breathe spontaneously on room air continuously and maintain a SaO_2 of 93% or greater on room air at rest.

♦ Impact on impairments

  • Airway clearance is improved to point where the patient's chest x-ray is clear.

  • Cough function is improved so that the patient is able to effectively clear excess pulmonary secretions independently.

  • Endurance is increased to point where the patient is able to tolerate sitting with minimal assistance without complaints of fatigue and maintain a SaO_2 of 93% or greater on room air while using rolling walker.

  • Optimal loading on a body part is achieved.

  • Postural control is improved with good axial extension achieved.

  • Ventilation and respiration/gas exchange are improved as respiratory muscle strength, power, and endurance are increased.

  • Work of breathing is decreased so that the patient is able to breathe spontaneously without complaints of shortness of breath.

♦ Impact on functional limitations

  • Patient is able to begin to assume or resume required self-care roles with minimal assistance.

  • Patient is able to perform physical actions, tasks, and activities related to self-care with minimal assistance.

  • Performance of and independence in ADL with or without devices and equipment are increased.

  • Tolerance of positions and activities is increased.

♦ Risk reduction/prevention

  • Family, significant others, and caregivers are able to safely care for the patient.

  • Pressure on body tissues is reduced.

  • Protection of body parts is increased.

  • Risk factors are reduced.

  • Risk of recurrence of the condition is decreased.

  • Risk of secondary impairment is reduced.

  • Safety is improved.

  • Self-management of symptoms is improved.

  • Wife's knowledge of body mechanics during wheelchair transfers is acquired.

♦ Impact on health, wellness, and fitness

  • Health status is improved.

  • Physical function is improved to point where the patient is able to perform bed mobility and transfers independently or with minimal assistance.

♦ Impact on societal resources

  • Cost of health care services is decreased.

  • Documentation occurs throughout patient management and across settings and follows APTA's *Guidelines for Physical Therapy Documentation.*[35]

  • Resources are utilized in a cost-effective way.

  • Utilization of physical therapy services results in efficient use of health care dollars, shorter length of stay, and appropriate discharge plan.

♦ Patient/client satisfaction

  • Access, availability, and services provided are acceptable to patient and address his concerns.

  • Care is coordinated with patient, family, significant others, caregivers, and other professionals.

  • Decision making is enhanced regarding patient health and the use of health care resources by patient family, significant others, and caregivers.

  • Intensity of care is decreased.

  • Interdisciplinary collaboration occurs through case conferences, patient care rounds, and patient family meetings.

  • Patient, family, significant others, and caregivers demonstrate knowledge and awareness of the diagnosis, prognosis, interventions, anticipated goals and expected outcomes.

  • Patient knowledge of personal and environmental factors associated with the condition is increased.

  • Referrals are made to other professionals or resources whenever necessary and appropriate.

  • Sense of well-being is improved with respect to consistent airway clearance, breathing, and relief of pressure areas.

- Stressors related to coughing and breathing are decreased.
- Stress on caregivers is decreased.

REEXAMINATION

Reexamination is performed daily throughout the episode of care.

DISCHARGE

Mr. Martinez is discharged from the acute care hospital to an inpatient rehabilitation facility after a total of 14 inpatient physical therapy sessions and progress toward his goals and expectations. These sessions have covered the entire episode of acute care. He is discharged because his pneumonia is cleared, and he is able to transfer out of the wheelchair and walk with minimal physical assistance. He no longer requires the support of an acute care setting and is ready to continue his rehabilitation in an inpatient rehabilitation setting. Since patients with GBS can take up to a year to fully recover their physical function, he may return to physical therapy as an outpatient for additional episodes of care. Adding a physical therapy plan for reduction of modifiable risk factors for coronary artery disease to Mr. Martinez's physical therapy in the rehabilitation period would also be indicated. Mr. Martinez has several of these risk factors including a sedentary lifestyle, being overweight, consuming high fat foods, smoking, and HTN.

PSYCHOLOGICAL ASPECTS

Mental health issues such as anxiety, anger, dependency, and depression are common for patients with GBS and their families.[118,119] GBS has a serious long-term impact on the work and private lives of patients and their partners.[119] These realities need to be considered by the physical therapist as part of the life experience for patients with GBS and their families. Psychological disturbances, including psychotic episodes, have been studied in severely compromised patients with GBS. These episodes were strongly associated with the presence of severe tetraparesis, mechanical ventilation, and multiple cranial nerve dysfunction.[114] Patients themselves report loss of the ability to communicate to be the most difficult aspect of the GBS experience.[114] Counseling and support services for families, psychopharmacological measures, and in-service education for health care providers may provide assistance in dealing with these important psychosocial concerns. The physical therapist may facilitate the implementation of these services by recognizing the signs of anxiety, depression, and extreme stress and making referrals to the appropriate mental health professionals (eg, social worker, psychiatrist, psychologist).

REFERENCES

1. Sadowsky HS. Anatomy of the cardiovascular and pulmonary systems. In Hillegass E, Sadowsky HS, eds. *Essentials of Cardiopulmonary Physical Therapy.* 2nd ed. Philadelphia, Pa: WB Saunders Co; 2001:2-47.
2. Watchie J. *Cardiopulmonary Physical Therapy A Clinical Manual.* Philadelphia, Pa: WB Saunders Co; 1995:35-39.
3. Mcardle WD, Katch FI, Katch WL. *Exercise Physiology, Energy, Nutrition and Human Performance.* 5th ed. Philadelphia, Pa: Lippincott Williams & Wilkins; 2001:358-382.
4. Leith DE. Cough. In Brain JD, Proctor D, Reid L, eds. *Lung Biology in Health and Disease: Respiratory Defense Mechanisms, Part 2.* New York, NY: Marcel Dekker; 1977:545-592.
5. Bach JR, Saporito LR. Criteria for extubation and tracheostomy tube removal for patients with ventilatory failure: a different approach to weaning. *Chest.* 1996;110:1566-1571.
6. Tzeng AC, Bach JR. Prevention of pulmonary morbidity for patients with neuromuscular disease. *Chest.* 2000;118:1390-1396.
7. Emery AE. The muscular dystrophies. *BMJ.* 1998;317:991-995.
8. Wagner KR. Genetic disease of muscle. *Neurol Clin.* 2002; 20:645-678.
9. Bach JR, Ishikawa Y, Kim H. Prevention of pulmonary morbidity for patients with Duchenne muscular dystrophy. *Chest.* 1997;112:1024-1028.
10. Bach JR. Disorders of ventilation weakness, stiffness, and mobilization (editorial). *Chest.* 2000;117:301-303.
11. Misuri G, Lanini B, Gigliotti F, et al. Mechanism of CO_2 retention in patients with neuromuscular disease. *Chest.* 2000;117:447-453.
12. Taivassalo T, Reddy H, Matthews PM. Metabolic myopathies: muscle response to exercise in health and disease. *Neurologic Clinics.* 2000;18:15-34.
13. Bach JR, Ishikawa Y, Tatara K. Pulmonary manifestations of neuromuscular disease (letter). *Pediatr Pulmonol.* 2001;31:89-90.
14. Kang SW, Bach JR. Maximum insufflation capacity. *Chest.* 2000;118:61-65.
15. Estenne M, Gevenois PA, Kinnear W, et al. Lung volume restriction in patients with chronic respiratory muscle weakness: the role of microatelectasis. *Thorax.* 1993;48:698-701.
16. Ward NS, Hill NS. Pulmonary function testing in neuromuscular disease. *Clin Chest Med.* 2001;22:769-781.
17. Phillips MF, Quinlivan RC, Edwards RH, Calverley PM. Changes in spirometry over time as prognostic marker in patients with Duchenne muscular dystrophy. *Am J Respir Crit Care Med.* 2001;164:2191-2194.
18. Gibson GJ, Pride NB, Davis JN, Loh LC. Pulmonary mechanics in patients with respiratory muscle weakness. *Am Rev Respir Dis.* 1977;115:389-395.
19. Bourke SC, Gibson GJ. Sleep and breathing in neuromuscular disease. *Eur Respir J.* 2002;19:1194-1201.
20. Suarez AA, Pessolano FA, Monteiro SG, et al. Peak flow and peak cough flow in the evaluation of expiratory muscle weakness and bulbar impairment in patients with neuromuscular disease. *Am J Phys Med Rehabil.* 2002;81:506-511.

21. Laghi F, Tobin MJ. Disorders of the respiratory muscles. *Am J Resp Crit Care Med.* 2003;168:10-48.

22. Chatwin M, Ross E, Hart N, et al. Cough augmentation with mechanical insufflation/exsufflation in patients with neuromuscular weakness. *Eur Respir J.* 2003;21:502-508.

23. Hoke A, Feasby TE. Disorders of the peripheral nervous system. In: Humes HD, ed in chief. *Kelly's Textbook of Internal Medicine.* 4th ed. Philadelphia, Pa: Lippincott Williams & Wilkins; 2000:2975-2987.

24. Winer JB, Hughes RAC, Anderson MJ, et al. A prospective study of acute idiopathic neuropathy. II. Antecedent events. *J Neurol Neurosurg Psychiatry.* 1998;51:613-618.

25. Winer JB, Hughes RAC, Osmond C. A prospective study of acute idiopathic neuropathy. I. Clinical failures and their prognostic value. *J Neurol Neurosurg Psychiatry.* 1998;51:605-612.

26. Moulin DE, Hagen N, Feasby TE, et al. Pain in Guillain-Barré syndrome. *Neurology.* 1997;48:328-331.

27. Singh NK, Jaiswal AK, Misra S, et al. Assessment in automomic dysfunction in Guillain-Barré syndrome and its prognostic implications. *Acta Neurol Scand.* 1987;75:101-105.

28. Seneviratne U. Guillain-Barré syndrome. *Postgrad Med J.* 2000;76:774-782.

29. Sharshar T, Boudain F, Raphaël J. Early predictors of mechanical ventilation in Guillain Barre syndrome. *Crit Care Med.* 2003;31(1):278-283.

30. Moffat M, ed. *Neuromuscular Essentials: Applying the Preferred Physical Therapist Practice Patterns.* Thorofare, NJ: SLACK Incorporated; 2007.

31. Ries M, Johnson T. Principles of chest x-ray interpretation. In: Frownfelter D, Dean E, eds. *Principles and Practice of Cardiopulmonary Physical Therapy.* 3rd ed. St. Louis, Mo: Mosby-Year Book; 1996:159-167.

32. DHHS. Caluculate your body mass index. Available at: http:// www.nhlbisupport.com. Accessed September 20, 2006.

33. Frownfelter D, Ryan J. Dyspnea: measurement and evaluation. *Cardiopulm Phys Ther.* 2000;11(1):7-15.

34. Moffat M, Rosen E, Rusnak-Smith S, eds. *Musculoskeletal Essentials: Applying the Preferred Physical Therapist Practice Patterns.* Thorofare, NJ: SLACK Incorporated; 2006.

35. American Physical Therapy Association. Guide to physical therapist practice. 2nd ed. *Phys. Ther.* 2001;81:9-744.

36. Martin AJ, Stern L, Yeates J, Lepp D, Little J. Respiratory muscle training in Duchenne muscular dystrophy. *Dev Med Child Neurol.* 1986;28:314-318.

37. Sharma KR, Mynhier MA, Miller RG. Muscular fatigue in Duchenne muscular dystrophy. *Neurology.* 1995;45:306-310.

38. Koessler W, Wanke T, Winkler G, et al. Two years' experience with inspiratory muscle training in patients with neuromuscular disorders. *Chest.* 2001;120:765-769.

39. Lanini B, Misuri G, Gigliotti F, et al. Perception of dyspnea in patients with neuromuscular disease. *Chest.* 2001;120:402-408.

40. Yasuma F, Kato T, Naya M. Adequate tidal volume with row-a-boat phenomenon in advanced Duchenne muscular dystrophy (letter). *Chest.* 2002;121:1726.

41. DiMarco A, Kelling J, DiMarco M, et al. The effects of inspiratory resistive training on respiratory muscle function in patients with muscular dystrophy. *Muscle Nerve.* 1985;8:284-290.

42. Wanke T, Toifl K, Merkle M, et al. Inspiratory muscle training in patients with Duchenne muscular dystrophy. *Chest.* 1994; 105:475-482.

43. Martin AJ, Stern L, Yeates J, et al. Respiratory muscle training in Duchenne muscular dystrophy. *Dev Med Child Neurol.* 1986;28:314-318.

44. Rodillo E, Noble-Jamieson CM, Aber V, et al. Respiratory muscle training in Duchenne muscular dystrophy. *Arch Dis Child.* 1989;64:736-738.

45. Stern LM, Martin AJ, Jones N, et al. Training inspiratory resistance in Duchenne dystrophy using adapted computer games. *Dev Med Child Neurol.* 1989;31:494-500.

46. Smith PE, Coakley JH, Edwards RH. Respiratory muscle training in Duchenne muscular dystrophy. *Muscle Nerve.* 1988;11:784-785.

47. Ungar, D, Gossler R, Toifl K, Wanke T. Innovative respiratory muscle training for patients with Duchenne muscular dystrophy—a psychological evaluation. *Wien Med Wochenschr.* 1996;146:213-216.

48. Vilozni D, Bar-Yishay E, Gur I, et al. Computerized respiratory muscle training in children with Duchenne muscular dystrophy. *Neuromuscul Disord.* 1994;4:249-255.

49. Gozal D, Thiriet P. Respiratory muscle training in neuromuscular disease: long-term effects on strength and load perception. *Med Sci Sports Exerc.* 1999;31:1522-1527.

50. Matecki S, Topin N, Hayot M, et al. A standardized method for the evaluation of respiratory muscle endurance in patients with Duchenne muscular dystrophy. *Neuromuscul Disord.* 2001;11:171-177.

51. Topin N, Matecki S, Le Bris S, et al. Dose-dependent effect of individualized respiratory muscle training in children with Duchenne muscular dystrophy. *Neuromuscul Disord.* 2002; 12:576-583.

52. Stefanutti D, Benoist MR, Scheinmann P, et al. Usefulness of sniff nasal pressure in patients with neuromuscular or skeletal disorders. *Am J Respir Crit Care Med.* 2000;162:1507-1511.

53. Stone AC, Nolan S, Abu-Hijelth M, et al. A novel form of manually assisted ventilation. *Chest.* 2003;123:949-952.

54. Tecklin JS. The patient with ventilatory pump dysfunction/failure-preferred practice pattern 6E. In: Irwin S, Tecklin JS, eds. *Cardiopulmonary Physical Therapy: A Guide to Practice.* 4th ed. St. Louis, Mo: Mosby; 2004:344-373.

55. Baydur A, Layne E, Aral H, et al. Long term non-invasive ventilation in the community for patients with musculoskeletal disorders: 46 year experience and review. *Thorax.* 2000;55:4-11.

56. Gomez-Merino E, Bach JR. Duchenne muscular dystrophy: prolongation of life by noninvasive ventilation and mechanically assisted coughing. *Am J Phys Med Rehabil.* 2002;81:411-415.

57. Bach JR. Pulmonary Rehabilitation in neuromuscular disorders. *Seminars Respir Med.* 1993;14:515-529.

58. JR, O'Brien J, Krotenberg R, Alba AS. Management of end stage respiratory failure in Duchenne muscular dystrophy. *Muscle Nerve.* 1987;10:177-182.

59. Bach JR. Update and perspectives on noninvasive respiratory muscle aids. Part 1: The inspiratory aids. *Chest.* 1994; 105:1230-1240.

60. Bach JR, Alba AS. Intermittent abdominal pressure ventilator in a regimen of noninvasive ventilatory support. Chest. 1991;99:630-636.

61. Hill NS, Redline S, Carskadon MA, et al. Sleepdisordered breathing in patients with Duchenne muscular dystrophy using negative pressure ventilators. Chest. 1992;102:1656-1662.

62. Guilleminault C, Philip P, Robinson A. Sleep and neuromuscular disease: bilevel positive airway pressure by nasal mask as a treatment for sleep disordered breathing in patients with neuromuscular disease. *J Neurol Neurosurg Psychiatr.* 1998; 65: 225-232.

63. Vianello A, Bevilacqua M, Salvador V, Cardaioli C, Vincenti E. Longterm nasal intermittent positive pressure ventilation in advanced Duchenne's muscular dystrophy. *Chest.* 1994;105:445-448.

64. Simonds AK, Muntoni F, Heather S, Fielding S. Impact of nasal ventilation on survival in hypercapnic Duchenne muscular dystrophy. *Thorax.* 1998;53:949-952.

65. Padman R, Lawless S, Von Nessen S. Use of BiPAP by nasal mask in the treatment of respiratory insufficiency in pediatric patients: preliminary investigation. *Pediatr Pulmonol.* 1994; 17:119-123.

66. Ellis ER, Bye PT, Bruderer JW, Sullivan CE. Treatment of respiratory failure during sleep in patients with neuromuscular disease: positive pressure ventilation through a nose mask. *Am Rev Respir Dis.* 1987; 135:148-152.

67. Barbe F, Quera-Salva MA, de Lattre J, Gajdos P, Agusti AG. Longterm effects of nasal intermittent positive-pressure ventilation on pulmonary function and sleep architecture in patients with neuromuscular diseases. *Chest.* 1996;110:1179-1183.

68. Rideau Y, Delaubier A, Guillou C, Renardel-Irani A. Treatment of respiratory insufficiency in Duchenne's muscular dystrophy: nasal ventilation in the initial stages. *Monaldi Arch Chest Dis.* 1995;50:235-238.

69. Smith PE, Edwards RH, Calverley PM. Oxygen treatment of sleep hypoxaemia in Duchenne muscular dystrophy. *Thorax.* 1989;44:997-1001.

70. Hukins CA, Hillman DR. Daytime predictors of sleep hypoventilation in Duchenne muscular dystrophy. *Am J Respir Crit Care Med.* 2000;161: 166-170.

71. Phillips MF, Smith PE, Carroll N, Edwards RH, Calverley PM. Nocturnal oxygenation and prognosis in Duchenne muscular dystrophy. *Am J Respir Crit Care Med.* 1999;160:198-202.

72. Eagle M, Baudouin SV, Chandler C, Giddings DR, Bullock R, Bushby K. Survival in Duchenne muscular dystrophy: Improvements in life expectancy since 1967 and the impact of home nocturnal ventilation. *Neuromuscul Disord.* 2002;12: 926-929.

73. Jeppesen J, Green A, Steffensen BF, Rahbek J. The Duchenne muscular dystrophy population in Denmark, 1977–2001: Prevalence, incidence, and survival in relation to the introduction of ventilator use. *Neuromuscul Disord.* 2003;13:804-812.

74. Calvert LK, McKeever TM, Kinnear WJ, Britton JR. Trends in survival from muscular dystrophy in England and Wales and impact on respiratory services. *Respir Med.* 2006;100:1058-1063.

75. Gozal D. Pulmonary manifestations of neuromuscular disease with special reference to Duchenne muscular dystrophy and spinal muscular atrophy. *Pediatr Pulmonol.* 2000; 29:141-150.

76. Bach JR, Rajaraman R, Ballanger F, et al. Neuromuscular ventilatory insufficiency: effect of home mechanical ventilator use vs. oxygen therapy on pneumonia and hospitalization rates. *Am J Phys Med Rehabil.* 1998;77:8-19

77. Meir-Jedrezejowicz A, Brophy C, Green M. Respiratory muscle weakness during upper respiratory tract infections. *Am Rev Respir Dis.* 1988;138:5-7.

78. American Thoracic Society Consensus Statement. Respiratory care of the patient with duchenne muscular dystrophy. *Am J Respir Crit Care Med.* 2004;170:456-465.

79. Sivasothy P, Brown L, Smith IE, Shneerson JM. Effect of manually assisted cough and mechanical insufflation on cough flow of normal subjects, patients with chronic obstructive pulmonary disease (COPD), and patients with respiratory muscle weakness. *Thorax.* 2001;56:438-444.

80. Szeinberg A, Tabachnik E, Rashed N, et al. Cough capacity in patients with muscular dystrophy. *Chest.* 1988;94:1232-1235.

81. King M, Brock G, Lundell C. Clearance of mucus by simulated cough. *J Appl Physiol.* 1985;58:1776-1782.

82. Bach JR. The assisted cough and neuromuscular disease. *Pulm Perspect.* 1997;14:4-6.

83. Bach JR. Mechanical insufflation-exsufflation. Comparison of peak expiratory flows with manually assisted and unassisted coughing techniques. *Chest.* 1993;104:1553-1562.

84. Segal M, Salomon A, Herschfus J. Alternating positive-negative pressures in mechanical respiration (the cycling valve device employing air pressures). *Dis Chest.* 1954;25:640-648.

85. Bach JR. Update and perspective on noninvasive respiratory muscle aids. Part 2: The expiratory aids. *Chest.* 1994;105:1538-1544.

86. Miske L, Hickey E, Kolb S, Weiner D, Panitch H. Use of the mechanical in-exsufflator in pediatric patients with neuromuscular disease and impaired cough. *Chest.* 2004;125:1406-1412.

87. Garstang SV, Kirshblum SC, Wood KE. Patient preference for in-exsufflation for secretion management with spinal cord injury. *J Spinal Cord Med.* 2000;23:80-85.

88. Dohna-Schwake C, Ragette R, Teschler H, et al. IPPB-assisted coughing in neuromuscular disorders. *Pediatr Pulm.* 2006;41: 551-557.

89. Birnkrant DJ, Pope JF, Eiben RM. Management of the respiratory complications of neuromuscular disease in the pediatric intensive care unit. *J Child Neurol.* 1999;14:139-143.

90. Stefanutti D, Benoist MR, Scheinmann P, et al. Usefulness of sniff nasal pressure in patients with neuromuscular or skeletal disorders. *Am J Respir Crit Care Med.* 2000;162:1507-1511.

91. Sciaky AJ. Patient education. In: Frownfelter D, Dean E, eds. *Principles and Practice of Cardiopulmonary Physical Therapy.* 3rd ed. St. Louis, Mo: Mosby Year-Book; 1996:453-465.

92. Bothwell JE, Dooley JM, Gordon KE, et al. Duchenne muscular dystrophy—parental perceptions. *Clin Pediatr (Phila).* 2002;41:105-109.

93. Harper DC. Personality correlates and degree of impairment in male adolescents with progressive and non-progressive physical disorders. *J Clin Psychol.* 1983;39:859-867.

94. Fitzpatrick C, Barry C, Garvey C. Psychiatric disorder among boys with Duchenne muscular dystrophy. *Dev Med Child Neurol.* 1986;28:589-595.

95. Witte RA. The psychosocial impact of a progressive physical handicap and terminal illness (Duchenne muscular dystrophy) on adolescents and their families. *Br J Med Psychol.* 1985;58:179-187.

96. Downie W, Leatham PA, Rhind VM, et al. Studies with pain rating scales. *Ann Rheum Dis.* 1978;37:378-381.

97. Jensen MP, Karoly P, Braver S. The measurement of clinical pain intensity: a comparison of six methods. *Pain.* 1986; 27(1):117-126.

98. Spitzer AR, Giancarlo T, Maher L, et al. Neuromuscular causes of prolonged ventilator dependency. *Muscle Nerve.* 1992;16:682-686.

99. Diehl JL, Lofaso F, Deleuze P, et al. Clinically relevant diaphragmatic dysfunction after cardiac operations. *J Thorac Cardiovasc Surg.* 1994;16:487-498.

100. Maher J, Rutledge F, Remtulla H, et al. Neuromuscular disorders associated with failure to wean from the ventilator. *Intensive Care Med.* 1995;16:737-743.

101. Alagesan K. Weaning from mechanical ventilation—present and future. Presented at the 8th World Congress of Intensive & Critical Care Medicine in Sydney, November 2001.

102. Martin AD, Davenport P, Harman E, et al. Use of inspiratory muscle training to facilitate weaning. *Chest.* 2002;122:192-196.

103. Horst HM, Mouro D, Hall-Jenssens RA, Pamukov N. Decrease in ventilation time with a standardized weaning process. *Arch Surg.* 1998;133:483-489.

104. Esteban A, Frutos F, Tobin MJ, et al. A comparison of four methods of weaning patients from mechanical ventilation. *N Engl J Med.* 1995;332:345-350.

105. Ely EW, Baker AM, Dunagan DP, et al. Effect on the duration of mechanical ventilation of identifying patients capable of breathing spontaneously. *N Engl J Med.* 1996;335:1864-1869.

106. Hall JB, Wood LD. Liberation of the patient from mechanical ventilation. *JAMA.* 1987;257:1621-1628.

107. Epstein SK. Controversies in weaning from mechanical ventilation. *J Intensive Care Med.* 2001;16:270-286.

108. Aldrich TK, Uhrlass RM. Weaning from mechanical ventilation: successful use of modified inspiratory resistive training in muscular dystrophy. *Crit Care Med.* 1987;16:247-249.

109. Aldrich TK, Karpel JP, Uhrlass RM, et al. Weaning from mechanical ventilation: adjunctive use of inspiratory muscle resistive training. *Crit Care Med.* 1989;16:143-147.

110. Tzeng AC, Bach JR. Prevention of pulmonary morbidity for patients with neuromuscular disease. *Chest.* 2000;118(5):1390-1396.

111. O'Sullivan SB. Strategies to improve motor control and motor learning. In: O'Sullivan SB, Schmitz TJ, eds. *Physical Rehabilitation Assessment and Treatment.* 4th ed. Philadelphia, Pa: FA Davis Co; 2001:363-410.

112. Fulgham JR, Wijdicks EF. Guillain-Barré syndrome. *Crit Care Clin.* 1997; 13(1):1-15.

113. Massery M. Manual breathing and coughing aids. *Phys Med Rehabil Clin North Am.* 1996;7:407-422.

114. Joseph SA, Tsao CY. Guillain-Barré syndrome. *Adolesc Med.* 2002;13(3): 487-494.

115. Sciaky A, Stockford J, Nixon E. Treatment of acute cardiopulmonary conditions. In: Hillegass EA, Sadowsky HS, eds. *Essentials of Cardiopulmonary Physical Therapy.* 2nd ed. Philadelphia, Pa: WB Saunders Co: 2001;647-675.

116. Eckmann DM, Gavriely N. Chest vibration redistributes intra-airway CO_2 during tracheal insufflation in ventilatory failure. *Crit Care Med.* 1996;24(3):451-457.

117. Gavriely N, Shabtai Y. The effect of tracheal bias flow on gas exchange during high-frequency chest compression. *J Appl Physiol.* 1987;63:303-308.

118. Shekelton M, Berry JK, Covey MK. Respiratory muscle weakness and training. In: Frownfelter D, Dean E, eds. *Principles and Practice of Cardiopulmonary Physical Therapy.* 3rd ed. St Louis, Mo: Mosby-Yearbook; 1996:447.

118. Cooke JF, Orb A. The recovery phase of Guillain-Barré syndrome: moving from dependency to independence. *Rehabil Nurs.* 2003;28(4):105-108, 130.

119. Bernsen RA, deJager AE, Schmitz PR, van der Meche FG. Long term impact on work and private life after Guillain-Barré syndrome. *J Neurol Sci.* 2002;201(1-2):13-17.

Impaired Ventilation and Respiration/Gas Exchange Associated With Respiratory Failure (Pattern F)

Steven Sadowsky, PT, RRT, PhD(c), CCS
Donna Frownfelter, PT, DPT, MA, CCS, FCCP, RRT
Marilyn Moffat, PT, DPT, PhD, FAPTA, CSCS

ANATOMY AND PHYSIOLOGY

The anatomy and physiology of the pulmonary system has been covered in Pattern A: Primary Prevention/Risk Reduction for Cardiovascular/Pulmonary Disorders and Pattern E: Impaired Ventilation and Respiration/Gas Exchange Associated With Ventilatory Pump Dysfunction or Failure.

PATHOPHYSIOLOGY

ACUTE RESPIRATORY FAILURE

Acute respiratory failure (ARF) accounts for more admissions to the ICU than any other organ failure.[1] In the earliest stage of respiratory dysfunction patients may have all, some, or none of the following signs and symptoms as a result of impaired ventilation and respiration/gas exchange: high respiratory rate, nasal flaring, cyanotic lips, abnormal chest movement, and use of the abdominal muscles. While there are innumerable factors that might contribute to the development of respiratory dysfunction, sepsis, aspiration pneumonitis, and trauma are implicated in the vast majority of clinical cases associated with respiratory failure (Table 6-1).[2-5]

When respiratory dysfunction does develop in patients with any of the commonly associated clinical disorders (see Table 6-1), it is generally rapid and progressive. Half of the patients that will go on to develop significant alveolar damage (acute lung injury [ALI], acute respiratory distress syndrome [ARDS], or ARF) will do so within 24 hours of the onset of the initiating event; 85% will do so by 72 hours.[3] When sepsis is the precipitating event, approximately 20% of patients will have already developed demonstrable lung injury at the time that the sepsis syndrome is identified. Yet, this finding is not quite as bleak as it seems since the ICU mortality is only slightly greater than 3% when the lungs are the only organs to fail.[6] Conversely, when ARF is associated with other failing organs, the ICU mortality rises with each additional organ failure to as much as 75% when more than five organs are involved.[1]

Respiratory dysfunction is not an all-or-none phenomenon; rather it presents as a continuum with variable degrees of severity. In its mildest form, respiratory dysfunction is characterized by tachypnea and hypoxemia. However, as lung injury progresses and respiratory function deteriorates, diffuse alveolar damage generates a breakdown in the respiratory and nonrespiratory functions of the lung that is manifested as increased work of breathing, hypercapnia, and worsening hypoxemia that can progress to the point of necessitating mechanical ventilatory support. The initial

Table 6-1

CLINICAL CONDITIONS ASSOCIATED WITH RISK FOR DEVELOPING ACUTE RESPIRATORY DYSFUNCTION

Most Common[a]	Less Common[b]
Sepsis	Acute neuromuscular dysfunction
Aspiration of gastric/oral contents	Anemia
Thoracic or multisystem trauma	Atelectasis
Pneumonia	Cardiothoracic surgery
	Chronic obstructive pulmonary disease
	Drug overdose
	Pneumothorax
	Pulmonary embolism
	Pre- and post-lung transplantation or rejection

The prevalence of any given risk condition varies considerably with geographical location and institution.

[a] Listed in order of prevalence.
[b] Not listed in order of prevalence.

lung injury arises from an unregulated acute inflammatory response that damages capillary endothelial and alveolar epithelial cells, and occurs largely as the consequence of increased alveolar capillary permeability and subsequent pulmonary edema. The development of clinically significant lung injury is typically described as occurring in distinct phases (Figure 6-1).

In the acute, or exudative, phase, a precipitating condition activates interstitial and alveolar macrophages and circulating neutrophils. The activated local macrophages secrete cytokines, interleukins (IL-1, 6, 8, and 10), and tumor necrosis factor α (TNF-α), which stimulate chemotaxis and activate neutrophils locally. Microvascular endothelial damage compounds the activation of circulating neutrophils through the release of lipopolysaccharide, TNF-α, IL-1, 6, and 8, platelet-activating factor, eicosanoids, and the enhanced expression of adhesion complexes.[7-9] The release of IL-1 also stimulates the production of an extracellular matrix by fibroblasts.[5] IL-6 plays a key role in the sequestration of neutrophils in the pulmonary microvasculature.[10,11] Ensuing damage to type I and type II alveolar epithelial cells contributes to alveolar flooding and impedes the removal of edema fluid from the alveolar spaces. In addition, the reduced production and turnover of surfactant contributes to ventilation/perfusion mismatching, atelectasis, and loss of lung compliance.[12,13] Together, these changes produce the characteristic protein-rich lung edema and hypoxemia that is unresponsive to supplemental oxygen therapy. The chest x-ray shows bilateral patchy infiltrates that are indistinguishable from cardiogenic pulmonary edema and may include pleural effusions.[14] Dependent on the severity of the damage, the lung injury will begin to either resolve or progress to a subacute fibroproliferative phase.

If the lung injury arising pursuant to the exudative phase does not resolve with initial therapeutic measures, a fibroproliferative phase ensues that can be seen histologically within about 5 days of the precipitant event.[15] Macrophagic and neutrophilic cytokines that facilitated damage to endothelial and epithelial cells during the exudative phase also play an early role in the process of fibrosis. Procollagens, released from activated interstitial fibroblasts, amplify the developing fibrosing alveolitis. Moreover, such extrinsic factors as mechanical ventilatory support can traumatize the injured lung by overdistending and repeatedly opening and closing damaged alveoli, contributing further to the fibroproliferative phase of lung injury.[16,17] Despite the fact that patients still have respiratory failure with continued poor or worsening lung compliance from fibrosing alveolitis, many will show morphological and radiographic evidence of reduced pulmonary edema 7 to 14 days following the initial onset of edema.[14,18,19]

Normally, squamous type I pneumocytes make up 90% to 95% of the alveolar surface area of the adult lung, and cuboidal type II pneumocytes make up the remainder.[20] However, it seems that type I pneumocytes are more susceptible to injury than type II pneumocytes.[5] Thus, the extent of the alveolar epithelial damage that develops in the acute (exudative) and subacute (fibroproliferative) phases plays a critically important role in the resolution phase. Cytokines and growth factors activated in the exudative and fibroproliferative processes initiate a reactive hyperplasia of remaining type II pneumocytes, which spread to cover the denuded basement membrane.[21] Many of these type II cells then differentiate into type I cells, restoring the normal alveolar epithelial conformation and facilitating the elimination of

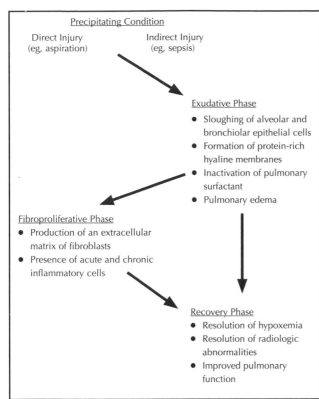

Precipitating Condition

Direct Injury   Indirect Injury
(eg, aspiration)   (eg, sepsis)

Exudative Phase
- Sloughing of alveolar and bronchiolar epithelial cells
- Formation of protein-rich hyaline membranes
- Inactivation of pulmonary surfactant
- Pulmonary edema

Fibroproliferative Phase
- Production of an extracellular matrix of fibroblasts
- Presence of acute and chronic inflammatory cells

Recovery Phase
- Resolution of hypoxemia
- Resolution of radiologic abnormalities
- Improved pulmonary function

Figure 6-1. Phases in the development of lung injury associated with acute respiratory dysfunction. A direct or indirect precipitating condition elicits an unregulated acute inflammatory response, which damages the pulmonary parenchyma. In the exudative phase, pathologic findings include diffuse alveolar damage, with a protein-rich edema fluid in the alveolar spaces, which may resolve or advance to the next phase. In the fibroproliferative phase, cellular debris and fibrin contribute to an evolving fibrosis. In the recovery phase there is a gradual improvement in lung compliance and hypoxemia as fibrosis and edema resolve.

pulmonary edema fluid.[22-24] Thus, the resolution phase is typified by a gradual lessening of hypoxemia and an improvement in lung compliance.

Asthma

Asthma is a chronic obstructive pulmonary disease, or COPD, of complex etiology involving external irritants and increased bronchial reactivity. The disease manifests itself by inflammation and edema of the airways, bronchospasm, and secretions. While the disease generally begins in early childhood, it may happen at any age. It has been estimated that 4 million children under the age of 18 years have had an asthma attack during the previous 12-month period.[25] The airways in patients with asthma may be hyperresponsive to both specific and nonspecific stimuli that result in their diffuse narrowing. The specific stimuli may include allergens

found in foods, chemicals, house dust, animal dander, fungi, molds, and the like. The nonspecific stimuli may include exercise, cold air, respiratory tract infections, or smoke, including passive smoke. Asthma is characterized by episodic airflow obstruction that leads to dyspnea and decreased activity tolerance. The disease is characterized by: hypertrophy of the smooth muscle in the airways; hypertrophy of the mucous glands leading to increased amounts of thick, tenacious mucus; infiltration of eosinophils and lymphocytes; edematous bronchial walls; and subepithelial fibrosis seen particularly in chronic asthma.[26,27]

Airway inflammation may be triggered by both known and unknown factors. Asthma does have a genetic component.[28] Anitgens are recognized as triggers in those with allergic asthma. Pollutants may also be triggers for asthma. Exercise-induced asthma (EIA) and asthma that occurs after a viral respiratory tract infection do not have recognizable triggers.[27] Asthma has also been found to worsen in the presence of other health-related conditions. These include: gastroesophageal reflux disease (GERD), which has been found to be common in patients with asthma and may be related to the asthma itself or its treatment; allergic rhinitis (hay fever), which has been considered a risk factor in asthma; and sinusitis, which when present appears to worsen the symptoms of asthma.[29]

An asthmatic attack is characterized by dyspnea, orthopnea, excessive use of the accessory muscles of respiration, hyperinflation of the lungs, diffuse musical rhonchi, rapid pulse, viscous sputum, and anxiousness.

Status asthmaticus is a life-threatening medical emergency in which asthma symptoms become refractory to bronchodilator therapy. Individuals who are admitted to the emergency department (ED) have complaints of chest tightness, rapidly progressing shortness of breath, wheezing, a dry cough, agitation, and hypoxemia. FEV_1 is significantly decreased. Status asthmaticus often may be seen following a viral infection or exposure to an inhalational irritant. It is more often seen in people with asthma who are not well controlled on their asthma medications.[27]

Medical management of asthma has included: avoidance of allergens, particularly aeroallergens; manipulation of the patient's diet, especially increasing the intake of antioxidants and decreasing the intake of fats; and pharmacological agents, including inhaled corticosteroids, long-acting beta-2 agonist inhalers, and leucotriene receptor antagonists. Based on increasing evidence of airway remodeling (hyperplasia of smooth muscle, proliferation of blood vessels, and deposition of collagen) as a basic component of the pathogenesis of asthma and not as a sequelae of inflammation, monitoring sputum eosinophils and airway hyperresponsiveness or inflammatory biomarkers may be incorporated into future management of asthma.[30]

Pharmacological management has been divided into five steps by the British Thoracic Society, and this guideline considers the management of children over 12 the same as an adult. Step 1 is for those patients with mild infrequent symptoms (treat as required with short-acting beta-2 adrenoceptor agonist bronchodilators); Step 2 is for those with mild persistent symptoms (treat with inhaled corticosteroids and short acting beta-2 agonist daily); Step 3 is for those with moderate persistent symptoms (treat with long-acting beta-adrenocepter agonist and increase inhaled steroid if the former does not work); and Steps 4 and 5 are for those with severe persistent symptoms (treat with high dose inhaled corticosteroids).[31]

One of the controversies in medical management of asthma is the need for and use of corticosteroids over long periods of time to manage the inflammatory issues in asthma. Inhaled corticosteroids are believed to avoid some effects associated with oral steroids, and they are frequently recommended and useful in newly detected disease. Inhaled corticosteroids reduce airway inflammation, airway hyperresponsiveness, and general asthma symptoms and improve pulmonary function.[32] However, the effect and efficacy of long-term corticosteroids is being questioned in asthma management, especially as they increase the risk of osteoporosis in women and in men. Jenkins and associates studied six children who were referred for difficult to control asthma and who underwent endobronchial biopsies. These biopsies revealed lung changes that were consistent with airway remodeling, including thickening of the basement membrane, hypertrophy of the smooth muscle, and a varying degree of hyperplasia of the goblet cells and submucous glands. In five of the six cases there was minimal to no histologic evidence of airway inflammation. Their conclusions suggest that there is a need to look at issues other than inflammation in severe asthma.[33] Gronke and colleagues observed that the issue of inflammation and treatment in asthma may be changed depending on the length of the disease process, such that inflammation may be more associated with hyperresponsiveness in acute asthma, while chronic asthma may have other functional characteristics.[34]

An acute life-threatening episode of asthma occurs when one of following three situations occur: acute severe asthma where the FEV_1 is 30% or less (normal FEV_1=75% to 80%); status asthmaticus where there is resistance to beta-adrenergic agonists and corticosteroids; or acute fulminant asthma which is very severe and rapid and the patient is obtunded. Management includes oxygen, inhaled salbutomol, and IV corticosteroids in order to control the acute episode. If this is not successful, the patient with status asthmaticus requires admission to the ICU for intubation, mechanical ventilation, and life support techniques.[35]

The incidence of status asthmaticus has been declining over the past 10 years. This is attributed to better education, improved medications, greater patient adherence, and improved access to care in the community.[36]

Emphysema

Emphysema is also a COPD of insidious onset that is characterized by irreversible overinflation and eventual destruction of the air spaces distal to the terminal bronchiole. Destruction of the alveolar walls leads to loss of parts of the capillary bed. Pulmonary emphysema has been associated with cigarette smoking, chronic bronchitis, fibrosing lung diseases, and a congenital deficiency of alpha1-antitrypsin (ATT). The types of emphysema are centriacinar, panacinar, paraseptal, and irregular. Centiacinar emphysema is most commonly found in smokers, affects the respiratory bronchioles in the middle of the acinus, spares the peripheral alveoli, and is found primarily in the upper lobes of the lungs. Panacinar emphysema is associated with an alpha1-antitrypsin deficiency, affects all of the alveoli, and is found more in the lower lobes. Paraseptal emphysema affects the outer part of the acinus, especially in the subpleural areas. Irregular emphysema is associated with several chronic destructive lung diseases that lead to scarring in the lung (eg, fibrosing lung diseases).[26,27,37]

Pathophysiologically the recurrent inflammation of the airways is associated with a release of proteolytic enzymes from the lung cells, which leads to the alveolar wall damage and eventual destruction. These changes lead to decreased elasticity of the lung and increased compliance. In addition, alveolar wall destruction leads to lesser lung surface area for gas exchange.[37] Cigarette smoking also destroys the cilia of the lungs, thus impairing the mucociliary transport. Consequently individuals with emphysema often can take in breaths, but they have difficulty in exhalation and emptying of the lungs. Some of the signs and symptoms that are found with long-standing emphysema include a barrel chest (due to the hyperinflation of the airways), use of the accessory muscles of respiration (due to the flattening of the diaphragm with the increasing barrel chest), dyspnea, weak cough, weight loss (the increased oxygen demands for digestion of foods makes the individual even more hypoxemic, which results in decreased food intake), pursed lip breathing (due to the effort to maintain the patency of the airways during expiration), and tachypnea (due to the hypoxemia and the body's attempt to maintain adequate levels of oxygenation to the cells).[37]

Complications of pulmonary emphysema include respiratory infections, cor pulmonale, and respiratory failure. The medical management of emphysema has included smoking cessation, vaccinations (flu and pneumonia), pharmacological agents (anticholinergic bronchodilators, beta-2 agonists, combination drug therapy, corticosteroids, antibiotics, mucolytics, and nonselective phosphodiesterase inhibitors, such as theophylline) oxygen therapy, respiratory support (noninvasive positive pressure ventilation [NPPV], traditional positive pressure ventilation, and invasive positive pressure ventilation), and heliox (a combination of helium and oxygen used for upper airway obstruction in stable severe emphysema).[38] The surgical management of patients with emphysema has included lung volume reduction surgery (LVRS), which has had positive results.[39] Other surgical interventions have included bullectomy and lung transplantation, the latter having shown increased survival, functional capability, and quality of life.[40]

Previously the patient with chronic long-standing emphysema who went into respiratory failure was placed on invasive positive pressure mechanical ventilation. The difficulty with this mechanical ventilation was the potential for even greater air trapping that occurred if the patient was not breathing synchronously with the ventilator. It has traditionally been very difficult to wean the patient from invasive ventilator support. The use of NPPV has proven to be superior with better outcomes than invasive ventilation in this population. This intervention can be started earlier than mechanical ventilation. If there is improvement and patient compliance, it can be effectively utilized to allow for time to reverse the failure and wean the patient entirely from the NPPV or continue to utilize the treatment at home as a supportive intervention.[41]

Innovative pharmacological approaches are being tried in the management of emphysema. These are directed toward the underlying pathophysiological processes of the disease, in addition to disease modification. These therapies include mediator agonists (eg, leukotriene B_4 inhibitors), new anti-inflammatories (eg, phosphdiesterase type 4 and type 5 inhibitors), and protease inhibitors.[38]

Acute Respiratory Distress Syndrome

ARDS, originally called adult respiratory distress syndrome, was first described in 1967 as encompassing the following clinical features: acute respiratory distress (eg, tachypnea, dyspnea), cyanosis that did not respond to oxygen therapy, decreased compliance of the lung, and diffuse fluffy infiltrates on the chest radiograph.[42] Because the syndrome was so poorly understood at the time, the diagnosis was made, as often as not, based on the postmortem findings of atelectasis, vascular congestion, hemorrhage, pulmonary edema, and hyaline membrane formation.

A definition that quantified respiratory impairment based on physiologic criteria using a four-point lung-injury scoring system was proposed for ARDS many years later.[43] Unfortunately, this scoring system lacked specific criteria to exclude a cardiogenic source for pulmonary edema and was not particularly effective in forecasting outcomes in the first 72 hours after onset. Therefore, in 1992, an American-European consensus committee proposed new definitions for ALI and ARDS, which encompassed varying degrees of respiratory dysfunction based upon sequential organ failure assessment (SOFA) score criteria.[44] Table 6-2 presents a paradigm for the classification of respiratory dysfunction based on the SOFA score criteria. The consensus definitions for ALI and ARDS have become the most used and recommended definitions worldwide of acute respiratory dysfunction involving diffuse alveolar damage.[2-5] To date, no consensus definition exists for ARF. However, in 1998, the SOFA score criteria were also proposed as the basis for a definition of ARF that has gained reasonably widespread acceptance.[45] This definition distinguishes ARF from ALI and ARDS by adding a requirement for some form of mechanical ventilatory support to the oxygenation, radiographic, and pulmonary wedge pressure criteria (see Table 6-2).

Despite presently well-accepted definitions for ALI, ARDS, and ARF (see Table 6-2), the incidence of these disorders remains unclear. The National Institutes of Health (NIH) first reported a consensus estimate for the incidence of ARDS at 150,000 cases per year.[46] Subsequent studies have suggested a much lower incidence of ALI/ARDS, with estimates ranging from 2,600 to 44,000 cases per year.[47-53] However, few of the investigators actually applied the SOFA score criteria when estimating incidences for ALI, ARDS, or ARF. Unfortunately, in the two studies that did employ SOFA score criteria, the screening period was limited to 8 weeks or less.[47,48] Nonetheless, the best estimates in the United States place the incidence of ALI at close to 128,000 cases per year[2] and ARDS at about 20,000 cases per year.[54] While there are no incidence estimates for ARF in the United States, the best guess places the incidence close to that originally stated by the NIH.[53]

Patients with ALI, ARDS, and ARF often have a high respiratory rate, nasal flaring, cyanotic lips, abnormal chest wall movement, and exaggerated use of the abdominal muscles as a consequence of bronchoconstriction, bronchial and alveolar edema, and lung inflammation. When compared with patients who do not have ARF, patients with ARF have substantially greater inspiratory resistance and markedly poorer lung/thorax compliance.[55,56] Lung involvement in cases of ALI, ARDS, or ARF is not homogeneous, and there are areas of aerated and appropriately functioning alveoli interspersed with areas of nonfunctional alveoli.[57] The chest radiographs of patients with ALI, ARDS, or ARF are characterized by bilateral pulmonary infiltrates. Too frequently, the distribution of lung injury is an outcome of the interventions administered in the intensive care unit. Typically, consolidation occurs in the lower and posterior regions of the lung, while cystic changes develop in the upper and anterior regions from overdistention secondary to positive pressure ventilation.[52] Impaired lung function is reflected in a reduced partial pressure of oxygen in the arterial blood (PaO_2) and/or an elevated partial pressure of carbon dioxide ($PaCO_2$). However, at the onset of respiratory disease, patients may be both hypoxemic and hypocapnic as they initially increase their minute ventilation in an effort to improve oxygen delivery. However, the work of breathing becomes too great and hypercapnia ensues. Ultimately, progression of the syndrome is evidenced by refractoriness to supplemental oxygen regardless of the $PaCO_2$. Consequently, the ratio of PaO_2 to the FiO_2 provides

Table 6-2

CLASSIFICATION OF THE SEVERITY OF LUNG INJURY BASED ON SOFA SCORE CRITERIA

Dysfunction	Criteria		
	Oxygenation	**Radiographic**	**Non-Cardiogenic Origin**
ALI	$PaO_2/FiO_2 \leq 300$	Bilateral infiltrates compatible with pulmonary edema	No clinical evidence of left atrial hypertension (if measured, PCWP ≤ 18 mmHg)
ARDS	$PaO_2/FiO_2 \leq 200$	Bilateral infiltrates compatible with pulmonary edema	No clinical evidence of left atrial hypertension (if measured, PCWP ≤ 18 mmHg)
ARF	$PaO_2/FiO_2 \leq 200$	Bilateral infiltrates compatible with pulmonary edema	No clinical evidence of left atrial hypertension (if measured, PCWP ≤ 18 mmHg)

Requires some form of mechanical ventilatory support

SOFA=sequential organ failure assessment; ALI=acute lung injury; ARDS=acute respiratory distress syndrome; ARF=acute respiratory failure; PCWP=pulmonary capillary wedge pressure; PaO_2=arterial partial pressure of oxygen; FiO_2=fraction of inspired oxygen

a sensitive and objective measurement of the degree to which oxygenation is impaired and is, therefore, a reliable measure of physiologic respiratory dysfunction.[4,6,58,59]

Overall, mortality rates are lowest in single organ ARF and increase dramatically with each additional organ failure.[1] Not surprisingly, the mortality rate for ARF also increases as the FiO_2 and the peak inspiratory pressure (PIP) required for positive pressure ventilation increase. In general, survivors of ARF are younger than nonsurvivors,[1,52,58,59] with mortality increasing exponentially beyond age 65. Survivors of ARF continue to show evidence of functional limitation even 1 year after discharge from the ICU.[60]

IMAGING

♦ Radiography or chest x-ray is the oldest and most widely available modality for imaging of the lungs

♦ Used to diagnose the site and progression or improvement of disorders of the lung, including pneumonia, infiltrates, hyperinflation, peribronchial thickening, and silhouette of the diaphragm

♦ CT scan
  • Used to detect masses, bronchiectasis, peribronchial wall thickening, and mucus plugging

PHARMACOLOGY

♦ Antianxiety
  • Examples: Lorazepam (Ativan)

  • Actions: Used to relieve anxiety
  • Administered: Orally as tablet or in liquid
  • Side effects: Drowsiness, dizziness, weakness, dry mouth, upset stomach, changes in appetite

♦ Antibiotic
  • Examples: Aminoglycocides (gentamicin [Garamycin, Jenamicin]), cephalosporins (Ancel, Defadyl, Keflex), ciprofloxacin (Cipro, Levaquin), lincomycins (Lincocin, Lincorex), penicillins (amoxicillin, ampicillin, pennicillin G), vancomycin (Vancocin)
  • Actions:
    ▪ Inhibit bacterial growth
    ▪ Aminoglycocides and lincomycins act by inhibiting protein synthesis of a broad spectrum of bacterial organisms
    ▪ Cephalosporins act by inhibiting cell wall synthesis and function of a broad spectrum of bacterial organisms
    ▪ Ciprofloxacin acts by inhibiting an enzyme called DNA gyrase in both gram-positive and gram-negative bacteria
    ▪ Lincomycins act by inhibiting protein synthesis of anaerobic organisms
    ▪ Penicillins act by inhibiting the formation of peptidoglycan cross links in the bacterial cell wall
    ▪ Vancomycin acts by interfering with the construction of cell walls in bacteria
  • Administered: Oral or parenteral
  • Side effects:

- Hypersensitivity reactions, gastrointestinal upset, secondary infections, ototoxicity, nephrotoxicity
- Ototoxicity and nephrotoxicity are rare

◆ Anti-inflammatory—Corticosteroids
- Examples: Fluticasone (Flovent), budesonide (Pulmicort), triamcinolone (Azmacort), flunisolide (Aerobid), beclomethasone (Qvar)
- Actions: Decrease airway inflammation
- Administered: Inhaled
- Side effects: Cough; hoarseness; oral yeast infections (thrush); long-term use may increase skin thinning, bruising, and osteoporosis

◆ Antiviral
- Examples: Imipenem-cilastatin or ganciclovir (Primaxin IV)
- Actions: Used to prevent cytomegalovirus (CMV) disease in high risk patients
- Administered: Intravenously
- Side effects: Stomach upset, diarrhea, constipation, dry mouth, depression, joint and muscle pain

◆ Bronchodilator—Inhaled—Short acting
- Examples: Beta$_2$ agonists (Albuterol, Alupent, Bronkaid Mist, Isuprel, Maxair, Proventil, Ventolin), anticholinergics (Atrovent, Bentyl, Levbid), tiotropium (Spiriva HandiHaler)
- Actions:
  - Open airways and optimize ventilation and airway clearance
  - Bronchomotor tone is mediated by cholinergic and adrenergic stimulation
  - Stimulation of adrenergic beta$_2$ receptors produces an increase in cyclic adenosine monophosphate and bronchodilation
  - Stimulation of cholinergic muscarinic receptors produces an increase in cyclic guanosine monophosphate and bronchoconstriction
- Administered: Oral inhalation
- Side effects: Dry mouth and throat, throat irritation, tachycardia, headache, nausea, hyperactivity, urinary retention, constipation, allergy

◆ Bronchodilators—Inhaled—Long acting
- Examples: Salmeterol (Serevent), formoterol (Foradil)
- Actions: Prevent bronchospasm during exercise by relaxing and opening airways
- Administered: Oral inhalation
- Side effects: Headache, dry mouth, cough, muscle pain, throat irritation, stuffed or runny nose, flu-like symptoms
- Note: In November 2005, the US Food and Drug Administration (FDA) issued an advisory that Foradil Aerolizer and Serevent Diskus may increase risk of severe asthma and possibly death

◆ Bronchodilators—Systemic
- Examples: Aminophylline and theophylline (Aerolate, Respbid, Theo-Dur)
- Actions: Open airways and relieve cough, wheezing, and dyspnea
- Administered: Oral or intravenously
- Side effects: Headache, tachypnea, increased urination, nausea, nervousness, trembling, trouble in sleeping, heartburn, vomiting, skin rash

◆ Central nervous system depressant
- Examples: Fentanyl (Duragesic)
- Actions: Used as an analgesic and central nervous system depressant
- Administered: Intravenously
- Side effects: Skin rash, swelling, dizziness, light-headedness, stomach upsets, constipation, difficulty urinating

◆ EIA suppressors
- Examples (conventional): Short-acting agonists, cromolyn sodium, nedocromil sodium, and leukotriene modifiers (montelukast [Singulair] and zafirlukast [Accolate])
- Examples (unconventional): Heparin, calcium channel blockers, furosemide (Lasix), terfenadine (Seldane)
- Actions: Effects bronchial vasculature to modulate both the cooling and/or rewarming phases of the EIA
- Administered: Metered dose inhalers
- Side effects: Insignificant to minimal for conventional suppressors

◆ Leukotriene modifiers
- Examples: Montelukast (Singulair), zafirlukast (Accolate)
- Actions: Reduce production of leukotrienes (released in lungs during asthma attack that lead to inflammation of lungs), as well as blocking their action to prevent asthma attack
- Administered: Oral
- Side effects: Headache, dizziness, upset stomach, nasal stuffiness, cough

◆ Mast cell stabilizer
- Example: Cromolyn sodium (Intal), nedocromil (Tilade)
- Action: Prevents wheezing and dyspnea, prevents inflammation of airways, prevent EIA
- Administered: Oral inhalation
- Side effects: Sore throat, stomach pain, cough, itching or burning of nasal passageways, headache

Case Study #1: Respiratory Failure

Susan Bradford is a 12-year-old female with asthma who was hospitalized due to an exacerbation that has resulted in status asthmaticus and respiratory failure.

PHYSICAL THERAPIST EXAMINATION

HISTORY

Because of the patient's condition, much of the history was obtained from her mother, Janet, from previous medical records, and from a discussion with her pediatrician.

- ♦ General demographics: Susan Bradford is a 12-year-old seventh grader in White Springs Junior High School. She is right-hand dominant. English is her native language.

- ♦ Social history: She lives with her parents, who are very protective of her and have shielded her from activities.

- ♦ Employment/work: She is a full-time student. She has done babysitting with her cousins on Saturday nights this year and wishes to continue to earn extra money for clothes and going to the movies.

- ♦ Living environment: She lives in a two-story single family home three blocks from her school. There are three steps to enter the house, five steps down to the recreation room, and 16 steps to the second floor bedrooms, all of which have handrails.

- ♦ General health status
  - General health perception: Susan and her mother feel her health has markedly declined this year. They would say her health is poor. She has missed several days from school because of her asthma and has had several "bad colds." Susan had stated that her medications "don't seem to help so I don't take them like I should."
  - Physical function: Susan has never consistently taken part in any after school or community center physical activities, as they made her short of breath with wheezing, which then made her stop the activity. On many occasions her mother had sent a note to school asking that she be excused from physical education since her asthma was "acting up." She often went to the school nurse's office to rest or asked to have her mother called so she could be taken home because she was short of breath and uncomfortable.
  - Psychological function: This current hospitalization was frightening to Susan and her family. Susan later stated that she felt very much out of control and thought she was "going to die."

- Role function: Daughter, student.
- Social function: Susan has not interacted with her peers as would be expected for her age due to her asthma and her reluctance to participate in any after school activities.

- ♦ Social/health habits: Neither Susan nor her parents smoke.

- ♦ Family history: Her mother also has asthma, which is controlled fairly well with medications. Her father has suffered from a variety of food and contact allergies.

- ♦ Medical/surgical history: Susan has a history of asthma that was originally diagnosed at age 3 following an upper respiratory tract infection. Of late, she has been noncompliant with her medications and activity recommendations.

- ♦ Prior hospitalizations: Susan has had several ED visits for exacerbations of her asthma. Two years ago she was also admitted to the hospital through the ED for pneumonia.

- ♦ Preexisting medical and other health-related conditions: Patient has had a 9-year history of asthma. She has been deconditioned over the past year and a half.

- ♦ Current condition(s)/chief complaint(s)
  - Susan had a "cold" for approximately 2 weeks prior to admission. She and her mother visited the pediatrician who felt it was a viral infection, and she was sent home with her usual asthma medication for relief of shortness of breath. Over the next week she became more distressed, missed a week of school, and her parents stated, "she had increased difficulty breathing, wheezing, and started to turn blue." She became difficult to arouse. Paramedics were called, and they administered aminophyllin intravenously, put her on oxygen by mask, and transported her to the hospital.
  - In the ED she was given bronchodilators and high flow oxygen at 50% FIO$_2$. Arterial blood gases initially were drawn (pH=7.26, pCO$_2$=55 mmHg, and pO$_2$=70 mmHg), and she was diagnosed with status asthmaticus and acute respiratory failure. She was intubated and placed on mechanical ventilation in an assist-control mode and transferred to the pediatric ICU.
  - Within 24 hours the medications had allowed Susan's acute exacerbation to stabilize, and she was extubated and removed from the mechanical ventilation and transferred out of the ICU 2 days later.
  - Susan was initially seen by the physical therapist in the ICU after she was extubated. She was in bed watching TV, looking tired. Her mother was sitting in a chair by her bed holding her hand.

- She remained in the hospital for 3 more days and then was seen for physical therapy as an outpatient.

♦ Functional status and activity level: Susan has led a very inactive life style since she did not like to take her metered dose inhalers, which would have made activity participation possible. Following the intubation and time on the ventilator she was very tired and is now even more fearful about participating in activity of any kind.

♦ Medications: Susan is currently on albuterol, atrovent, prednisone, beclamethosone, aminophyllin, and intol (chromolyn sodium).

♦ Other clinical tests:
  - ABG analyses were used to follow her clinical course in the ICU
    - Following 24 hours on mechanical ventilation, her ABGs on O_2 at 24% FiO_2 indicated the following:
      - pH: 7.35 (below 7.35=acidosis and above 7.45=alkalosis)
      - pCO_2=45 mmHg (normal=35 to 45 mmHg and above 45=hypercapnea and below 35=hypocapnea)
      - pO_2=80 mmHg (normal=80 to 100 mmHg and below 80=hypoxemia)
    - Her ABGs were WNL with supplemental O_2
    - On the third ICU day, her ABGs were WNL, and she was taken off oxygen
  - Oxygen saturation (SO_2) was used to follow her clinical course after the ICU
    - Initially her SaO_2 was 93% (normal=typically 98%)
    - During activity and exercise her O_2 sat levels were to be maintained above 91% since therapy is usually contraindicated in most clinics when values fall below 90%
  - Blood chemistry: Results first day out of ICU
    - Hgb: 14 gm/dL=WNL (normal for females=13 to 16 gm/dL)
    - Hct: 42%=WNL (normal for females=37% to 48%)
    - No bacterial infection
  - Chest radiograph: Results first day out of ICU
    - Indicated scattered haziness throughout the lungs and mild hyperinflation (most likely due to dynamic hyperinflation with shortness of breath and rapid respiratory rate)
  - Postdischarge from the ICU, Susan may have the following tests:
    - Spirometry to determine her vital capacity (maximum air inhaled and exhaled), peak expiratory flow rate (also known as peak flow rate and is the maximum flow rate generated during a forced exhalation), and FEV_1
    - A Challenge Test to determine if airway obstruction and asthma symptoms are triggered through an airway constricting chemical (eg, methacholine), and a positive test is defined as a decrease from the baseline of FEV_1 or of the postdiluent FEV_1 value of 20%
    - A Challenge Test may also be used to determine if airway obstruction and asthma symptoms are triggered through breaths of cold air or through an exercise bout of sufficient intensity to trigger symptoms
    - Nitric oxide, which is a marker of asthma, is measured in exhaled air

SYSTEMS REVIEW

♦ Cardiovascular/pulmonary
  - BP: 118/78 mmHg
  - Edema: None
  - HR: 110 bpm at rest
  - RR: 24 bpm

♦ Integumentary
  - Presence of scar formation: None
  - Skin color: WNL
  - Skin integrity: Small areas of redness on cheeks from tape from endotracheal tube

♦ Musculoskeletal
  - Gross range of motion: WFL
  - Gross strength: WFL considering her deconditioning
  - Gross symmetry: Slight pectus excavatum, slumped posture, shoulders protracted, slightly forward head and neck
  - Height: 5'3" (1.6 m)
  - Weight: 100 lb (45.36 kg)

♦ Neuromuscular
  - Balance: Not able to assess at this time
  - Locomotion, transfers, and transitions:
    - Able to come to sit on the side of the bed
    - Able to come to stand with minimal assist
    - Able to walk 25 feet with moderate assistance, but with great difficulty (see Tests and Measures, Aerobic Capacity/Endurance)

♦ Communication, affect, cognition, language, and learning style
  - Susan understands and responds appropriately to verbal commands
  - She is frightened about the incident and becoming short of breath again

- She is concerned about her asthma in that it seems to be getting worse, and she feels helpless and does not want to die having another bad asthma attack
- Learning preference is not determined at this time

TESTS AND MEASURES

- ◆ Aerobic capacity/endurance
  - Susan walked 25 feet, coughed, and became short of breath
  - HR was 110 bpm at rest and rose to 132 bpm following the walk
  - BP was 118/78 mmHg at rest and rose to 132/80 mmHg following the walk
  - RR was 24 bpm at rest and rose to 26 bpm following the walk
  - Vertical visual analogue scale for dyspnea: 3 cm at rest to 8 cm following walk (on 10 cm scale where 0=no dyspnea and 10=worst dyspnea)[61]
  - She also had mild to moderate inspiratory wheezing following the short walk
- ◆ Anthropometric characteristics
  - BMI: 17.7 which is considered underweight[62]
- ◆ Arousal, attention, and cognition
  - Alert and oriented x3
- ◆ Circulation
  - Auscultation revealed S_1 and S_2 heart sounds, but no S_3 or S_4
  - HR at rest 110 bpm considered tachypnea (normal=60 to 100 bpm)
  - Pulses easily palpable
- ◆ Ergonomics and body mechanics
  - Poor body mechanics with transfers and ambulation
  - Sits slumped in chair
- ◆ Gait, locomotion, and balance
  - Single leg stance: Difficulty standing on one foot for 20 seconds
  - Tends to use stairs with use of handrail only if necessary as it makes her short of breath
  - Does not do any activities that challenge her balance
  - Ambulates independently but slowly and with dyspnea and moderate inspiratory wheezing at the end of 25 feet
- ◆ Muscle performance
  - Overall 4/5 muscle strength in UEs and LEs
  - Decreased core muscle strength 3+/4
  - Flaring of lower ribs
  - Accessory muscle use to breathe at rest that increases with activity
- ◆ Posture
  - Mild forward head and neck

- Slight lordosis
- Shoulders protracted bilaterally
- Moderate kyphosis
- Minimal pectus excavatum
- ◆ Range of motion
  - ROM all peripheral joints: WNL
  - Chest wall mobility decreased at upper, middle, and lower chest
    - Upper chest: ¾" expansion at 2nd rib
    - Mid chest: 1" at 4th rib
    - Lower chest: 1½" at xiphoid
- ◆ Self-care and home management
  - Prior to this episode
    - Susan was independent in all ADL, but did become short of breath when cleaning her room, going up and down stairs, and carrying laundry or groceries
    - With chores that required more physical exertion, she had to take rest breaks and was also affected by dust and molds
  - At this time
    - Her heart rate increased to 116 bpm and her respiratory rate increased to 25 bpm with positional change from supine to sit
    - Susan was able to come to sit at side of the bed, but she became fearful and more short of breath
    - With instruction in pursed lip breathing, she was able to calm down and achieve the seated position
    - When seated in a chair, she pushes up on armrests of the chair to stand
- ◆ Ventilation and respiration/gas exchange
  - Auscultation revealed
    - Significantly decreased breath sounds throughout the lung fields
    - Inspiratory wheezing bilaterally in the upper anterior chest
    - Coarse scattered crackles in both lower lung bases
  - Breathing pattern
    - Susan tends to be an upper chest breather using accessory muscles (especially the sternocleidomastoid, scalenes, pectoralis major, and trapezius muscles) at rest with increased use of these muscles with talking and activity
    - Inspiration/expiration ratio revealed prolongation of the expiratory phase
    - She speaks in short three- or four-word sentences
  - Cough is productive of small to moderate amounts of thick, clear to slightly yellow mucus
  - 15-count breathlessness score was 4

♦ Work, community, and leisure integration or reintegration
  • Susan has become short of breath when carrying school bag
  • Susan has not participated in any community or school physical activity outside of physical education and even here she has sat out of many classes secondary to shortness of breath
  • She has not done any sport activities where balance is needed
  • She expresses a desire to be more like the other kids, but she is concerned her asthma will not allow her to do the activities in which she would be interested (eg, dancing in a jazz group at school or running with the track team)
  • She has also tried swimming but found the local pool had so much chlorine she became wheezy and could not swim

EVALUATION

Susan is a 12-year-old junior high student with a long-standing history of asthma that became refractory to medication and consequently she was admitted with status asthmaticus and respiratory failure. She is beginning to have improved medication management, but she continues to have inspiratory wheezing and congestion. Her activity tolerance is fair but limited by dyspnea and fear. Her family is frightened that her asthma may get worse and after this episode she may die. They have been very protective and shielded her from activities that could cause her shortness of breath. Consequently she is very deconditioned and not sure if she can or wants to increase her physical activity and fitness level. Her nutrition and hydration status are also a concern. She is discouraged and is having difficulty motivating herself to perform physical activity because she is afraid of another "asthma attack."

DIAGNOSIS

Susan is a patient admitted to the ED with status asthmatics in respiratory failure. She is deconditioned secondary to lack of exercise and an inactive lifestyle, which was limited by shortness of breath and noncompliance with her medication management. She has impaired: aerobic capacity/endurance; anthropometric characteristics; ergonomics and body mechanics; gait, locomotion, and balance; muscle performance; posture; and ventilation and respiration/gas exchange. She is functionally limited in self-care, home management school, community, and leisure actions, tasks, and activities. These findings are consistent with placement in Pattern F: Impaired Ventilation and Respiration/Gas Exchange Associated With Respiratory Failure and Pattern

B: Impaired Ventilation and Respiration/Gas Exchange Associated With Deconditioning.[63]

PROGNOSIS AND PLAN OF CARE

Over the course of visits, the following mutually established acute care outcomes have been determined:
♦ Ability to perform self-care activities is improved
♦ Aerobic capacity and endurance is increased
♦ Airway clearance is improved
♦ Balance is increased
♦ Energy expenditure for a given workload is decreased
♦ Fitness is improved
♦ Functional independence in ADL and IADL is increased
♦ Knowledge of behaviors that foster healthy habits, wellness, and prevention is increased
♦ Muscle performance is increased
♦ Physical capacity is improved
♦ Physical function is improved
♦ Posture is improved
♦ Risk of increased exacerbations is decreased
♦ ROM is improved
♦ Self-management of medications and symptoms is improved
♦ Work of breathing is decreased

To achieve these outcomes, the appropriate interventions for this patient will include: coordination, communication, and documentation; patient/client-related instruction; therapeutic exercise; functional training in self-care and home management; functional training in school, community, and leisure or reintegration; and airway clearance techniques.

Based on the diagnosis, Susan will receive six visits twice daily for the 3 days in the hospital on the pediatric floor. She will then have 8 to 12 outpatient visits over a 4- to 6-week period with a follow-up visit every 2 months for the next 6 months to upgrade her exercise program and monitor her progression and adherence to medication and activity regimens. Susan's prognosis is good secondary to her motivation and the concern of her parents to have her enjoy a healthier lifestyle without the need for life-saving interventions.

INTERVENTIONS

RATIONALE FOR SELECTED INTERVENTIONS

The goals of treating asthma in young individuals have traditionally been to improve symptoms and normalize lung function. Today's goals include reduction in frequency and severity of asthma exacerbations, decreased potential for mortality, normalization of the hyper-responsiveness of the airways, normal development of lung function, and normal psychosocial development. These goals are achieved by improved patient/parent education, exercise training, compliance with drug regimens, and easy access to health care.[64]

Therapeutic Exercise

Exercise conditioning in people with asthma demonstrates that exercise can be performed safely and can significantly improve cardiovascular fitness levels and quality of life. These changes are important in the short-term management of patients with asthma, but also in the long-term outcomes of living a healthier life. An appropriate exercise program for the child with asthma will enhance physical activity and lead to more normal growth and self-concept.[65] Research has reported reduced school absenteeism, hospitalizations, wheezing, need for medications, doctor consultations, and asthma attacks and improved peer social interaction, aerobic fitness, and functional capacity in children with asthma who exercised vigorously and regularly.[66-68] Cambach and associates found that patients with asthma who underwent an intensive physical therapy training program consisting of exercise, breathing retraining, pulmonary hygiene, relaxation techniques, education, leisure activities, and drug treatment had significant improvements in their exercise tolerance and quality of life.[69] Of interest is the fact that about 10% of athletes from the United States who have participated in the Olympics have been individuals with asthma.[70]

About one-third of children with asthma miss the opportunity for exercise in physical education or sports about once a week because of their condition. In the United Kingdom a program called "Out There & Active" aims to promote more understanding about the benefits of exercise for asthma in parents, children, and teachers through the use of posters, booklets, and other means of education.[71]

Education and experience with exercise are the keys to turning around the pattern of deconditioning seen in many children with asthma. Minute ventilation and oxygen consumption are both improved in patients with asthma with exercise, while blood lactate is decreased.[72] In addition to these changes, physical fitness activities have also been shown to raise exercise tolerance and exercise capacity and decrease the ventilatory requirement and cardiac frequency.[73]

The intensity of exercise is dependent upon the patient's symptoms and previous conditioning. Most patients with asthma who have engaged in exercise should be able to safely exercise at intensities of 50% to 60% of their age-predicted maximum heart rate (MHR). Patients who wish to exercise at higher intensities should consider alternating the intensity of the activity between high and moderate while training and should also consider their symptoms on any given day and exercise at higher intensities on symptom-free days.[74]

Patients with mild asthma who participated in a 10-week aerobic conditioning program had increases in maximum voluntary ventilation, maximum oxygen consumption, anaerobic threshold, and the amount of air moved in and out of the lungs as compared to the normal controls. In addition, they had decreases in their: minute ventilation for each level of work; ventilatory equivalent; exercise-induced rapid breathing; and dyspnea index at both submaximal and maximal exercise.[75] In a study of an 8-week basketball training program as an alternative exercise program for children with asthma, beneficial effects were shown in quality of life and exercise capacity.[76]

The type of exercise prescribed is very important. Lighter aerobic activity, such as walking, bicycling, or swimming, will usually be better tolerated than running. Weight training is usually well tolerated, but one must make sure to prevent breath holding. Sports that have some "down time," such as baseball, bowling, gymnastics, wrestling, golf, volleyball, and tennis may be better tolerated since all of these sport activities have more built in rest periods than other sport activities. If the person decides he or she wants to run, then consideration of the environment is important. For example running outdoors generally will potentially be more difficult than running inside on a track, especially during cold weather, during hay fever and pollen seasons, and in more polluted environments. An indoor treadmill, bicycle, or skiing machine may be tolerated better in bad weather. Swimming, which occurs in a warm, moist environment, has been found to be an optimal exercise and generally causes less bronchospasm and is less asthmogenic than running.[77,78] Yet a pool with strong chlorine fumes can also cause bronchospasm; so many factors need to be evaluated in choosing an exercise program.[79] Sport activities that should generally be avoided may include basketball, soccer, distance running, field hockey, ice hockey, cross country skiing, and ice skating.

Exercises to improve ventilation and chest wall motion are integral in the exercise program. Pursed lip breathing and ventilatory strategies are integrated into movement patterns to decrease shortness of breath with activity.[80] Breathing strategies pair trunk extension with inspiration and trunk flexion with exhalation to improve ventilation and oxygenation and reduce exertional dyspnea. From a theoretical viewpoint it might seem that training inspiratory muscles may be beneficial but there is a lack of evidence to strongly recommend this intervention. Esteve and associates provided 30 training sessions for patients with asthma in a breathing retraining program that was aimed at having the patient adjust each breath to a target breath using video feedback. Patients had significant improvements in FEV_1 and FVC.[81]

Slader and associates also trained 57 people with asthma between the ages of 15 and 80 years in two different types of breathing exercises through use of a video tape (group 1 was taught shallow nasal breaths with slow exhalation and group 2 was taught postural alignment, UE exercises, relaxation, and breath control through the nose or mouth). All participants had used a preventer inhaler and also required a rescue inhaler at least four times a week prior to the study. The exercises were done twice daily for a period of 30 weeks, and the videotape was used for at least one session each day. Patients were also instructed to perform their breathing exercises for 3 to 5 minutes before they used any rescue inhalers (drugs taken for an asthma attack). The results were similar in both groups and showed an 86% reduction in use of the rescue inhalers and a 50% drop in use of preventer drugs. No changes in lung function, airway responsiveness, or quality of life scores were noted.[82]

Buteyko breathing techniques, originally proposed by Russian scientist Konstantin Buteyko, are based on his philosophy that one of the major pathophysiological causes of asthma is the result of hyperventilation that leads to both airway and alveolar hypocapnia. Thus, the Buteyko treatment attempts to normalize breathing so that the patient with asthma breathes less. The breathing exercises are aimed at reducing both the depth and the frequency of respiration.[83] Bowler and associates evaluated the effect of Buteyko breathing techniques in patients with asthma and found a significant reduction in beta-2 agonist dosage and a trend toward a decrease in minute volume and steroid use and an increase in quality of life.[84]

A yoga training program for patients with bronchial asthma resulted in improved peak expiratory flow rates and number of asthma attacks and decreased drug use. Individuals who practiced yoga regularly had the greatest changes.[85,86] Yoga breathing exercises consisting of deep breathing for 15 minutes performed twice daily over a 2-week period of time improved airway hypersensitivity to histamine in patients with mild asthma.[87] Children with asthma who were trained in yoga were shown to have significant increases in exercise capacity and pulmonary function which continued to show reduced symptoms and decreased drug use over a 2-year period of time.[88] A yoga therapy program performed by patients with chronic bronchial asthma resulted in increased exercise tolerance as measured by the 12-Minute Walk test and a modified Harvard Step test and decreased symptoms as measured by the Exercise Liability Index. These same patients 1 year later still had reduced symptom scores and decreased drug use.[89] A 1-week yoga training program for patients with bronchial asthma resulted in decreased RHR and sympathetic reactivity leading to relaxation of the voluntary muscles of inspiration and expiration.[90] In a randomized control trial, patients with moderate to severe asthma who underwent 4 months of 2-hour Sahaja yoga sessions once a week had improved level of airway responsiveness to methacholine (an aerosolized chemical that triggers a hyperresponsive reaction) and increased mood scores on quality of life measures.[91]

One study had looked at the effect of yoga and naturopathy (nonpharmacological approach to treatment) on patients with bronchial asthma. Significant improvement in pulmonary function (PEFR, VC, FVC, FEV_1, FEV/FEC %, maximum voluntary ventilation) and in erythrocyte sedimentation rate (ESR) and absolute eosinophil count were noted, as well as an increased feeling of well-being.[92]

Coordination of exercise and activity with medication has been shown to produce optimal outcomes. Short-acting beta agonists, such as Alupent metered dose inhalers, have been shown to be effective in preventing bronchoconstriction with exercise.[93]

McCleary and associates studied 21 patients with asthma who participated in a 24-week pulmonary rehabilitation program that consisted of aerobic conditioning, strength training, and education. These patients had improved workload (VO_2 max) and anaerobic threshold. In addition, they had improved quality of life as determined by the SF-36 and Asthma Quality of Life Questionnaire.[94]

Exercise Prescription

The important considerations in exercise prescription for patients with asthma are to slowly increase the exercise tolerance starting with smaller increments and building up the time and distance of walking, bicycling, or swimming. The warm-up period will be extended prior to exercise incorporating easy walking coordinated with breathing exercises and stretching of the chest wall and UEs and LEs. In the same way, the cool-down period will be extended to allow the airways to rewarm. Pacing during exercise at lower levels of intensity in appropriately warm, more moist environments will initially be used to begin to develop aerobic conditioning. As conditioning improves, the intensity of the activity will be increased. Patients with asthma have been shown to benefit from aerobic conditioning exercise at 60% to 85% of their MHR over a period of 20 to 30 minutes with a frequency of several times a week.[95] The exercise prescription will take into account the patient's personal preferences and what activities she finds more enjoyable and fun, which should enhance participation in a long-term program of physical activity.

Barriers to Exercise

Negative attitudes about exercise for patients with asthma have been shown to exist in those patients with more severe disease, those with less self-efficacy, those with less knowledge, and those with more negative attitudes toward their disease. Internal and external barriers have been reported by patients with asthma as to why they either limited their exercise or did not participate in exercise at all. These barriers included time constraints, lack of intrinsic motivation, and weather conditions that made their asthma worse and thus decreased participation. On the other hand, a desire to be healthy and the patient's social supports were given as items that facilitated physical activity.[96]

Exercise-Induced Asthma (EIA)

EIA occurs in many children who are asthmatic. EIA is believed to be the result of reduced temperature and water content of inspired air in the lower respiratory tract during exercise, which then results in increased airway resistance and bronchospasm.[97] While this has been the traditionally held basis of EIA, McFadden postulated that the severity of EIA depends on the usual cooling and drying of the airways, but also depends on the rate of rewarming and rehydration of the airways after the exercise has stopped.[98,99] The symptoms of EIA include dyspnea, wheezing, chest tightness or pain, cough, and facial distress, and they follow a fairly short period of bronchodilation that occurs early in exercise.[100] EIA usually requires an exercise workload that is at an intensity of about 80% of the patient's maximum oxygen consumption. However, in patients with severe asthma, exercise at a very minimal level may be sufficient to produce EIA symptoms.[101] McFadden has stated that all patients with asthma will experience EIA if the exercise challenge is of sufficient magnitude.[102]

Bronchospasm may occur within 10 to 15 minutes of the start of exercise, may peak 8 to 15 minutes after exercise cessation, and usually resolves about 1 hour later.[103] EIA has been observed to occur immediately after short bouts of intense exercise or may occur 6 to 8 hours after submaximal exercise.[100]

Treatment of Exercise-Induced Asthma

EIA may be minimized through several different approaches. The patient should be taught to breathe through the nose rather than through the mouth so that the air entering the respiratory passageways is warmed, filtered, and humidified. In addition, the use of a facemask may help to reduce the loss of heat and moisture during exercise.[104,105] A prolonged warm-up period with brief periods of intense activity may also help to minimize EIA.[106,107] The cool down period should be gradual to increase the rate of rewarming of the airways and decrease the bronchospasm.[108] Options of activities (eg, walking, bicycling, swimming) should be given as it has been noted that EIA tends to be increased in cold dry air and fewer problems are noted in humid air. Consequently, time of the year, allergies, and cold weather will play a part in decisions about outdoor aerobic activity versus indoor aerobic activity.[78]

Although the data do not support a decrease in EIA with consistent exercise or a change in pulmonary function, consistent exercise has been shown to allow patients to increase their exercise load before they reach the EIA threshold.[73,108,109]

EIA symptoms can be controlled by using an inhaled bronchodilator prior to exercise ("reliever" inhalers). If this is not enough to prevent EIA, then a "preventor" medication, such as Intal (chromolyn sodium), can also be used. "Rescue" inhalers (eg, beta agonists) would be used in the case of an asthma attack. The drug guidelines for prevention of EIA issued by the National Heart Lung and Blood Institute include the use of short-acting agonists and salmeterol, nedocromil, and cromolyn.[110] Another consideration is that the nasal passages should be clear if they are to act as filters and humidifiers to filter out pollutants, allergens, and keep the air at body temperature and humidity. Nasal infections and rhinitis are very common in this population and can affect the lower airways and cause more irritability. Some precipitants to EIA include cold air, tobacco smoke, stress, infections, laughing, GERD, and some medications that contain respiratory irritants, and therefore these precipitants should be avoided as much as possible.

COORDINATION, COMMUNICATION, AND DOCUMENTATION

Communication will occur with all individuals concerned with Susan's health and wellness. Coordination of activities must occur between Susan's physician, her parents, the teachers in her school, the physical education teacher or any other personnel involved in physical activity programs at school, the school nurse, and the school counselor so that there is follow through on recommendations for exercise and physical activity and for her medications. Of particular importance will be the appropriate use of preventer medications prior to participation in physical education classes and any other physical activity in which she may participate. In addition school personnel can support her need to rest as necessary until her aerobic conditioning and breathing control is developed.

A referral to a dietitian may be helpful if her low weight continues to be a concern. Susan's eating may be typical of junior high school girls, who want to be thin, or it can be the result of her asthma. A referral to a psychologist may also be appropriate to help her deal with her fears about increasing activity and the difficulties encountered with this recent episode. All elements of the patient's management will be documented.[111]

PATIENT/CLIENT-RELATED INSTRUCTION

Susan had a short course of mechanical ventilation following status asthmaticus following a viral infection. She has had numerous exacerbations due to her poor compliance with medications and general health and lack of exercise and fitness. She will need a coordinated approach of the health care team so that instruction is provided on asthma self-management, the necessity of self-monitoring, and the need for being proactive in achieving a positive healthy lifestyle. Emphasis will be placed on adherence to medications, breathing exercises, aerobic conditioning, strength training, and increasing leisure and community activities. She will be instructed in correct use of her inhaler. Her parents will also be instructed to take a proactive role in facilitating Susan's weight gain by finding food she enjoys and encouraging good nutrition and hydration.

Many people with asthma feel that exercise is harmful to them. This concern needs to be addressed with Susan and her parents through education and positive experiences with exercise.[96]

The physical therapist will need to work with Susan's family to address issues of medication compliance, improved nutrition and hydration, and increased activity and participation in after school activities or classes. The parents need to change their behavior towards her shortness of breath and participate in making sure she uses her medication properly and help her understand the importance of becoming more physically active and fit. They can be encouraged to be more involved as a family in physical activities and help their daughter build more confidence in her ability to be more active without experiencing shortness of breath limiting her function. The mother in particular, who also has mild asthma, can be supportive in sharing how she has managed her asthma, yet recognizing that her daughter's asthma may be worse and needs additional treatment, attention, and support. They will need to receive information on asthma and current treatment and can be directed to support groups and educational offerings through the American Lung Association. The American Lung Association has asthma training programs that can be conducted in local schools for education and support for children with asthma.

THERAPEUTIC EXERCISE

- ◆ Aerobic capacity/endurance conditioning
  - • In hospital
    - ▪ Susan will begin with a very gentle walking program to start developing a positive attitude to increasing aerobic conditioning
    - ▪ Gentle warm-up exercises of breathing coordinated with UE activity will allow the airways to begin to adjust to increasing demand
    - ▪ Gentle cool down will then allow the airways to rewarm after the walking program
  - • Outpatient
    - ▪ At all times she will make sure that her asthma is under control before beginning any aerobic conditioning
    - ▪ Preventive medications of cromolyn (Intal) or bronchodilators may be taken 15 to 20 minutes before exercise
    - ▪ She will warm up at least 10 minutes
    - ▪ Initially she will start at lower levels (eg, recumbent bicycle, treadmill, indoor skiing machine, water walking, or swimming) and increase her time and workload (eg, add intermittent inclines on the treadmill)
    - ▪ If symptoms occur during exercise, Susan will be instructed to stop and rest and if necessary, take her rescuer medication
    - ▪ She will cool down to allow the bronchial tree to rewarm

  - ▪ She will use the Ventilatory Response Index to monitor her exertion, stopping to rest if it takes more than three breaths to count to 15[112] and the Borg dyspnea scale[113]
  - ▪ Susan will progress to aerobic activities four to five times per week for 30 to 40 minutes
  - ▪ She will avoid exercising in cold weather (if outdoors, she should cover nose and mouth with a scarf), in dry environments, or in heavily polluted environments
  - ▪ She will be fully instructed in EIA and aerobically trained to increase the exercise load before she reaches the EIA threshold
  - ▪ Susan can listen to CDs or music videos and dance for continuous aerobic activity
- • Balance, coordination, and agility training
  - ▪ In hospital
    - ▶ Begin balance activities on one foot for 10 seconds, alternating feet
    - ▶ Then rise up on toes and lift one foot off the floor and balance for 5 seconds
  - ▪ Outpatient
    - ▶ Susan will progress to standing on one foot up to 30 to 60 seconds then progress to standing on a foam surface, roller, balance board, or rocker
    - ▶ UE movements will be added to balancing on one foot to further challenge her balance
    - ▶ Tandem walking on a line will be performed
    - ▶ Carioca, grapevine, and line dancing steps may be utilized as fun activities to enhance balance, coordination, and agility
    - ▶ Yoga Tree Position balancing on one foot with arms up overhead
- • Body mechanics and postural stabilization
  - ▪ In hospital
    - ▶ Initial instruction on postural alignment stressing axial extension and relaxed shoulders
  - ▪ Outpatient
    - ▶ Instruction in proper body mechanics for home and school stressing good upright alignment with the chest open to facilitate breathing
    - ▶ Postural awareness training using a mirror for visual input as needed
    - ▶ Avoid any Valsalva maneuver during exercises
    - ▶ Begin bridging to increase core stabilization and progress by decreasing the base of support
    - ▶ Increase strengthening of abdominals and back extensor muscles being sure to coordinate with breathing (eg, backlying knees up, breathe in through the nose as reach hands to knees, blow out through pursed lips as raise head and shoulders up and lower back down; on hands

and knees, breathe in though nose as raise right arm and left leg our in air and blow out through pursed lips as lower back to starting position)

▶ Seated balance on gymnastic ball making it a fun activity for core stabilization

■ Flexibility exercises
▶ In hospital
  ○ Initial warm up and breathing prior to stretching
  ○ Gentle flexibility exercises to include trunk flexion, extension, rotation, and lateral trunk flexion
  ○ Raise arms overhead as breathe in through nose and blow out through pursed lips as lower back down
  ○ Hands behind head with elbows forward, breathe in through nose as press elbows back, and blow out through pursed lips as bring elbows forward
▶ Outpatient
  ○ Stretching exercises should be done after warming up, using a slow and steady stretch accompanied by deep breathing, and building hold up to 15 to 30 seconds
  ○ Done two to three times a day, at least two to three repetitions
  ○ Stretching of the chest wall by standing with right side near the wall and reaching left hand up and over head to touch wall to increase lateral flexion of the trunk and reverse sides
  ○ Trunk rotation with arms out to shoulder height
  ○ Trunk flexion and extension with arms overhead
  ○ UE (eg, Back Scratch Test position) and LE (eg, straight leg raises, hip flexor stretch) stretches
  ○ Yoga stretching exercises (eg, Side Stretch—standing, arms up with one hand on top of the other in front of body, breathe in with elongation of spine and rotate to one side as breathe out; Full Bend—standing or sitting, breathe in with elongation of spine and breathe out with spinal flexion; The Butterfly—sitting with soles of feet together, knees toward floor; The Cobra—prone push up on hands with extended spine; Spine Twist—seated one leg crossed over other and twist spine to other side)

■ Gait and locomotion training

▶ In hospital
  ○ Instruction in pacing ambulation coordinated with breathing (expiration twice as long as inspiration, thus ratio of 1 inspiration to 2 expiration) so that breathe in for count of 1 or 2 or 3 and blow out for count of 2 or 4 or 6 respectively
▶ Outpatient
  ○ Instruction in pacing and breathing strategies for stair climbing

■ Relaxation
▶ In hospital
  ○ Breathing strategies to increase relaxation (diaphragmatic breathing, pursed lip breathing, Jacobsen's relaxation exercises)
  ○ Relaxation of accessory muscles using mirror for feedback
▶ Outpatient
  ○ Continue relaxation training especially during periods of shortness of breath
  ○ Teach diaphragmatic action using shallow nasal breaths with slow exhalation and decreased accessory muscle use during periods of stress
  ○ Teach her to use relaxation with breathing exercises for 3 to 5 minutes before using any rescue inhalers
  ○ Yoga relaxation techniques (eg, Shoulder rolls, arm rolls, head rolls, Baby pose)

■ Strength, power and endurance training
▶ Outpatient
  ○ Avoid any Valsalva maneuver during exercises
  ○ General strengthening exercises for UEs and LEs coordinated with breathing so that when possible, if the exercise opens up the chest, it should be coordinated with inspiration, and if the exercise compresses the chest, it should be coordinated with expiration
  ○ Practice sit to stand without using arms
  ○ Chair push-ups using armrests coordinated with breathing
  ○ Back extensor and trunk flexor muscle strengthening exercises using Swiss Ball coordinated with breathing (eg, partial sit-ups on the ball coordinated with breathing as indicated in core stabilization exercises, back extension over the ball to neutral with inspiration on extension and expiration on return to starting position over the ball)
  ○ Yoga strengthening (eg, Easy Bridge with arms flat on floor, Downward Dog on hands

and knees with buttocks up in air; Plank position on hands and knees with body perfectly straight; The Triangle with feet wider than shoulders as slide right hand down right leg to ankle and left hand stretches out over head to the right)

FUNCTIONAL TRAINING IN SELF-CARE AND HOME MANAGEMENT

♦ In hospital
  • Instruction in self-care activities using ventilatory strategies (eg, pursed lip breathing, breathing paced with movements)
♦ Outpatient
  • Continued instruction in self-care and home chores using ventilatory strategies
  • Instruction in use of proper posture and body mechanics during self-care and home chore activities
  • Injury prevention or reduction
  • Instruction in efficiency and energy conservation while performing ADL and IADL

FUNCTIONAL TRAINING IN SCHOOL, COMMUNITY, AND LEISURE INTEGRATION OR REINTEGRATION

♦ Outpatient
  • School
    ▪ Only carry necessary books to class or encourage use of a rolling backpack to decrease dyspnea
    ▪ Communication with physical education teacher and school nurse on appropriate steps to increase her activity
    ▪ Participate in any activity in which Susan can find enjoyment (eg, softball, gymnastics, volleyball)
    ▪ Participate in before or after school programs of her choice keeping in mind appropriate guidelines for physical education activities (eg, longer warm-up and cool-down periods, progressively increasing the demand of the activity, appropriate use of medications, use of rest when needed, breathing strategies if shortness of breath occurs, adequate hydration)
  • Community
    ▪ Susan and family should find a community activity to increase activity
    ▪ Contact the local pool regarding the levels of chlorine
    ▪ Other community sport activities which Susan should try to see if she can find enjoyment and eventual increased fitness may include bowling, golf, or tennis

AIRWAY CLEARANCE TECHNIQUES

♦ In hospital
  • Breathing strategies
    ▪ Active cycles of breathing technique for more effective secretion clearance
      ► Three to four thoracic expansions using diaphragmatic breathing at normal TV
      ► Three to four deep thoracic expansions to the inspiratory reserve volume (may use breathe hold or sniff) at end of expansion
      ► Forced expiratory technique using huffing interspersed with breathing control—May use one or two huffs after medium-sized breath to mobilize secretions in the peripheral airways and one or two huffs after a deep breath to mobilize secretions in the proximal airways
      ► Pause for breathing control after one or two huffs
    ▪ Cough techniques for more effective secretion clearance
      ► Adequate inspiration associated with trunk extension
      ► Closure of the glottis
      ► Build up of both intra-abdominal and intra-thoracic pressures
      ► Glottis opening and expulsion associated with trunk flexion
  • Mechanical techniques
    ▪ Acapella™ device which provides oscillation and positive pressure to facilitate airway clearance when secretions are present
  • Positioning
    ▪ Positioning to alter work of breathing (eg, seated and using trunk extension to facilitate inspiration and flexion to facilitate expiration; sidelying to facilitate inspiration in the uppermost lung segments) and to maximize ventilation and perfusion (eg, use of gravity in lower most segments of lungs to facilitate perfusion)
♦ Outpatient
  • Breathing strategies
    ▪ Active cycles of breathing technique for more effective secretion clearance
    ▪ Cough techniques for more effective secretion clearance
    ▪ Yoga breathing techniques (eg, Arched Breath—sitting on feet, arch back as breathe in through nose and round back as breathe out through nose; Complete Breath—sitting legs crossed with hands on lower abdomen, diaphragmatic breathing, then move hands up rib cage and expand mid chest,

and finally upper chest; Standing 8-Count—deep breath and elongate spine, breathe out for count of 8 using complete breath technique from lower chest to upper chest; Alternate nostril breath)

- As she increases her respiratory and aerobic capabilities, practice breathing exercises for 3 to 5 minutes before use of any rescue inhaler
- Try Buteyko breathing exercises to reduce the depth and the frequency of respiration

- Mechanical techniques
  - Acapella™ device which provides oscillation and positive pressure to facilitate airway clearance when secretions are present

- Positioning
  - Positioning to alter work of breathing and to maximize ventilation and perfusion

Anticipated Goals and Expected Outcomes

- ◆ Impact on pathology/pathophysiology
  - Acute exacerbations are markedly decreased.
  - Episodes of dyspnea are decreased.
  - Incidence of pneumonias is decreased.

- ◆ Impact on impairments
  - Aerobic capacity is increased to 20 to 30 minutes of walking or bicycling with minimal dyspnea in 4 weeks.
  - Balance is improved so patient can stand on one leg unsupported for 40 seconds.
  - Chest wall mobility is improved.
  - Effort expenditure per unit of work is decreased.
  - Endurance is increased, and she is more active in physical education, in after school activities, and in community activity programs.
  - Muscle performance is increased so extremity strength is 4+/5 and core strength is 4/4+.
  - Posture is improved, head is more axially extended, shoulders are back and down, and lumbar lordosis is reduced.
  - Posture is improved with use of rolling backpack.
  - Relaxation is increased.
  - Ventilation/respiration and gas exchange are improved.
  - Work of breathing is decreased.

- ◆ Impact of functional limitations
  - Susan's ability to perform and find enjoyment in physical activity at school, at home, and in the community is improved in 4 weeks.

- ◆ Risk reduction/prevention
  - Parents will cooperate with more active family outings together.

- Parents will encourage Susan to be adherent to her medication regimen and become more active and participatory at school and in the community.
- Susan will find satisfaction and pride in self-management of her asthma and her ability to lead a more normal life.

- ◆ Impact on societal resources
  - Documentation occurs throughout the patient management and follows APTA's *Guidelines for Physical Therapy Documentation*.[111]

- ◆ Impact on health, wellness, and fitness
  - Susan has improved health status through improved activity, nutrition, and hydration.
  - Physical capacity is increased.
  - Physical function is improved.

REEXAMINATION

Reexamination is performed throughout the episode of care.

DISCHARGE

Susan is discharged from physical therapy after a total of six inpatient visits over 3 days in the hospital and 10 outpatient visits over 6 weeks. She will have follow-up visits scheduled in 1 month, 3 months, and 5 months to monitor progress and attainment of goals and expectations. A letter will be sent to her pediatrician discussing follow-up in the future as needed. She will continue to need monitoring, but for this episode of care she has completed her goals and expected outcomes.

PSYCHOLOGICAL ASPECTS

The family has been through a frightening time with this exacerbation and Susan's hospitalization and need for mechanical ventilation. They are very concerned and want to prevent this from happening again. They now realize that trying to protect and limit Susan's activity level to prevent shortness of breath was the wrong approach and are willing to try the regimen of medication, exercise, and increased physical activity and fitness. They are willing to support Susan and become more active as a family.

Since Susan was frightened by this exacerbation, she is at a point where she can take on responsibility for the self-management of her asthma with supervision from her parents. This responsibility will allow her to be more independent and to function at an improved level.

A referral to a school guidance counselor may help Susan discuss issues of concern and help monitor her progress. The school may be able to work with the American Lung

Association to bring their Asthma 101 program into the school so Susan can meet with others in the school with asthma and can learn more about the disease and strategies of management. This could form a support group for her as well.

Susan and her parents feel encouraged and hopeful that their new understanding of asthma and the need for more exercise and conditioning will make a significant difference in Susan's life. The more active lifestyle and adherence to her medication regimen will make a significant difference in her ability to lead a more normal and productive life. As a junior high student, Susan wants to be "like the rest of the kids" and increasing activity with more breathing control will allow her to do that.

Case Study #2: Acute Respiratory Failure

Wally Maier is an 84-year-old male with long-standing end-stage chronic obstructive pulmonary disease who was hospitalized due to an acute lower respiratory tract infection which led to ventilatory failure.

PHYSICAL THERAPIST EXAMINATION

HISTORY

- General demographics: Wally Maier is an 84-year-old white male who is right-hand dominant. His native language is English.

- Social history: He was widowed 16 years ago. He has three children who live across the country and visit only on holidays or special occasions. He has four grandchildren, none living nearby. He has few friends because so many have died, and he has not made close friends at the assisted living residence.

- Employment /work: Mr. Maier was an auto painter and retired 17 years ago.

- Living environment: Mr. Maier has been living in a senior assisted-living center for the past 9 years.

- General health status
  - General health perception: He considers himself to be in poor to fair health at this time.
  - Physical function: Mr. Maier can typically walk to meals (less than 150 feet) using his rolling walker and supplemental O_2 at 3 liters per minute, but occasionally requires minimal to moderate assistance for balance loss due to fatigue and weakness. He often needs to stop three or four times to rest while walking to meals.

- Psychological function: He has occasional mild depression (appropriate for his medical condition). He does not feel his family visits often enough and is sad that many friends have died.

- Role function: Father, grandfather, friend, patient.

- Social function: Mr. Maier's social activity has been diminishing over the past few years. Recently he gave up organizing the checkers and card games in his assisted living residence. He has acquaintances and infrequent family visits. He occasionally participates in social activities that are not "too strenuous," such as cards, checkers, group TV or movies, and chair exercises depending on how he feels on a given day. He does not do these activities on any regular basis.

- Social/health habits: Mr. Maier has an 80 pack-a-year smoking history, and he quit smoking 25 years ago. He enjoys an occasional beer (but he misses the shots of whiskey that he used to have with his buddies).

- Family history: His father died in World War II, and his mother died 20 years ago secondary to a MI. He had a younger brother, who died 10 years ago in a motor vehicle accident.

- Medical/surgical history: Mr. Maier has had: a tonsillectomy/adenectomy at age 7, an appendectomy at age 19, a fractured left ulna and left radius following a motorcycle accident at age 29, numerous bouts of pneumonia, and numerous acute exacerbations of his COPD. Most recently, Mr. Maier experienced an acute lower respiratory infection initially treated with broad-spectrum antibiotics. Four days ago, he complained of dyspnea, malaise, fever, and chills. He was seen by his pulmonologist and referred to the local community hospital, where he was admitted for sputum culture and sensitivity and definitive antibiotic therapy. However, on hospital day 1 he complained of difficulty breathing. Because of his age and diagnosis, and in keeping with his advanced directive, the decision was made not to intubate, but rather to attempt to provide noninvasive mechanical ventilatory assistance.

- Prior hospitalizations: He has had numerous bouts of pneumonia requiring hospitalizations: the first bout was at age 44 "in the right lung"; the second and third bouts were at age 46 in the right lung and in both lungs, respectively; the fourth bout was at age 47 in the left lung (at which time he was diagnosed with COPD, which was initially managed by his general practitioner); the fifth bout of bilateral pneumonia was at age 53; and the sixth episode of pneumonia was in the right lung at age 62. His case management was shifted to a pulmonologist during the sixth bout. He also was hospitalized for his COPD at ages 56,

58, 63, 65, 68, 71, 72, 74, and 75. At age 75, his son placed him in the senior assisted living center at the recommendation of the pulmonologist. Since moving into the assisted-living center and being monitored more closely by nursing and medical staff, the number of exacerbations has diminished, but their severity has continued to increase. He has been hospitalized twice since moving into the assisted living residence for pneumonia and COPD exacerbation.

- Preexisting medical and other health-related conditions: He has had long-standing COPD.
- Current condition(s)/chief complaint(s): Mr. Maier has general weakness and severe shortness of breath with any activity, and he complains about the bilevel positive airway pressure (BIPAP) mask.
- Functional status and activity level: He is currently dependent for assisted bed mobility and transfer skills (bed to chair; bed to commode, etc) due to shortness of breath, weakness (especially LE), and depression.
- Medications: He is currently receiving ciprofloxacin (Cipro) and tiotropium (Spiriva).
- Other clinical tests:
  - ABGs
    - pH: 7.21 (normal pH 7.35 to 7.45)
    - pCO_2: 68 mmHg (normal 35 to 45 mmHg)
    - pO_2: 58 mmHg (normal 80 to 100 mmHg)
    - HCO_3^-: 34 mEq/L (normal 21 to 28 mEq/L)
    - SaO_2: 85% on room air
    - Above values indicating a significant respiratory acidosis (partially compensated) with ventilatory failure and severe oxygenation deficit
  - Hct: 48% (normal=37% to 47%) slightly elevated
  - Hgb: 19 (normal=12 to 18) slightly elevated
  - Imaging: X-ray revealed:
    - Hyperinflation
    - Flat hemidiaphragms
    - Bullous changes
  - Pulmonary function tests (PFTs) percent predicted (liters)
    - FEV_1: 27% predicted (0.62)
    - FVC: 55% predicted (1.73)
    - FEV_1/FVC ratio: 36%
    - TLC: 90% predicted (5.11)
    - RV: 148% (3.22)
    - $DLCO_2$: 60% (12.7 ml/min/mmHg) indicating severe end-stage COPD with dynamic hyperinflation and marked reduction in diffusing capacity

SYSTEMS REVIEW

- Cardiovascular/pulmonary
  - BP: 138/86 mmHg
  - Edema: None
  - HR: 118 bpm
  - RR: 26 bpm
- Integumentary
  - Presence of scar formation: Old, well-healed appendectomy scar in right lower abdominal quadrant
  - Skin color: WNL, but ecchymoses noted on both forearms and hands
  - Skin integrity: Intact, but fragile with ecchymoses noted above
- Musculoskeletal
  - Gross range of motion: UEs and LEs WFL with slight hip and knee flexion contractures
  - Gross strength: Generalized weakness with LE>UE (difficult to adequately assess due to shortness of breath and fatigue)
  - Gross symmetry: Symmetrical with barrel chest
  - Height: 5'11" (1.80 m)
  - Weight: 168 lbs (76.4 kg)
- Neuromuscular
  - Balance: Difficulty with balance noted
  - Locomotion, transfers, and transitions:
    - Locomotion not tested at this time due to BIPAP
    - Transfers to/from bed/chair with contact guarding
- Communication, affect, cognition, language, and learning style
  - Communication: Responds appropriately to direct questions, able to follow simple commands, shortness of breath limits communication, able to speak in three- or four-word sentences
  - Affect: Flat
  - Cognition: Grossly intact
  - Learning preferences: Unable to assess at this time

TESTS AND MEASURES

- Aerobic capacity/endurance
  - Unable to assess at this time due to inability to perform 6-Minute Walk test or any continuous activity secondary to shortness of breath and BIPAP
  - In time, as Mr. Maier increases his activity upon return to home, a 6-Minute Walk test may be used to assess his aerobic capacity using his rating of shortness of breath to monitor his exercise intensity
  - Eventually a symptom limited exercise test using a treadmill or bicycle may be used to determine his training HR and perceived exertion

♦ Anthropometric characteristics
- BMI for his age=weight (lbs) ÷ height (inches) ÷ height (inches) x 703
- Mr. Maier's BMI was 23.4, which is within normal range[62]

♦ Arousal, attention, and cognition
- Alert and oriented x3
- Distracted due to shortness of breath

♦ Circulation
- Pulse is 118 bpm at rest, indicating significant tachycardia
- Pulse is regular
- Auscultation of heart revealed presence of S_1 and S_2, but no S_3 or S_4
- Dorsalis pedis pulse is diminished and difficult to palpate

♦ Gait, locomotion, and balance
- Unable to assess secondary to acute status
- Patient was independently using rolling walker (with seat) for ambulation at the assisted living center
- Ambulation was previously limited by shortness of breath after about 30 feet (rate of perceived exertion=12[112] and 15-Count Breathlessness Score [also known as the Ventilatory Response Index]=2 to 3)[113]
- Needed to make several stops walking to meals or activities to "catch his breath"
- Recently he had been doing less as he was more congested

♦ Integumentary integrity
- Assessment of skin integrity of the nose and face revealed no breakdown or pressure wounds as a result of using the BIPAP

♦ Muscle performance
- Overall strength: Generalized weakness with LE > UE (difficult to adequately assess due to shortness of breath and fatigue)

♦ Posture
- Forward head and neck position
- Barrel chest
- Kyphosis
- Slight flexion hips and knees

♦ Range of motion
- Decreased chest wall mobility in lateral planes
- Decreased use of diaphragm
- 10-degree right hip flexion contracture and 5-degree flexion contractures in left hip and both knees

♦ Reflex integrity: Slightly diminished in both UE and LE

♦ Self-care and home management
- Currently Mr. Maier needs help with bathing and ADL secondary to BIPAP and weakness

- Nursing staff positioning him well and turning frequently
- At his residence Mr. Maier needed help with homemaking
- He has a cleaning service in two times a week
- Meals are served in the dining room, but he has a refrigerator and microwave and likes to have snacks between meals that he can prepare

♦ Ventilation and respiration/gas exchange
- Auscultation of lungs revealed
  - Crackles heard in both lower lobes, R>L
  - Audible upper airway congestion
- Breathing pattern
  - Primarily upper chest with accessory muscles
  - Accessory muscles at rest and increased use with activity
- Cough productive of thick yellow mucous, which is difficult to mobilize

♦ Work, community, and leisure integration or reintegration
- Mr. Maier has been participating less in social activities prior to this hospitalization
- He feels somewhat isolated and this may contribute to his depression

EVALUATION

Mr. Maier has had long standing COPD with numerous exacerbations and hospitalizations. Since he has been under the care of a pulmonologist, the nursing and medical staff at the assisted living facility have monitored him carefully and have treated his pneumonias on site rather than allowing for progression of congestion to pneumonia and hospitalization. He is a widower, none of his sons or grandchildren live nearby and only visit on occasion. He participates socially only in low-level activities and lately has decreased participation due to shortness of breath. He has expressed feeling depressed and sad. He appears weak and is currently on a BIPAP by nasal mask for assisted ventilation in the Respiratory Care Floor of the hospital.

DIAGNOSIS

Mr. Maier has COPD with acute respiratory failure. He has impaired: aerobic capacity/endurance; anthropometric characteristics; gait, locomotion, and balance; muscle performance; posture; range of motion; and ventilation/respiration/gas exchange. He is functionally limited in self-care and home management and in work, community, and leisure actions, tasks, and activities. He is currently on bilevel positive airway pressure. These findings are consistent with placement in Pattern F: Impaired Ventilation and Respiration/

Gas Exchange Associated With Respiratory Failure. He may also be classified in Pattern C: Impaired Ventilation, Respiration/Gas Exchange, and Aerobic Capacity/Endurance Associated With Airway Clearance Dysfunction and Pattern B: Impaired Aerobic Capacity/Endurance Associated With Deconditioning.

Prognosis and Plan of Care

Over the course of the visits, the following mutually established outcomes have been determined:

♦ Aerobic capacity and endurance is improved

♦ Affect is improved and social interaction in assisted living is resumed

♦ Energy expenditure per unit of work is decreased

♦ Functional independence in ADL and IADL is increased

♦ Gait, locomotion, and balance are improved and independent ambulation is achieved

♦ Hydration status is improved

♦ Independence in ADL continues

♦ Muscle performance is increased

♦ Physical and psychological status will be improved

♦ Physical capacity is improved

♦ Physical function is improved

♦ Risk factors are reduced

♦ ROM is improved

To achieve these outcomes, the appropriate interventions for this patient are determined. These will include: coordination, communication, and documentation; patient/client-related instruction; therapeutic exercise; functional training in self-care and home management; functional training in work, community, and leisure integration or reintegration; prescription, application, and, as appropriate, fabrication of devices and equipment; airway clearance techniques; and electrotherapeutic modalities.

Based on the diagnosis and prognosis, Mr. Maier will be seen for 20 to 24 visits, 10 to 12 in the acute care during his 7-day hospitalization and 10 to 12 in the skilled care unit over 3 weeks. Mr. Maier has little social support, but he is somewhat motivated to get back to more social activity and will follow through with his exercise program.

Interventions

RATIONALE FOR SELECTED INTERVENTIONS

The American Lung Association has found that the majority of patients with COPD find their disease limits their ability to work, perform household chores, engage in family and social activities, physically exert themselves, and even sleep.[114] Thus, it is incumbent upon physical therapists to provide interventions that will enhance independence in self-care, home management, work, community, and leisure actions, task, and activities, as well as enhance quality of life and physical performance. The primary interventions for maximizing cardiovascular and pulmonary function and oxygen transport in patients with COPD include patient education, exercises, support devices and equipment, and airway clearance techniques. Energy conservation is essential to simplify tasks and to decrease oxygen demands of everyday tasks and ADL. Smoking cessation is an essential part of the education process for these patients.[115,116]

Therapeutic Exercise

Aerobic Conditioning/Endurance and Strength Training

The benefits of aerobic and strength training in people with COPD is well established for the long-term management of air flow limitations to optimize oxygen transport.[117-120] Even people with COPD, who cannot achieve significant workloads, will have improvement with lower level activity. This improvement may be the result of desensitization of dyspnea, greater efficiency of movement, and improved anaerobic capacity, muscle strength, and endurance. Motivation may also be enhanced with increasing activity and is an important parameter of the exercise prescription for these patients.[117,121,122]

Increasing shortness of breath in patients with emphysema leads to a more sedentary life, a decline in functional capacity, and often more social isolation and depression. With decreasing ability to perform aerobic conditioning/endurance activities and strength training exercises, a viscous cycle occurs of increased shortness of breath with exertion → increased fatigue within the muscles → progressive loss of functional capacity → increasing disability → increased shortness of breath. Thus, physical therapist's interventions must seek to reverse this decline.

Increasing exercise training and physical activity with patients with COPD has been shown to reverse the deconditioning cycle by increasing: exercise tolerance and endurance, physical capacity, quality of life, functional improvements and independence in ADL, and ability to perform work, community, and leisure actions, tasks, and activities. Increasing exercise training and physical activity has also been shown to decrease: dyspnea, fatigue, anxiety about breathlessness, number of hospitalizations, and health care utilization. Exercise has been shown to stimulate the nervous system in patients with COPD leading to benefits in cognitive performance. In addition, such increased activity may also improve survival.[118,123-132] Even after an acute exacerbation, patients with COPD are excellent candidates for a progressive exercise training program.[131] Physiologically exercise results in several training effects for patients with emphysema, including faster uptake of oxygen following the beginning of exercise,[132] higher tidal volumes, lower ventilatory requirement for exercise,[133] decreased heart rate for given work load, decreased lactic acidosis, increased trained muscle capillary density, and enhanced mitochondrial enzyme activity.[134-136] It is important to translate the physiological changes that result from exercise training into improvements in ADL, and therefore exercise prescriptions for both aerobic capacity/endurance training and resistive strengthening exercises must be rigorous and scientifically based in accordance with the patient's abilities.[137]

Exercise prescriptions for patients with emphysema must incorporate the basic principles of mode, intensity, frequency, duration, and suitable progression. Patients who have severe chronic emphysema have been shown to be capable of attaining and sustaining the training intensity and duration necessary for adaptation of the skeletal muscles.[138,139] A combination of both aerobic conditioning/endurance training and strength training are probably best suited to treat the peripheral muscle dysfunction found in patients with chronic emphysema, because they lead to improvements in total body endurance and muscle strength.[140] The joint statement of the American College of Chest Physicians and the American Association of Cardiovascular and Pulmonary Rehabilitation (ACCP/AACVPR) recommends an exercise program that incorporates LE training to improve exercise tolerance and UE training of strength and endurance to improve arm function.[141] The American Thoracic Society (ATS) and the European Respiratory Society (ERS) have put forth the following guidelines for exercise programs for patients with COPD based upon the evidence available:[142]

1. A minimum of 20 sessions should be given at least three times per week to achieve physiologic benefits; twice-weekly supervised plus one unsupervised home session may also be acceptable.[143]

2. High-intensity exercise produces greater physiologic benefit and should be encouraged; however, low-intensity training is also effective for those patients who cannot achieve this level of intensity.[134,142]

3. Interval training (repeated high-intensity exercise interspersed with rest or light exercise) may be useful in promoting higher levels of exercise training in the more symptomatic patients.[144-147]

4. Both UE (eg, arm cycle ergometer, free weights, elastic bands) and LE (eg, treadmill, stationary cycle ergometer) training should be utilized.[148]

5. The combination of endurance and strength training generally has multiple beneficial effects and is well tolerated; strength training would be particularly indicated for patients with significant muscle atrophy (eg, 50% to 85% of 1 RM for 6 to 12 repetitions and for two to four sets).[149,150]

The ATS/ERS guidelines also indicate that an exercise intensity exceeding 60% of peak exercise capacity is deemed enough to achieve a training effect, although higher percentages will produce greater benefits and are tolerated. Symptoms of dyspnea or fatigue are usually used as the targets for exercise and a Borg dyspnea score of between 4 and 6 is considered an appropriate target for exercise performance.[141]

Patients with COPD who were strength trained significantly increased their strength, those who were endurance trained significantly increased their submaximal exercise capacity, and those who were both strength and endurance trained significantly increased both parameters. These patients also had significant improvements in breathlessness scores and dyspnea.[149]

Muscle function and walking endurance has also been found to increase in patients with COPD, who were on a combined program of aerobic capacity exercise and progressive resistance strengthening exercises.[151]

Exercise has been shown to have positive effects on mental health in particular in the elderly. Aerobic exercise has been shown to significantly reduce depression in older individuals.[142]

Muscle wasting has been shown to be a common clinical finding in patients with advanced emphysema,[152] and gains in strength and muscle mass have been shown to result in increased exercise tolerance and survival.[153-155] Thus, exercise programs for patients with emphysema should incorporate activities aimed at improving peripheral muscle strength.

Inspiratory Muscle Training

Diaphragmatic breathing and decreased use of the accessory muscles of respiration have been historically advocated in the management of patients with emphysema. While patients trained in diaphragmatic breathing are able to change their pattern of breathing,[156-158] asynchronous and paradoxical breathing movements may be increased,[156-160] while no changes appear to occur in ventilation distribution.[158] In addition, no changes were found in exercise capacity or pulmonary function with diaphragmatic breathing.[160] In patients with severe COPD, dyspnea was found to increase with diaphragmatic breathing.[156,161] Diaphragmatic breathing was also found to reduce the efficiency of breathing, increase the work of breathing, and increase the oxygen demands of breathing.[156,159,161] Thus, it appears that there is scant support for the use of diaphragmatic breathing training in patients with emphysema.

Slow deep breathing has also been advocated in the management of patients with emphysema. On the one hand, this breathing pattern has been shown to have positive benefits of increasing TV, increasing PaO_2, and decreasing respiratory frequency, but on the other hand has shown that diaphragmatic fatigue occurred faster.[162]

Since both inspiratory muscle strength and endurance are compromised in patients with emphysema, respiratory muscle training has been advocated. This training has included: inspiratory resistive breathing or inspiratory muscle training (patient breathes through a mouthpiece with an adjustable diameter mouthpiece providing flow-dependent resistance); threshold loading (patient breathes though a mouthpiece with flow-independent resistance); and normocapnic hyperpnea ([NCH] patient breathes maximally for 15 to 20 minutes through a simple partial rebreathing system). Well-controlled inspiratory muscle training (at least 30% of the MIP for 30 minutes per day) has been shown to increase MIP, the endurance of the inspiratory muscles, exercise performance, and the proportion of type I fibers and the size of type II fibers in the external intercostals muscles, while it has been shown to decrease dyspnea and nocturnal desaturation time.[163-172] The combination of inspiratory muscle training with exercise training enhanced exercise capacity more than exercise training alone.[164,165,168,170] Threshold loading has been shown to increase the speed of shortening on the inspiratory muscles.[172] An 8-week program of NCH resulted in improvements in maximum oxygen uptake, respiratory muscle endurance, 6-Minute Walk test, and health-related quality of life.[173,174]

Ten medically complex patients who had failed weaning from the ventilator by conventional means for 7 days or more were placed on an inspiratory muscle strength training (IMST) program at low repetitions and high intensity with a threshold device. Daily IMST consisted of four sets of six breaths at a setting that yielded a perceived exertion rating of 6 to 8 on a maximal scale of 10. The duration of the spontaneous breathing periods increased, and 9 of the 10 patients were weaned from mechanical ventilation. Inspiratory muscle pressure initially was measured as 7 ± 3 cm H_2O and was increased to 18 ± 7 cm H_2O. This study needs to be done on a larger scale with patients on invasive and noninvasive mechanical ventilation.[175]

Relaxation Training

Relaxation exercises taught to patients with emphysema have been shown to result in decreases in dyspnea, HR, RR, and anxiety, although only respiratory rate significantly decreased over time.[176] Kolaczkowski and associates found that the combination of relaxation exercises and manual compression of the thorax significantly increased oxygen saturation and thoracic excursion in patients with emphysema.[177]

Prescription, Application, and, as Appropriate, Fabrication of Devices and Equipment

Noninvasive Ventilation

BIPAP is a form of noninvasive ventilation (NIV) that uses a tightly fitting nasal or facial mask to deliver positive pressure (pressure above atmospheric pressure) at two different levels, one for inspiration and another for exhalation. It may also be referred to as pressure relief ventilation. Indications for BIPAP include respiratory failure in patients with severe COPD, with increased work of breathing, and with neuromusculoskeletal impairments that limit ventilation. BIPAP will improve oxygenation by improving ventilation.

In many countries invasive positive pressure mechanical ventilation is still very much the norm. Concerns with invasive mechanical ventilation are the need for an endotracheal or tracheostomy tube connection to the positive pressure ventilator and the complications that can occur with their use. The trend in North American seems to be growing acceptance of NIV mechanical ventilation using a nasal or facial mask versus invasive mechanical ventilation.[178-180]

Because NIV provides improved ventilation and oxygenation, it will improve the patient's function and endurance.[181] NIV is growing in use primarily for patients with acute hypercapnic ventilatory failure, especially for acute exacerbations of COPD. The benefits of NIV include a reduction in the need for intubation, a decrease in complication rates, a reduced length of hospitalization, and a decrease in mortality. One factor specifically noted for the success of NIV is the early delivery of ventilation in patients with respiratory failure.[182-186]

Early BIPAP ventilation is now recognized as being more successful than invasive ventilation.[182] Its use has improved the patient outcomes in terms of decreased daytime fatigue and improved activity levels. Other benefits may include improved sleep, increased quality of life, and reduced hospitalization.[41] It may also be used as a bridge for patients, such as those with end stage cystic fibrosis who need lung transplants[187,188] or those with COPD who are awaiting lung reduction or lung transplant surgery.

The efficacy of NIV is jeopardized at times by poor compliance. Predictors of good compliance for successful use are the ability of the patient to protect his airway, the acuity of the illness, and a good initial response within the first couple of hours of use of BIPAP. Barriers to use of BIPAP include discomfort produced by the nosepiece or facemask, lack of patient-ventilator synchrony, increased sternocleidomastoid activity, altered vital signs, prolonged hours of ventilator use, problems with adaptation, increasing respiratory symptoms, and imbalances in gas exchange.[41]

Low flow oxygen with BIPAP has been shown to increase alveolar ventilation during sleep in a group of patients with cystic fibrosis.[189]

Supplemental Oxygen

The use of supplemental oxygen has been noted to be both advantageous for patients with mild to moderate hypoxemia[190] and disadvantageous to patients with mild hypoxemia.[191] In those studies that have shown the benefits of use of supplemental oxygen for patients with COPD, they have included a decrease in dyspnea and an increase in exercise tolerance by reducing the hypoxic stimulation of the carotid bodies, increasing the arterial oxygen content, and increasing the vasodilitation of the pulmonary circulation.[192-196] Patients with severe COPD, who were nonhypoxemic, were put on a cycle ergometer program with progressively increasing work loads for a duration of 45 minutes with a frequency of three times/week over a period of 7 weeks. This double blind study had one group given supplemental oxygen (3 L min-1) via nasal cannula and the other group given air (3 L min-1) via cannula. While both groups increased their exercise tolerance, the results of this study supported the use of supplemental oxygen with exercise training and revealed significantly greater increase in exercise endurance and more rapid increase in exercise training intensity.[197] In contrast, Serres and associates found that patients with COPD, who underwent high intensity training, increased their oxygen uptake without supplemental oxygen.[198] Palange and associates had patients with COPD breathe heliox (a mixture of 79% helium and 21% oxygen) while cycling at a rate of 50 rpm at 80% of their max rate until exhaustion. They found these patients more than doubled their cycling time, had decreased dyspnea, had decreased dynamic lung hyperinflation, and had increased inspiratory capacity.[199]

Airway Clearance Techniques

Controlled breathing in patients with emphysema relieves dyspnea by increasing the strength and endurance of the respiratory muscles, facilitating correct thoracic/abdominal movement, and reducing the hyperinflation of the rib cage and enhancing gas exchange.[200]

Pursed lip breathing is a technique utilized by many people with COPD to create positive pressure in the airways to prolong exhalation and prevent collapse of the airways.[201] The patient actively exhales through pursed lips generally inducing expiratory mouth pressures around 5 cm H_2O pressure.[202] Pursed lip breathing has been shown to be effective in increasing TV and gas exchange and thus oxygen saturation and in reducing dyspnea, RR, arterial pressure of carbon dioxide (PCO_2), and the activation of the diaphragm.[200,202-207]

Active expiration using abdominal contraction decreases the functional residual capacity (FRC) and increases the transdiaphragmatic pressure and during bicycle ergometry has been shown to increase maximum oxygen uptake.[208,209] Reybrouck and associates combined electromyographic feedback with active expiration and found that it significantly decreased the FRC and increased the MIP more than without the feedback.[210]

Evidence for other breathing pattern changes, other than pursed lip breathing and active expiration, in people with COPD is not well supported.[211] However in clinical practice and anecdotally in case studies many physical therapists and their patients have felt it has been effective.

Body positioning can affect pulmonary mechanics. Patients can assume positions that facilitate breathing. Often the upright and sidelying positions have been found to be particularly helpful.[212] A forward leaning position is often assumed by patients with COPD. This forward leaning position can increase intra-abdominal pressure and intrathoracic pressure, which can elevate the diaphragm and increase the expiratory flow and cough maneuvers and relieve dyspnea.[213-216] The benefit of this position seems unrelated to the severity of airway obstruction,[214] changes in minute ventilation,[213] or improved oxygenation.[214] Forward leaning has also been shown to significantly reduce the electromyographic activity of the sternocleidomastoid and scalene muscles, improve thoracoabdominal movements, and increase the transdiaphragmatic pressure.[214-216] In addition, the forward leaning position coupled with arm support enables greater rib cage elevation by the pectoralis major and minor.

Electrotherapeutic Modalities

Neuromuscular Electrical Stimulation

Evidence is growing that supports the use of neuromuscular electrical stimulation (NMES) in patients with systemic diseases with exercise intolerance and functional skeletal muscle deficits.[217-220] Patients with advanced COPD underwent a 6-week quadriceps femoris NMES home training program and had significant improvements in dyspnea (Chronic Respiratory Disease Questionnaire), maximal exercise, endurance exercise tolerance, and muscle function.[221] Stable patients with COPD received a 6-week LE transcutaneous electrical muscle stimulation for a duration of 20 minutes and a frequency of three times a week. These patients not only had significantly improved quadriceps and hamstring muscle strength, but also increased performance in the shuttle walk test.[222] Bed-bound patients with COPD, who had chronic hypercapnic respiratory failure, were on mechanical ventilation, and had significant peripheral muscle atrophy and hypotonia, performed active limb motions and also received 30 minutes of NMES twice a day over a 28-day period of time while the control group only performed the active movements. These patients who received the NMES had significantly improved muscle strength and functionally they had decreased number of days needed to transfer from bed to chair as compared to the controls. An additional finding in this study was improved respiratory rate for the patients receiving NMES.[223] While NMES may allow passive muscle activity without ventilatory stress, studies have also shown no significant changes in aerobic ability or clinical status with electrotherapeutic modalities.[224,225] Therefore, additional studies in this area are needed.

COORDINATION, COMMUNICATION, AND DOCUMENTATION

Mr. Maier will require the coordination of the entire intensive care team, the step down unit, and a coordinated plan for return home with a progressive home exercise program. Coordination with nurses, respiratory care practitioners, and other therapists will be important to establish a schedule where the patient is able to exercise and also find time to rest and gain strength. Communication will include hydration needs to promote airway clearance and caloric intake needs to support exercise. A consultation with a social worker may be indicated to address his depression.

Discussions with the team to assess possible placement in a skilled care setting rather than his current assisted living setting will depend on his progress. All elements of the patient's management will be documented.

PATIENT/CLIENT-RELATED INSTRUCTION

Mr. Maier will initially be instructed in simple activity and exercise and the importance of being up in the chair and moving rather than staying recumbent. In addition, if BIPAP will be prescribed for the home, he and the staff in the residence need to be instructed in the use of the noninvasive mechanical ventilator.

Upon his return to the residence, he will be encouraged to be active in social and light physical activity. Nursing staff and aides will be instructed to encourage him to resume walking to meals and other activities. The staff will also be instructed to allow him to stop while walking to enable him to regain his breathing control as needed.

THERAPEUTIC EXERCISE

- ◆ Aerobic capacity/endurance conditioning
  - Mr. Maier will have close monitoring of vital signs during all exercise including determining his rate of perceived exertion using the Borg scale[111]
  - Exercises to increase aerobic capacity may be performed while the patient is on NIV and may progress from bed positioning to bed mobility, sitting up in the chair, standing balance, and short walks in the room
  - Initially in the ICU bed mobility and supine to sit maneuvers will be used to evaluate his physiological responses to exercise
  - When he tolerates sitting and sitting exercise, he will be progressed to standing and walking short distances monitoring his vital signs, pulse oximetry, and perceived exertion
  - When he returns to the residence, the goal will be to have him walk to one meal with a staff member taking pauses as necessary to control his breathing and eventually building his walking to 1 hour per day
  - Begin a recumbent bicycle program starting with no resistance and for whatever time he can pedal taking pauses as necessary to control his breathing gradually building to 20- to 30-minute sessions three times per week
  - As he progresses in his outpatient program, the program will aim to include:
    - Aerobic and strength exercise program three times per week

- High-intensity exercise within his capabilities
- Interval training (repeated high-intensity exercise interspersed with rest or light exercise)
- Both UE (eg, arm cycle ergometer, free weights, elastic bands) and LE (eg, treadmill, stationary cycle ergometer) training

- ◆ Balance, coordination, and agility training
  - Initially sitting balance dangling at the bedside
  - Progress to standing balance, shifting weight, and marching in place
  - Standing on one leg with walker
  - Side stepping holding on to hall railing

- ◆ Body mechanics and postural stabilization
  - Body mechanics training
    - Appropriate sitting posture
    - Utilize lumbar roll to get more anterior pelvic tilt to open chest
    - Sit in chair with lateral support or use rolls of blanket or towels to support trunk
    - Appropriate use of body mechanics with ADL and activities
  - Postural control training
    - Proper position of head, cervical and thoracic spines, shoulders, pelvis, hips, knees, and ankles while in bed and sitting in a chair
    - Scapular retraction and depression
    - Chicken wing position (hands behind head, horizontal abduction of shoulders)
    - Postural control when transitioning positions from supine to sit, sit to stand, and walking with rolling walker
  - Postural stabilization activities
    - Avoid Valsalva maneuver
    - Increase strengthening of abdominals and back extensor muscles being sure to coordinate with breathing (eg, backlying knees up, breathe in through the nose as reach hands to knees, blow out through pursed lips as raise head and shoulders up and lower back down; on hands and knees, breathe in though nose as raise right arm and left leg out in air and blow out through pursed lips as lower back to starting position)
    - Bridging
    - Unsupported sitting
    - Standing with walker support

- ◆ Flexibility exercises
  - Minimal at this time, but may include trunk rotation and lateral flexion to mobilize trunk assisted by the physical therapist
  - Cervical ROM in all directions
  - Shoulder ROM in all directions

- Scapular adduction and depression
- Hip, knee, and ankle ROM in all directions

♦ Gait and locomotion training
- Will occur with transfer to the step down unit and continue at the residence

♦ Relaxation
- Pursed lip breathing and ventilatory strategies to be combined with activity and movement patterns to facilitate relaxation
- Frequent rest periods as needed
- Encourage imagery (imagine a calm place, breathe and allow for times of peace) several times a day for relaxation

♦ Strength, power, and endurance training
- Vital signs, pulse oximetry, and perceived exertion will be monitored closely with all exercise
- Caution to avoid breath holding during strength, power, and endurance training that will cause a Valsalva maneuver
- Exercise in an upright seated position in a good supporting chair offers trunk support so UE and LE exercises can be performed
- UE and LE strength training beginning with active assistive to active exercise
- Progression to include social and physical activity in the residence
- Inspiratory resistive training
  - Inspiratory muscle training—Patient breathes at least 30% of the MIP for 30 minutes per day through a mouthpiece with an adjustable diameter mouthpiece providing flow-dependent resistance
  - Threshold loading—Patient breathes though a mouthpiece with flow-independent resistance
  - NCH—Patient breathes maximally for 15 to 20 minutes through a simple partial rebreathing system
  - Combine inspiratory muscle training with exercise training

FUNCTIONAL TRAINING IN SELF-CARE AND HOME MANAGEMENT

♦ Self-care
- Mr. Maier previously was independent in self-care, but he currently needs moderate to maximal assistance with bathing, dressing, and other self-care activity secondary to shortness of breath, weakness, all tubes and connections, and the BIPAP
- Progress to return to independent self-care in all ADL using ventilatory strategies (eg, pursed lip breathing, paced activity with 1:2 breathing ratio of inspiration to expiration) and energy conservation techniques

- If his strength and endurance are not adequate at time of discharge to handle his self-care, consideration should be given to discharge to a skilled nursing facility

♦ Home management
- Although Mr. Maier has assistance with his housekeeping and with meals at the assisted living facility, he will probably need increased help until his strength and endurance improve
- If his strength and endurance are not adequate at time of discharge to handle his assisted living residence, consideration should be given to discharge to a skilled nursing facility until transfer to assisted living can be made

FUNCTIONAL TRAINING IN WORK, COMMUNITY, AND LEISURE INTEGRATION OR REINTEGRATION

♦ Leisure
- Previously Mr. Maier attended only occasional social activities that involved little physical activity, such as cards, checkers, or watching the group television or movies
- Upon return to assisted living residence, he should be encouraged to resume these activities and also participate in some group physical exercise or movement activities
- The recreation therapy department or social activities department may have suggestions of other programs he could attend
- In addition there may be some activities he may enjoy in the area of crafts or planning events that would give him a chance to be more involved socially and keep his mind on positive things and events in the future to help his depression and feeling of isolation
- He could learn computer skills that would enable him to e-mail his sons and grandchildren, which would challenge him intellectually and create a positive connection with his family, who he misses and only sees when they occasionally visit

PRESCRIPTION, APPLICATION, AND, AS APPROPRIATE, FABRICATION OF DEVICES AND EQUIPMENT

♦ Support devices
- BIPAP
  - Inspiration 16 cm H_2O
  - Exhalation 8 cm H_2O pressure
  - Continuous use at this time

- Wean from continuous BIPAP to night use and use as needed to facilitate rest of the respiratory muscles and improve sleep
- Supplemental oxygen
  - Initially as needed to keep O_2 saturation at rest at 94% to 95% above 90% with activity
  - As he progresses use supplemental oxygen 3 L min via nasal cannula while aerobic training on cycle ergometer

Airway Clearance Techniques

- Breathing strategies
  - Cough techniques, such as active cycles of breathing
  - Paced breathing
  - Pursed lip breathing
  - Lateral costal expansion to facilitate full diaphragmatic motion
  - Active expiration using abdominal contraction
- Body positioning to facilitate breathing
  - Upright and sidelying positions
  - Forward leaning position to increase intra-abdominal pressure and intrathoracic pressure, elevate the diaphragm, and increase the expiratory flow and cough maneuvers

Electrotherapeutic Modalities

- NMES: 30 minutes twice a day for 28 days

Anticipated Goals and Expected Outcomes

- Impact on pathology/pathophysiology
  - Energy expenditure per unit of work is decreased.
  - Indicators of O_2 transport are improved as evidenced by decreased shortness of breath with exertion.
  - Nutrition and hydration status are improved.
  - Physiological response to exacerbation of COPD and ventilatory failure is improved.
  - Self-mastery of his symptoms and physiologic responses to physical activity and exercise are increased.
  - Symptoms associated with ventilatory failure are decreased.
- Impact on impairments
  - Ability to sleep is improved to 4 consecutive hours.
  - Endurance is increased, and HR and BP are decreased during exercise.
  - Gait, locomotion, and balance are improved, and independent ambulation in the residence with a rolling walker is achieved.
  - Posture is improved in bed and while sitting, standing, and walking.
  - Strength and endurance are improved so all WFL.
  - Ventilation and oxygenation are improved.
- Impact on functional limitations

- Ability to pursue more social and community activities is enhanced.
- Going to meals (150 feet) is resumed with rest breaks as needed.
- Participation in physical and social activities is increased under the frequent guidance and interventions of the pulmonologist and the physical therapist in the residence.
- Performance of all ADL is achieved initially with minimal to moderate assistance and with mild to moderate shortness of breath and progressed to minimal to no assistance with mild shortness of breath.
- Shortness of breath at rest and with activity is reduced with ventilatory strategies, pursed lip breathing, and energy conservation techniques.
- Risk reduction/prevention
  - Further exacerbations are prevented possibly through a higher skilled nursing level of care with closer monitoring of his condition.
  - Further frequent hospitalizations are decreased with use of the BIPAP at home in the evening and at times during the day if necessary.
- Impact on health, wellness, and fitness
  - Behaviors that promote healthy nutrition, physical activity, and wellness are acquired.
  - Fitness is improved.
  - Health status is improved.
  - Physical capacity is increased.
  - Physical function is improved.
- Impact on societal resources
  - Documentation occurs throughout the patient management and follows APTA's *Guidelines for Physical Therapy Documentation*.[111]
- Patient/client satisfaction
  - Attitude is more positive.
  - Capacity to relax is improved.
  - Care is coordinated with family and other professionals.
  - Patient's and family's knowledge and awareness of the diagnosis, prognosis, interventions, and understanding of anticipated goals and expected outcomes are increased.
  - Sense of well-being is improved.

REEXAMINATION

Reexamination is performed throughout the episode of care. It is anticipated that patients placed in this pattern may require multiple episodes of care over the lifetime. Periodic reexamination and initiation of new episodes of care should occur as the patient's functional limitations or disability change.

DISCHARGE

Mr. Maier is discharged from physical therapy after a total of 20 visits, 10 in the acute care during his 7-day hospitalization stay and 10 in the skilled care unit over 3 weeks. He will then be seen weekly for the next 3 months to further increase his aerobic conditioning/endurance and his strength.

PSYCHOLOGICAL ASPECTS

Mr. Maier has had numerous exacerbations of his COPD. This episode was the worst in that he suffered ventilatory failure and needed BIPAP. However, if he is compliant with the BIPAP at the residence, his condition may stabilize or improve from his current status. He should be able to sleep better. When he is getting more supervision and support either as an outpatient or in a skilled unit, his depression should lessen, and he should feel more positive about his condition and ability to function.

As his strength and endurance increases, he will feel more independent and confident in his ability to breathe and ability to use the BIPAP for support as needed. His family may be able to make more of an effort to visit, and they may desire to be in more communication with him, both personally and online.

In addition, more social opportunities may allow Mr. Maier to connect with his fellow residents and enjoy mutually pleasant activities.

Case Study #3: Respiratory Failure

Dr. Mary Taylor is a 38-year-old female with acute respiratory failure post surgical revision of a continent ileostomy who developed a pneumothorax and is on mechanical ventilation.

PHYSICAL THERAPIST EXAMINATION

HISTORY

Because of her condition at the time of the initial examination, Dr. Taylor's history was obtained from a review of the medical record and discussions with her husband, physicians, and nurses.

- General demographics: Dr. Taylor is a 38-year-old white female, who is left-hand dominant. Her native language is English, but she is fluent in Spanish and French and has a working knowledge of Italian.

- Social history: Dr. Taylor lives with her spouse, who is a management consultant at a computer firm. They have no children.

- Employment/work: Dr. Taylor is a professor in a nearby college, teaching in the Department of Romance Languages.

- Living environment: She lives in a two-story home with four steps to enter with a handrail and 14 steps to the second floor with a handrail.

- General health status
  - General health perception: Dr. Taylor had rated her health as fair to good in light of her problems.
  - Physical function: Prior to this planned hospitalization for revision of a continent ileostomy, Dr. Taylor had been independent in all self-care and moderate intensity activities.
    - Continent ileostomy (Koch pouch)—construction of an internal reservoir by refashioning the small intestine. A one-way valve, also made from the small intestine, prevents the flow of waste to the outside until the patient inserts a small tube to overcome the valve. This surgery eliminates the need for an external pouch.)
  - Psychological function: Normal.
  - Role function: Professor, wife.
  - Social function: She has enjoyed hiking and bird watching.

- Social/health habits: Dr. Taylor does not smoke and drinks wine socially.

- Family history: Her family history is noncontributory. Dr. Taylor is the first in her family to express this genetic disorder.

- Medical/surgical history: The current hospitalization for revision of her continent ileostomy was unremarkable until hospital day 3, when Dr. Taylor developed an acute episode of dyspnea. Her chest x-ray showed bibasilar haziness with patchy bilateral perihilar infiltrates in comparison with her preoperative film. Six hours later, her chest x-ray showed diffuse patchy opacities throughout both lung fields with silhouetting of both hemidiaphragms. She was given 100% O_2 via high-flow facemask and was transferred to the ICU. Six hours later, her ventilatory status had deteriorated further, and she was orally intubated and mechanically ventilated. Her chest x-ray showed diffuse patchy opacities throughout both lung fields with silhouetting of both hemidiaphragms. Because it became progressively more difficult to control her oxygenation and ventilation, Dr. Taylor was sedated. On hospital day 4, she developed a left pneumothorax, for which a thoracostomy tube was placed in the left anterolateral 5th intercostal space. On hospital day 5, physical therapy was initiated.

- Prior hospitalizations: Fifteen years prior to this admission, she was diagnosed with familial adenomatous polyposis. Thirteen years ago, Dr. Taylor had a colectomy and ileostomy, which was complicated by hepatitis C following a blood transfusion. Twelve years ago she underwent a hysterectomy and right oophrectomy, and a year later she had an exploratory laparotomy, left oophrectomy, and ileostomy revision. The following year Dr. Taylor had a transabdominal revision and replacement of a stenotic ileostomy with a continent ileostomy. The continent ileostomy was revised 5 ½ years ago.

- Familial adenomatous polyposis is an inherited condition that primarily affects the large intestine (colon and rectum), with large numbers of polyps developing on the inner lining of the bowel. Familial adenomatous polyposis is a premalignant disease, meaning that if left untreated, it will invariably develop into cancer.

♦ Preexisting medical and other health related conditions: She has familiar adenomatous polyposis and has had a colectomy, a continent ileostomy, and bilateral oophrectomies.

♦ Current condition(s)/chief complaint(s): Dr. Taylor is in acute respiratory failure. An oral endotracheal tube (OETT) is secured at the left side of her mouth. A NG tube is secured in her left nostril and connected to suction. An indwelling arterial line is secured in the right radial artery. A multilumen IV catheter is noted at the right internal jugular vein. A thoracostomy tube protrudes from the left anterolateral 5th intercostal space and is connected to a water-sealed, negative-pressure, fluid collection device. A Foley catheter, connected to a urine drainage bag, is evident.

♦ Functional status and activity level: At the time of initial evaluation, Dr. Taylor was dependent for all care because she was sedated and mechanically ventilated. Prior to this episode she had been active in school and enjoyed hiking and bird watching.

♦ Medications: Dr. Taylor's medications at the time of initial assessment were as follows:
- Imipenem-cilastatin (Primaxin IV): 500 mg over 30 minutes (min), every (q) 6 hours (h)
- Vancomycin (Vancocin): 1 g, q12h
- Lorazepam (Ativan): 2 mg, q4h as needed (PRN)
- Fentanyl (Duragesic): 100 µg/hr

♦ Other clinical tests:
- X-rays: Diffuse patchy opacities throughout both lung fields with silhouetting of both hemidiaphragms
- Laboratory test results that were taken most proximate to the time of the initial examination are detailed in Table 6-3.
- From the patient's routine blood chemistry, the physical therapist should infer that there is no real anion gap[226,227] but should also recognize a potential risk

of protein or hydration deficiency (suggested by the low BUN/Cr ratio). The patient's blood count results indicate the likely presence of an infection (elevated WBC) and a reduced oxygen carrying capacity (low Hgb and Hct). The arterial blood gas results show a PaO_2/FiO_2 ratio of less than 200 mmHg. Dr. Taylor also exhibits a significant hypoxemia (PaO_2 171 mmHg) despite an adequate alveolar ventilation ($PaCO_2$ 44 mmHg) and 100% oxygen. Because of the high FiO_2, the risks of oxygen toxicity cannot be ignored for this patient.

- Pressure readings
  - CVP or right atrial pressure (RAP): 13 mmHg
  - PIP: 33 to 47 cm H_2O
    - PIP indicates the amount of force required to distend the lung/thorax during delivery of a tidal volume breath from the mechanical ventilator
    - A normal PIP is between 25 and 35 cmH_2O; the higher the PIP, the poorer the compliance of the lung/thorax complex

SYSTEMS REVIEW

Dr. Taylor was initially observed in a supine position with the head of the bed elevated to 30 degrees.

♦ Cardiovascular/pulmonary
- BP: 111/66 mmHg at rest
- Edema: Negligible
- HR: 107 bpm at rest
- RR: 12 to 38 depending on agitation state

♦ Integumentary
- Presence of scar formation: Scars observed on abdomen from previous surgeries
- Skin color: WNL
- Skin integrity: Disrupted with an OETT, a NG tube, an indwelling arterial line in the right radial artery, a multilumen intravenous catheter in the right internal jugular vein, and a thorocostomy tube in the 5th left intercostals space

♦ Musculoskeletal
- Gross range of motion: WFL passively
- Gross strength: Not able to adequately assess
- Gross symmetry: Not able to adequately assess
- Height: 5'6" (167.6 cm)
- Weight: 130 lbs (59.1 kg)

♦ Neuromuscular
- Balance: Not able to assess at this time
- Locomotion, transfers, and transitions: Not able to adequately assess

♦ Communication, affect, cognition, language, and learning style

Table 6-3
LABORATORY TEST RESULTS

Chemistry

	Value	Unit	Normal range
Sodium	136	mEq/L	(135 to 147)
Potassium	3.7	mEq/L	(3.5 to 5.0)
Chloride	104	mEq/L	(95 to 105)
Bicarbonate	26	mEq/L	(22 to 28)
Blood urea nitrogen (BUN)	6.6	mg/dL	(7 to 18)
Creatinine	1.6	mg/dL	(0.6 to 1.2)
Glucose	122	mg/dL	(75 to 110)
Calcium	8.6	mg/dL	(8.4 to 11)
Magnesium	2.0	mg/dL	(1.5 to 2.0)
Phosphorus	4.2	mg/dL	(3.0 to 4.4)

Blood count

	Value	Unit	Normal range
WBC	15.4	k/µL	(4.5 to 11.0)
Hgb	10.6	g/dL	(12.0 to 16.0)
Hct	31.1	%	(36% to 46%)
Platelet count	896	k/mm³	(150 to 400)

ABG (obtained within 1 hour of the physical therapist's examination)

pH	7.41 (normal=7.35 to 7.45)
pCO_2	44 (normal=35 to 45 mmHg or Torr)
pO_2	171 (normal=80 to 100 mmHg or Torr)
HCO_3	28 (normal=24 to 28)
SaO_2	100% (normal=97.5%)

- Dr. Taylor responds appropriately to single-level commands
- She is sedated and lethargic, but arousable
- Her expected emotional/behavioral response is as expected for the level of sedation
- Learning preference not determined at this time

TESTS AND MEASURES

♦ Aerobic capacity/endurance
  - Unable to assess at this time
♦ Anthropometric characteristics
  - BMI for her age=weight (lbs) ÷ height (inches) ÷ height (inches) x 703
  - BMI: 21.0 which is considered normal weight[62]
♦ Arousal, attention, and cognition
  - Difficult to fully determine at this time, because the patient is receiving strong prophylactic pharmocologic agents (imipenem and vancomycin), and she is being sedated (fentanyl and loreazepam) in order to promote her comfort and reduce agitation

- The sedatives may also prolong the duration of her mechanical ventilation and interfere with the assessment of her neurologic status
- Responds appropriately to single-level instructions
  - Glasgow Coma Score (GCS)[230]=9, eye response=3, verbal response=1, motor response=5
  - GCS is scored between 3 and 15 with 3 the worst and 15 the best
  - GCS composed of three parameters
    ▸ Best eye response (4): 1=No eye opening, 2=Eye opening to pain, 3=Eye opening to verbal command, 4=Eyes open spontaneously
    ▸ Best verbal response (5): 1=No verbal response, 2=Incomprehensible sounds, 3=Inappropriate words, 4=Confused, 5=Orientated
    ▸ Best motor response (6): 1=No motor response, 2=Extension to pain, 3=Flexion to pain, 4=Withdrawal from pain, 5=Localizing pain, 6=Obeys commands
- The physical therapist should be aware of a heightened potential for nephrotoxicity, tinnitus, seizures, and arrhythmias because of the medications

- ◆ Circulation
  - Capillary refill essentially within normal parameters
- ◆ Cranial and peripheral nerve integrity
  - Sensation: Grossly intact
- ◆ Gait, locomotion, and balance
  - She is bedridden and unable to ambulate at this time
- ◆ Integumentary integrity
  - Scars observed on abdomen from previous surgeries
  - Skin integrity is disrupted with an OETT, a NG tube, an indwelling arterial line in the right radial artery, a multilumen IV catheter in the right internal jugular vein, and a thorocostomy tube in the 5th left intercostals space
- ◆ Motor performance
  - Maximally assisted bed mobility assessment resulted in acceptable BP and peak inspiratory pressures (122/69 mmHg; < 50 cmH$_2$0, respectively), but her minute ventilation (RR x Vt) more than doubled (from 7.2 L/min^{-1} to 14.7 L/min^{-1}), and her HR rose to 122 bpm, thus any more vigorous assessment was not done at this time
- ◆ Orthotic, protective, and supportive devices and equipment
  - Mechanical ventilator is providing her breathing unless she is stimulated
  - Mechanical ventilator settings
    - Mode: SIMV
    - Set tidal volume (V$_t$): 600 mL
    - Set rate: 12 bpm
    - FiO$_2$: 1.0
    - PEEP: +5 cm H$_2$O (relative to atmospheric)
    - Pressure support: +5 cm H$_2$O (relative to atmospheric)
    - Observed respiratory rate: 12 to 38 (stimulation dependent)
    - Spontaneous tidal volume: 175 to 230 mL (stimulation dependent)
- ◆ Pain
  - Not assessed at this time due to sedation medications
- ◆ Range of motion
  - Extremities: WNL passively
  - Diminished diaphragmatic displacement of the abdomen (decreased inferolateral costal excursion)
  - Reduced thoracic expansion of the lower chest wall and abdomen on inhalation
- ◆ Self-care and home management
  - Dependent in all self-care activities at this time
- ◆ Ventilation and respiration/gas exchange

- • Auscultation
  - Decreased aeration and diffuse position-independent (noncardiogenic) crackles, especially over the posterior- and lateral-basal segments of the lower lobes, bilaterally
- • Breathing pattern
  - Diminished diaphragmatic displacement of the abdomen (decreased inferolateral costal excursion)
  - Reduced thoracic expansion of the lower chest wall and abdomen on inhalation, resulting in upper chest pattern of motion

EVALUATION

Dr. Taylor is a patient with familial adenomatous, who was hospitalized for a revision of a continent ileostomy and developed ARF 3 days postop. She is presently sedated, on a ventilator with multiple tubes in place. When the findings are considered in their entirety, the PaO$_2$/FiO$_2$ ratio of less than 200 mmHg, the bilateral patchy infiltrates on the chest x-ray, the lack of clinical signs of left atrial hypertension, and the rapidity of the onset of symptoms, they are suggestive of a problem of even greater impact than impaired ventilation and respiration/gas exchange associated with respiratory failure. When considered in their entirety, the above findings are most consistent with a diagnosis of ARDS associated with very poor activity tolerance.

DIAGNOSIS

Dr. Taylor is a patient with familial adenomatous, who was hospitalized for a revision of a continent ileostomy and is ventilator dependent. She has impaired aerobic capacity/endurance; circulation; gait, locomotion, and balance; motor performance; range of motion; and ventilation and respiration/gas exchange. She is functionally limited in self-care and home management. She is in need of supportive ventilatory devices and equipment. These findings are consistent with placement in Pattern F: Impaired Ventilation and Respiration/Gas Exchange Associated With Respiratory Failure. The identified impairments and functional limitations will be addressed in determining the prognosis and the plan of care.

PROGNOSIS AND PLAN OF CARE

Over the course of the visits, the following mutually established outcomes have been determined.

- ◆ Bed mobility with thoracic rotation and breathing control is increased
- ◆ Care is coordinated with patient, family, and other professionals
- ◆ Case is managed throughout episode of care

♦ Chest wall ROM is enhanced

♦ Integumentary integrity is improved

♦ Knowledge of behaviors that foster healthy habits is gained

♦ Muscle performance is improved

♦ Respiratory muscles are strengthened

♦ Risk factors are reduced

♦ Risk of secondary impairment is reduced

♦ Stress is decreased

To achieve these outcomes, the appropriate interventions for this patient are determined. These will include: coordination, communication, and documentation; patient/client-related instruction; therapeutic exercise; functional training in self-care and home management; prescription, application, and, as appropriate, fabrication of devices and equipment; and airway clearance techniques.

Based on the diagnosis and prognosis, Dr. Taylor is expected to require between 25 and 35 visits. She is severely ill, but her previous history indicates that she has good social support and should be motivated when she stabilizes.

INTERVENTIONS

RATIONALE FOR SELECTED INTERVENTIONS

At the present time, the treatment for any of the forms of acute respiratory disease is nonspecific. Therapeutic intervention is palliative in the hope that the patient will spontaneously recover. Unfortunately, there is disagreement about what constitutes the best support.

Therapeutic Exercise and Functional Training in Self-Care and Home Management

In overcoming the still-too-persistent refrain of "They're too sick, they're in the ICU," physical therapists are frequently required to act as agents of change and advocates for the preservation or restoration of the patient's functional capabilities (eg, bed mobility, transfers, ADL, balance, etc). Nevertheless, physical therapists often participate in the clinical management of patients with impaired ventilation and respiration/gas exchange associated with respiratory failure. In today's health care environment, physical therapy is more often than not instituted as some form of early mobilization as opposed to bronchial hygiene.

The case for early physical therapy intervention is supported by at least one randomized study of patients admitted to the ICU for the treatment of ARF.[229] Patients were divided into two groups: one group given early mobilization (eg, bed mobility training, respiratory muscle training, active gravity-dependent ROM training, and progressive ambulation) plus standard medical therapy and the other group given standard medical therapy alone. While complaints of dyspnea (as reflected by visual analog scale) were reduced in both groups, only patients in the early mobilization group exhibited significant improvements in 6-Minute Walk test distance ($p<0.001$) and maximal inspiratory force ($p<0.05$). Additional support comes from a recent multicenter longitudinal study in which the authors concluded that survivors of ARF have functional disability 1 year after discharge from the ICU primarily because of muscle wasting and weakness.[230]

Understandably, the question of what physiologic parameter(s) the physical therapist should monitor when treating patients with ALI, ARDS, or ARF has no widely accepted answer. While heart rate and blood pressure are closely observed and often continuously displayed on a bedside monitor, these parameters are most useful as end-point markers. For the patient receiving mechanical ventilatory assistance, minute ventilation and pulse oximetry (SpO_2) may provide more immediately useful information about the patient's activity tolerance. Normal resting minute ventilation approximates 4 to 5 L/min with a respiratory rate less than 18 bpm. Typically, a minute ventilation greater than 20 L/min is suggestive of the patient's ventilatory intolerance of the early mobilization activity. Additionally, if patients remain hypoxemic despite optimization of ventilatory support, it may be necessary to accept SpO_2 values as low as 80%.

In considering the effect of positioning on patients with ARF, there is no evidence to support increased oxygenation or other benefits from the semirecumbent or sidelying positions when both lungs are involved.[231] Additionally, although placing patients with ARF in a prone position does improve their oxygenation, it does not improve survival.[232] Some authors advocate calculating the alveolar-arterial oxygen difference ($Aa\text{-}DO_2$) to distinguish between hypoxemia due to hypoventilation and hypoxemia due to impaired gas exchange.[233] However, this measurement may be an unreliable indicator of abnormal gas exchange in the presence of alveolar hypoventilation ($PaCO_2 \geq 50$ mmHg) or in the absence of steady-state conditions.[234,235] According to this author, it is more informative from a clinical standpoint to estimate the severity of any hypoxemia in the face of oxygen supplementation by calculating the "room-air equivalent" of the patient's oxygen-supplemented PaO_2 (room-air equivalent=[{measured $PaO_2 \div F_IO_2$} • 0.21] - 5). For example, if a patient was receiving an F_IO_2 of 0.5 (50% oxygen) and exhibited a PaO_2 of 100 mmHg, the room-air equivalent would be approximately 37 mmHg—a severely hypoxemic state (Table 6-4).

Although there is little if any evidence beyond anecdote to support their use, physical therapists often employ rate-reduction interventions, bed mobility training, respiratory muscle training, chest wall and active gravity-dependent ROM training, and progressive ambulation in their attempts

Table 6-4 CLASSIFICATION OF THE SEVERITY OF HYPOXEMIA WHEN BREATHING ROOM AIR (FiO$_2$=0.21)	
PaO$_2$ (mmHg)	**Severity of Hypoxemia**
≥60 but <80	Mild
≥40 but <60	Moderate
<40	Severe

to preserve or restore their patients' functional capabilities as they recover from ALI, ARDS, and ARF.

Prescription, Application, and, as Appropriate, Fabrication of Devices and Equipment

Endotracheal intubation and positive pressure ventilation constitute the mainstay of support for critically ill patients with respiratory failure.[236] PEEP is almost always employed to optimize oxygenation. Serendipitously, PEEP may also decrease the accumulation of interstitial fluid. Because ventilation with large TVs and high PIPs has been shown to contribute to the advancement of lung injury,[16,237] it is now common practice to use pressure-controlled ventilation, low TV (~6 mL/kg), inverted inspiration-to-expiration ratio, decelerating inspiratory flow curve, or permissive hypercapnia.[238-240] Although endotracheal intubation and positive-pressure ventilation are the most often utilized methods for delivering ventilatory support to critically ill patients with respiratory failure, noninvasive positive-pressure ventilation is quickly becoming an accepted initial treatment for patients with ARF.[241,242]

COORDINATION, COMMUNICATION, AND DOCUMENTATION

Communication will occur with both Dr. Taylor and her husband regarding all components of her care and to engender support for her program. This will take place in the hospital. Bed positioning options will be discussed with the nursing staff to facilitate the prevention of loss of ROM of the extremities and aeration of the posterior and basal lung segments. All elements of the patient's management will be documented. The plan of care will be developed and discussed with the patient and her family. Discharge planning will be provided.

PATIENT/CLIENT-RELATED INSTRUCTION

Education regarding Dr. Taylor's current condition, impairments, and functional limitations will be discussed. The patient will be instructed in appropriate body mechanics, proper posture, and core stabilization to ensure adequate respiratory function and proper breathing mechanics. As feasible, the patient will be instructed in proper self-care techniques. Risk factors will be discussed.

THERAPEUTIC EXERCISE

- ◆ Flexibility exercises
  - AAROM for all extremities
  - Chest wall mobility including trunk rotation
- ◆ Strength, power, and endurance training
  - Hospital day 5
    - Any activities will be nonvigorous at this time since the patient's minute ventilation (minute ventilation; RR x Vt) more than doubled (from 7.2 L/min^{-1} to 14.7 L/min^{-1}) and her HR rose to 122 bpm during the tests and measures
    - Bed mobility with emphasis on thoracic rotation and breathing control exercises will be a basic means of strength training for this patient at this time
    - Ventilatory muscle strength
      - ▶ Breathing control activities in conjunction with functional bed mobility exercises to facilitate weaning from mechanical ventilation
      - ▶ Use of side-to-side rolling and controlled inhalation and inspiratory hold techniques
        - ○ The primary goal for these interventions is to maximize the patient's participation in functional activities while maintaining physiological indices (eg, HR, BP, PIP, minute ventilation) within clinically acceptable limits
  - Hospital day 7
    - Dr. Taylor was able to tolerate gentle chest wall mobility (trunk rotation) and UE AROM/AAROM in conjunction with localized thoracic expansion
    - At rest, her breath sounds were still diminished at both bases with diffuse crackles and with activity, the aeration sounds were clearer and louder
    - Her HR response to the activity varied between 104 and 112 bpm, which was stable and appropriate
    - Her PIP was lower during activity
    - The mechanical RR and FiO$_2$ are now lower than the initial settings
    - With activity, she improved basilar aeration and reduced the intensity of the crackles
  - Hospital day 8
    - The left thoracostomy tube was clamped and disconnected from suction prior to physical therapy
    - The mechanical ventilator settings were changed as follows: Rate at 7 bpm and fraction of inspired oxygen (FiO$_2$) at 0.3

- Activities included:
  ▶ Bed mobility activities
  ▶ Dangling at the edge of the bed, using the mechanical ventilator's tidal volume and minute ventilation visual displays to facilitate breathing control
- During her treatment her HR varied between 95 and 116 bpm; her RR was 12 at rest and 19 with activity; and her PIPs peaked during activity at 31 cm H_2O
- ABG (obtained with in 1 hour of treatment) results were: pH=7.38; pCO_2=42; pO_2=99; HCO_3=30; and SaO_2=99%
- The FiO_2 and mechanical RR have been reduced and despite a mild hypoxemia (supplemental O_2 of 30%, with PaO_2 of 97), she tolerated increased activity with appropriate HR and RR responses, and she was able to carry the bulk of her ventilatory demand with reduced mechanical assistance (reduced tidal volume and set rate)
- Hospital day 9
  - The left thoracostomy tube was removed
  - The pretreatment ABG results were: pH=7.35; pCO_2=38; pO_2=98; HCO_3=30; and SaO_2= 99%
  - Activities included:
    ▶ Minimally assisted mobility activities
    ▶ Sitting at the edge of the bed
    ▶ Standing with minimal assistance/contact guarding four times for 1 to 2 minutes each time
  - During treatment, her PIPs never exceeded 29 cm H_2O; her RR peaked at 19; and her HR never exceeded 118 bpm
  - Despite continued mild hypoxemia, Dr. Taylor showed excellent activity tolerance and breathing control
- Hospital day 10
  - The mechanical ventilator settings were changed to the following: Pressure +10 cm H_2O pressure; FiO_2 0.28, and PEEP +5 cm H_2O
  - ABG results obtained 30 minutes after the mode change where deemed acceptable by the ICU team
  - Activities included:
    ▶ Minimally assisted mobility activities
    ▶ Sitting at the edge of the bed
    ▶ Standing with minimal assistance/contact guarding four times for 2 to 4 minutes each time
  - During treatment her HR never exceeded 114 bpm and her RR never exceeded 22 bpm
  - The posttreatment ABG results were: pH= 7.41; pCO_2=44; pO_2=98; HCO_3=28; and SaO_2= 99%
  - With minimal mechanical assist (PS +10), she

maintained adequate alveolar ventilation and acceptable oxygenation throughout the increased activity level
- Hospital day 11
  - She was removed from pressure support and placed on a tracheostomy collar with 28% oxygen
  - She demonstrated only intermittent crackles at the initiation of her treatment session and no crackles at the conclusion
  - Activities included:
    ▶ Independent sitting at the edge of the bed
    ▶ Independent transfer to a chair at bedside using a walker for support
    ▶ Stand and ambulate 50 feet with a wheeled walker and a Venturi device connected to an E-cylinder (oxygen in a compressed form) to maintain her supplemental O_2
  - Her RR remained under 28 bpm and HR never exceeded 118 bpm indicating that she was tolerating spontaneous breathing during low-moderate intensity activity with reasonably well-controlled RR and HR
- Hospital day 12
  - Dr. Taylor was transferred to the general care floor on the tracheostomy collar at 28% oxygen
  - Activities included:
    ▶ Active standing exercises
    ▶ Independent ambulation 200 feet on level surfaces using a cane
  - Her RR remained below 24 bpm and her HR stayed below 114 bpm
- Hospital day 13
  - Her tracheostomy was capped and a nasal cannula at 3 L/min was used
  - Breath sounds remained clear to auscultation
  - Activities included:
    ▶ Same as HD 12: Active standing exercises and independent ambulation 200 feet on level surfaces using a cane
    ▶ Stair climbing was deferred
  - Her HR was 126 bpm after ambulating the 200 feet with a cane
- Hospital day 14
  - Dr. Taylor was transferred to an inpatient rehabilitation facility

FUNCTIONAL TRAINING IN SELF-CARE AND HOME MANAGEMENT

- ♦ Functional bed mobility exercises in conjunction with breathing control activities to facilitate weaning from mechanical ventilation

♦ ADL training
  ● Bathing
  ● Transfer training to chair
  ● Self-care and home management activities
    ▪ Injury prevention education during self-care and home management
    ▪ Safety during activities

PRESCRIPTION, APPLICATION, AND, AS APPROPRIATE, FABRICATION OF DEVICES AND EQUIPMENT

♦ Hospital day 5
● Mechanical ventilation: See settings above in Tests and Measures
♦ Hospital day 7
  ● Incentive spirometry begun using the TV display on the mechanical ventilator in coordination with her spontaneous breaths
♦ Hospital day 11
  ● Tracheostomy collar with 28% oxygen
  ● Venturi device connected to an E-cylinder to maintain supplemental O_2
  ● Walker for standing support
  ● Wheeled walker for ambulation
♦ Hospital day 12
  ● Cane
♦ Hospital day 13
  ● Nasal cannula at 3 L/min

AIRWAY CLEARANCE TECHNIQUES

♦ Breathing strategies
  ● Active cycle of breathing or forced expiratory techniques
  ● Assisted cough/huff techniques
  ● Techniques to maximize ventilation (eg, pursed lip breathing, incentive spirometer)
♦ Positioning
  ● Positioning to alter work of breathing (eg, seated and using trunk extension to facilitate inspiration and flexion to facilitate expiration; sidelying to facilitate inspiration in the uppermost lung segments)
  ● Positioning to maximize ventilation and perfusion (eg, use of gravity in lowermost segments of lungs to facilitate perfusion)

ANTICIPATED GOALS AND EXPECTED OUTCOMES

♦ Impact on pathology/pathophysiology
  ● Nutrient delivery to tissue is increased.

● Physiological responses to increased oxygen demand are improved.
● Symptoms associated with increased oxygen demand are decreased.
● Tissue perfusion and oxygenation are enhanced.
♦ Impact on impairments
  ● Aerobic capacity/endurance is increased to point where patient can ambulate 200 feet with a cane while on supplemental oxygen via nasal cannula.
  ● Airway clearance is improved as demonstrated by a clear chest x-ray.
  ● Balance is improved as evidenced by standing on each leg for 5 seconds.
  ● Cough is improved with increased vital capacity and good abdominal contraction.
  ● Energy expenditure per unit of work is decreased.
  ● Gait, locomotion, and balance are improved, and patient is independent in locomotion and balance while on supplemental oxygen via nasal cannula.
  ● Integumentary integrity is improved, lines are removed, and scar is well healed.
  ● Motor function is improved.
  ● Muscle performance (strength, power, and endurance) is increased, and she is able to perform all ADL.
  ● Relaxation is increased.
  ● ROM is normal.
  ● Ventilation and respiration/gas exchange are improved, and supplemental oxygen via nasal cannula is at 3 L/min.
  ● Work of breathing is decreased.
♦ Impact on functional limitations
  ● Ability to assume or resume required self-care and home management roles is improved.
  ● Ability to perform physical actions, tasks, and activities related to self-care is increased with supplemental oxygen.
  ● Level of supervision required for task performance is decreased.
  ● Tolerance to positions and activities is increased.
♦ Risk reduction/prevention
  ● Communication enhances risk reduction and prevention.
  ● Protection of body parts is increased.
  ● Risk factors are reduced.
  ● Risk of recurrence of condition is reduced.
  ● Risk of secondary impairment is reduced.
  ● Safety is improved.
  ● Self-management of symptoms is improved.
♦ Impact on health, wellness, and fitness
  ● Behaviors that foster healthy habits, wellness, and prevention are acquired.

- Fitness is improved.
- Health status is improved.
- Intensity of care is decreased.
- Physical capacity is increased.
- Physical function is improved.

♦ Impact on societal resources
  - Available resources are maximally utilized.
  - Documentation occurs throughout the client management and follows APTA's *Guidelines for Physical Therapy Documentation.*[111]
  - Utilization and cost of health care services are decreased.
  - Utilization of physical therapy services is optimized.

♦ Patient/client satisfaction
  - Care is coordinated with patient/client, family, significant others, and other professionals.
  - Case is managed throughout the episode of care.
  - Patient and family knowledge and awareness of the diagnosis, prognosis, interventions, and anticipated goals and expected outcomes are increased.
  - Patient knowledge of personal and environmental factors associated with the condition is increased.
  - Referrals are made to other professionals or resources whenever necessary and appropriate.
  - Sense of well-being is improved.
  - Stressors are decreased.

REEXAMINATION

Reexamination is performed throughout the entire episode of care each time the patient is seen and each time a new activity is started.

DISCHARGE

Dr. Taylor is discharged from physical therapy after a total of 30 physical therapy sessions and attainment of her goals and expectations. These sessions have covered her entire episode of care. She is discharged because she has achieved her goals and expected outcomes.

REFERENCES

1. Flaatten H, Gjerde S, Guttormsen AB, et al. Outcome after acute respiratory failure is more dependent on dysfunction in other vital organs than on the severity of the respiratory failure. *Crit Care.* 2003;7(4):R72.
2. Goss CH, Brower RG, Hudson LD, Rubenfeld GD. Incidence of acute lung injury in the United States. *Crit Care Med.* 2003;31(6):607-1611.
3. Hudson LD, Steinberg KP. Epidemiology of acute lung injury and ARDS. *Chest.* 1999;116(1 Suppl):74S-82S.
4. Vincent JL, Sakr Y, Ranieri VM. Epidemiology and outcome of acute respiratory failure in intensive care unit patients. *Crit Care Med,* 2003;31(4 Suppl):S296-299.
5. Ware LB, Matthay MA. The acute respiratory distress syndrome. *N Engl J Med.* 2000;342(18):1334-1349.
6. Lewandowski K. Contributions to the epidemiology of acute respiratory failure. *Crit Care.* 2003;7(4):288-290.
7. Doerschuk CM. Mechanisms of leukocyte sequestration in inflamed lungs. *Microcirculation.* 2001;8(2):71-88.
8. Downey GP, Worthen GS, Henson PM, Hyde DM. Neutrophil sequestration and migration in localized pulmonary inflammation. Capillary localization and migration across the interalveolar septum. *Am Rev Respir Dis.* 1993;147(1):168-176.
9. Mantovani A, Bussolino F, Introna M. Cytokine regulation of endothelial cell function: from molecular level to the bedside. *Immunol Today.* 1997;18(5):231-240.
10. Downey GP, Dong Q, Kruger J, et al. Regulation of neutrophil activation in acute lung injury. *Chest.* 1999;116(1 Suppl):46S-54S.
11. Moraes TJ, Chow CW, Downey GP. Proteases and lung injury. *Crit Care Med.* 2003;31(4 Suppl):S189-S194.
12. Eisner MD, Parsons P, Matthay MA, et al. Plasma surfactant protein levels and clinical outcomes in patients with acute lung injury. *Thorax.* 2003;58(11):983-988.
13. Martin TR, Nakamura M, Matute-Bello G. The role of apoptosis in acute lung injury. *Crit Care Med.* 2003;31(4 Suppl):S184-S188.
14. Aberle DR, Wiener-Kronish JP, Webb WR, Matthay MA. Hydrdostatic versus increased permeability pulmonary edema: diagnosis based on radiographic criteria in critically ill patients. *Radiology.* 1988;168(1):73-79.
15. Bachofen M, Weibel ER. Structural alterations of lung parenchyma in the adult respiratory distress syndrome. *Clin Chest Med.* 1982;3(1):35-56.
16. Pinhu L, Whitehead T, Evans T, Griffiths M. Ventilator-associated lung injury. *Lancet.* 2003;361(9354):332-340.
17. Ranieri VM, Suter PM, Tortorella C, et al. Effect of mechanical ventilation on inflammatory mediators in patients with acute respiratory distress syndrome: a randomized controlled trial. *JAMA.* 1999;282(1):54-61.
18. Bachofen M, Weibel ER. Alterations of the gas exchange apparatus in adult respiratory insufficiency associated with septicemia. *Am Rev Respir Dis.* 1977;116(4):589-615.
19. Matthay MA. Fibrosing alveolitis in the adult respiratory distress syndrome. *Ann Intern Med.* 1995;122(1):65-66.
20. Crapo JD, Barry BE, Gehr P, et al. Cell number and cell characteristics of the normal human lung. *Am Rev Respir Dis.* 1982;126(2):332-337.
21. Ware LB, Matthay MA. Alveolar fluid clearance is impaired in the majority of patients with acute lung injury and the acute respiratory distress syndrome. *Am J Respir Crit Care Med.* 2001;163(6):1376-1383.
22. Adamson IY, Young L. Alveolar type II cell growth on a pulmonary endothelial extracellular matrix. *Am J Physiol.* 1996;270(6 Pt 1):L1017-L1022.
23. Folkesson HG, Nitenberg G, Oliver BL, et al. Upregulation of alveolar epithelial fluid transport after subacute lung injury in rats from bleomycin. *Am J Physiol.* 1998;275(3 Pt 1):L478-L490.

24. Matthay MA, Folkesson HG, Clerici C. Lung epithelial fluid transport and the resolution of pulmonary edema. *Physiol Rev.* 2002;82(3):569-600.

25. National Center for Health Statistics. Raw Data from the National Health Interview Survey, U.S., 1982-1996, 2001-2004. Available at: http://www.lungusa.org/site/pp.aspx=dvL UK9O0E&b=22782. Accessed October 4, 2006.

26. Kent TH, Hart MN. *Introduction to Human Disease.* Norwalk, Conn: Appleton & Lange; 1993.

27. West JB. *Pulmonary Pathophysiology: The Essentials.* 6th ed. Philadelphia, Pa: Lippincott Williams & Wilkins; 2003.

28. Kim H, Tsai P, Oh C. The genetics of asthma. *Curr Opin Pulmonary Med.* 1998;4:46-48.

29. Smith M, ed. Asthma Complexities. Available at: http://www.webmd.com/content/article/105/107728.htm. Accessed October 1, 2006.

30. Currie GP, Devereux GS, Lee DKC, Ayers JG. Recent developments in asthma management. *BMJ.* 2005;330:585-589.

31. Grigg J. Management of paediatric asthma. *Postgrad Med J.* 2004;80:535-540.

32. Barnes PJ. Current issues for establishing inhaled corticosteroids as the anti-inflammatory agents of choice in asthma. *J Allergy Clin Immunol.* 1998;101(4 Pt 2):S427-S433.

33. Jenkins HA, Cool C, Szeffler SJ, et al. Histopathology of severe childhood asthma: a case series. *Chest.* 2003;124(1):32-41.

34. Gronke L, Kanniess F, Holz O, et al. The relationship between airway hyper-responsiveness, markers of inflammation and lung function depends on the duration of the asthmatic disease. *Clin Exp Allergy.* 2002;32(1):57-63.

35. Hegde RM, Worthely LT. Acute asthma and the life threatening episode. *Crit Care Resusc.* 1999;1(4):371-387.

36. Han P, Cole RP. Evolving differences in the presentation of severe asthma requiring intensive are unit admission. *Respiration.* 2004;71(5);458-462.

37. *Professional Guide to Diseases.* 7th ed. Springhouse, Pa: Springhouse Corp; 2001.

38. Chitkara RK, Sarinas PSA. Recent advances in diagnosis and treatment of chronic bronchitis and emphysema. *Curr Opinion Pulm Med.* 2002;8:126-136.

39. Mineo TC, Pompeo E, Roglianai P, et al. Effect of lung volume reduction surgery for severe emphysema on right ventricular function. *Amer J Crit Care Med.* 2002;165:489-494.

40. Bennett LE, Keck BM, Daily OP, et al. Worldwide thoracic organ transplantation: a report from UNOS/SHLT international registry for thoracic organ transplantation. *Clin Transplant.* 2000;31-34.

41. Frownfelter D, Dean E. *Cardiovascular and Pulmonary Physical Therapy Evidence and Practice.* 4th ed. St. Louis, Mo: Mosby Elsevier; 2006.

42. Ashbaugh, DG, Bigelow DB, Petty TL, Levine BE. Acute respiratory distress in adults. *Lancet.* 1967;2(7511):319-323.

43. Murray JF, Matthay MA, Luce JM, Flick MR. An expanded definition of the adult respiratory distress syndrome. *Am Rev Respir Dis.* 1988;138(3):720-723.

44. Bernard GR, Artigas A, Brigham KL, et al. The American-European consensus conference in ARDS: definitions, mechanisms, relevant outcomes, and clinical trial coordination. *Am J Respir Crit Care Med.* 1994;149(3 Pt 1):818-824.

45. Vincent JL, de Mendonca A, Cantraine F, et al. Use of the SOFA score to assess the incidence of organ dysfunction/failure in intensive care units: results of a multicenter, prospective study. *Crit Care Med.* 1998;26(11):1793-1800.

46. Bersten AD, Edibam C, Hunt T, Moran J. Incidence and mortality of acute lung injury and the acute respiratory distress syndrome in three Australian States. *Am J Respir Crit Care Med.* 2002;165(4):443-448.

47. Conference report: mechanisms of acute respiratory failure. *Am Rev Respir Dis.* 1977;115(6):1071-1078.

48. Luhr OR, Antonsen K, Karlsson M, et al. Incidence and mortality after acute respiratory failure and acute respiratory distress syndrome in Sweden, Denmark, and Iceland. The ARF Study Group. *Am J Respir Crit Care Med.* 1999;159(6):1849-1861.

49. Nolan S, Burgess K, Hopper L, Braude S. Acute respiratory distress syndrome in a community hospital ICU. *Intensive Care Med.* 1997;23(5):530-538.

50. Roupie E, Lepage E, Wysocki M, et al. Prevalence, etiologies and outcome of the acute respiratory distress syndrome among hypoxemic ventilated patients. SRLF Collaborative Group on Mechanical Ventilation. Societe de Reanimation de Langue Francaise. *Intensive Care Med.* 1999;25(9):920-929.

51. Thomsen GE, Morris AH. Incidence of the adult respiratory distress syndrome in the state of Utah. *Am J Respir Crit Care Med.* 1995;152(3):965-971.

52. Valta P, Uusaro A, Nunes S, et al. Acute respiratory distress syndrome: frequency, clinical course, and costs of care. *Crit Care Med.* 1999;27(11):2367-2374.

53. Villar J, Slutsky AS. The incidence of the adult respiratory distress syndrome. *Am Rev Respir Dis.* 1989;140(3):814-816.

54. Roupie E. Incidence of ARDS. *Intensive Care Med.* 2000;26(6): 816-817.

55. Jubran A, Tobin MJ. Pathophysiologic basis of acute respiratory distress in patients who fail a trial of weaning from mechanical ventilation. *Am J Respir Crit Care Med.* 1997; 155(3):906-915.

56. Laghi F, Tobin MJ. Disorders of the respiratory muscles. *Am J Respir Crit Care Med.* 2003;168(1):10-48.

57. Gattinoni L, Bombino M, Pelosi P, et al. Lung structure and function in different stages of severe adult respiratory distress syndrome. *JAMA.* 1994;271(22):1772-1779.

58. Behrendt CE. Acute respiratory failure in the United States: incidence and 31-day survival. *Chest.* 2000;118(4):1100-1105.

59. Rubenfeld GD. Epidemiology of acute lung injury. *Crit Care Med.* 2003;31(4 Suppl):S276-S284.

60. Herridge MS, Cheung AM, Tansey, CM, et al. One-year outcomes in survivors of the acute respiratory distress syndrome. *N Engl J Med.* 2003;348(8):683-693.

61. Gift AG. Validation of a vertical visual analog scale as a measure of clinical dyspnea. *Rehab Nurse.* 1989;14:323-325.

62. DHHS. Calculate Your Body Mass Index. Available at: http://www.nhlbisupport.com/bmi. Accessed September 20, 2006.

63. American Physical Therapy Association. Guide to Physical Therapist Practice. 2nd ed. *Phys Ther.* 2001;81:9-744.

64. Pedersen S. What are the goals of treating pediatric asthma? *Pediatr Pulmonol Suppl.* 1997;15:22-26.

65. Chiang LC, Huang JL, Fu LS. Physical activity and physical self concept: comparison between children with and without asthma. *J Adv Nurs.* 2006;54(67):653-662.

66. Szentagothai K, Gyene I, Szocska M, Osvath P. Physical exercise program for children with bronchial asthma. *Pediatr Pulmonol.* 1987;3(3):166-172.

67. Lucas SR, Platts-Mills TA. Physical activity and exercise in asthma: relevance to etiology and treatment. *J Allergy Clin Immunol.* 2005;115(5):928-934.

68. Welsh L, Kemp JG, Roberts RG. Effects of physical conditioning on children and adolescents with asthma. *Sports Med.* 2005;35(2):127-141.

69. Cambach W, Chadwick-Straver RV, Wagenaar RC, et al. The effects of a community-based pulmonary rehabilitation programme on exercise tolerance and quality of life: a randomized controlled trial. *Eur Respir J.* 1997;10(1):104-113.

70. University of Maryland Medical Center. What are Ways to Manage Asthma and Reduce the Allergic Response? Available at: http://www.umm.edu/patiented/doc04manage.html. Accessed September 14, 2006.

71. Asthma UK. Exercise. Available at: http://www.asthma.org.uk/all_about_asthma/healthy_lifestyles/exercise.html. Accessed September 21, 2006.

72. Cypcar D, Lemanske R. Asthma and exercise. *Chest.* 1994;15(2):351-365.

73. Carroll N, Sly P. Exercise training as an adjunct to asthma management. *Thorax.* 1999;54:190-191.

74. Morton AR, Fitch KD, Hahn AG. Physical activity and the asthmatic. *Phys Sportsmed.* 1981;9(3):51-64.

75. Hallstrand TS, Bates PW, Schoene RB. Aerobic conditioning in mild asthma decreases the hyperpnea of exercise and improves exercise and ventilatory capacity. *Chest.* 2000;118:1460-1469.

76. Basaran S, Guler Uysal F, Ergen N, et al. Effects of physical exercise on quality of life and exercise capacity in children with asthma. *J Rehabil Med.* 2006;38(2):130-135.

77. Sly RM. Exercise-related changes in airway obstruction: frequency and clinical correlates in asthmatic children. *Ann Allergy.* 1970;28(1):1-16.

78. Stensrud T, Berntsen S, Carlsen KH. Humidity influences exercise capacity in subjects with exercise induced bronchoconstriction (EIB). *Respir Med.* 2006;100(9):1633-1641.

79. American Lung Association. Childhood Asthma Overview. Available at: http://www.lungusa.org/site/pp.asp?c=dvLUK9O0E&b=22782. Accessed September 20, 2006.

80. Frownfelter DL. Massery M. Facilitating ventilation patterns and breathing strategies. In: Frownfelter DL, Dean E, eds. *Cardiovascular and Pulmonary Physical Therapy: Evidence and Practice.* St. Louis, Mo: Mosby Elsevier; 2006.

81. Esteve F, Blanc-Gras N, Gallego J, Benchetrit G. The effects of breathing pattern training on ventilatory function in patients with COPD. *Biofeedback Self Regul.* 1996;21(4):311-321.

82. Slader, C, Reddel HK, Spencer LM, et al. Double blind randomized controlled trial of two different breathing techniques in the management of asthma. *Thorax.* 2006;61:651-656.

83. Stalmatski A. *Freedom from Asthma—Buteyko's Revolutionary Treatment.* London: Kyle Cathie Ltd; 1997.

84. Bowler SD, Green A, Mitchell CA. Buteyko breathing techniques in asthma: a blinded randomised controlled trial. *Med J Australia.* 1998;169:575-578.

85. Nagarathna R, Nagendra HR. Yoga for bronchial asthma: a controlled study. *Brit Med J Clin Res Ed.* 1985;291:1077-1079.

86. Nagendra HR, Nagarathna R. An integrated approach of yoga therapy for bronchial asthma: a 3-54-month prospective study. *J Asthma.* 1986;23:123-137.

87. Singh V, Wisniewski A, Britton J, Tattesfield A. Effect of yoga breathing exercises (Pranayama) on airway reactivity in subjects with asthma. *Lancet.* 1990;335:1381-1383.

88. Jain SC, Rai L, Valecha A, et al. Effect of yoga training on exercise tolerance in adolescents with childhood asthma. *J Asthma.* 1991;28:437-442.

89. Jain SC, Talukdar B. Evaluation of yoga therapy programme for patients of bronchial asthma. *Singapore Med J.* 1993;34:306-308.

90. Khanam AA, Sachdeva U, Guleria R, Deepak KK. Study of pulmonary and autonomic functions of asthma patients after yoga training. *Indian J Physiol Pharm.* 1996;40:318-324.

91. Manocha R, Marks GB, Kenchington P, et al. Sahaja yoga in the management of moderate to severe asthma: a randomised controlled trial. *Thorax.* 2002;57:110-115.

92. Sathyaprabha TN, Murthy H, Murthy BT. Efficacy of naturopathy and yoga in bronchial asthma—a self controlled matched scientific study. *Indian J Physiol Pharm.* 2001;4:80-86.

93. Preston J, Cucuzzella M, Jamieson B. Clinical inquiries: what prevents exercise induced bronchoconstriction for a child with asthma? *J Fam Pract.* 2006;55(7):631-633.

94. McCleary JL, Samuelson WM, Pazos WJ, et al. A RN evaluation of exercise tolerance and quality of life in asthma patients who attend a pulmonary rehabilitation program. *Chest.* 1999;116(4):Supplement 2:292S.

95. Disabella V, Sherman C. Exercise for asthma patients: little risk, big rewards. *Phys Sportsmed.* 1998;26(6):75.

96. Mancuso CA, Sayles W, Robbins L, et al. Barriers and facilitators to healthy physical activity in asthma patients. *J Asthma.* 2006;43(2):137-143.

97. Deal EC Jr, McFadden ER Jr, Ingram RH Jr, et al. Role of respiratory heat exchange in production of exercise-induced asthma. *J Appl Physiol.* 1979;46:467-475.

98. McFadden ER Jr, Lenner KA, Strohl KP. Postexertional airway rewarming and thermally induced asthma. New insights into pathophysiology and possible pathogenesis. *J Clin Invest.* 1986;78:18-25.

99. McFadden ER Jr, Gilbert IA. Exercise-induced asthma. *N Engl J Med.* 1994;330:1362-1367.

100. Cypcar D, Lemanske R. Asthma and exercise. *Chest.* 1994;15(2):351-365.

101. Mehta H, Busse WW. Prevalence of exercise-induced asthma in the athlete. In: Weiler JM, ed. *Allergic and Respiratory Disease in Sports Medicine.* New York, NY: Marcel Dekker, Inc; 1997:81-86.

102. McFadden ER. Exercise-induced asthma. Assessment of current etiologic concepts. *Chest.* 1987;91:151S-157S.

103. Tan RA, Spector SL. Exercise-induced asthma. *Sports Med.* 1998;25:1-6.

104. Shturman-Ellstein R, Zeballos RJ, Buckley JM, Souhrada JF. The beneficial effect of nasal breathing on exercise-induced bronchoconstriction. *Am Rev Respir Dis.* 1978;118:65-73.

105. Stewart EJ, Cinnamond MJ, Siddiqui R, et al. Effect of a heat and moisture retaining mask on exercise induced asthma. *BMJ.* 1992;304:479-480.

106. Godfrey S. Clinical and physiological features. In: McFadden ER Jr, ed. *Exercise-Induced Asthma.* Vol 130. New York, NY: Marcel Dekker, Inc; 1999:11-45.

107. Parry DE, Lemanske RF Jr. Prevention and treatment of exercise-induced asthma. In: McFadden ER Jr, ed. *Exercise-Induced Asthma.* Vol 130. New York, NY: Marcel Dekker, Inc; 1999:387-317.

108. McFadden ER. Respiratory heat exchange. In: McFadden ER, ed. *Exercise-Induced Asthma.* Vol 130. New York, NY: Marcel Dekker, Inc; 1999:47-76.

109. Matsumoto I, Araki H, Tsuda K. Effects of swimming training on aerobic capacity and exercise induced bronchoconstriction in children with bronchial asthma. *Thorax.* 1999;54:196-201.

110. National Asthma Education and Prevention Program. *Highlights of the Expert Panel Report 2: Guidelines for the Diagnosis and Management of Asthma.* Bethesda, Md: US Department of Health and Human Services, Public Health Service, National Institutes of Health, National Heart, Lung, and Blood Institute, 1997. Publication No. 97-4051A.

111. American Physical Therapy Association. Guidelines for physical therapy documentation. In: Guide to Physical Therapist Practice. 2nd ed. *Phys Ther.* 2001;81:703-705.

112. Prasad SA, Randall SD, Balfour-Lynn IM. Fifteen-count breathlessness score: an objective measurement for children. *Pediatr Pulmonol.* 2000;30(1):56-62.

113. Borg G. *Borg's Perceived Exertion and Pain Scales.* Champaign, Ill: Human Kinetics; 1998.

114. American Lung Association. Chronic Obstructive Pulmonary Disease (COPD) Fact Sheet. Available at: http://www.lungusa.org/site/pp.asp?c=dvLUK9O0E&b=35020. Accessed October 14, 2006.

115. Anthonisen NR, Connett JE, Kiley JP, et al. Effects of smoking intervention and the use of an inhaled anticholinergic bronchodilator on the rate of decline of FEV1. The Lung Health Study. *JAMA.* 1994;272:1497-1505.

116. Anthonisen NR, Connett JE, Murray RP. Smoking and lung function of lung health study participants after 11 years. The Lung Health Study Research Group. *Am J Respir Crit Care Med.* 2002;166:675-679.

117. Dean E. Oxygen transport: a physiologically based conceptual framework for the practice of cardiopulmonary physiotherapy. *Physiother.* 1994;(80):347-355.

118. Niederman MS, Clemente PH, Fein AM, et al. Benefits of a multidisciplinary pulmonary rehabilitation program. Improvements are independent of lung function. *Chest.* 1991;99:798-804.

119. Ries AL. Pulmonary rehabilitation in COPD. *Semin Respir Crit Care Med.* 2005;(7):133-141.

120. Zu Wallack RL, Patel K, Reardon JZ, et al. Predictors of improvement in 12-minute walking distance following a pulmonary rehabilitation program. *Chest.* 1991;99(4):805-808.

121. Belman MJ, Kengregan BA. Exercise training fails to increase skeletal muscle enzymes in patients with chronic obstructive lung disease. *Amer Rev Respir Dis.* 1981;123(3): 256-261.

122. Belman MJ, Wasserman K. Exercise training and testing in patients with chronic obstructive pulmonary disease. *Basic Respir Dis.* 1981;10:1-6.

123. Wijkstra PJ, van Altena R, Kraan J, et al. Quality of life in patients with chronic obstructive pulmonary disease improves after rehabilitation at home. *Eur Respir J.* 1994;7: 269-273.

124. Berry MJ, Adair NE, Sevensky KS, et al. Inspiratory muscle training and whole-body reconditioning in chronic obstructive pulmonary disease. *Am J Respir Crit Care Med.* 1996;153:1812-1816.

125. ACCP/AACVPR Pulmonary Rehabilitation Guidelines Panel. Pulmonary rehabilitation: joint ACCP/AACVPR evidence-based guidelines. American College of Chest Physicians. American Association of Cardiovascular and Pulmonary Rehabilitation. *Chest.* 1997;112:1363-1396.

126. Hirata K, Otsuka T, Okamoto T. Exercise therapy of respiratory insufficiency. *Nippon Naika Gakkai Zasshi.* 1999;88(1):70-76.

127. Bowen JB, Votto JJ, Thrall RS, et al. Functional status and survival following pulmonary rehabilitation. *Chest.* 2000;118: 697-703.

128. Connor MC, O'Shea FD, O'Driscoll MF, et al. Efficacy of pulmonary rehabilitation in an Irish population. *Ir Med J.* 2001;94:46-48.

129. Emery CF, Honn VJ, Frid DJ, et al. Acute effects of exercise on cognition in patients with chronic obstructive pulmonary disease. *Am J Respir Crit Care Med.* 2001;164(9):1624-1627.

130. Griffiths TL, Phillips CJ, Davies S, et al. Cost effectiveness of an outpatient multidisciplinary pulmonary rehabilitation programme. *Thorax.* 2001;56:779-784.

131. Puhan MA, Scharplatz M, Troosters T, Steurer J. Respiratory rehabilitation after acute exacerbation of COPD may reduce risk for readmission and mortality: a systematic review. *Respir Res.* 2005;6:54.

132. Casaburi R, Porszasz J, Burns MR, et al. Physiologic benefits of exercise training in rehabilitation of severe COPD patients. *Am J Respir Crit Care Med.* 1997;155:1541-1551.

133. Casaburi R. Mechanisms of the reduced ventilatory requirement as a result of exercise training. *Eur Respir Rev.* 1995; 5:25,42-46.

134. Casaburi R, Patessio A, Ioli F, et al. Reduction in exercise lactic acidosis and ventilation as a result of exercise training in patients with obstructive lung disease. *Am Rev Respir Dis* 1991;143:9-18.

135. Gosselink R, Troosters T, Decramer M. Exercise training in COPD patients: the basic questions. *Eur Respir J.* 1997; 10:2884-2891.

136. Maltais F, LeBlanc P, Jobin J, et al. Intensity of training and physiologic adaptation in patients with chronic obstructive pulmonary disease. *Am J Respir Crit Care Med.* 1997;155:555-561.

137. Cooper CB. Exercise in chronic pulmonary disease: limitations and rehabilitation. *Med Sci Sports Exerc.* 2001;33(7 Suppl): S643-S646.

138. Maltais F, LeBlanc P, Simard C, et al. Skeletal muscle adaptation to endurance training in patients with chronic obstructive pulmonary disease. *Am J Respir Crit Care Med.* 1996;154:442-447.

139. Whittom F, Jobin J, Simard PM, et al. Histochemical and morphological characteristics of the vastus lateralis muscle in

patients with chronic obstructive pulmonary disease. *Med Sci Sports Exerc.* 1998;30:1467-1474.

140. Bernard S, Whittom F, LeBlanc P, et al. Aerobic and strength training in patients with chronic obstructive pulmonary disease. *Am J Respir Crit Care Med.* 1999;159:896-900.

141. Ries AL, ACCP/AACVPR Pulmonary Rehabilitation Guidelines Panel. Pulmonary rehabilitation: joint ACCP/AACVPR evidence-based guidelines. *Chest.* 1997;112:1363-1396.

142. Nici L, Donner D, Wouters E, et al. American Thoracic Society/European Respiratory Society Statement on Pulmonary Rehabilitation. *Amer J Resp Crit Care Med.* 2006;173: 1390-1413.

143. Fuchs-Climent D, Le Gallais D, Varray A, et al. Quality of life and exercise tolerance in chronic obstructive pulmonary disease: effects of a short and intensive inpatient rehabilitation program. *Am J Phys Med Rehabil.* 1999;78:330-335.

144. Vogiatzis I, Nanas S, Roussos C. Interval training as an alternative modality to continuous exercise in patients with COPD. *Eur Respir J.* 2002;20:12-19.

145. Coppoolse R, Schols AM, Baarends EM, et al. Interval versus continuous training in patients with severe COPD: a randomized clinical trial. *Eur Respir J.* 1999;14:258-263.

146. Gosselink R, Troosters T, Decramer M. Effects of exercise training in COPD patients: interval versus endurance training. *Eur Respir J.* 1998;12:2S.

147. Vallet G, Ahmaidi S, Serres I, et al. Comparison of two training programmes in chronic airway limitation patients: standardized versus individualized protocols. *Eur Respir J.* 1997;10:114-122.

148. Lake FR, Henderson K, Briffa T, et al. Upper-limb and lower-limb exercise training in patients with chronic airflow obstruction. *Chest.* 1990;97:1077-1082.

149. Ortega F, Toral J, Cejudo P, et al. Comparison of effects of strength and endurance training in patients with chronic obstructive pulmonary disease. *Am J Respir Crit Care Med.* 2002;166(5):669-674.

150. Clark CJ, Cochrane LM, Mackay E, Paton B. Skeletal muscle strength and endurance in patients with mild COPD and the effects of weight training. *Eur Respir J.* 2000;15(1):92-97.

151. Panton LB, Golden J, Broeder CE, et al. The effects of resistance training on functional outcomes in patients with chronic obstructive pulmonary disease. *Eur J Appl Physiol.* 2004;91(4):443-449.

152. American Thoracic Society/European Respiratory Society. Skeletal muscle dysfunction in chronic obstructive pulmonary disease. *Am J Respir Crit Care Med.* 1999;159:S1-S40.

153. Schols AMWJ, Slangen J, Volovics L, Wouters EFM. Weight loss is a reversible factor in the prognosis of chronic obstructive pulmonary disease. *Am J Respir Crit Care Med.* 1998;157:1791-1797.

154. Musaro A, McCullagh K, Paul A, et al. Localized Igf-1 transgene expression sustains hypertrophy and regeneration in senescent skeletal muscle. *Nat Genet.* 2001;27:195-200.

155. Debigarè R, Còtè CH, Maltais F. Peripheral muscle wasting in chronic obstructive pulmonary disease. Clinical relevance and mechanisms. *Am J Respir Crit Care Med.* 2001;164:1712-1717.

156. Gosselink RA, Wagenaar RC, Sargeant AJ, et al. Diaphragmatic breathing reduces efficiency of breathing in chronic obstructive pulmonary disease. *Am J Respir Crit Care Med.* 1995;151:1136-1142.

157. Sackner MA, Gonzalez HF, Jenouri G, Rodriguez M. Effects of abdominal and thoracic breathing on breathing pattern components in normal subjects and in patients with COPD. *Am Rev Respir Dis.* 1984;130:584-587.

158. Grimby G, Oxhoj H, Bake B. Effects of abdominal breathing on distribution of ventilation in obstructive lung disease. *Clin Sci Mol Med.* 1975;48:193-199.

159. Willeput R, Vachaudez JP, Lenders D, et al. Thoracoabdominal motion during chest physiotherapy in patients affected by chronic obstructive lung disease. *Respiration.* 1983;44:204-214.

160. Williams IP, Smith CM, McGavin CR. Diaphragmatic breathing training and walking performance in chronic airways obstruction. *Br J Dis Chest.* 1982;76:164-166.

161. Vitacca M, Clini E, Bianchi L, Ambrosino N. Acute effects of deep diaphragmatic breathing in COPD patients with chronic respiratory insufficiency. *Eur Respir J.*1998;11:408-415.

162. Bellemare F, Grassino A. Force reserve of the diaphragm in patients with chronic obstructive pulmonary disease. *J Appl Physiol.* 1983;55:8-15.

163. Belman MJ, Shadmehr R. Targeted resistive ventilatory muscle training in chronic pulmonary disease. *J Appl Physiol.* 1988;65:2726-2735.

164. Wanke T, Formanek D, Lahrmann H, et al. The effects of combined inspiratory muscle and cycle ergometer training on exercise performance in patients with COPD. *Eur Respir J.* 1994;7:2205-2211.

165. Dekhuijzen PNR, Folgering HThM, van Herwaarden CLA. Target-flow inspiratory muscle training during pulmonary rehabilitation in patients with COPD. *Chest.* 1991;99:128-133.

166. Heijdra YF, Dekhuijzen PNR, van Herwaarden CLA, Folgering HThM. Nocturnal saturation improves by target-flow inspiratory muscle training in patients with COPD. *Am J Respir Crit Care Med.* 1996;153:260-265.

167. Preusser BA, Winningham ML, Clanton TL. High- vs low-intensity inspiratory muscle interval training in patients with COPD. *Chest.* 1994;106:110-117.

168. Larson JL, Kim MJ, Sharp JT, Larson DA. Inspiratory muscle training with a pressure threshold breathing device in patients with chronic obstructive pulmonary disease. *Am Rev Respir Dis.* 1988;138:689-696.

169. Lisboa C, Munoz V, Beroiza T, et al. Inspiratory muscle training in chronic airflow limitation: comparison of two different training loads with a threshold device. *Eur Respir J.* 1994;7:1266-1274.

170. Lisboa C, Villafranca C, Leiva A, et al. Inspiratory muscle training in chronic airflow limitation: effect on exercise performance. *Eur Respir J.* 1997;10:537-542.

171. Patessio A, Rampulla C, Fracchia C, et al. Relationship between the perception of breathlessness and inspiratory resistive loading: a report on a clinical trial. *Eur Respir J.* 1989;7:587S-591S.

172. Villafranca C, Borzone G, Leiva A, Lisboa C. Effect of inspiratory muscle training with intermediate load on inspiratory power output in COPD. *Eur Respir J.* 1998;11:28-33.

173. Boutellier U, Piwko P. The respiratory system as an exercise limiting factor in normal sedentary subjects. *Eur J Appl Physiol.* 1992;64:145-152.

174. Scherer TA, Spengler C, Owassapian D, et al. Respiratory muscle endurance training in chronic obstructive pulmonary disease. Impact on exercise capacity, dyspnea, and quality of life. *Am J Respir Crit Care Med*. 2000;162:1709-1714.

175. Martin AD, Davenport PD, Franceschi AC, Harman E. Use of inspiratory muscle strength training to facilitate ventilator weaning. *Chest*. 2002;122:192-196.

176. Renfroe KL. Effect of progressive relaxation on dyspnea and state of anxiety in patients with chronic obstructive pulmonary disease. *Heart Lung*. 1988;17:408-413.

177. Kolaczkowski W, Taylor R, Hoffstein V. Improvement in oxygen saturation after chest physiotherapy in patients with emphysema. *Physiother Canada*. 1989;41:18-23.

178. Antonelli M, Pennisi MA, Conti G. New advances in the use of noninvasive ventilation for acute hypoxaemic respiratory failure. *Eur Respir J*. 2003;22:65S-71S.

179. Wysocki M, Antonelli M. Noninvasive mechanical ventilation in acute hypoxaemic respiratory failure. *Eur Respir J*. 2001;18:209-220.

180. Casanova C, Celli BR, Tost L, et al. Long-term controlled trial of nocturnal nasal positive pressure ventilation in patients with severe COPD. *Chest*. 2000;118(6):1582-1590.

181. Schonhofer B, Wallstein S, Weise C, Kohler D. Noninvasive mechanical ventilation improves endurance performance in patients with chronic respiratory failure due to thoracic restriction. *Chest*. 2001;119;1371-1378.

182. Brochard L. Mechanical ventilation: invasive versus noninvasive. *Eur Respir J*. 2003;22:31S-37S.

183. Kramer N, Meyer TJ, Meharg J, et al. Randomized, prospective trial of noninvasive positive pressure ventilation in acute respiratory failure, *Am J Respir Crit Care Med*. 1995;151:1799-1806.

184. Poponick JM, Renston JP, Bennett RP, Emerman CL. Use of a ventilatory support system (BIPAP) for acute respiratory failure in the emergency department. *Chest*. 1999;116:166-171.

185. Antonelli M, Conti G, Rocco M, et al. A comparison of noninvasive positive-pressure ventilation and conventional mechanical ventilation in patients with acute respiratory failure. *N Engl J Med*. 1998;339:429-435.

186. Brochard L, Mancebo J, Wysocki M, et al. Noninvasive ventilation for acute exacerbations of chronic obstructive pulmonary disease. *N Engl J Med*. 1995;333:817-822.

187. Padman R, Lawless S, Van Nessen S. Use of BIPAP by nasal mask in the treatment of respiratory insufficiency in pediatric patients: a preliminary investigation. *Pediatr Pulmonol*. 1994;17(2):119-123.

188. Hill NS. Noninvasive ventilation for chronic obstructive pulmonary disease. *Respir Care*. 2004;49(1):72-87.

189. Milross MA, Piper AJ, Norman M, et al. Low-flow oxygen and bilevel ventilatory support. *Am J Respir Crit Care Med*. 2001;163(1):129-134.

190. Somfay A, Porszasz J, Lee SM, Casaburi R. Effect of hyperoxia on gas exchange and lactate kinetics following exercise onset in non-hypoxemic COPD patients. *Chest*. 2002; 121:393-400.

191. Terrados N, Jansson E, Sylven C, Kaijser L. Is hypoxia a stimulus for synthesis of oxidative enzymes and myoglobin? *J Appl Physiol*. 1990;68:2369-2372.

192. Somfay A, Porszasz J, Lee SM, Casaburi R. Effect of oxygen on hyperinflation and exercise endurance in non-hypoxemic COPD patients. *Eur Respir J*. 2001;18:77-84.

193. Stein DA, Bradley BL, Miller W. Mechanisms of oxygen effects on exercise in chronic obstructive pulmonary disease. *Chest*. 1982;81:6-10.

194. Bradley BL, Garner AE, Billiu K, et al. Oxygen-assisted exercise in chronic obstructive lung disease: the effect on exercise capacity and arterial blood gas tensions. *Am Rev Respir Dis*. 1978;118:239-243.

195. Dean NC, Brown JK, Himelman RB, et al. Oxygen may improve dyspnea and endurance in patients with chronic obstructive pulmonary disease and only mild hypoxemia. *Am Rev Respir Dis*. 1992;148:941-945.

196. O'Donnell DE, Bain DJ, Webb KA. Factors contributing to relief of exertional breathlessness during hyperoxia in chronic airflow limitation. *Am J Respir Crit Care Med*. 1997;155:530-535.

197. Emtner M, Porszasz J, Burns M, et al. Benefits of supplemental oxygen in exercise training in non-hypoxemic COPD patients. *Am J Respir Crit Care Med*. 2003; 68:1034-1042.

198. Serres I, Varray A, Vallet G, et al. Improved skeletal muscle performance after individualized exercise training in patients with chronic obstructive pulmonary disease. *J Cardiopulm Rehabil*. 1997;17:232-238.

199. Palange P, Valli G, Onorati P, et al. Effect of heliox on lung dynamic hyperinflation, dyspnea, and exercise endurance capacity in COPD patients. *J Appl Physiol*. 2004;97:1637-1642.

200. Gosselink R. Controlled breathing and dyspnea in patients with chronic obstructive pulmonary disease (COPD). *J Rehabil Res Devel*. 2003;40(5 Supp 2):25-34.

201. Mueller, R, Petty, T, Filley, G. Ventilation and arterial blood gas changes induced by pursed-lips breathing. *J Appl Physiol*. 1970;28:784-789.

202. van der Schans CP, De Jong W, Kort E, et al. Mouth pressures during pursed lip breathing. *Physioth Theory Pract*. 1995; 11:29-34.

203. Breslin EH. The pattern of respiratory muscle recruitment during pursed-lips breathing in COPD. *Chest*. 1992;101:75-78.

204. Tiep BL, Burns M, Kao D, et al. Pursed lips breathing training using ear oximetry. *Chest*. 1986;90:218-221.

205. Petty TL, Guthrie A. The effects of augmented breathing maneuvres on ventilation in severe chronic airway obstruction. *Respir Care*. 1971;16:104-111.

206. Ingram RH, Schilder DP. Effect of pursed lips breathing on the pulmonary pressure-flow relationship in obstructive lung disease. *Am Rev Respir Dis*. 1967;96:381-388.

207. Thoman, RL, Stoker GL, Ross JC. The efficacy of pursed-lips breathing in patients with chronic obstructive pulmonary disease. *Am Rev Respir Dis*. 1966;93:100-106.

208. Erpicum B, Willeput R, Sergysels R, De Coster A. Does abdominal breathing below FRC give a mechanical support for inspiration? *Clin Respir Physiol*. 1984;20:117.

209. Casciari RJ, Fairshter RD, Harrison A, et al. Effects of breathing retraining in patients with chronic obstructive pulmonary disease. *Chest*. 1981;79:393-398.

210. Reybrouck T, Wertelaers A, Bertrand P, Demedts M. Myofeedback training of the respiratory muscles in patients with chronic obstructive pulmonary disease. *J Cardiopulm Rehabil*. 1987;7:18-22.

211. Dechman G, Wilson CR. Evidence underlying breathing retraining in people with stable chronic obstructive pulmonary disease. *Phys Ther*. 2004;84(12):1189-1197.

212. Badr C, Elkins MR, Ellis ER. The effect of body position on maximal expiratory pressure and flow. *Aust J Physiother.* 2002; 48(2):95-102.

213. Barach AL. Chronic obstructive lung disease: postural relief of dyspnea. *Arch Phys Med Rehabil.* 1974;55:494-504.

214. Sharp JT, Druz WS, Moisan T, et al. Postural relief of dyspnea in severe chronic obstructive pulmonary disease. *Am Rev Respir Dis.* 1980;122:201-211.

215. O'Neill S, McCarthy DS. Postural relief of dyspnoea in severe chronic airflow limitation: relationship to respiratory muscle strength. *Thorax.* 1983;38:595-600.

216. Delgado HR, Braun SR, Skatrud JB, et al. Chest wall and abdominal motion during exercise in patients with COPD. *Am Rev Respir Dis.* 1982;126:200-205.

217. Maillefert JF, Eicher JC, Walker P, et al. Effects of low-frequency electrical stimulation of quadriceps and calf muscles in patients with chronic heart failure. *J Cardiopulm Rehabil.* 1998;18:277-282.

218. Vaquero AF, Chicharro JL, Gil L, et al. Effects of muscle electrical stimulation on peak VO_2 in cardiac transplant patients. *Int J Sports Med.* 1998;19:17-22.

219. Quittan M, Sochor A, Wiesinger GF, et al. Strength improvement of knee extensor muscles in patients with chronic heart failure by neuromuscular electrical stimulation. *Artif Organs.* 1999;23:432-435.

220. Quittan M, Wiesinger GF, Sturm B, et al. Improvement of thigh muscles by neuromuscular electrical stimulation in patients with refractory heart failure: a single-blind, randomized, controlled trial. *Am J Phys Med Rehabil.* 2001;80:206-214.

221. Neder JA, Sword D, Ward SA, et al. Home based neuromuscular electrical stimulation as a new rehabilitative strategy for severely disabled patients with chronic obstructive pulmonary disease (COPD). *Thorax.* 2002;57:333-337.

222. Bourjeily-Habr G, Rochester CL, Palermo F, et al. Randomised controlled trial of transcutaneous electrical muscle stimulation of the lower extremities in patients with chronic obstructive pulmonary disease. *Thorax.* 2002;57:1045-1049.

223. Zanotti E, Felicetti G, Maini M, Fracchia C. Peripheral muscle strength training in bed-bound patients with COPD receiving mechanical ventilation. Effect of electrical stimulation. *Chest.* 2003;124:292-296.

224. Engelen MP, Shols AM, Lamers RJ, Wouters E. Different patterns of chronic tissue wasting among patients with chronic obstructive pulmonary disease. *Clin Nutr.* 1999;18:275-280.

225. Vengust R, Strojnik V, Pavlovic V, et al. The effect of electrostimulation and high load exercises in patients with patellofemoral joint dysfunction. A preliminary report. *Pflugers Arch.* 2001;442(Suppl 1):153-154.

226. Casaletto JJ. Differential diagnosis of metabolic acidosis. *Emerg Med Clin North Am.* 2005;23(3):771-787.

227. Jurado RL, del Rio C, Nassar G, et al. Low anion gap. *South Med J.* 1998;91(7):624-629.

228. Teasdale G, Jennett B. Assessment of coma and impaired consciousness. *Lancet.* 1974;ii:81-83.

229. Nava S. Rehabilitation of patients admitted to a respiratory intensive care unit. *Arch Phys Med Rehabil.* 1998;79(7):849-854.

230. Herridge MS, Cheung AM, Tansey CM, et al. One-year outcomes in survivors of the acute respiratory distress syndrome. *N Engl J Med.* 2003;348(8):683-693.

231. Gattinoni L, Tognoni G, Pesenti A, et al. Effect of prone positioning on the survival of patients with acute respiratory failure. *N Engl J Med.* 2001;345(8):568-573.

232. Behrendt CE. Acute respiratory failure in the United States: incidence and 31-day survival. *Chest.* 2000;118(4):1100-1105.

233. Wong WP. Physical therapy for a patient in acute respiratory failure. *Phys Ther.* 2000;80(7):662-670.

234. Gray BA, Blalock JM. Interpretation of the alveolar-arterial oxygen difference in patients with hypercapnia. *Am Rev Respir Dis.* 1991;143(1):4-8.

235. Story DA. Alveolar oxygen partial pressure, alveolar carbon dioxide partial pressure, and the alveolar gas equation. *Anesthesiology.* 1996;84(4):1011.

236. Parker JC, Hernandez LA, Peevy KJ. Mechanisms of ventilator-induced lung injury. *Crit Care Med.* 1993;21(1):131-143.

237. Ranieri VM, Giunta F, Suter PM, Slutsky AS. Mechanical ventilation as a mediator of multisystem organ failure in acute respiratory distress syndrome. *JAMA.* 2000;284(1):43-44.

238. Derdak S, Mehta S, Stewart TE, et al. High-frequency oscillatory ventilation for acute respiratory distress syndrome in adults: a randomized, controlled trial. *Am J Respir Crit Care Med.* 2002;166(6):801-808.

239. Hickling KG, Walsh J, Henderson S, Jackson R. Low mortality rate in adult respiratory distress syndrome using low-volume, pressure-limited ventilation with permissive hypercapnia: a prospective study. *Crit Care Med.* 1994;22(10):1568-1578.

240. Laffey JG, Tanaka M, Engelberts D, et al. Therapeutic hypercapnia reduces pulmonary and systemic injury following in vivo lung reperfusion. *Am J Respir Crit Care Med.* 2000;162(6):2287-2294.

241. Peter JV, Moran JL, Phillips-Hughes J, Warn D. Noninvasive ventilation in acute respiratory failure--a meta-analysis update. *Crit Care Med.* 2002;30(3):555-562.

242. Sinuff T, Cook DJ, Randall J, Allen CJ. Evaluation of a practice guideline for noninvasive positive-pressure ventilation for acute respiratory failure. *Chest.* 2003;123(6):2062-2073.

CHAPTER SEVEN

Impaired Ventilation, Respiration/ Gas Exchange, and Aerobic Capacity/Endurance Associated With Respiratory Failure in the Neonate (Pattern G)

Mary Rahlin, PT, MS, PCS

ANATOMY/PHYSIOLOGY

Development of the heart begins with the formation of two endocardial tubes starting on the 19th gestational day[1] and their subsequent fusion into a primitive heart tube in the 4th gestational week.[1,2] While contractions of the heart begin on day 22, blood flow starts by the 24th gestational day.[1] By the end of the 8th gestational week, the heart possesses the definitive structures of the adult heart with slight modifications and is a functioning part of the circulatory system.[1] Fetal circulation differs from adult circulation in that blood is oxygenated not by the lungs, but by the placenta and the maternal circulation.[2,3] The foramen ovale between the right and left atria allows blood to pass from the right to the left atrium, thus bypassing the pulmonary circulation. Blood then flows to the left ventricle and to the ascending aorta of the fetus. The ductus arteriosus, an opening between the pulmonary artery and the aorta, also allows blood to bypass the lungs by leaving the pulmonary artery and flowing directly into the descending aorta.[2,3] The foramen ovale closes with the first breath of the newborn infant.[2] Its anatomical closure is usually complete in 2 to 3 months after that.[3] Functionally, the ductus arteriosus closes within 15 to 72 hours after birth, which is followed by a complete anatomical closure a few weeks later.[2,3]

Development of the lungs begins during the 4th gestational week with the formation of a lung bud,[4,5] which bifurcates into two primary bronchial buds on the 26th to 28th gestational days.[4] In the 5th week, further branching leads to the formation of five secondary bronchial buds (two on the left and three on the right), which later develop into the lobes of the lungs. The branching process continues until the 28th gestational week.[4] First primitive alveoli or terminal sacs begin to form in weeks 26 to 28, and respiratory vasculature also develops at that time.[4,5] Alveolar cells that are responsible for the production of surfactant appear by the end of the 6th gestational month.[5] Surfactant is a lipoprotein that serves to lower the surface tension of the fluid lining the alveoli and allows them to expand. The amount of produced surfactant continues to increase and peaks during the last 2 prenatal weeks.[5] Before birth, only 20 to 70 million alveoli are present in each lung as compared to 300 to 400 million in the lung of an adult.[4] Formation of alveoli continues until approximately 8 years of age.[4,5]

Of note is the fact that significant anatomical differences exist in the infant's pulmonary system as compared to the adult's.[3,6] The diameter of the infant's airway is smaller; the larynx is higher facilitating feeding, but necessitating nasal breathing; the resistance to airflow is increased; there are fewer alveoli and therefore less surface area; the rib cage is primarily composed of cartilage making it very compliant; the ribs are aligned more horizontally decreasing movement efficiency of the chest wall; and the diaphragm has less fatigue-resistant fibers. These differences result in increased work of breathing for the infant as compared to the adult.[3,6]

The anatomy and physiology of the adult heart and lungs are covered in Pattern A: Primary Prevention/Risk Reduction for Cardiovascular/Pulmonary Disorders; Pattern C: Impaired Ventilation, Respiration/Gas Exchange, and Aerobic Capacity/Endurance Associated With Airway Clearance Dysfunction; and Pattern E: Impaired Ventilation and Respiration/Gas Exchange Associated With Ventilatory Pump Dysfunction or Failure.

PATHOPHYSIOLOGY

RESPIRATORY FAILURE IN THE PRETERM NEONATE

Advances in health care over the past two decades have made it possible for neonates born as early as 23 to 25 weeks of gestational age,[7] with a birth weight as low as 500 to 800 grams, to survive.[8] Infants born prematurely (below 37 weeks gestation) are hospitalized in the neonatal intensive care units (NICU) designed to decrease the rates of neonatal mortality and morbidity.[7] Pathophysiologic problems observed in these infants are largely associated with the immaturity of their respiratory and central nervous systems[7-9] and are related to their birth weight[7,8] (Table 7-1) and gestational age at birth.[7-9] Medical complications of prematurity, such as apnea, bradycardia, respiratory distress syndrome, and bronchopulmonary dysplasia, are discussed below.

The American Academy of Pediatrics defines apnea as "cessation of breathing for 20 seconds or longer, or as a briefer episode if associated with bradycardia, cyanosis, or pallor."[10] Three types of apnea have been identified.[9] They include central apnea characterized by a pause in breathing movement and airflow, obstructive apnea described as cessation of airflow with continuation of respiratory efforts, and mixed apnea that constitutes a combination of central and obstructive apneas. Apnea may affect blood oxygenation causing cyanosis and hypoxemia defined as a PO_2 <40 mmHg. According to Poets and associates,[9] severe hypoxemia and recurrent cyanosis with a decrease in SaO_2 below 80% may develop in preterm infants without cessation of airflow or respiratory movements. Eichenwald and associates[11] have demonstrated that apnea and bradycardia in infants born at 24 to 28 weeks gestation frequently persist beyond 36 to 38 weeks postconceptional age (PCA). They described bradycardia as a HR below 100 bpm for infants younger than 34 to 35 weeks PCA and below 80 bpm for infants at 34 to 35 weeks PCA and older. In most infants, episodes of apnea and bradycardia that require intervention disappear first, followed by self-resolved observed apnea and bradycardia, and then by self-resolved bradycardia without observed apnea. The amount of time to the resolution of recurrent episodes of apnea and bradycardia has been found to be inversely related to the gestational age at birth.[11]

Table 7-1	
CLASSIFICATION OF NEONATES BASED ON BIRTH WEIGHT—DATA FROM KAHN-D'ANGELO AND UNANUE[7]	
Category	**Birth Weight**
Low birth weight (LBW)	1501-2500 g
Very low birth weight (VLBW)	1000-1500 g
Extremely low birth weight (ELBW)	Below 1000 g

Another serious complication of premature birth is respiratory distress syndrome (RDS) or hyaline membrane disease that remains the primary cause of neonatal mortality and morbidity.[7,12] Its incidence increases with lower birth weight. Approximately one-fifth of the low birth weight and two-thirds of the very low birth weight infants are diagnosed with RDS.[12] Respiratory failure in these neonates results from the immaturity of the lungs and other organs and from the deficiency of surfactant.[7,12] In the preterm infant, the alveoli are deficient in number, thus producing less surfactant than is needed to prevent the alveoli from collapsing during expiration.[12] Upon expiration, the lung volume decreases, and the subsequent increase in surface tension causes atelectasis followed by ventilation/perfusion mismatching and respiratory failure. In addition, other problems of prematurity, such as hypothermia, acidosis, and hypoxia, may further reduce the synthesis of surfactant and contribute to respiratory dysfunction.[12] As-Sanie and associates[13] have demonstrated that there is an association between RDS at 34 to 36 weeks PCA and increased morbidity, including apnea, bradycardia, pneumonia, and suspected sepsis as compared to preterm infants without RDS. These morbidities, in turn, increase the length of the NICU and hospital stays and the need for neonatal interventions.[13]

Mechanical ventilation and oxygen supplementation that are used as interventions for RDS in infants born prematurely[7,14] may lead to injury of the lung or exacerbate respiratory problems initially exhibited by the neonates.[14-16] Mechanical ventilation may cause structural damage to the alveoli of the premature lungs and produce pulmonary edema, inflammation, and fibrosis.[14-16] Oxygen toxicity and mechanical injury have been implicated in causing bronchopulmonary dysplasia (BPD), one of the most common complications of prematurity.[7,15-18] Northway and associates[17] were the first to describe BPD in 1967[15,17] in preterm infants born at 31 weeks gestation or older, with a birth weight of 1474 grams or greater, who developed this condition after severe RDS.[17] Since that time, as the rate of survival of the very premature infants increased, the incidence of BPD increased as well,[15] but its clinical presentation changed.[15,16,18] Currently, this condition is rarely seen in infants born at gestational age higher than 30 weeks and with a birth weight over 1200 grams.[16] In many infants, BPD occurs after mild or no RDS, when they do not necessarily require continuous administration of supplemental oxygen in the first weeks of life.[15,16] Instead of being exposed to high airway pressures and high oxygen concentration, they may initially require low-pressure ventilation and minimal or no need for oxygen supplementation.[15] However, after prolonged mechanical ventilation, these infants may demonstrate deterioration in function of the lungs and may require increased ventilatory and oxygen support due to the development of respiratory failure.[15] This may be related to immaturity and disrupted development of the alveoli and vasculature of the lungs,[14-16,18] perinatal infection,[15,18] inflammation,[15,16,18] and patent ductus arteriosus (PDA).[15] At the same time, oxygen toxicity and mechanical trauma continue to be crucial in the pathogenesis of BPD, and infants who have more severe RDS are at a higher risk for developing the disease.[15]

The new clinical course of BPD has prompted the need for change in its definition.[15,16] The diagnostic criteria for this condition proposed by Corcoran and associates in 1993[19] included oxygen dependency for more than 28 days and areas of increased densities on chest radiographs in low birth weight infants after their exposure to intermittent positive pressure ventilation (IPPV) for longer than 12 hours. A workshop organized by the National Institute of Child Health and Human Development (NICHD), the National Heart, Lung, and Blood Institute (NHLBI), and the Office of Rare Diseases (ORD) provided the new definition and diagnostic criteria for BPD that are summarized in Table 7-2.[16,17] The reported inconsistencies in interpretation of chest radiographs in BPD contributed to the exclusion of radiographic findings from the new definition of this condition.[16]

Several authors[20-22] reported lung function changes in infants with BPD. These changes included air trapping and moderate obstruction of the airflow,[20] increased airway resistance and work of breathing,[21] decreased lung compliance,[20-22] hypoventilation, and retention of carbon dioxide.[21] Robin and associates[20] obtained baseline lung function measurements from 28 infants with a history of BPD. They found decreased forced expiratory volume in 0.5 seconds and decreased forced expiratory flow at 25% to 75% and at 75% of expired forced vital capacity. In addition, infants with a history of BPD demonstrated increased residual volume, an increased ratio of residual volume to total lung capacity, and increased functional residual capacity values as compared to normally developing infants.[20] Tortorolo and associates[22] have measured pulmonary mechanics in preterm infants and used respiratory flow, TV, and airway pressure data to calculate respiratory system compliance and lung resistance. They found that ventilated infants exhibiting lower lung compliance values had a significantly higher probability of developing severe BPD than infants with higher lung compliance.[22]

Supplemental oxygen, in addition to its negative effects on the immature lungs, interferes with normal development of vasculature in prematurely born infants.[23-25] This, in turn, leads to the development of retinopathy of prematurity (ROP).[23,24] ROP develops in two phases. In the first phase, exposure to supplemental oxygen causes hyperoxia leading to vasoconstriction and cessation of retinal vascularization in an infant with incomplete vascular development of the retina. In the second phase, as the infant matures, metabolic activity of the nonvascularized retina increases and causes hypoxia that is followed by rapid growth of new blood vessels.[23,24] Consequently, retinal detachment may occur that may lead to blindness.[24]

The incidence of ROP increases with lower gestational age at birth and lower birth weight.[25] It is associated with other morbidities, such as BPD, necrotizing enterocolitis, and intraventricular hemorrhage (IVH)[23] and is considered to be one of the major causes of blindness in children.[23,24] York and associates,[24] who conducted a retrospective study of 231 infants, reported that fluctuations in partial pressure of dissolved arterial oxygen (PaO$_2$) lead to increased risk of ROP in very low birth weight infants. In addition, Kim and associates[25] implicated apnea, surfactant therapy, and prolonged ventilator use as being significant risk factors for ROP.

Germinal matrix-intraventricular hemorrhage (GM-IVH) is another characteristic complication of prematurity that is related to immaturity of the vasculature in the germinal matrix.[7,26] As with ROP,[25] its incidence increases with lower gestational age at birth and lower birth weight. Volpe[26] described grading the severity of GM-IVH using ultrasonography. Grade I was given to a germinal matrix hemorrhage without or with a minimal intraventricular hemorrhage. Grade II was an IVH involving 10% to 50% of the ventricular area, and Grade III was an IVH that involved more than 50% of the ventricular area, with ventricular dilation.[26] Instead of describing Grade IV as other authors did,[7] Volpe designated a separate category to IVH complicated by periventricular hemorrhagic infarction that was diagnosed by periventricular echodensity on the ultrasound scan.[26]

The pathogenesis of IVH is complex and includes: fluctuating cerebral blood flow; abrupt increases in arterial blood pressure and blood flow; increases in cerebral venous pressure;[7,26] respiratory disturbances, such as RDS;[26] and platelet and coagulation disturbances.[7,26] Decreases in cerebral blood flow associated with hypoxic-ischemic events,[26] such as those caused by meconium aspiration,[27] may also be an important factor in the pathogenesis of IVH in full-term infants.[26]

Note: Depending on the level of severity of IVH, the physical therapist may determine that the neonate with respiratory failure would be more appropriately managed through classification in both Pattern G and an additional pattern, such as Neuromuscular Pattern C: Impaired Motor Function and Sensory Integrity Associated With Nonprogressive

Table 7-2

DEFINITION OF BRONCHOPULMONARY DYSPLASIA: DIAGNOSTIC CRITERIA

Gestational Age	<32 wk	≥ 32 wk
Time point of assessment	36 wk PMA or discharge to home, whichever comes first	> 28 d but < 56 d postnatal age or discharge to home, whichever comes first
	Treatment with oxygen > 21% for at least 28 d **plus**	
Mild BPD	Breathing room air at 36 wk PMA or discharge, whichever comes first	Breathing room air by 56 d postnatal age or discharge, whichever comes first
Moderate BPD	Need[*] for < 30% oxygen at 36 wk PMA or discharge, whichever comes first	Need for < 30% oxygen at 56 d postnatal age or discharge, whichever comes first
Severe BPD	Need[*] for ≥ 30% oxygen and/or positive pressure, (PPV or NCPAP) at 36 wk PMA or discharge, whichever comes first	Need for ≥ 30% oxygen and/or positive pressure (PPV or NCPAP) at 56 d postnatal age or discharge, whichever comes first

Definition of abbreviations: BPD=bronchopulmonary dysplasia; NCPAP=nasal continuous positive airway pressure; PMA =postmenstrual age; PPV=positive-pressure ventilation.

[*]A physiologic test confirming that the oxygen requirement at the assessment time point remains to be defined. This assessment may include a pulse oximetry saturation range. BPD usually develops in neonates being treated with oxygen and positive pressure ventilation for respiratory failure, most commonly respiratory distress syndrome. Persistence of clinical features of respiratory disease (tachypnea, retractions, rales) are considered common to the broad description of BPD and have not been included in the diagnostic criteria describing the severity of BPD. Infants treated with oxygen > 21% and/or positive pressure for nonrespiratory disease (eg, central apnea or diaphragmatic paralysis) do not have BPD unless they also develop parenchymal lung disease and exhibit clinical features of respiratory distress. A day of treatment with oxygen > 21% means that the infant received oxygen > 21% for more than 12 h on that day. Treatment with oxygen > 21% and/or positive pressure at 36 wk PMA, or at 56 d postnatal age or discharge, should not reflect an "acute" event, but should rather reflect the infant's usual daily therapy for several days preceding and following 36 wk PMA, 56 d postnatal age, or discharge. (Reproduced with permission from: Jobe AH, Banclari E. Bronchopulmonary dysplasia. *Am J Respir Crit Care Med.* 2001;163:1723-1729. Official Journal of the American Thoracic Society. © American Thoracic Society.)

Disorders of the Central Nervous System—Congenital Origin or Acquired in Infancy or Childhood.

RESPIRATORY FAILURE IN THE FULL-TERM NEONATE

Respiratory failure may occur not only in infants born prematurely, but also in full-term neonates. It may be due to meconium aspiration through meconium-stained amniotic fluid (MSAF) that is seen in approximately 5% of deliveries performed.[28,29] At the time of delivery, MSAF is seen in 10% to 15% of pregnancies.[28] Meconium aspiration syndrome (MAS) is a form of respiratory distress[28] seen in a neonate born through MSAF whose symptoms do not have any other explanation.[29] MAS is associated with long-term respiratory sequelae. In addition, infants with this condition may develop neonatal seizures and chronic seizure disorders. Five percent of all perinatal deaths are related to meconium aspiration.[29]

The pathophysiology of MAS is complex.[28,29] Meconium aspiration may occur with the first breath after birth or in utero with fetal gasping.[28,29] Aspiration is followed by a mechanical obstruction of the airway that is usually incomplete and causes a "ball-valve" phenomenon, when inspiration is possible but is followed by air trapping distally to the meconium during expiration.[28,29] This affects lung function by increasing functional residual capacity, expiratory lung resistance, and the anterior-posterior chest diameter.[29] Small airways may be completely obstructed, which leads to atelectasis and ventilation-perfusion mismatching. If the adjacent areas of the airway are overexpanded due to a partial obstruction, pneumothorax may develop. Atelectasis, pneumothorax, and lung hyperexpansion are common radiographic findings in MAS.[29]

Aspiration is followed by an intense inflammatory response in the lungs (pneumonitis) caused by chemotactic cytokines contained in meconium.[29] Polymorphonuclear leukocytes and macrophages infiltrate the lung parenchyma and the airways and cause a local injury to the lung. This injury may lead to the formation of hyaline membranes and may cause pulmonary hemorrhage and vascular necrosis.[29] Many components of meconium, such as bile salts, may be toxic to the tissue of the lungs and to blood vessels.[28] Fatty acids and proteins in aspirated meconium may inhibit the function of surfactant and intensify such symptoms of MAS as atelectasis, hypoventilation, and decreased lung compliance.[29]

Note: Due to the high risks associated with the provision of routine care for fragile and physiologically and behaviorally sensitive neonates, physical therapy for this patient population is considered to be an advanced, highly specialized area of practice.[30] Precepted training is recommended for physical therapists who would like to work in the NICU.[30]

IMAGING

NEONATAL LUNG DISEASE

All of the methods used to assess the severity of lung disease in neonates measure the lung density.

- ◆ Plain film radiography: Uses radiation to identify the areas and location of opacities and cystic "bubbly" changes in the infant's lungs.[31,32]
  - These findings are scored on a six-point scale[31,32] and have been reported to be used to:
    - Diagnose BPD[31]
      - ▸ Moya and associates[31] reported an "unacceptably low" interrater reliability of this method when used for the diagnosis of BPD.
      - ▸ The reported inconsistencies in interpretation of chest radiographs in BPD contributed to the exclusion of radiographic findings from the new definition of this condition.[16]
    - Predict which of the high-risk infants will develop this disease[32]
      - ▸ Clark and associates[32] successfully used chest radiographs taken at 9 to 16 days of age to predict the development of BPD in infants born prematurely.
- ◆ Ultrasonography (US): Uses ultrasound waves to identify the areas of hyperechogenicity in the infant's lungs interspersed with areas of unaffected lung tissue.[33] This US pattern signifies hyaline membrane disease. US may be used to predict the development of BPD.[33]
- ◆ High resolution computed tomography (HRCT): Uses a radiographic beam and a computerized analysis of the variance in absorption to produce images[34] of the lungs and to identify the areas of parenchymal alterations signifying atelectasis, consolidation, increased thickness of bronchial wall, formation of cysts, and other abnormalities seen in the lungs of infants with BPD.[35]

GERMINAL MATRIX-INTRAVENTRICULAR HEMORRHAGE

All of the methods used to assess GM-IVH in neonates measure the extent of the hemorrhage and identify its site.[26]

- ◆ US
  - Effectively demonstrates the severity of hemorrhage (see Pathophysiology for the description of grading system suggested by Volpe[26]).
  - Serial US scans may be used to identify the time of hemorrhage onset.[26]
- ◆ CT scan
  - Identifies the site and the severity of hemorrhage but is more expensive than US and exposes the premature infant to radiation.[26]
  - Is used to identify lesions complicating IVH, such as cerebral parenchymal abnormalities, posterior fossa lesions, and subdural hemorrhage.[26]
- ◆ MRI
  - Is useful in identification of IVH after the first several days of hemorrhage.[26]
  - Is expensive and prohibits the use of metal parts of monitoring equipment.[26]
- ◆ PET
  - Is used to assess periventricular hemorrhagic infarction.[26]

PHARMACOLOGY

The following pharmacological agents are used in the management of neonatal patients with respiratory failure and associated problems.

- ◆ Management of apnea and bradycardia of prematurity
  - Methylxanthines: Theophylline (1-3-dimethylxanthine) and caffeine (1-3-7 trimethylxanthine)[36,37]
    - Stimulate central nervous system leading to an increased output of respiratory centers and, therefore, promoting increased ventilation
    - Increase sensitivity of chemoreceptors to CO_2
    - Improve metabolic homeostasis
    - Enhance contractility of respiratory muscles[36,37]
    - Increase catecholamine response[36]
    - Decrease episodes of hypoxia[37]
    - Caffeine is reported to be more effective in stimulating central nervous system and respiratory system than theophylline.[36,37] Side effects are few and may include jitteriness, irritability, convulsions, and rarely gastrointestinal intolerance and tachycardia.[37]
    - Theophylline has a higher incidence of adverse effects, including tachycardia, irritability, jitteriness,

feeding intolerance,[36,37] hyperglycemia, electrolyte imbalance, and seizures[37]

- Doxapram (derivative of pyrrolidinone)[36,37]
  - Stimulates respiratory system
  - May be used together with theophylline[36] or alone, when methylxanthine effects on apnea are insufficient[37]
  - Adverse effects may be severe and are similar to those of theophylline[36,37]

♦ Management of neonatal lung disease and RDS
  - Antenatal corticosteroid administration in women at risk for premature birth[38,39]
    - Betamethasone is the most recommended corticosteroid drug that induces fetal maturation[38]
    - Repeated doses of prenatal corticosteroids may be given, because a single course does not benefit infants born more than 7 days after the drug has been administered[39]
    - Effects on mother
      - Crowther and Harding[39] reported finding little evidence of harm or benefit to the mother from repeated doses of corticosteroids
    - Effects on infants born preterm
      - Significant increase in Apgar scores at 1 minute[38]
      - Reduced incidence of RDS by 19%[39] to 50%[38]
      - Reduced mortality[38,39]
      - Reduced risk of IVH[38,39]
      - Reduced need for surfactant therapy[39]
      - Reduced length of stay and costs associated with neonatal care
      - Insufficient evidence for other benefits and risks
      - No data regarding the infants' outcomes in neurodevelopmental status[39]
  - Surfactant therapy for RDS
    - Types of surfactants[40]
      - Synthetic surfactants
        - Protein-free
        - With synthetic/recombinant proteins
      - Animal-derived surfactants
        - Lavaged from intact lungs
        - Extracted from minced lungs
      - Human surfactant
        - Derived from amniotic fluid[40]
    - Effects of surfactant therapy on infants born preterm[40-43]
      - Reduced neonatal mortality[40-43]
      - No significant effect on the incidence of chronic lung disease[40,41]

- Improved gas exchange[42]
- Improved SaO_2
- Decreased mean airway pressure
- Decreased incidence of pneumothorax and pulmonary interstitial emphysema
- Increased functional residual capacity[42]
- If administered within 15 minutes of birth as compared to 16 to 180 minutes[43]
  - Decreased incidence of RDS, pulmonary interstitial emphysema, and periventricular leukomalacia
  - Lower ventilator setting for peak inspiratory pressure
  - Shorter duration of oxygen administration[43]
  - Effects of surfactant therapy on full-term infants with MAS[44]
    - No effect on overall mortality
    - Reduced severity of respiratory disease
    - Decreased number of infants requiring extracorporeal membrane oxygenation (ECMO)[44]

Case Study #1:
Neonatal Respiratory Distress

Maria Lopez is a 1-week-old (29 weeks PCA) baby girl, twin A, born at 28 weeks gestation with a birth weight of 750 grams and hospitalized in the NICU.

A decision-making algorithm for neonatal physical therapy included in the *Practice Guidelines for the Physical Therapist in the Neonatal Intensive Care Unit*[30] will be used to describe the physical therapy management of this patient.

PHYSICAL THERAPIST EXAMINATION

HISTORY

The history provides the first information that will be obtained from Maria's mother, Mrs. Lopez, and from Maria's nurse and other members of the primary care team. The history is a crucial first step in the clinical decision-making process as it enables the physical therapist to form an early hypothesis that helps guide the remainder of the clinical exam. The interview with Mrs. Lopez and the nurse and a review of other available information received from the primary care team provide the initial facts that will be used to determine parental concerns, generate the primary care team and family identified problem list (PFPL), and formulate the examination strategy (Figure 7-1).[30] Observations of the patient and caregivers will allow the physical therapist to generate the infant problem list (IPL) and to plan further examination procedures. Further testing will be performed to produce the therapist problem list (TPL). After merging and refining the problem lists (PFPL, IPL, and TPL), the physical therapist will establish the goals of intervention, and develop the physical therapy intervention plan (Figures 7-1 and 7-2).[30]

♦ General demographics: Maria is a 1-week-old (29 weeks PCA) Hispanic baby girl.

♦ Social history: Maria's father is 26 years old, and her mother is 24 years old. This was Mrs. Lopez's first pregnancy. Maria's twin sister is also hospitalized in the NICU. Mrs. Lopez spends all day in the unit every day. Her husband works night shifts and is able to visit his children in the afternoon. Both parents speak English but need an interpreter when complex medical issues are discussed. Mrs. Lopez has a twin sister who is married and lives close by. Both parents have extended family in Mexico but no other family members live in the United States.

♦ Employment/work: Maria's father is a factory worker, and her mother is a homemaker.

♦ Living environment: Maria's parents have just moved from a one-bedroom into a two-bedroom apartment on the second floor of an apartment building with an elevator.

♦ General health status
  • Maria is currently hospitalized in the NICU due to prematurity and respiratory failure.
  • Both parents report being in good health.

♦ Social/health habits: Maria's mother states that her husband smokes cigarettes but "never in the house."

♦ Family history: Neither parent has any family members who were born prematurely or had developmental problems.

♦ Medical/surgical history: Mrs. Lopez states that she had frequent emesis throughout her pregnancy and was hospitalized due to premature contractions at 27 weeks. Corticosteroids were administered to the mother prenatally. Maria and her twin sister were delivered vaginally at 28 weeks gestational age. Maria's birth weight was 750 grams. Her Apgar scores were 3 and 7 at 1 and 5 minutes, respectively. After birth, the neonate was intubated and ventilated due to respiratory distress, with subsequent surfactant administration in the delivery room. The infant was transferred to the NICU and placed on a PEEP ventilator, with oxygen supplementation. Maria was diagnosed with apnea and bradycardia of prematurity, mild RDS confirmed by radiography, and perinatal sepsis.

♦ Prior hospitalizations: N/A.

♦ Preexisting medical and other health-related conditions: Mrs. Lopez had prenatal care, and all uterine US examinations performed during prenatal visits were normal.

♦ Current condition(s)/chief complaint(s): Mrs. Lopez states that she is afraid to touch her daughters, "because they are so small," she is nervous that she might "break something" if she holds them; they look "so much smaller and thinner" than her sister's son did when he was born. She is also concerned that her children will not know who she is, because they are supposed to remain in isolettes most of the time.

♦ Functional status and activity level: Maria is currently positioned in an isolette on monitoring equipment and on low-pressure ventilation with low oxygen requirements. She receives nasogastric (NG) tube feedings and has an IV line in her right forearm. Maria's nurse reports that the infant is in a drowsy state most of the time and sometimes demonstrates transient bradycardia during routine handling.

♦ Medications: Patient is receiving IV antibiotics for perinatal sepsis, caffeine for apnea and bradycardia of prematurity, and repeated administrations of surfactant.

♦ Other clinical tests: Two head US examinations performed since birth have been negative for IVH.

SYSTEMS REVIEW

The systems review is performed by observation of the infant and the caregivers that will allow the physical therapist to generate the IPL and to plan further the examination procedures while following the decision-making algorithm for neonatal physical therapy (see Figure 7-1).[30]

♦ Cardiovascular/pulmonary
  • BP: 55/28 mmHg
  • Edema: N/A
  • HR: 140 bpm
    ▪ Observed HR decrease to 105 bpm during a diaper change performed by the nurse, but the episode resolved spontaneously once the infant was repositioned
  • RR: 50 bpm

♦ Integumentary
  • Presence of scar formation: N/A
  • Skin color: Pink, reddish
  • Skin integrity
    ▪ Patient has dry skin
    ▪ Redness noted in the areas where NG tube is taped to the face
    ▪ Red "dots" observed on the left heel (site where blood was drawn)
    ▪ IV board is taped to right forearm

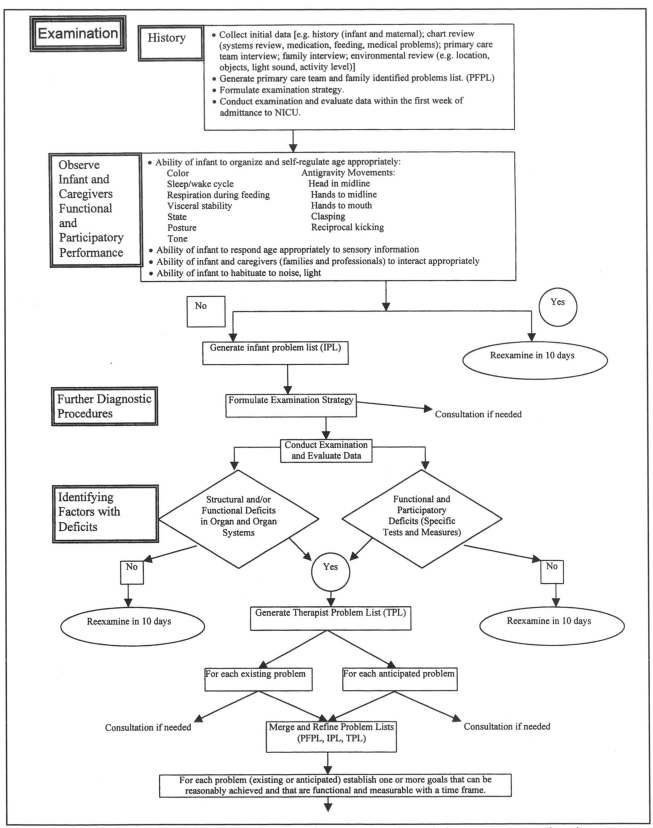

Figure 7-1. Examination decision-making algorithm for neonatal physical therapy. (Reprinted with permission from Sweeney JK, Heriza CB, Reilly MA, Smith C, VanSant AF. Practice guidelines for the physical therapist in the Neonatal Intensive Care Unit (NICU). *Pediatr Phys Ther.* 1999;11:119-132.)

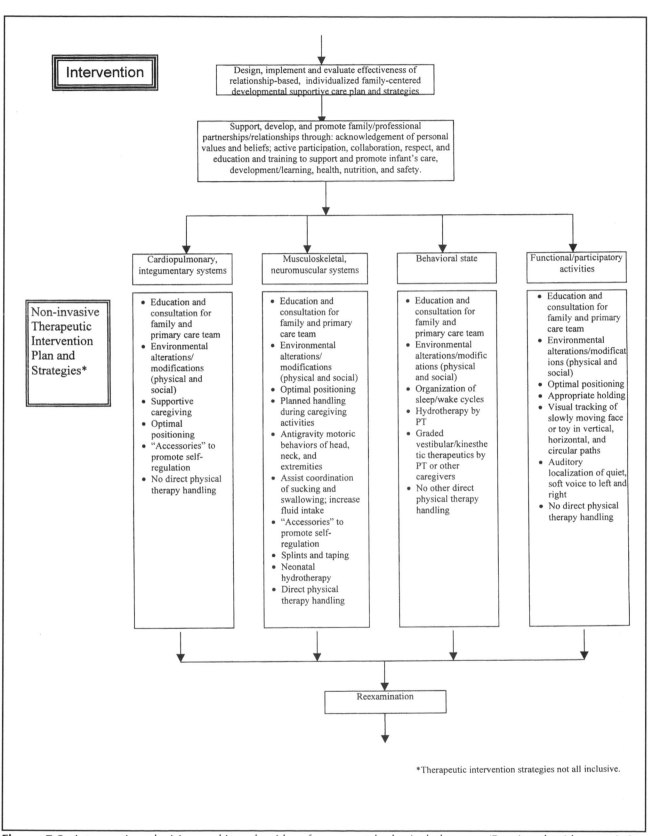

Figure 7-2. Intervention decision-making algorithm for neonatal physical therapy. (Reprinted with permission from Sweeney JK, Heriza CB, Reilly MA, Smith C, VanSant AF. Practice guidelines for the physical therapist in the Neonatal Intensive Care Unit (NICU). *Pediatr Phys Ther.* 1999;11:119-132.)

- Musculoskeletal
  - Gross range of motion
    - Excessive hip abduction and lateral rotation bilaterally with knee extension noted in supine
    - UEs widely abducted, with elbows extended (observed during routine change of baby's position performed by the nurse)
  - Gross strength
    - Minimal infant movement noted
    - No reciprocal kicking or hand-to-mouth movement observed
  - Gross symmetry: Infant tends to maintain head rotated to the right (toward the ventilator) with neck in hyperextension
  - Height: 13.39" (34 cm)
  - Weight: 1.70 lbs (770 g)
- Neuromuscular
  - Balance: N/A
  - Locomotion, transfers, and transitions: As expected, infant is fully dependent on caregiver for position changes
- Communication, affect, cognition, language, and learning style
  - Communication, affect, and cognition: Maria briefly opened her eyes during the diaper change but did not focus on the caregiver's face and quickly transitioned to the light sleep state once repositioned
  - Learning preferences: N/A

TESTS AND MEASURES

Selection of specific tests and measures for this patient was based upon the results of history taking and systems review. Maria's parents were present during this examination, and all procedures and findings were explained to them through an interpreter.

- Arousal, attention, and cognition
  - Infant's behavioral state was monitored and recorded throughout the examination as recommended for the Neurological Assessment of the Preterm and Full-Term Newborn Infant[45] (see Neuromotor Development and Sensory Integration below)
  - Orientation and behavior were also assessed as a part of this test[45] (see Neuromotor Development and Sensory Integration below)
- Circulation
  - Infant's vital signs were carefully monitored using the monitoring equipment readings
  - Vital signs remained WNL, except
    - Observed a brief episode of decreased heart rate and SaO_2 in supported sitting

- Neuromotor development and sensory integration
  - The Neurological Assessment of the Preterm and Full-Term Newborn Infant[45] was selected for Maria for the following reasons:
    - This neuromotor assessment tool is used with preterm infants from the first days of life to 40 weeks PCA
    - Only 15 to 20 minutes are required to administer this test
    - Examination may be shortened if the infant does not tolerate all the items[45]
  - Infant's behavioral state was monitored and recorded throughout examination using the six categories of the Brazelton Scale[46] as recommended by Dubowitz and associates:[45]
    - State 1: Deep sleep[46]
    - State 2: Light sleep
    - State 3: Drowsy
    - State 4: Quiet alert
    - State 5: Active alert
    - State 6: Crying[46]
  - The test was administered in the isolette as recommended by Maria's nurse, because of the infant's poor thermoregulation, and the order of items described below follows the test record form:[45]
    - Posture and tone
      - In supine, infant displayed UE extension and slight flexion of both knees, with hip abduction and external rotation
      - Hands were open and toes straight most of the time
      - No resistance was felt to arm or leg traction, and arm and leg recoil was minimal
      - Popliteal angle ROM was 180 degrees bilaterally
      - In supported sitting, infant did not attempt to elevate head against gravity from either hyperextended or hyperflexed positions
      - During the administration of this section of the test, infant remained in a light sleep state until transitioned by the physical therapist into supported sitting, at which point she briefly assumed a drowsy state, with eyes partially open
      - When head control was being tested from the hyperflexed position of the head, Maria displayed a HR drop from 135 to 108 bpm and SaO_2 decrease from 99% to 91%
      - She was repositioned into supine, with subsequent HR increase to normal
      - As a result, several items of this section of the test were not administered

■ Muscle tone patterns
  ▸ Infant demonstrated equally low tone in all UE and LE muscles
■ Reflexes
  ▸ Placing and Moro reflexes were excluded from this examination due to Maria's low tolerance to position change resulting in transient tendency toward bradycardia
  ▸ Palmar and plantar grasp reflexes were present but weak
  ▸ Infant displayed weak and irregular non-nutritive suck
  ▸ She demonstrated three beats of clonus, left ankle
  ▸ No ankle clonus response was noted on the right
■ Movements
  ▸ When in a drowsy state, Maria displayed only stretches and short isolated movements
  ▸ Ability to elevate head against gravity in prone was not tested
■ Abnormal signs/patterns
  ▸ No abnormal signs were noted
  ▸ No tremors were observed
  ▸ A startle response to a sudden noise was observed
■ Orientation and behavior
  ▸ While in a drowsy state, infant opened her eyes only partially
  ▸ There was no true orientation to sound, only a startle response was observed to the sound of a rattle
  ▸ Maria did not focus on visual stimuli
  ▸ She remained quiet and did not cry during the examination; therefore, consoling was not required
♦ Ventilation and respiration/gas exchange
  • Infant's vital signs were carefully monitored using the monitoring equipment readings
  • HR
    ■ 135 bpm
    ■ Observed a brief decrease in HR to 108 bpm accompanying decrease in SaO_2 described above
  • Respiratory vital signs remained WNL
  • SaO_2
    ■ 99%
    ■ Observed a brief decrease in SaO_2 to 91% accompanying decrease in HR described above

EVALUATION

Maria is a baby girl born prematurely and hospitalized in the NICU due to respiratory distress. Maria has been diagnosed with apnea and bradycardia of prematurity, mild RDS, and perinatal sepsis. She is currently on low-pressure mechanical ventilation with low oxygen requirements. Her respiratory status, combined with perinatal infection, extremely low birthweight (ELBW), and low gestational age at birth put her at risk for the development of BPD, ROP, and developmental delays. Based on the results of her examination, Maria's strengths include: 1) ability to tolerate standardized testing for 15 minutes with only one episode of decreased HR and with a spontaneous return to normal when repositioned; 2) no abnormal signs, postures, or movement patterns observed; 3) appropriate responses to auditory stimuli; 4) no crying and no consoling required; and 5) parental interest in learning intervention strategies that would allow them to help their baby's development.

The PFPL includes the following:

♦ ELBW
♦ Need for assisted ventilation and O_2 supplementation
♦ Need for NG feeding
♦ Bonding concerns
♦ Bradycardia during routine handling
♦ Excessive drowsiness

The IPL includes the following:

♦ Excessive UE and LE extension ROM with hip abduction and external rotation in supine
♦ Asymmetrical head position with neck hyperextension
♦ Transient bradycardia during routine handling
♦ Lethargy

The TPL includes the following based on the results of neuromotor testing:[30]

♦ Hypotonia throughout body appropriate for the age of 28 weeks PCA or less
♦ Excessive extension in all extremities for the patient's PCA
♦ Poor head control for the infant's PCA
♦ Excessive drowsiness during handling
♦ Decreased responses to visual stimuli
♦ Weak and irregular nonnutritive suck
♦ Transient decrease in HR in supported sitting

The problem list developed by merging and refining the PFPL, IPL, and TPL (see Figure 7-1)[30] included the following:

♦ Need for NG feeding and weak, irregular non-nutritive suck

♦ Excessive hypotonia and limb extension ROM for PCA

♦ Asymmetrical posture with neck hyperextension in supine

♦ Muscle weakness throughout body

♦ Poor head control for PCA

♦ Excessive drowsiness and inability to transition to a quiet alert state

♦ Decreased responses to visual stimuli that may be related to the baby's behavioral state

♦ Tendency toward transient decrease in HR and SaO_2 in supported sitting

♦ Parental difficulty bonding with the infant

DIAGNOSIS

Maria is an infant born prematurely, with ELBW, who exhibits respiratory failure. She displays the following impairments: arousal, attention, and cognition; circulation; neuromotor development and sensory integration; and ventilation and respiration/gas exchange. These findings are consistent with placement in Pattern G: Impaired Ventilation, Respiration/Gas Exchange, and Aerobic Capacity/Endurance Associated With Respiratory Failure in the Neonate.[47] Maria's impairments will be addressed in determining her prognosis and plan of care while taking into account the refined problem list.

PROGNOSIS AND PLAN OF CARE

Based on the results of physical therapy examination and evaluation, the following outcomes have been determined for Maria to be achieved during this episode of care (Figure 7-3):[30]

♦ Infant is at appropriate level of development for PCA[30]

♦ Infant is nipple fed

♦ Infant's sleep/wake cycles are well established

♦ Infant's family is ready to care for her at home

♦ Infant and her family successfully transition from the hospital to the community[30]

To achieve these outcomes, the appropriate interventions for this patient are determined. These will include: coordination, communication, and documentation; patient/client-related instruction; developmentally supportive care; therapeutic exercise; functional training and home management training for caregivers; manual therapy techniques; and airway clearance techniques.

Based on the diagnosis and prognosis, over the course of 6 to 12 months, several episodes of care may be required for the patient to demonstrate optimal ventilation, respiration/gas exchange, and aerobic capacity/endurance and the highest level of age-appropriate functioning. During this episode of care, Maria will be seen by physical therapy two to three times per week over the course of 22 to 33 visits (11 weeks).

INTERVENTIONS

RATIONALE FOR SELECTED INTERVENTIONS

Developmentally Supportive Care

A developmentally supportive approach to neonatal intensive care referred to as Newborn Individualized Developmental Care and Assessment Program (NIDCAP)[48] was developed as a clinical framework for developmental care. This approach suggests that care for each infant should be designed based on the caregiver's observations of the baby's self-regulatory strategies and stress behaviors.[48-50] NIDCAP guidelines for care include consistent caregiving, individualized scheduling of the infant's day, pacing caregiving based on the infant's behavioral reactions, individualized positioning and feeding, Kangaroo care, soothing environment that promotes parent-infant bonding, collaborative care, discharge planning, and linking the infant and family to the community.[49] The positive effects of NIDCAP implementation reported in the research literature include decreased duration of mechanical ventilation and oxygen supplementation, increased weight gain,[50,51] earlier transition to nipple feedings,[49,50] improved neurobehavioral functioning, and reduced length of stay and cost of care.[50]

Results of NIDCAP implementation reported by several authors[52-54] vary across the studies. Westrup and associates[52] found that the use of the NIDCAP approach with VLBW infants does not have a significant effect on the amount of quiet sleep. However, the authors[52] acknowledged that their results should be treated with caution because of the small sample size (12 infants in the NIDCAP group and 13 infants in the conventional care group). Kleberg and associates[53] reported significantly higher scores on the Mental Developmental Index of the Bailey Scales of Infant Development at 1 year of corrected age for infants in the NIDCAP group as compared to the control group. However, they found no significant difference between the groups in their scores on the Psychomotor Developmental Indices.[53] Jacobs and associates[54] performed a systematic review of the effectiveness of NIDCAP as compared to conventional care in improving short- and long-term neurodevelopmental outcomes and short-term medical outcomes in preterm infants. They reported a statistically significant decrease in supplemental oxygen requirement and earlier acquisition of oral feeding skills in infants participating in NIDCAP, but the evidence regarding their average daily weight gain was

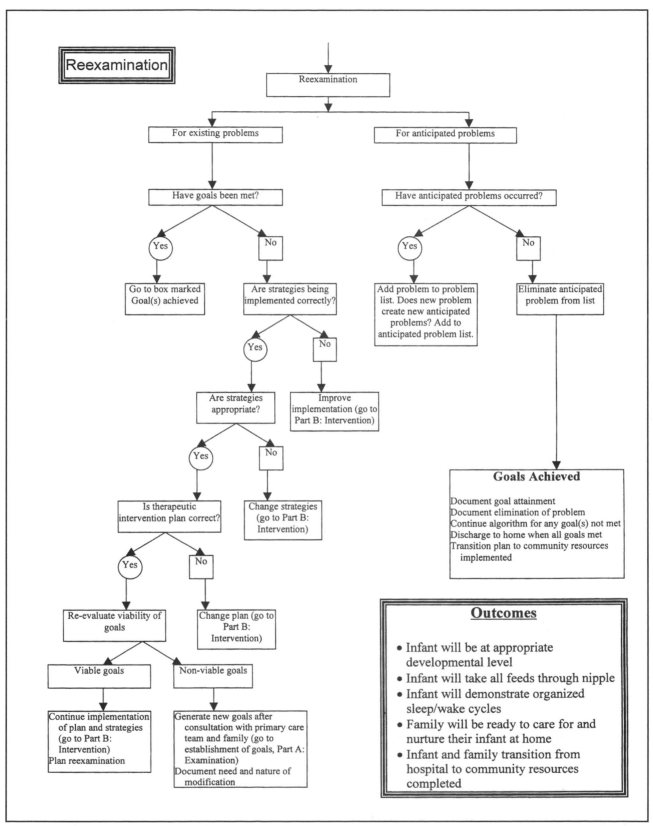

Figure 7-3. Reexamination decision-making algorithm for neonatal physical therapy. (Reprinted with permission from Sweeney JK, Heriza CB, Reilly MA, Smith C, VanSant AF. Practice guidelines for the physical therapist in the Neonatal Intensive Care Unit (NICU). *Pediatr Phys Ther.* 1999;11:119-132.)

conflicting. In addition, this systematic review revealed that these infants showed improved neurodevelopmental outcomes at 9 to 12 months of age but not at 2 years.[54]

As stated above, NIDCAP includes recommendations to enhance self-regulation in preterm infants.[48-50,55] Grenier and associates[55] compared self-regulatory and stress behaviors observed in 15 infants born at mean age of 32 weeks gestation across different body positions, including prone, sidelying, and supine, both nested and unnested. The authors defined nesting as the use of blanket rolls, blanket boundaries, a heat shield, or "any other detectable boundary" for the infant's body[55] (Figure 7-4). Results of this study indicated that infants demonstrated the fewest number of stress behaviors in prone, both nested and unnested, and in sidelying nested positions.[55] Therefore, these positions may assist in conserving these babies' energy for growth.[55]

Among other interventions, neurodevelopmental care in the NICU includes Kangaroo care that involves mother-infant skin-to-skin contact.[56-58] The naked infant is placed against the mother's bare chest in an upright[56] or reclined[58] prone position for several hours to promote thermoregulation and provide stimulation and nutrition.[56] This intervention may assist in decreasing the incidence of infection, increasing daily weight gain, and improving parent satisfaction with medical care in the NICU.[56] Other reported benefits include increased survival, earlier discharge from the hospital, prolonged maternal lactation, and decreased behavioral problems.[57]

Bohnhorst and associates[57] observed unexpected adverse effects of Kangaroo care in preterm infants born at 24 to 31 weeks gestation. These effects included a significant increase in combined frequency of hypoxemia and bradycardia and decreased proportion of the regular breathing pattern. The researchers reported that these negative changes might be associated with heat stress and suggested that the infant's body temperature, oxygenation, and HR should be carefully monitored during Kangaroo care.[57] Ludington-Hoe and associates[58] suggested safe criteria and procedures for skin-to-skin care with ELBW infants on mechanical ventilation. They reported no adverse events after implementing a protocol that included the following elements: 1) using a head cap if the infant's temperature fell below 36.0° C; 2) covering the baby's body with a standard receiving blanket folded in fourths; 3) positioning the infant prone on the mother's chest at a 40-degree upright incline; 4) supporting the mother's feet on a footrest or a footstool; 5) providing the mother with a cup of fluid every hour to prevent overheating and to support lactation; 6) checking the infant's temperature to prevent overheating if the mother felt that he or she was perspiring; 7) using a safe procedure for a standing transfer of the infant by the caregiver into Kangaroo care; 8) monitoring the baby for 10 to 15 minutes after the transfer was completed to assess physiological signs for a possible need for intervention; 9) performing suctioning during skin-to-skin care instead of removing the infant from the mother for this procedure; 10) draping the ventilator tubing over the mother's shoulder without attaching it to her clothing; and 11) using a safe procedure for a standing transfer by the caregiver back to the incubator.[58]

Therapeutic Exercise

Graded vestibular/kinesthetic stimulation is one of the methods suggested for improvement of behavioral state control.[30] Kahn-D'Angelo and Unanue[7] recommended using swaddling, positioning in supported sitting, and facilitating of trunk and neck flexor musculature to help a hypotonic and lethargic infant reach and maintain an alert state. For a patient who responds well to these interventions, graded arrhythmic rocking may also be used. Once the infant is able to maintain a quiet alert state, sensory stimulation may be initiated. Care should be taken to introduce one stimulus at a time, and the baby's responses should be constantly monitored, as recommended by the NIDCAP,[48-50] to maintain physiologic stability.[7] The physical therapist's or caregiver's face, and red and black-and-white pictures or toys can be used for visual stimulation. If the infant is able to focus on the object, visual tracking may be initiated.[7] Auditory stimulation may include introducing the sound of a soft rattle, calling the baby's name,[7,46] and classical instrumental music.[7,59,60]

Direct physical therapist handling may consist of encouraging midline and antigravity head control and hand-to-mouth, hand-to-hand, hand-to-knee, and hand-to-foot movement through appropriate positioning and graded facilitation of antigravity movement of UEs and LEs.[7,30,61] These interventions should be initiated only when the infant is able to tolerate handling, and her responses to these techniques should be closely monitored.[7,30,61] A neurodevelopmental treatment (NDT) protocol including movement facilitation in supine, prone, sidelying, and supported sitting has been

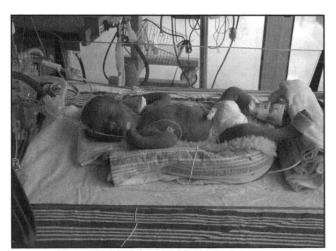

Figure 7-4. Example of nested positioning.

reported to be effective in improving postural control in infants born prematurely who are hospitalized in the NICU and are considered to be at high risk for developmental disabilities.[61] Girolami and Campbell[61] in a randomized, controlled clinical trial found that infants selected for intervention because of their poor motor performance did not demonstrate a significant improvement in behavioral state, reflexes, muscle tone, or autonomic regulation. However, the NDT protocol was shown to be safe for their physiological stability when they reached 34 to 37 weeks PCA.[61]

Functional Training in Self-Care and Home Management and Functional Training in Work, Community, and Leisure Integration or Reintegration

Perkins and associates[62] evaluated the effects of various forms of nurses' education on their abilities to perform developmentally supportive positioning of neonates and investigated the nurses' perceptions of effectiveness of these educational methods in enhancing their positioning skills. Formal education provided to nurses by the physical therapists, including conferences, workshops, in-services, and bedside consultations, improved their positioning skills and was perceived by nurses as more helpful than such educational methods as general hospital in-services, independent reading, and the use of audiovisual resources. However, because the nurses' performance declined when formal education was terminated, the authors concluded that the physical therapists should provide ongoing bedside consultation and formal instruction to the nursing staff to maintain the quality of developmentally supportive positioning.[62] This study supports training Maria's caregivers in positioning techniques.

Another area of functional training is supporting the infant's transition from tube to oral feedings. Infants born prematurely have difficulty coordinating sucking, swallowing, and breathing, until they reach approximately 32 to 34 weeks PCA.[63,64] Therefore, until that time, they are usually fed via an oro-gastric or a NG tube. To support the future transition to oral feedings and to assess the patient's readiness for it, Lemons and Lemons[63] recommended offering the infant a pacifier during tube feedings to initiate rhythmic non-nutritive sucking and swallowing of oral secretions. It is important to educate caregivers in recognizing warning signs that indicate that the baby is not ready for the transition to nipple feedings. These warning signs observed during non-nutritive sucking may include bradycardia, tachycardia, and apnea.[63]

When the baby is ready for the transition to oral feedings, it becomes necessary to train the caregiver in appropriate positioning and handling techniques supporting this process.[63] The patient should be held in a relatively upright position, with the back supported in a straight alignment, with shoulders in forward flexion and head positioned in midline. Swaddling may assist in maintaining proper positioning and help the infant focus on the task of oral feeding. In addition, the caregiver may be trained to place a finger between the baby's chin and neck to provide support to the base of the tongue and to stabilize the lower jaw, so that the infant could initiate effective sucking. Supporting the baby's cheeks may also be helpful to maintain the seal around the nipple. It is important to avoid increasing pressure on the cheeks if the infant is attempting to break the seal, because this may be a sign of an attempt to breathe around the nipple. Lemons and Lemons[63] reported that preventing the patient from catching her breath in this situation might lead to apnea and bradycardia. Other precautions during oral feedings include: 1) allowing the infant to establish an individualized feeding pace; 2) avoiding frequent changes in position; 3) monitoring vital signs to identify changes that may lead to apnea and bradycardia; 4) monitoring behavioral state and motor changes as the possible signs of distress related to the infant's difficulty coordinating sucking, swallowing, and breathing; 5) and minimizing visual, auditory, and vestibular stimulation during feeding.[63]

Manual Therapy Techniques

Sweeney and associates[30] include oral-motor techniques addressing the infant's ability to coordinate sucking, swallowing, and breathing for effective, safe feeding into the list of clinical proficiencies required for the physical therapists working in the NICU. A prefeeding stimulation program[65] may be used for these purposes. Gaebler and Hanzlik[65] conducted a small, randomized experimental study investigating the effects of such a program on growing, healthy preterm infants born at 30 to 34 weeks gestation. Nine infants in the experimental group received stroking and perioral and intraoral stimulation prior to feeding, while nine infants in the control group received only the stroking intervention. The stroking protocol included positioning the baby prone and firmly but gently stroking the head, neck, and shoulders, then stroking down the legs and arms in supine. The oral-motor protocol consisted of perioral and intraoral stimulation. It included rubbing the area from the ear to the corner of the infant's mouth and around the mouth, alternating with the application of gentle pressure under the chin, followed by rubbing the upper and lower gums and the upper palate, and holding the therapist's small finger against the baby's upper palate. Gentle pressure under the chin was applied again after the intraoral stimulation on each side of the mouth was completed. Infants in the experimental group obtained higher scores on the Revised Neonatal Oral Motor Assessment nutritive suck scale as compared to the control group. In addition, they required a smaller number of gavage feedings, demonstrated a greater weight gain, and were hospitalized for a shorter period of time.[65]

Another manual therapy technique that may be successfully used with infants hospitalized in the NICU is soft tissue mobilization in the form of modified infant massage.[30,66,67] Field[66] developed a 15-minute, standardized protocol of tactile-kinesthetic stimulation to apply three times a day for 10 days with medically stable infants born prematurely.[66,67] This protocol started and ended with a 5-minute period of stroking provided to the baby's head, neck, back, legs, and arms in prone using gentle but firm touch to avoid adverse effects that might be caused by the "tickle stimulus"[66] of light stroking.[66,67] During the second 5 minutes of stimulation, the infant was positioned supine for UE and LE passive flexion/extension movements. The patients' reactions to tactile-kinesthetic input were carefully monitored. This protocol was demonstrated to be safe for medically stable preterm infants.[66,67] Some of the reported benefits of this technique included significantly higher weight gain (28% to 53%) in massaged patients as compared to infants in control groups and improved ability to assume and maintain the active alert state.[66,67] Dieter and associates[67] conducted this protocol with healthy, low-risk preterm infants and found that after only 5 days of massage intervention, patients in the experimental group slept less and gained more weight as compared to the control group. Other reported benefits of modified infant massage were improved performance on the Neonatal Behavioral Assessment Scale[66,67] possibly leading to enhanced parent-infant interaction and bonding[66] and decreased length of hospital stay.[66,67]

Airway Clearance Techniques

Chest physical therapy is used for infants born prematurely who are at risk for or have already developed airway clearance problems.[3] Therapists should select appropriate bronchial drainage techniques and apply their knowledge of precautions and contraindications for these procedures to each individual patient. Positional rotation programs for infants should be structured to affect all lung lobes, and the baby's change in position should occur every 2 hours. Using mechanical nursery beds that produce positional oscillation may help minimize disruption of physiological homeostasis in the premature infant that may be induced by excessive handling. Some of the guidelines for positional rotation suggested by Moerchen and Crane[3] include: 1) coordinating manual repositioning of the infant with other nursing procedures to decrease the amount of unnecessary stimulation; 2) performing manual repositioning slowly to maintain the infant's physiological homeostasis; 3) never leaving patients in a head-down position unattended and avoiding that position for 1 hour after feeding; 4) closely monitoring vital signs and auscultating the baby's chest after positioning; 5) applying suctioning in a drainage position for no longer than 5 seconds at a time while monitoring transcutaneous oxygen saturation; and 6) modifying postural drainage positions for patients with unstable vital signs or suspected intracranial hemorrhage.[3]

For infants weighing less than 800 grams, slightly elevated or horizontal head position is recommended as a precaution for IVH Grades I and II, CHF, apnea and bradycardia, abdominal distension, acute respiratory distress, hydrocepha-

lus, and some other conditions.[3] Head-down positioning is contraindicated if the patient has untreated tension pneumothorax, recent repair of a tracheoesophageal fistula, IVH Grades III and IV, recent intracranial or eye surgery, cor pulmonale, or acute CHF. For prone positioning, precautions for arterial catheters, chest tubes, and other lines should be closely followed, and it is contraindicated if the infant has an untreated tension pneumothorax.[3]

Moerchen and Crane[3] discussed using percussion and vibration techniques in combination with postural drainage to move secretions in a preterm infant. Tenting three fingers or using four fingers, small anesthesia masks or small percussion devices have been suggested for chest percussion. Some of the precautions for this technique are unstable vital signs, IVH, coagulopathy, and subcutaneous emphysema. Percussion over a healing thoracotomy incision is contraindicated. Other contraindications include irritability and respiratory distress in response to this intervention. Vibration may be performed manually or using a mechanical vibrator. Because infants tend to demonstrate lower tolerance to this intervention as compared to percussion, precautions for vibration include increased irritability, bradycardia, and respiratory distress.[3]

COORDINATION, COMMUNICATION, AND DOCUMENTATION

Communication will occur with Maria's parents and her primary care team members, such as the neonatologist, nurse, pulmonologist, respiratory therapist, nutritionist, social worker, discharge planner, and others. The physical therapist will participate in patient care rounds and interdisciplinary case conferences with and without family members present, as appropriate. In addition, the physical therapist will maintain ongoing communication with Maria's parents regarding her plan of care, goal attainment, and interventions she will receive. When required, interpreter services will be requested for the meetings with the family. Prior to the infant's discharge from the hospital, her further needs for continuation of care will be determined and referrals will be made to the NICU Developmental Follow-Up Clinic, Early Intervention Services, or both, and medical specialists, if needed. All elements of the patient's management will be documented.

PATIENT/CLIENT-RELATED INSTRUCTION

The patient's parents will be educated regarding Maria's current condition, including the results of her physical therapy examination/evaluation. They will be instructed in the risk factors related to the infant's prematurity and respiratory status in terms of impact they may have on her overall development. Issues associated with the development of Maria's cardiovascular/pulmonary, integumentary, musculoskeletal, and neuromuscular systems will be addressed (see Figure 7-

2).[30] Infant behavioral states will be described.[30] Plan of care addressing primary impairments and functional limitations, and prevention of secondary impairments and functional limitations will be discussed. Dangers of secondary smoke for the infant's health will be outlined. Parental concerns about Maria's discharge to home and her transition to appropriate services in the community will be addressed.

DEVELOPMENTALLY SUPPORTIVE CARE

Developmentally supportive care for this patient will include environmental modifications, such as reducing noise in the NICU and dimming lights for scheduled sleep times, grouping caregiving tasks together to promote uninterrupted sleep, nested positioning, and skin-to-skin holding (Kangaroo care). These interventions will address the establishment of a sleep-wake cycle, help maintain stable vital signs, promote normal musculoskeletal and neuromuscular development, support the development of age-appropriate functional skills, and enhance parent-infant bonding.

THERAPEUTIC EXERCISE

- ◆ Graded sensory motor stimulation
  - Activities to develop appropriate state control and responses to visual, auditory, vestibular, and tactile stimuli, for example:
    - ■ Graded vestibular/kinesthetic stimulation in the form of arrhythmic rocking to increase alertness
    - ■ Visual tracking of the caregiver's face in supine or reclined supported sitting (if tolerated)
    - ■ Auditory stimulation using a soft rattle to encourage head turning to the source of sound
- ◆ Neuromotor development training
  - Activities to improve head control and increase muscle strength in order to develop functional movement appropriate for the infant's PCA, for example:
    - ■ Graded facilitation of antigravity movement of UEs and LEs to encourage hand-to-mouth, hand-to-hand, hand-to-knee, and hand-to-foot movement[61] in a supine nested position
    - ■ Movement facilitation through graded anterior-posterior and lateral weight shifting in supported sitting (if tolerated) to encourage midline and antigravity head control[61]

FUNCTIONAL TRAINING IN SELF-CARE AND HOME MANAGEMENT AND FUNCTIONAL TRAINING IN WORK, COMMUNITY, AND LEISURE INTEGRATION OR REINTEGRATION

- ◆ Ongoing ADL/IADL training for nurses and Maria's parents will include:

- Developmentally supportive positioning promoting flexion, midline orientation and postural symmetry
- Use of pacifier during tube feeding
- Positioning and safety precautions during oral feeding

MANUAL THERAPY TECHNIQUES

- ◆ Oral-motor stimulation
- ◆ Soft tissue mobilization in the form of modified infant massage following the protocol suggested by Field[66]
  - Stroking provided to the baby's head, neck, back, legs, and arms in prone using gentle but firm touch, followed by UE and LE passive flexion/extension ROM exercise in supine[66]

AIRWAY CLEARANCE TECHNIQUES

- ◆ Manual techniques
  - Depending on changes in her medical condition, respiratory status, and tolerance to handling in the course of her hospital stay, manual techniques may be used, including chest percussion and vibration
  - Airway suctioning may also be performed
- ◆ Positioning
  - To alter the work of breathing and maximize ventilation and perfusion
    - ■ Nested positioning in prone, supine, and sidelying with manual repositioning every 2 hours
    - ■ Slightly elevated or horizontal head position is recommended for Maria because her weight is less than 800 grams[3]
  - Depending on changes in her medical condition, respiratory status, and tolerance to handling in the course of her hospital stay, pulmonary postural drainage may be used

ANTICIPATED GOALS AND EXPECTED OUTCOMES

- ◆ Impact on pathology/pathophysiology
  - Patient's weight gain is increased.
  - Stability of patient's vital signs is improved.
  - Tissue perfusion and oxygenation are enhanced.
- ◆ Impact on impairments
  - Ability to perform age-appropriate visual tracking is improved.
  - Ability to recognize and respond to auditory stimuli is improved.
  - Airway clearance is improved.
  - Coordination of sucking, swallowing, and breathing is improved.
  - Duration of mechanical ventilation and oxygen supplementation is decreased.

- Earlier transition to nipple feeding is implemented.
- Muscle performance is increased.
- Number of patient's self-regulatory behaviors is increased.
- Number of patient's stress behaviors is decreased.
- Patient's head and neck hyperextension are decreased.
- Patient's midline orientation and postural symmetry are improved.
- Patient's non-nutritive suck is improved.
- Patient's sleep-wake cycle is established.
- Patient's state control is improved.
- Quality and quantity of movement between and across body segments are improved.
- Ventilation and respiration/gas exchange are improved.
- Work of breathing is decreased.

◆ Impact on functional limitations
  - Tolerance to position change and to developmental activities is increased.

◆ Impact on disabilities
  - Disability associated with acute or chronic illness is reduced.

◆ Risk reduction/prevention
  - Behaviors that foster prevention are acquired.
  - Caregiver positioning skills are improved.
  - Communication enhances risk reduction, prevention of secondary impairments and functional limitations, and prevention of fragmentation of care during the infant's transition from the NICU to the community.[30]
  - Risk of secondary impairment is reduced.

◆ Impact on health, wellness, and fitness
  - Behaviors that foster healthy habits and wellness are acquired.
  - Patient's physical function is improved.

◆ Impact on societal resources
  - Awareness and use of community resources by family are improved.
  - Cost of health services is decreased.
  - Documentation occurs throughout patient management and follows APTA's *Guidelines for Physical Therapy Documentation*.[47]
  - Interdisciplinary collaboration occurs through case conferences, patient care rounds, and meetings with the family.
  - Patient placement needs after discharge from the hospital are determined.
  - Referrals are made to other professionals or resources whenever necessary and appropriate.
  - The length of NICU stay is decreased.

◆ Patient/client satisfaction
  - Caregiver's sense of well-being is improved.
  - Caregiver's stressors are decreased.
  - Care is coordinated with the family, caregivers, and other professionals.
  - Decision making by family regarding patient's health and health care resources is enhanced.
  - Family knowledge and awareness of the diagnosis, prognosis, interventions, and anticipated goals and expected outcomes are increased.
  - Parent-infant bonding is improved.

REEXAMINATION

According to the decision-making algorithm suggested by Sweeney and associates,[30] reexamination of the infants hospitalized in the NICU should be scheduled if: 1) in the process of the initial examination, the physical therapist does not observe any problems in functional and participatory performance of the infant and caregiver; and 2) these problems or structural or functional deficits in organ systems are not found during further diagnostic procedures (see Figure 7-1). After the patient's goals are set and physical therapy intervention strategies are implemented, the physical therapist should also reexamine the patient for existing and newly anticipated problems. The appropriateness of the therapeutic intervention plan should be assessed and modified if needed (see Figure 7-3).[30]

DISCHARGE

Maria is discharged from physical therapy in the NICU after a total of 28 physical therapy sessions and attainment of her goals and expectations. These sessions have covered her entire episode of care. She is discharged because she has achieved goals and expected outcomes for her transition to home. Maria has been referred to the NICU Developmental Follow-Up Clinic for an appointment for a multidisciplinary evaluation scheduled in 8 weeks. This evaluation will be conducted to reassess her medical and developmental status and to determine whether a referral for Early Intervention services will be needed.

PSYCHOLOGICAL ASPECTS

It is necessary for physical therapists to understand the unique psychological aspects of their clinical practice in the NICU, such as:

◆ Families of infants who require intensive care often feel stressed and separated from their children.[68]

◆ Although measures are being taken to improve family-centered care by including parents in making major decisions about their infants, medical personnel continue to be largely in control of the decision-making process.

♦ Changing hospital guidelines for parent participation in their child's care may be a difficult and lengthy process.[68]

Family-centered care may be enhanced through the process of quality improvement by implementing potentially better practices as discussed by several authors.[68,69] These practices may include but are not limited to the following:

♦ Families need to be viewed not as visitors to the NICU but as the members of the care team capable of making decisions for their infants.[68]

♦ Families are given the necessary education and support to participate in their infant's care at the level with which they are comfortable[68] (Figure 7-5).

♦ Families are encouraged to serve as advisors on family advisory boards and family-steering committees, participate in orientation and training activities for other parents, and serve on other hospital committees.[68,69]

♦ The quality of family-centered care is evaluated based on the feedback received from the families.[69]

♦ Staff members are encouraged to participate in developing ideas to improve the NICU experience and outcomes for families and their infants.

♦ Staff members are provided with support, education, and resources to implement a change in family-centered care.[69]

PATIENT/FAMILY SATISFACTION

Because of the complexity of care provided to the infants and their families in the NICU, using the standard Patient/Client Satisfaction Questionnaire found in the back of the

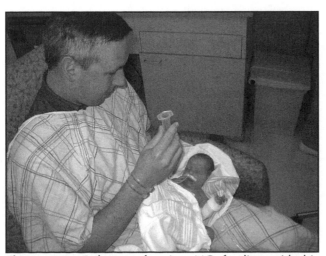

Figure 7-5. Father performing NG feeding with his son.

Guide[47] to determine parent or family satisfaction with physical therapy management may not be appropriate. A parent satisfaction questionnaire developed to assess the quality of medical care in the NICU may need to be used instead. The Neonatal Index of Parent Satisfaction (NIPS)[70] is an example of such a questionnaire. It contains 27 items scored on a seven-point ordinal scale, including questions related to satisfaction with care rated by the mother and the father, medical caregiver's perception of parental satisfaction with care, and the infant's health status as perceived by the parents. The NIPS was validated for assessment of medical care provided by nurses, neonatologists, resident physicians, nutritionists, social workers, and other clinicians and was found to be reliable with an ICC=0.71.[70] To validate this questionnaire for use with physical therapy services, additional research may be needed.

Case Study #2: Meconium Aspiration Syndrome

Kevin Jones is a 2.5-week-old baby boy, born at 41 weeks gestation with a birth weight of 3200 grams and hospitalized in the NICU.

A decision-making algorithm for neonatal physical therapy included into the *Practice Guidelines for the Physical Therapist in the Neonatal Intensive Care Unit*[30] will be used to describe the physical therapy management of this patient.

PHYSICAL THERAPIST EXAMINATION

HISTORY

The interview with Mrs. Jones and the nurse and a review of other available information received from the primary care team provide the initial facts that will be used to determine parental concerns, generate the PFPL, and formulate the examination strategy (see Figure 7-1).[30] Observations of the patient and caregivers will allow the physical therapist to generate the IPL and to plan further examination procedures. Further testing will be performed to produce the TPL. After merging and refining the problem lists (PFPL, IPL, and TPL), the physical therapist will establish the goals of intervention and develop the physical therapy intervention plan (see Figures 7-1 and 7-2).[30]

♦ General demographics: Kevin is a 2.5-week-old white baby boy.

♦ Social history: Kevin's mother is 34 years old, and his father is 37 years old. Their older son is 4 years old; he currently attends preschool. Mrs. Jones spends most of the day with Kevin in the NICU. Her husband is able to visit his son in the evenings and on weekends. Maternal grandparents live in the area and come to visit one or two times per week. They also help Kevin's parents with caring for their older son.

♦ Employment/work: Kevin's father has a plumbing business. His mother is a school secretary, and she is currently on maternity leave.

♦ Living environment: Kevin's parents own a single-family home.

♦ General health status

• Kevin is currently hospitalized in the NICU due to perinatal meconium aspiration and respiratory failure.

• Mr. Jones recently injured his knee at work and underwent an anterior cruciate ligament (ACL) reconstruction surgery. Otherwise, both parents report being in good health.

♦ Social/health habits: Neither parent smokes.

♦ Family history: Kevin's aunt has a daughter who was born with Down syndrome.

♦ Medical/surgical history: Mrs. Jones reports that she did not have any complications during pregnancy, but at 41 weeks, because the baby was overdue, the labor was induced. During labor, there was a sudden drop in fetal HR that warranted an emergency C-section. Kevin's birth weight was 3200 grams. He did not cry at birth, and his Apgar scores were 1 and 4 at 1 and 5 minutes, respectively. After birth, the neonate required suctioning and resuscitation. According to the neonatology admission note entered in the infant's chart, presence of meconium below the vocal cords indicated meconium aspiration that was later confirmed by radiographic findings of aspiration pneumonitis. In the delivery room, Kevin was intubated and placed on mechanical ventilation with oxygen supplementation. The infant was then transferred to the NICU, where he remained for the next 48 hours. In his second day of life, he developed neonatal seizures that were manifested as apneic spells and were confirmed by an EEG. At that time, phenobarbital treatment was initiated. Because of continued respiratory distress due to persistent pulmonary hypertension of the newborn (PPHN), Kevin required ECMO and remained on it for 4 days. He was successfully weaned from ECMO to a high-frequency ventilator with oxygen supplementation, then a week later, transitioned to continuous positive airway pressure (CPAP) with decreased oxygen requirement, and 2 days ago, transitioned to oxygen supplementation via nasal cannula.

♦ Prior hospitalizations: N/A.

♦ Preexisting medical and other health-related conditions: Mrs. Jones had prenatal care, and all uterine US examinations performed during prenatal visits were normal.

♦ Current condition(s)/chief complaint(s): Mrs. Jones states that she is concerned about her son's seizures and the impact they may have on his overall development. She is also worried about his continuous need for oxygen and whether he would still need it when he goes home.

♦ Functional status and activity level: Kevin is currently positioned in an open crib on monitoring equipment and on low oxygen requirements. Oxygen is delivered via nasal cannula. The infant receives NG tube feedings and has an IV line in his left ankle. Kevin's nurse reports that she has tried to feed the infant orally but he appears to have a very weak suck and fatigues very quickly.

♦ Medications: Patient is receiving phenobarbital to control seizures.

♦ Other clinical tests: A head US examination performed after transition from ECMO has been negative for IVH.

SYSTEMS REVIEW

The systems review is performed by observation of the infant and the caregivers that will allow the physical therapist to generate the IPL and to plan further the examination procedures (see Figure 7-1).[30]

♦ Cardiovascular/pulmonary
• BP: 75/52 mmHg
• Edema: N/A
• HR: 125 bpm
• RR: 40 bpm

♦ Integumentary
• Presence of scar formation: N/A
• Skin color: Pink
• Skin integrity
  ▪ Some redness noted in the areas where NG tube is taped to the face
  ▪ Red "dots" observed on the right heel (site where blood was drawn)
  ▪ IV line is taped to left lower leg

♦ Musculoskeletal
• Gross range of motion
  ▪ LE PROM WNL bilaterally
  ▪ UE PROM WNL bilaterally
• Gross strength
  ▪ Observed single spontaneous kicking (active hip and knee flexion and extension) movements performed by each LE; no reciprocal kicking noted
  ▪ Ankles remained plantarflexed during kicking; no active ankle dorsiflexion observed
• Gross symmetry
  ▪ Infant tended to maintain head partially rotated to the right or to the left with neck hyperextension
  ▪ Did not actively bring head to midline

- Observed left elbow extension and opening of the left hand when the nurse turned the infant's head to the left to clean his neck; right elbow remained flexed with hand fisted that was consistent with asymmetrical tonic neck reflex
  - Height: 20.47" (52 cm)
  - Weight: 7.05 lbs (3300 g)
- Neuromuscular
  - Balance: N/A
  - Active gross coordinated movement: Infant displays atypical movement patterns and postures
    - Persistent ankle plantarflexion with LE extension and hip adduction
    - Head consistently partially rotated away from midline
    - Elbow flexion and strong hand fisting with thumb adduction on the skull side of the head
  - Locomotion, transfers, and transitions: As expected, infant is fully dependent on caregiver for position changes
- Communication, affect, cognition, language, and learning style
  - Communication, affect, and cognition
    - Kevin was awake during this observation
    - He briefly focused on the nurse's face during her attempt to feed him orally but quickly became fatigued and transitioned to a drowsy state
    - Kevin became irritable and cried briefly when the nurse was cleaning his neck after feeding; however, he quickly calmed down when she picked him up from the crib, held him in her arms in a horizontal position, and used a pacifier
  - Learning preferences: N/A

TESTS AND MEASURES

Kevin's parents were absent during the first part of this examination, and the physical therapist discussed all procedures and findings with Mrs. Jones after she arrived in the unit. She observed the second part of the examination.

- Arousal, attention, and cognition
  - Infant's behavioral state was monitored throughout this examination using the six categories of the Brazelton Scale[46]
  - The items on the Test of Infant Motor Performance (TIMP)[71] were administered only if the infant was able to maintain state 3, 4, or 5, as recommended by Campbell[71] (see Neuromotor Development and Sensory Integration below)
- Circulation
  - Infant's vital signs were carefully monitored using the monitoring equipment readings

- Cardiac vital signs remained WNL, except for an episode of decreased SaO_2 with crying during pull to sit that necessitated an interruption in standardized testing described below
- Neuromotor development and sensory integration
  - The TIMP[71] was selected for Kevin for the following reasons:
    - The TIMP is an assessment tool that, besides its application with preterm infants, is appropriate for use with full-term high-risk infants from birth to 4 to 5 months of age[71]
    - The test items assess the infant's postural control required for functional performance of everyday motor tasks typical for that age
    - The TIMP helps the physical therapist to identify infants who display atypical motor performance[71]
    - Using the TIMP at this time would allow the physical therapist to establish a baseline for future reassessments and to make recommendations for intervention during Kevin's hospitalization in the NICU and upon his discharge
    - The TIMP has been shown to be a good predictor of motor performance on the Alberta Infant Motor Scale (AIMS)[72] at 12 months of age[73] and on the Peabody Developmental Motor Scales (PDMS-2)[74] at preschool age[75] when the infant is tested on the TIMP at 3 months.[71,73,75] This information will assist the physical therapist in making recommendations regarding the timing of Kevin's first appointment at the NICU follow-up clinic upon his future discharge from the hospital (assuming the TIMP is used in the Follow-Up Clinic).
    - It takes on average approximately 30 minutes to administer and score the TIMP[71]
    - Because Kevin demonstrated stable vital signs during observation of his interaction with the caregiver, 30 minutes appeared to be acceptable amount of time required for testing
    - If the examination needs to be interrupted, the remaining items may be administered later, within 24 hours of the first testing session[71]
  - The test was administered in the open crib
  - As stated above, the infant's behavioral state was monitored throughout this examination using the six categories of the Brazelton Scale,[46] and the items were administered only if the infant was able to maintain state 3, 4, or 5, as recommended by Campbell[71]
  - Observed items
    - Kevin was not able to bring head within 15 degrees of midline

- He displayed individual finger movement in the right hand but not with the left (at the time of observation, his head was partially rotated to the right)
- He fingered his blanket with the right hand but not with the left (at the time of observation, his head was partially rotated to the right)
- Kevin displayed ballistic movement of the RUE
- He did not display bilateral hip and knee flexion to clear feet off of the supporting surface of the crib
- The infant did not demonstrate:
  - Isolated movement of either ankle
  - Reciprocal kicking of his LEs
  - Fidgety or oscillating movement
  - Reaching for any objects presented to him in midline in supine or supported sitting
- Kevin received a score of 3 for the observed items

- Elicited items
  - On head control items, Kevin was able to rotate his head to 15 to 20 degrees for visual tracking to each side from midline in reclined sitting, with head supported by the examiner
  - On the other head control items performed in sitting when support was provided to the baby's trunk but not to the head, he displayed no upright head control
  - In supine, Kevin was not able to maintain his head in midline even with visual stimulation but attempted to bring it to midline from the position of full rotation to either side while tracking a red ball
  - In response to passive rotation of the head to the side, the infant lifted the opposite shoulder, scapula, and pelvis off support, but did not roll to the side
  - He displayed similar responses when rolling was elicited from the legs and from the arms to both sides
  - Kevin demonstrated a neck stretch and turned his head to the right within 10 seconds when his eyes were covered with a soft cloth but did not use his hands to attempt to remove the cloth when it was used to cover his entire face and upper chest
  - The infant started crying and displayed a SaO_2 decrease from 97% to 89% when handled for pull to sit for the assessment of activity in neck and UE muscles
    - The testing session was interrupted, and the infant was allowed to rest
    - The physical therapist resumed the examination within 2 hours, before the next feeding.

At that time, Mrs. Jones arrived to the unit and was able to observe the rest of this examination

- During the second part of this examination, Kevin demonstrated bilateral elbow flexion and full head lag upon pull to sit, but his vital signs remained stable, and he did not cry
- In prone suspension, the infant aligned the head with the trunk and demonstrated activity in cervical and thoracic extensor muscles
- On prone head control items, he was able to lift his head, clear the supporting surface, and turn the head to the side
  - He attempted to turn his head from either side toward midline in response to sound but was not able to complete this movement
  - Kevin demonstrated insufficient head control and LE movement in response to stimulation for crawling
- When held in vertical suspension, the infant was unable to right his head against gravity in response to the lateral tilt of the trunk
- When placed in supported standing, he displayed neck hyperextension and extension of both LEs and trunk that he maintained for 3 to 4 seconds, and then started crying
  - Kevin quickly calmed down with a pacifier and displayed a strong non-nutritive suck
- Two test items had to be omitted because of the baby's lack of upright head control
- Kevin received a score of 38 for the elicited items
- The infant's total raw score on the TIMP was 42 that was greater than 2 standard deviations below the mean for his age of 2.5 weeks

- Ventilation and respiration/gas exchange
  - Infant's vital signs were carefully monitored using the monitoring equipment readings
  - Respiratory vital signs remained WNL
  - SaO_2: 96% to 97%
    - Displayed a SaO_2 decrease from 97% to 89% when handled for pull to sit as described above

EVALUATION

Kevin is a baby boy born at 41 weeks gestation and hospitalized in the NICU due to respiratory distress. He has been diagnosed with MAS and neonatal seizures. He currently continues to require oxygen supplementation that he receives via nasal cannula. The baby's total raw score of 42 on the TIMP is far below average for his age of 2.5 weeks and is more than 2 standard deviations below the mean. His respiratory status combined with neurological sequelae and low score on the TIMP put him at risk for developmental delays. However, based on the results of his examination, Kevin displays the following strengths: 1) his gross PROM of both UE joints and both ankles were WNL; 2) he was able to tolerate standardized testing for the total of 30 minutes in two sessions, with only one episode of decreased SaO_2; 3) he was able to visually track the therapist's face to 15 to 20 degrees to each side from midline in reclined sitting, with head supported; 4) he was able to initiate rolling toward side-lying position in response to stimulation at the head, arm, or leg; 5) he was able to elevate head against gravity to clear the supporting surface while turning his head to the side in prone; 6) he was able to respond to auditory stimuli; 7) he exhibited a calming response to the use of a pacifier; and 8) he has concerned and supportive parents.

The PFPL includes the following:

♦ Need for O_2 supplementation
♦ Need for NG feeding
♦ Neonatal seizures
♦ Weak nutritive suck

The IPL includes the following:

♦ Asymmetrical head position with neck hyperextension in supine
♦ Elbow flexion and hand fisting with thumb adduction on the skull side of the head
♦ Persistent ankle plantarflexion with hip and knee extension and hip adduction
♦ Absent reciprocal kicking
♦ Difficulty staying alert during attempted oral feeding

The TPL includes the following based on the results of neuromotor testing[30]:

♦ Clinical impression of atypical development derived from observation and handling during testing
♦ Strong LE extension and UE flexion with resistance to passive movement indicative of increased muscle tone
♦ Decreased isolated movement in LE and UE joints
♦ Poor antigravity head control with inactive neck flexors
♦ Inability to bring head to midline or maintain midline head position when placed
♦ Decrease in SaO_2 during pull to sit, possibly due to fatigue with handling

The problem list developed by merging and refining the PFPL, IPL, and TPL (see Figure 7-1)[30] includes the following:

♦ Need for O_2 supplementation
♦ Need for NG feeding
♦ Weak nutritive suck and difficulty staying alert during oral feeding
♦ Asymmetrical head position with neck hyperextension in supine and supported sitting

♦ Inability to bring head to midline or maintain midline head position when placed
♦ Poor antigravity head control with inactive neck flexors
♦ Increased muscle tone in LE extensors and UE flexors
♦ Persistent ankle plantarflexion bilaterally
♦ Decreased active movement, including isolated movement in UE and LE joints and absent reciprocal kicking
♦ Tendency toward decrease in SaO_2 with prolonged handling, possibly due to fatigue

DIAGNOSIS

Kevin is a patient with MAS and neonatal seizures. He has impaired: arousal, attention, and cognition; circulation; neuromotor development and sensory integrity; and ventilation and respiration/gas exchange. These findings are consistent with placement in Pattern G: Impaired Ventilation, Respiration/Gas Exchange, and Aerobic Capacity/Endurance Associated With Respiratory Failure in the Neonate. Kevin's impairments will be addressed in determining his prognosis and the plan of care while taking into account the refined problem list.

PROGNOSIS AND PLAN OF CARE

Based on the results of the physical therapy examination and evaluation, the following outcomes have been determined for Kevin to be achieved during this episode of care (see Figure 7-3):[30]

♦ Infant is at appropriate developmental level[30] or demonstrates progress toward appropriate developmental level
♦ Infant is nipple fed[30]
♦ Infant demonstrates organized sleep/wake cycles
♦ Infant's family is ready to care for him at home
♦ Infant and his family successfully transition from hospital to the community[30]

To achieve these outcomes, the appropriate interventions for this patient are determined. These will include: coordination, communication, and documentation; patient/client-related instruction; developmentally supportive care; therapeutic exercise; functional training and home management training for caregivers; manual therapy techniques; prescription, application, and, as appropriate, fabrication of devices and equipment and airway clearance techniques.

Based on the diagnosis and prognosis, over the course of 6 to 12 months, several episodes of care may be required for the patient to demonstrate optimal ventilation, respiration/gas exchange, and aerobic capacity/endurance and the highest level of age-appropriate functioning. During this episode of care Kevin will be seen by physical therapy four to five times per week over the course of 12 to 15 visits (3 weeks).

INTERVENTIONS

RATIONALE FOR SELECTED INTERVENTIONS

See Case Study #1 for applicable information on developmentally supportive care; therapeutic exercise; functional training and home management training for caregivers; manual therapy techniques; and airway clearance techniques. In addition, to address prevention of ankle plantarflexion contractures, ankle splinting may be indicated as suggested by Sweeney and associates.[30]

COORDINATION, COMMUNICATION, AND DOCUMENTATION

Communication will occur with Kevin's parents and his primary care team members, such as the neonatologist, nurse, pulmonologist, respiratory therapist, nutritionist, social worker, discharge planner, and others. The physical therapist will participate in patient care rounds and interdisciplinary case conferences with and without family members present, as appropriate. In addition, the physical therapist will maintain ongoing communication with Kevin's parents regarding his plan of care, goal attainment, and interventions he will receive. Prior to the infant's discharge from the hospital, his further needs for continuation of care will be determined, and referrals will be made to the NICU Developmental Follow-Up Clinic, Early Intervention Services, and medical specialists, if needed. All elements of the patient's management will be documented.

PATIENT/CLIENT-RELATED INSTRUCTION

The patient's parents will be educated regarding Kevin's current condition, including the results of his physical therapy examination/evaluation. They will be instructed in the risk factors related to the infant's respiratory and neuromotor status in terms of impact they may have on his overall development. Issues associated with the development of Kevin's cardiovascular/pulmonary, integumentary, musculoskeletal, and neuromuscular systems will be addressed (see Figure 7-2).[30] Infant behavioral states will be described.[30] Plan of care addressing primary impairments and functional limitations, and prevention of secondary impairments and functional limitations, will be discussed. Parental concerns about Kevin's discharge to home and his transition to appropriate services in the community will be addressed.

DEVELOPMENTALLY SUPPORTIVE CARE

Developmentally supportive care for this patient will include environmental modifications, such as reducing noise in the NICU and dimming lights for scheduled sleep times; grouping caregiving tasks together to promote uninterrupted sleep; and nested positioning. These interventions will address the establishment of a sleep-wake cycle, help maintain stable vital signs, promote normal musculoskeletal and neuromuscular development, and support the development of age-appropriate functional skills.

THERAPEUTIC EXERCISE

♦ Graded sensory motor stimulation
  • Activities to develop appropriate state control and responses to visual, auditory, vestibular, and tactile stimuli, for example:
    ▪ Graded vestibular/kinesthetic stimulation in the form of arrhythmic rocking to increase alertness prior to feedings
    ▪ Visual tracking of a red ball to encourage bringing the infant's head to midline while swaddled and positioned supine or in reclined supported sitting, with head support provided by the therapist
    ▪ Auditory stimulation using a rattle to promote head rotation toward midline
♦ Neuromotor development training
  • Activities to improve head control and increase muscle strength in order to develop functional movement appropriate for the infant's age, for example:
    ▪ Graded movement facilitation in sidelying to promote active neck flexion and bringing hands to midline
    ▪ Movement facilitation through graded posterior weight shifting in supported sitting (while swaddled with hip and knee flexion and hands brought to midline) to encourage active chin tuck
    ▪ Movement facilitation through graded lateral weight shifting in supported sitting (while swaddled with hip and knee flexion and hands brought to midline) to encourage midline head alignment and antigravity head control

FUNCTIONAL TRAINING IN SELF-CARE AND HOME MANAGEMENT AND FUNCTIONAL TRAINING IN WORK, COMMUNITY, AND LEISURE INTEGRATION OR REINTEGRATION

♦ Ongoing ADL/IADL training for nurses and Kevin's parents will include:
  • Developmentally supportive positioning promoting flexion, midline orientation, and postural symmetry
  • Use of pacifier during tube feeding
  • Positioning and safety precautions during oral feeding
  • PROM exercise to UEs and LEs performed during dressing/undressing and diaper changing

MANUAL THERAPY TECHNIQUES

♦ Oral-motor stimulation
♦ Soft tissue mobilization in the form of modified infant massage
  • Stroking provided to the baby's head, neck, back, legs, and arms in prone using gentle but firm touch to be performed prior to PROM exercise to UEs and LEs in supine[66]
  • Gentle but firm stroking
    ▪ Over the thenar eminence and the dorsum of the hand to facilitate hand opening
    ▪ Over the dorsum of the foot and over the lateral side of the plantar surface of the foot to facilitate active ankle dorsiflexion
♦ PROM exercise to UEs and LEs
  • Will be initiated by the physical therapist and taught to Kevin's nurse and parents
  • Will assist in prevention of the development of contractures in the UE and LE joints

PRESCRIPTION, APPLICATION, AND, AS APPROPRIATE, FABRICATION OF DEVICES AND EQUIPMENT

♦ Orthotic devices
  • Intermittent use of ankle splints
♦ Protective devices
  • Apnea monitor for home use

AIRWAY CLEARANCE TECHNIQUES

♦ Manual techniques
  • Depending on changes in his medical condition, respiratory status, and tolerance to handling in the course of his hospital stay, manual techniques may be used, including chest percussion and vibration
  • Airway suctioning may also be performed
♦ Positioning
  • To alter the work of breathing and maximize ventilation and perfusion
  • Depending on changes in his medical condition, respiratory status, and tolerance to handling in the course of his hospital stay, pulmonary postural drainage may be used

ANTICIPATED GOALS AND EXPECTED OUTCOMES

♦ Impact on pathology/pathophysiology
  • Patient's weight gain is increased.
  • Stability of patient's vital signs is improved.
  • Tissue perfusion and oxygenation are enhanced.
♦ Impact on impairments
  • Ability to perform age-appropriate visual tracking and auditory tracking is improved.
  • Ability to recognize and respond to auditory stimuli is improved.
  • Airway clearance is improved.
  • Coordination of sucking, swallowing, and breathing is improved.
  • Duration of oxygen supplementation is decreased.
  • Muscle performance is increased.
  • Number of patient's self-regulatory behaviors is increased.
  • Patient's head and neck control is increased.
  • Patient's midline orientation and postural symmetry are improved.
  • Patient's nutritive suck is improved.
  • Patient's sleep-wake cycle is established.
  • Patient's state control is improved.
  • Quality and quantity of movement between and across body segments are improved.
  • Ventilation and respiration/gas exchange are improved.
  • Work of breathing is decreased.
♦ Impact on functional limitations
  • Tolerance to position change and to developmental activities is increased.
♦ Impact on disabilities
  • Disability associated with acute or chronic illness is reduced.
♦ Risk reduction/prevention
  • Behaviors that foster prevention are acquired.
  • Caregiver positioning skills are improved.
  • Communication enhances risk reduction, prevention of secondary impairments and functional limitations, and prevention of fragmentation of care during the infant's transition from the NICU to the community.[30]
  • Risk of secondary impairment is reduced.
♦ Impact on health, wellness, and fitness
  • Behaviors that foster healthy habits and wellness are acquired.
  • Patient's physical function is improved.
♦ Impact on societal resources
  • Awareness and use of community resources by family are improved.
  • Cost of health care services is decreased.
  • Documentation occurs throughout patient management and follows APTA's *Guidelines for Physical Therapy Documentation*.[47]

- Interdisciplinary collaboration occurs through case conferences, patient care rounds, and meetings with the family.
- Length of NICU stay is decreased.
- Patient placement needs after discharge from the hospital are determined.
- Referrals are made to other professionals or resources whenever necessary and appropriate.

♦ Patient/client satisfaction
- Caregiver's sense of well-being is improved.
- Caregiver's stressors are decreased.
- Care is coordinated with the family, caregivers, and other professionals.
- Decision making by family regarding patient's health and health care resources is enhanced.
- Family knowledge and awareness of the diagnosis, prognosis, interventions, and anticipated goals and expected outcomes are increased.
- Parent-infant bonding is improved.

REEXAMINATION

Reexamination is performed throughout the episode of care to evaluate progress and to modify or redirect interventions. See Case Study #1 for further information.

DISCHARGE

Kevin is discharged from physical therapy in the NICU after a total of 14 physical therapy sessions and attainment of his goals and expectations. These sessions have covered his entire episode of care. He is discharged because he has achieved goals and expected outcomes for his transition to home. Kevin is currently breathing room air but requires an apnea monitor for home use. He has been referred to the NICU Developmental Follow-Up Clinic, with an appointment for a multidisciplinary evaluation scheduled at 3 months of age. This evaluation will be conducted to reassess his medical and developmental status. At that time, the TIMP will be readministered for predictive purposes.[73,75] In addition, because of his continued neuromotor problems, Kevin has been referred for Early Intervention services.

PSYCHOLOGICAL ASPECTS

It is necessary for physical therapists to understand the unique psychological aspects of their clinical practice in the NICU. See Case Study #1 for further information.

PATIENT/FAMILY SATISFACTION

Because of the complexity of care provided to the infants and their families in the NICU, using the standard *Patient/Client Satisfaction Questionnaire*[47] found in the back of the *Guide* to determine parent or family satisfaction with physical therapy management may not be appropriate. See Case Study #1 for further information.

REFERENCES

1. Larsen WJ. Development of the heart. In: *Human Embryology.* 3rd ed. New York, NY: Churchill Livingstone; 2001:157-193.
2. Sadler TW. Cardiovascular system. In: *Langman's Medical Embryology.* 8th ed. Philadelphia, Pa: Lippincott Williams & Wilkins; 2000:208-259.
3. Moerchen VA, Crane LD. The neonatal and pediatric patient. In: Frownfelter D, Dean E, eds. *Cardiovascular and Pulmonary Physical Therapy.* 4th ed. Philadelphia, Pa: Mosby, Inc; 2006:657-683.
4. Larsen WJ. Embryonic folding. In: *Human Embryology.* 3rd ed. New York, NY: Churchill Livingstone; 2001:133-155.
5. Sadler TW. Respiratory system. In: *Langman's Medical Embryology.* 8th ed. Philadelphia, Pa: Lippincott Williams & Wilkins; 2000:260-269.
6. Crane LD. Physical therapy for the neonate with respiratory disease. In: Irwin S, Tecklin JS, eds. *Cardiopulmonary Physical Therapy.* 3rd. ed. St. Louis, Mo: Mosby; 1995:486-515.
7. Kahn-D'Angelo L, Unanue RA. The special care nursery. In: Campbell SK, ed. *Physical Therapy for Children.* 2nd ed. Philadelphia, Pa: WB Saunders Co; 2000:840-880.
8. Harper RG, Rehman KU, Sia C, et al. Neonatal outcome of infants born at 500 to 800 grams from 1990 through 1998 in a tertiary care center. *J Perinatol.* 2002;22:555-562.
9. Poets CF, Samuels MP, Southall DP. Epidemiology and pathophysiology of apnoea of prematurity. *Biol Neonate.* 1994;65:211-219.
10. American Academy of Pediatrics. Task Force on Prolonged Apnea. Prolonged apnea. *Pediatrics.* 1978;61(4):651-652.
11. Eichenwald EC, Aina A, Stark AR. Apnea frequently persists beyond term gestation in infants delivered at 24 to 28 weeks. *Pediatrics.* 1997;100(3):354-359.
12. Crowley P, Roberts D, Dalziel S, Shaw BNJ. Antenatal corticosteroids to accelerate fetal lung maturation for women at risk of preterm birth (Protocol for a Cochrane Review). In: *The Cochrane Library.* Chichester, UK: John Wiley & Sons, Ltd; 2004:Issue 1.
13. As-Sanie S, Mercer B, Moore J. The association between respiratory distress and nonpulmonary morbidity at 34 to 36 weeks' gestation. *Am J Obstet Gynecol.* 2003;189:1053-1057.
14. Attar M, Donn S. Mechanisms of ventilator-induced lung injury in premature infants. *Semin Neonatol.* 2002;7(5):353-360.
15. Bancalari E, Claure N, Sosenko IRS. Bronchopulmonary dysplasia: changes in pathogenesis, epidemiology and definition. *Semin Neonatol.* 2003;8:63-71.

16. Jobe AH, Bancalari E. Bronchopulmonary dysplasia. *Am J Respir Crit Care Med.* 2001;163:1723-1729.

17. Northway WH Jr, Rosan RC, Porter DY. Pulmonary disease following respirator therapy of hyaline-membrane disease: bronchopulmonary dysplasia. *N Engl J Med.* 1967;276(7):357-368.

18. Jobe AH, Ikegami M. Prevention of bronchopulmonary dysplasia. *Curr Opin Pediatr.* 2001;13:124-129.

19. Corcoran JD, Patterson CC, Thomas PS, Halliday HL. Reduction in the risk of bronchopulmonary dysplasia from 1980-1990: results of a multivariate logistic regression analysis. *Eur J Pediatr.* 1993;152(8):677-681.

20. Robin B, Kim YJ, Huth J, et al. Pulmonary function in bronchopulmonary dysplasia. *Pediatr Pulmonol.* 2004;37:236-242.

21. Carey B, Trotter C. Bronchopulmonary dysplasia. *Neonatal Netw.* 2000;19(3):45-49.

22. Tortorolo L, Vento G, Matassa P, et al. Early changes of pulmonary mechanics to predict the severity of bronchopulmonary dysplasia in ventilated preterm infants. *J Matern Fetal Neonatal Med.* 2002;12(5):332-337.

23. Smith L. Pathogenesis of retinopathy of prematurity. *Semin Neonatol.* 2003;8:469-473.

24. York J, Landers S, Kirby R, et al. Arterial oxygen fluctuation and retinopathy of prematurity in very-low-birth-weight infants. *J Perinatol.* 2004;24:82-87.

25. Kim T, Sohn J, Pi S, Yoon Y. Postnatal risk factors of retinopathy of prematurity. *Paediatr Perinat Epidemiol.* 2004;18:130-134.

26. Volpe JJ. Intracranial hemorrhage: germinal matrix-intraventricular hemorrhage of the premature infant. In: *Neurology of the Newborn.* 3rd ed. Philadelphia, Pa: WB Saunders Co; 1995:403-463.

27. Volpe JJ. Hypoxic-ischemic encephalopathy: intrauterine assessment. In: *Neurology of the Newborn.* 3rd ed. Philadelphia, Pa: WB Saunders Co; 1995:260-278.

28. Wiswell TE. Advances in the treatment of the meconium aspiration syndrome. *Acta Paediatr Suppl.* 2001;90(436):28-30.

29. Klingner MC, Kruse J. Meconium aspiration syndrome: pathophysiology and prevention. *J Am Board Fam Pract.* 1999; 12:450-466.

30. Sweeney JK, Heriza CB, Reilly MA, et al. Practice guidelines for the physical therapist in the Neonatal Intensive Care Unit (NICU). *Pediatr Phys Ther.* 1999;11:119-132.

31. Moya MP, Bisset GS, Auten RL Jr, et al. Reliability of CXR for the diagnosis of bronchopulmonary dysplasia. *Pediatr Radiol.* 2001;31(5):339-342.

32. Clark PW, Bloomfield FH, Harding JE, Teele RL. Early chest radiographs in very low birth weight babies receiving corticosteroids for lung disease. *Pediatr Pulmonol.* 2001;31:297-300.

33. Pieper CH, Smith J, Brand EJ. The value of ultrasound examination of the lungs in predicting bronchopulmonary dysplasia. Pediatr Radiol [serial online]. Dec 17, 2003.

34. *Taber's Cyclopedic Medical Dictionary* [computer program]. Version: 4.0.33. Philadelphia, Pa: FA Davis Co; 2001.

35. de Mello RR, Dutra MV, Ramos JR, et al. Lung mechanics and high-resolution computed tomography of the chest in very low birth weight premature infants. *Sao Paulo Med J.* 2003;121:167-172.

36. Hascoet JM, Hamon I, Boutroy MJ. Risks and benefits of therapies for apnoea in premature infants. *Drug Saf.* 2000; 23:363-379.

37. Bhatia J. Current options in the management of apnea of prematurity. *Clin Pediatr.* 2000;39:327-336.

38. Meneguel JF, Guinsburg R, Miyoshi MH, et al. Antenatal treatment with corticosteroids for preterm neonates: impact on the incidence of respiratory distress syndrome and intrahospital mortality. *Sao Paolo Med J.* 2003;121:45-52.

39. Crowther CA, Harding J. Repeat doses of prenatal corticosteroids for women at risk of preterm birth for preventing neonatal respiratory disease (Cochrane Review). In: *The Cochrane Library.* Chichester, UK: John Wiley & Sons, Ltd; 2004:1.

40. Ainsworth S, Milligan D. Surfactant therapy for respiratory distress syndrome in premature neonates. A comparative review. *Am J Respir Med.* 2002;1:417-433.

41. Shah PS. Current perspectives on the prevention and management of chronic lung disease in preterm infants. *Pediatr Drugs.* 2003;5:463-480.

42. Dinger J, Töpfer A, Schaller P, Schwarze R. Functional residual capacity and compliance of the respiratory system after surfactant treatment in premature infants with severe respiratory distress syndrome. *Eur J Pediatr.* 2002;161:485-490.

43. Bevilacqua G, Parmigiani S. An observational study of surfactant treatment in infants of 23-30 weeks' gestation: comparison of prophylaxis and early rescue. *J Matern Fetal Neonatal Med.* 2003;14:197-204.

44. Soll RF, Dargaville P. Surfactant for meconium aspiration syndrome in full term infants. *Cochrane Database Syst Rev.* 2000;(2):CD002054.

45. Dubowitz LMS, Dubowitz V, Mercuri E. *The Neurological Assessment of the Preterm and Full-term Newborn Infant.* 2nd ed. London, UK: Mac Keith Press; 1999.

46. Brazelton TB, Nugent JK. *Neonatal Behavioral Assessment Scale.* 3rd ed. London, UK: Mac Keith Press; 1995.

47. American Physical Therapy Association. Guide to physical therapist practice. 2nd ed. *Phys Ther.* 2001;81:9-744.

48. Als H, Gibes R. *Newborn Individualized Developmental Care and Assessment Program (NIDCAP).* Boston, Mass: Children's Hospital; 1986.

49. Als H, Gilkerson L. The role of relationship-based developmentally supportive newborn intensive care in strengthening outcome of preterm infants. *Semin Perinatol.* 1997;21:178-189.

50. Robinson L. An organizational guide for an effective developmental program in the NICU. *J Obstet Gynecol Neonatal Nurs.* 2003;32:379-386.

51. Westrup B, Kleberg A, von Eichwald K, et al. A randomized, controlled trial to evaluate the effects of the newborn individualized developmental care and assessment program in a Swedish setting. *Pediatrics.* 2000;105:66-72.

52. Westrup B, Hellström-Westas L, Stjernqvist K, Lagercrantz H. No indications of increased quiet sleep in infants receiving care based on the Newborn Individualized Developmental Care and Assessment Program (NIDCAP). *Acta Paediatr.* 2002;91(3):318-322.

53. Kleberg A, Westrup B, Stjernqvist K, Lagercrantz H. Indications of improved cognitive development at one year of age among infants born very prematurely who received care based on the Newborn Individualized Developmental Care and Assessment Program (NIDCAP). *Early Hum Dev.* 2002;68:83-91.

54. Jacobs SE, Sokol J, Ohlsson A. The Newborn Individualized Developmental Care and Assessment Program is not supported by meat-analyses of the data. *J Pediatr.* 2002;140:699-706.

55. Grenier I, Bigsby R, Vergara E, Lester B. Comparison of motor self-regulatory and stress behaviors of preterm infants across body positions. *Am J Occup Ther.* 2003;57:289-297.

56. Aucott S, Donohue P, Atkins E, Allen M. Neurodevelopmental care in the NICU. *Ment Retard Dev Disabil Res Rev.* 2002;8:298-308.

57. Bohnhorst B, Heyne T, Peter CS, Poets CF. Skin-to-skin (kangaroo) care, respiratory control, and thermoregulation. *J Pediatr.* 2001;138:193-197.

58. Ludington-Hoe SM, Ferreira C, Swinth J, Ceccardi JJ. Safe criteria and procedure for Kangaroo care with intubated preterm infants. *J Obstet Gynecol Neonatal Nurs.* 2003;32:579-588.

59. Burke M, Walsh J, Oehler J, Gingras J. Music therapy following suctioning: four case studies. *Neonatal Netw.* 1995;14(7):41-49.

60. Kaminski J, Hall W. The effect of soothing music on neonatal behavioral states in the hospital newborn nursery. *Neonatal Netw.* 1996;15(1):45-54.

61. Girolami GL, Campbell SK. Efficacy of a neuro-developmental treatment program to improve motor control in infants born prematurely. *Pediatr Phys Ther.* 1994;6:175-184.

62. Perkins E, Ginn L, Fanning JK, Bartlett DJ. Effect of nursing education on positioning of infants in the Neonatal Intensive Care Unit. *Pediatr Phys Ther.* 2004;16:2-12.

63. Lemons PK, Lemons JA. Transition to breast/bottle feedings: the premature infant. *J Am Coll Nutr.* 1996;15(2):126-135.

64. Gewolb IH, Vice FL, Schweitzer-Kenney EL, et al. Developmental patterns of rhythmic suck and swallow in preterm infants. *Dev Med Child Neurol.* 2001;43:22-27.

65. Gaebler CP, Hanzlik JR. The effects of a prefeeding stimulation program on preterm infants. *Am J Occup Ther.* 1996;50: 184-92.

66. Field T. Preterm infant massage therapy studies: an American approach. *Semin Neonatol.* 2002;7:487-494.

67. Dieter JNI, Field T, Hernandez-Reif M, et al. Stable preterm infants gain more weight and sleep less after five days of massage therapy. *J Pediatr Psychol.* 2003;28: 403-411.

68. Cisneros Moore KA, Coker K, DuBuisson AB, et al. Implementing potentially better practices for improving family-centered care in Neonatal Intensive Care Units: successes and challenges. *Pediatrics.* 2003;111:e450-e460.

69. Saunders RP, Abraham MR, Crosby MJ, et al. Evaluation and development of potentially better practices for improving family-centered care in Neonatal Intensive Care Units. *Pediatrics.* 2003;111:e437-e449.

70. Mitchell-DiCenso A, Guyatt G, Paes B, et al. A new measure of parent satisfaction with medical care provided in the Neonatal Intensive Care Unit. *J Clin Epidemiol.* 1996;49:313-318.

71. Campbell S. *The Test of Infant Motor Performance. Test User's Manual Version 1.4.* Chicago, Ill: Suzanne K. Campbell; 2001.

72. Piper MC, Darrah J. *Motor Assessment of the Developing Infant.* Philadelphia, Pa: WB Saunders Co; 1994.

73. Campbell SK, Kolobe TH, Wright BD, Linacre JM. Validity of the Test of Infant Motor Performance for prediction of 6-, 9- and 12-month scores on the Alberta Infant Motor Scale. *Dev Med Child Neurol.* 2002;44:263-272.

74. Folio MR, Fewell RR. *Peabody Developmental Motor Scales.* 2nd ed. Austin, Tex: Pro-Ed Inc; 2000.

75. Kolobe THA, Bulanda M, Susman L. Predicting motor outcomes at preschool age for infants tested at 7, 30, 60, and 90 days after term age using the Test of Infant Motor Performance. *Phys Ther.* 2004;84:1144-1156.

Impaired Circulation and Anthropometric Dimensions Associated With Lymphatic System Disorders (Pattern H)

Antoinette P. Sander, PT, DPT, MS, CLT-LANA

ANATOMY

The lymphatic system provides a one-way path for the movement of lymph to the cardiovascular system. The lymphatic capillaries work alongside the blood capillaries and postcapillary venules of microcirculation in absorbing fluid from the interstitial space. The lymph capillaries are located throughout the body in the superficial fascia tissue layer. Variations in tissue pressure through muscle contraction, joint movement, respiration, and pulsation of adjacent blood vessels facilitate venous return and also increase lymph flow per unit time. Lymph then moves into collecting vessels that have valves and smooth muscle contractions to control the direction and quantity of lymph flow. The functional segment of the lymph vessel between two valves is called a lymphangion.[1] The frequency of the lymphangion contraction at rest is 6 to 10 contractions per minute. This increases 10-fold when increased transport capacity is needed, creating a lymphatic functional reserve.[1] The distribution of the collecting vessels creates watersheds which determine quadrants of lymphatic drainage throughout the body.[2] Watersheds are areas where the deeper collecting vessels are decreased, but the lymph capillaries remain present. For fluid to cross a watershed, it must move into the capillary network. The dorsal and ventral vertical watersheds divide the trunk into right and left drainage areas. The horizontal watershed at the level of the umbilicus directs drainage superiorly into the axillary nodes or inferiorly into the inguinal nodes.[3]

Lymph moves through the collecting vessels into the lymph nodes. From the regional nodes, lymph is transported through trunks back into the venous circulation. The right lymphatic duct drains the right upper quadrant of the body and the right head and neck; the thoracic duct drains both LEs, the left upper quadrant, and the left head and neck. Fluid enters the venous circulation at the venous angles located between the subclavian and the internal jugular veins. Lymph is thus transported through both a superficial and a deep lymphatic system.[4]

PHYSIOLOGY

The pertinent physiology for this pattern relates to Starling's law of the capillaries[5] that describes the movement of fluids in microcirculation between the capillaries and the interstitial space. The rate and direction of fluid exchange are determined by the hydrostatic and colloid osmotic pressures of the fluids in the capillaries and the interstitial space. In normal circulation, the capillary hydrostatic and colloid osmotic pressures dictate fluid exchange, with the interstitial pressures having minimal input. Filtration at the arterial end of the capillary occurs when capillary hydrostatic pressure is greater than plasma osmotic pressure; absorption at the venous end of the capillary occurs when capillary hydrostatic pressure is less than plasma osmotic pressure. The lymphatic capillaries have an obligatory load of approximately 4 L a day in maintaining fluid balance.[5] This lymphatic fluid has a high protein concentration, with proteins that are too large to be carried in the venous circulation.[6]

PATHOPHYSIOLOGY

LYMPHEDEMA

Lymphedema is a high protein edema that results when lymphatic load exceeds the lymphatic transport capacity.[6] Primary lymphedema is caused by impaired lymph vessel or lymph node development, and secondary lymphedema results from damage to lymphatic structures.[1] Treatment for cancer that includes lymph node dissection and radiation are primary risk factors for development of lymphedema.[7,8] The advancement in surgical techniques to sentinel lymphadenectomy has improved, but not eliminated the incidence of lymphedema in breast cancer survivors.[9] Radiation directly affects the lymph nodes by scarring and shrinking the nodal tissue and indirectly affects the lymphatic vessels by entrapping them with scarred surrounding tissues.[8] The transport capacity of the lymphatic system is regionally altered within the quadrant affected by surgery or radiation.

A change in the ability to transport lymphatic fluid will result in an increase of high protein fluid in the interstitial space.[6] The protein concentration of the fluid will alter the interstitial osmotic pressure, promoting decreased absorption and thus edema. Initially, the lymphatic functional reserve mechanism will work to control the edema by increasing the rate of lymphangion contraction. During this time, a person may experience feelings of heaviness or tightness in the affected limb, but not visible swelling. Eventually, the functional reserve mechanism will be exhausted and lymphedema will develop. Because of the anatomical watersheds that dictate quadrants of lymphatic drainage, secondary lymphedema is located within the trunk and/or extremity with reduced transport capacity.

Lymphedema is classified by stages (I, II, III) that are based on the amount of swelling and grades (1, 2, elephantiasis) that are based on the amount of pitting edema in the tissues.[10] Early stages of lymphedema have pitting edema, but later stages develop tissue fibrosis due to the accumulation of proteins in the interstitial space.[11] The surplus of fluid and accumulated proteins result in a propensity for recurrent infection in the limb with lymphedema.[11]

CHRONIC VENOUS INSUFFICIENCY

Chronic venous insufficiency results in an increase in venous capillary hydrostatic pressure in the superficial and/or deep vein systems.[12] This increase in venous pressure changes the Starling equilibrium with a resultant decrease in absorption. Fluid then accumulates in the interstitial space giving the clinical picture of unilateral or bilateral lower leg edema.

The lymphatic functional reserve mechanism will be activated to absorb the increase in fluid. When the accumulation of fluid overwhelms the lymphatic system, the long-standing edema will develop a high protein component similar to lymphedema.[3]

IMAGING

The methods used to assess lymphedema measure the anatomical arrangement of lymph vessels and nodes, the rate of lymph fluid movement, the lymph node uptake speeds, and the changes in the soft tissue.[1,3,13]

♦ Lymphoscintigraphy: This test assesses superficial and deep lymph transport of the extremities. A radioactive medium is injected into the hand or foot. The time it takes the radioactive substance to be transported from the injection site to the axillary or inguinal lymph nodes is determined and compared to established norms. The test also produces a visual picture of the lymph collectors and nodes.

♦ MRI: Due to the ability to depict tissue contrast, MRI is used to diagnose edematous soft tissue alterations, including the skin. In lymphedema, increased volume of the subcutaneous tissue and a honeycomb pattern between the muscle and subcutis can be identified. MRI is also used for tumor diagnosis.

♦ CT: In chronic lymphedema, CT shows the accumulations of fibrous connective tissue structures. It is also used for tumor diagnosis and can image the lymphatic pathways of the pelvis, retroperitoneum, and mediastinum.

♦ US: This test is used for the noninvasive depiction of enlarged iliac and axillary lymph nodes. It also can depict cutaneous and subcutaneous edema in the extremities.

PHARMACOLOGY

There is no effective drug therapy for treatment of lymphedema that has FDA approval within the United States.[10]

♦ Benzopyrones have been used in Europe and Australia and current studies are underway in North America. The National Lymphedema Network strongly advises patients not to take benzopyrones outside of a clinical trial.

♦ Diuretics are commonly used to control peripheral edema but are ineffective for the treatment of lymphedema because diuretics do not address the protein component of the edema.

Case Study #1: Lymphedema

Mrs. Martha Johnson is a 56-year-old female, 2 years postlumpectomy and axillary dissection for right breast cancer who has developed secondary lymphedema in her right UE.

PHYSICAL THERAPIST EXAMINATION

HISTORY

♦ General demographics: Mrs. Johnson is a 56-year-old black American female. She is right-hand dominant. She is a college graduate with a BS in nursing.

♦ Social history: Mrs. Johnson is married and the mother of a daughter, who is 20 years of age and away at college. She states that her family has been very supportive during her cancer treatment.

♦ Employment/work: She works full time as a pediatric nurse at a local hospital.

♦ Living environment: She lives in a one-story house with her husband.

♦ General health status
  • General health perception: Mrs. Johnson reports the status of her health to be good.
  • Physical function: She reports difficulty sleeping because hot flashes awaken her frequently through the night.
  • Psychological function: Mrs. Johnson sees herself as a breast cancer survivor. She is frustrated and anxious about the development of lymphedema following all of the breast cancer treatment that she has received. She is embarrassed by the look of her arm and has decreased her social engagements.
  • Role function: Wife, mother, nurse.
  • Social function: She is active in her church and often counsels other women who are newly diagnosed with breast cancer.

♦ Social/health habits: Mrs. Johnson has never smoked, and she drinks socially two to three times a week. She has never exercised on a regular basis.

♦ Family history: Her mother died from breast cancer at the age of 57. Her father is living and has elevated BP and Type 2 diabetes.

♦ Medical/surgical history: Mrs. Johnson was diagnosed with Stage II breast cancer that was estrogen positive following a lumpectomy and axillary dissection 2 years ago. Eleven lymph nodes were removed and two nodes were positive for metastasis. Cancer treatment consisted of chemotherapy with adriamycin, cytoxan, and taxol followed by 6 weeks of radiation to the breast and axillary regions. Chemotherapy resulted in menopause, and she states she has multiple incidents of hot flashes daily, difficulty sleeping at night, and osteopenia. She has no history of CHF. Biannual follow-up with her oncologist shows no indications of cancer recurrence.

♦ Prior hospitalizations: She was hospitalized for the birth of her daughter 20 years prior and for her cancer surgery 2 years ago.

♦ Preexisting medical and other health-related conditions: She has a mild increase in BP and cholesterol that are controlled with medication. She is overweight.

♦ Current condition(s)/chief complaint(s): Mrs. Johnson states that she noticed some swelling in her arm a year ago, but that the arm always returned to normal size when she elevated it. Swelling seemed to occur when she did a lot of house or garden work using her right arm. The current episode of swelling began 6 months ago during the summer months, when she was doing a lot of garden work for long hours in the hot sun. Toward the end of the summer, she got a mosquito bite on her right arm and states that the swelling increased following this. Over the past 6 months swelling has gradually increased, and the arm has not returned to normal size. Mrs. Johnson wants the swelling in her arm to decrease so that she can better fit into her clothes and resume her social activities. She has had no prior treatment for her lymphedema.

♦ Functional status and activity level: Mrs. Johnson reports stiffness in her shoulder and elbow from swelling. Her arm feels heavy when she tries to use it during daily activities. She has difficulty donning and doffing shirts and has a problem finding clothing that fits over her edematous arm. She is independent in all ADL and IADL. At work she has difficulty with lifting the children, and she feels tiredness in her arm at the end of the work day. She does not exercise regularly.

♦ Medications: Mrs. Johnson is taking tamoxifen (10 mg bid) as an anti-estrogen; diovan (160 mg daily) for high BP; actonel (35 mg weekly) for osteopenia; lipitor (10 mg daily) for cholesterol; daily multivitamin; and calcium.

♦ Other clinical tests: DEXA found femoral neck bone mineral density of 0.814 g/cm² yielding a t Score of -1.35. Lumbar spine bone mineral density was 0.856 g/cm², yielding a t Score of -1.74. Osteoporosis is defined as at least 2.5 standard deviations (SD) below the young normal mean, taken as ages between 25 and 30 years old; while osteopenia is defined as more than 1 SD but less than 2.5 SDs below the young normal mean. The t Score represents this standard deviation.[14] Mrs. Johnson's tests indicate that she is osteopenic.

SYSTEMS REVIEW

- ◆ Cardiovascular/pulmonary
  - BP: 120/80 mmHg (with medication)
  - Edema: Present in hand, forearm, and upper arm of RUE
  - HR: 75 bpm
  - RR: 14 bpm
- ◆ Integumentary
  - Presence of scar formation: Lumpectomy scar in the right lower/outer breast quadrant, axillary scar from node dissection
  - Skin color: Mild erythemia over the dorsum of the right forearm
  - Skin integrity: Skin is intact and smooth
- ◆ Musculoskeletal
  - Gross range of motion: Limited in right shoulder and elbow
  - Gross strength: Decreased in RUE
  - Gross symmetry: RUE larger than LUE
  - Height: 5'7" (1.702 m)
  - Weight: 200 lbs (90.72 kg)
- ◆ Neuromuscular
  - Balance: WNL
  - Locomotion, transfers, and transitions: WNL
- ◆ Communication, affect, cognition, language, and learning style
  - Communication, affect, and cognition: WNL
  - Learning preferences: Visual learner

TESTS AND MEASURES

- ◆ Aerobic capacity/endurance
  - 6-Minute Walk test[15]
    - Walked 1270 feet (387.1 meters) with dyspnea on Borg Scale[16] that increased from none at rest to 9/20 after walk (range is reported to be from 1312 to 2297 feet [400 to 700 m] in healthy adults, and approximately 1640 feet [500 m] for healthy women)
    - HR at rest was 75 bpm and increased to 86 bpm after walk
    - BP was 120/80 mmHg at rest and increased to 132/82 mmHg after walk
    - Vital signs recovery time after walk to baseline was 8 minutes
- ◆ Anthropometric characteristics
  - BMI[17]=weight (kg) divided by height^2 (meters)= 90.7 kg/2.89
    - Her BMI=31.38, which is considered to be overweight

- Arm volume determined from girth measurements, using a frustum formula to determine segmental volume, and then summing the segmental volumes[18]:
  - Volume of one segment=1/3 π h (a^2 + ab + b^2) where: h=height of the segment; a=girth of one end of segment; and b=girth of other end of segment
  - Right hand and arm=3500 mL, L hand and arm=2800 mL
- Pitting edema 2+ over dorsum of right hand
- Nonpitting edema with moderate fibrosis present in right forearm and upper arm[10]
- Stemmer skin fold sign present (thickened cutaneous folds on the dorsum of the fingers when compared to the opposite side)[1]

- ◆ Arousal, attention, and cognition: WNL
- ◆ Circulation
  - Impaired lymphatic circulation in RUE as evidenced by pitting hand edema, fibrotic forearm and upper arm edema, and observation of mild forearm erythemia
- ◆ Cranial and peripheral nerve integrity
  - Peripheral nerve integrity
    - Decreased sensation to light touch over the right medial upper arm and lateral chest wall secondary to surgical incision
- ◆ Ergonomics and body mechanics
  - Observation of lifting strategies during work revealed poor body mechanics in bending knees and getting close to the child being lifted
- ◆ Gait, locomotion, and balance: WNL
- ◆ Integumentary integrity
  - Skin characteristics
    - Skin is intact and smooth
    - Both breast and axillary scar are well healed with mild hypomobility on palpation
    - Mild erythemia is present over the dorsum of the forearm
    - No heat noted on palpation
- ◆ Muscle performance
  - Manual muscle tests revealed the following deviations from normal:
    - Scapula adduction and depression: R=3/5, L=4/5
    - Shoulder elevation and abduction: R=4/5
    - Elbow flexion and extension: R=4/5
  - Grip strength: R=15 kg, L=21 kg (normal=23 kg)
- ◆ Pain
  - She had no complaints of pain in the RUE
- ◆ Posture
  - Observational assessment revealed:
    - Increased thoracic kyphosis

- Bilateral shoulder protraction
- Forward head
- Trunk side bent to the right
- RUE held close to the body

♦ Range of motion
- Right shoulder flexion AROM and PROM=0 to 165 degrees, firm end feel, no pain, stretching at end range
- Right shoulder abduction AROM and PROM=0 to 160 degrees, firm end feel, no pain, stretching at end range
- Right elbow flexion AROM and PROM=0 to 100 degrees, early soft tissue end feel due to swelling, no pain

♦ Self-care and home management
- Mrs. Johnson reports stiffness in her shoulder and elbow, and the arm feels heavy when she tries to use it during daily activities
- She has difficulty donning and doffing shirts
- She is independent in all ADL and IADL

♦ Work, community, and leisure integration or reintegration
- She has difficulty with lifting the children at work as a pediatric nurse
- She feels tiredness in her arm at the end of the work day
- She is unable to do her gardening at this time
- Mrs. Johnson is still able to participate in her church activities and counsel other women with breast cancer

EVALUATION

Her history and risk factors previously outlined indicated that she is a 56-year-old female, 2-year breast cancer survivor with a 6-month onset of secondary lymphedema. In addition to node dissection and radiation, the high BMI may have contributed to the development of lymphedema.[19,20] There is 2+ pitting edema in the hand and nonpitting edema with moderate fibrosis in the forearm and upper arm. Her secondary lymphedema is classified as Stage II, Grade 2, or moderate (nonpitting on pressure; not reduced with elevation; moderate to severe clinical fibrosis; and 3 to 5 cm differential between the affected and the unaffected limb).[10] There is a decrease in ROM in the right elbow and shoulder secondary to edema and soft tissue stiffness. She has weakness throughout the RUE and scapula that may contribute to the tiredness in her arm at the end of the workday. Erythemia in the forearm could be due to chronic inflammation.[1] She has had no previous treatment for lymphedema. There are no contraindications for manual lymphatic drainage (MLD) or compression therapy.

DIAGNOSIS

Mrs. Johnson is a patient who is a 2-year breast cancer survivor with a 6-month onset of secondary lymphdema. She has impaired: aerobic capacity/endurance; anthropometric characteristics; circulation; ergonomics and body mechanics; muscle performance; posture; and range of motion. She is functionally limited in work, community, and leisure actions, tasks, and activities. Because of the chronic nature of lymphedema, she is at risk for infection in the RUE and integumentary disorders. These findings are consistent with placement in Pattern H: Impaired Circulation and Anthropometric Dimensions Associated With Lymphatic System Disorders.[21] These impairments will be addressed in determining the prognosis and the plan of intervention.

PROGNOSIS AND PLAN OF CARE

Over the course of the visits, the following mutually established outcomes have been determined:

♦ Ability to perform physical activities related to dressing, home management, work, and leisure is improved

♦ Integumentary integrity is improved

♦ Lymphedema is reduced

♦ Muscle strength and endurance are improved

♦ Risk factors are reduced

♦ Risk of recurrence of condition is reduced

♦ Risk of secondary impairment is reduced

♦ ROM is increased

♦ Self-management of symptoms is improved

♦ Sense of well-being is improved

♦ Stressors are decreased

To achieve these outcomes, the appropriate interventions for this patient are determined. These will include: coordination, communication, and documentation; patient/client-related instruction; therapeutic exercise; functional training in self-care and home management; functional training in work, community, and leisure integration or reintegration; manual therapy techniques; and physical agents and mechanical modalities.

Based on the diagnosis and prognosis, Mrs. Johnson will be seen for 16 visits over 4 weeks. Mrs. Johnson has good social support, is motivated, and will follow through with her home exercise program. She may require multiple episodes of care for lymphatic management over her lifetime.

INTERVENTIONS

RATIONALE FOR SELECTED INTERVENTIONS

Therapeutic Exercise

All schools that teach management of lymphedema acknowledge the importance of exercise,[22-26] although the specific parameters of exercise that may safely reduce swelling have not been fully defined.[27,28] The schools of lymphedema management emphasize that exercise must be tailored to individual patient tolerance. The rationale for the use of exercise with patients with lymphedema is based on the premise that muscle contraction and joint motion promote lymphatic flow.[29] With muscle relaxation, the lymphatic capillaries open, allowing interstitial fluid to enter. When the muscle contracts, the lymphatics are compressed, propelling the lymph fluid forward. Lymph flow is also increased by intrathoracic pressure changes associated with respiration.[5]

Aerobic exercise promotes lymphatic flow through changes in respiration. Aerobic exercise has been found to improve depressive and anxiety symptoms,[30] improve body image,[31] and increase quality of life in breast cancer survivors.[32] Aerobic exercise has the additional advantage of cardiovascular fitness and weight control.

Axillary dissection and radiation may compromise shoulder mobility, and flexibility exercises have resulted in improvement in arm movements.[33] Flexibility exercises are initiated immediately postoperatively and continued until full ROM is achieved, within 2 to 6 months postsurgery. A long-term decrease in shoulder mobility may result in decreased use of the involved arm that would decrease lymphatic flow in that extremity.

Strength and endurance training is controversial for patients with lymphedema. Exercise increases blood flow in the arm, thereby increasing lymph production and the need for lymph transport. Precautions, based on anecdotal reports, include avoidance of vigorous, repetitive movements against resistance.[33-35] However, women with lymphedema have been able to safely participate in upper extremity resistive exercise without increase in arm volume.[36-39] This controversy regarding strength training emphasizes the need for individual instruction and gradual progression based on exercise tolerance. Improvement in strength and endurance will improve the ability to perform work and recreational activities, and potentially decrease the risk of injury. Strength and endurance exercise is performed wearing compression bandages or garments to provide external support to the potentially stretched skin and to facilitate the muscle pump that enhances lymphatic flow.[27]

Manual Therapy Techniques

MLD stimulates the lymphatic capillaries to absorb fluid by increasing the frequency of lymph vessel contraction, the volume of lymph fluid transported, and the pressure in the lymph collector vessels. The manual techniques break up protein stasis and help to move fluid across the watersheds.[1,10] MLD utilizes functioning lymph pathways adjacent to regions that have developed lymphedema. Lymph is moved from congested areas into noncongested regions for absorption into the venous circulation. MLD is part of a complete decongestive therapy program that includes patient education, skin care, compression, and exercise. MLD has been found to be effective in managing postbreast cancer lymphedema.[40] The frequency and duration of treatment sessions is not consistent across studies,[41] but seems to be related to the severity of symptoms and the amount of fibrosis.

Physical Agents and Mechanical Modalities

Compression in the form of bandages or garments supports the skin and provides a working force with the muscles to stimulate the lymphatic capillaries to absorb fluid. Short stretch bandages are used in layers, sometimes with the addition of foam padding, and this combination softens fibrotic areas and promotes protein absorption. Short stretch bandages have a high working pressure to facilitate the absorption of fluid during muscle contraction, and a low resting pressure so that the bandages do not constrict during rest and can be worn overnight. Laplace's law[3] states that bandage pressure is defined as the ratio of the tension on the bandage to the radius of the bandaged limb. A smaller limb circumference will receive more pressure than a large circumference, if the bandages are applied with equal tension. This creates an appropriate pressure gradient from distal to proximal. However, care must be taken over bony prominences because the bandage is stretched more in this area. Additional padding is needed to distribute the pressure equally. Overall bandage strength is achieved by using several layers of bandages. Bandages are used during active treatment to maintain the effects of MLD and to provide support to tissues that have lost elasticity due to edema. Garments are ordered when the edema reduction is stabilized. They are generally more cosmetically pleasing to the patient than bandages and are easier to don and doff. For patients with long-term compression needs, bandages are recommended for nighttime use and garments for daytime use.

Vasopneumatic compression pumps provide a repetitive, graded, sequential compression to assist in edema control. The majority of the fluid removed from the interstitium using a compression pump treatment is water, leaving behind the proteins that constitute lymphedema. To achieve maximum protein and water absorption into the lymphatic system, MLD to adjacent trunk areas should accompany pump interventions.

Evidence for compression therapies in the management of lymphedema supports the use of compression garments.[27,42] Controversy exists over the parameters and use of compression pumps,[27] with one randomized trial indicating no significant benefit for pumps when compared with no treatment.[43] The use of pumps as an isolated modality is now rare.[44]

COORDINATION, COMMUNICATION, AND DOCUMENTATION

Communication will occur with family members, equipment suppliers for compression supplies, and the physician. Referral will be made for nutritional counseling. All elements of the client's management will be documented.

PATIENT/CLIENT-RELATED INSTRUCTION

The patient will be instructed in the pathophysiology of lymphedema as it relates to home management. With or without the assistance of family members, she will be independent in performing self-MLD, compression bandaging, exercise, and in donning and doffing her compression garment. Risk factors for infection and for worsening of lymphedema will be discussed. Specific risk factors for developing and worsening of lymphedema include obesity and HTN.[20,45] Scrupulous skin care is recommended, including avoidance of cuts, insect bites, burns, having blood drawn, vaccinations, and application of a BP cuff on the affected arm. Lymphedema may be exacerbated by use of hot tubs, saunas, hot weather, and air travel.[40,46] Precautions are designed to reduce the risk of infection and consequent inflammation that would increase the lymphatic load, decrease trauma to the lymphatic system, and limit activities that may increase arterial blood flow.

Therapeutic Exercise

- ◆ Aerobic capacity/endurance conditioning
  - Mode
    - Walking, treadmill, elliptical, climbing machine, bicycle
    - Aerobics classes
  - Duration
    - 15 minutes or more
  - Intensity
    - 60% to 80% of THR; 12 to 16 range on Borg scale of perceived exertion
  - Frequency
    - Three to five times a week
  - Precautions
    - Patients on active chemotherapy need to monitor blood counts to determine exercise parameters
- ◆ Flexibility exercises
  - Stretching exercises should be done after warming up, using a slow and steady stretch accompanied by deep breathing, and building hold up to 30 seconds

- Active and passive exercises for shoulder ROM with emphasis on flexion and abduction
- Supine sagittal plane flexion and frontal plane abduction
- Anterior chest stretch for postural correction
- Precautions include stretching radiated skin

- ◆ Strength, power, and endurance training
  - Any movement performed while wearing compression bandages or sleeve has a decongestive effect on lymphedema
  - Stimulation of the axillary lymph nodes through self-MLD techniques and diaphragmatic breathing prior to exercise will facilitate the decongestive effect
  - Exercises may be repetition of functional movements or specific to the muscles of the UE: Shoulder flexion, abduction, overhead press, scapular retraction, latissimus pull down, elbow flexion, elbow extension, wrist flexion, wrist extension
  - Exercises to strengthen grip
    - Ball squeezes
    - Functional activities requiring grip strength
  - Active movements may progress to resistive exercises beginning with low weights and progressing as tolerated
    - Duration: Two sets of 12 repetitions
    - Frequency: Functional exercises may be done daily, resistive exercises two to three times per week
    - Precautions: Monitor subjective changes in arm such as increased heaviness, pain, fullness, throbbing,[47] and increase in arm volume

FUNCTIONAL TRAINING IN SELF-CARE AND HOME MANAGEMENT

- ◆ Self-care and home management
  - Review all activities and postural alignment for self-care and home management
  - Review of appropriate dressing techniques

FUNCTIONAL TRAINING IN WORK, COMMUNITY, AND LEISURE INTEGRATION OR REINTEGRATION

- ◆ Work
  - Mrs. Johnson will be instructed in lifting strategies during work that improve body mechanics and maximize use of the uninvolved LUE
  - She will wear a compression sleeve on the RUE during work hours
- ◆ Leisure
  - Decrease in edema may promote improvement in body image

- This may encourage Mrs. Johnson to resume social and leisure activities

MANUAL THERAPY TECHNIQUES

♦ MLD
  - Precautions for use of MLD include untreated acute infections, untreated malignancies, uncontrolled bronchial asthma, cardiac edema, renal edema, acute DVT, and aortic aneurysm
  - MLD is directed to the superficial fascia tissue layer with a light stretching pressure on the skin
    - The strokes have a working "pressure on" stage and a resting "pressure off" stage
    - Treatment initiates centrally with diaphragmatic breathing and specific MLD strokes to the venous angles to open the central lymph channels
    - The contralateral axillary nodes and ipsilateral inguinal nodes are treated next, followed by specific strokes to move fluid from the right (congested) axilla across the trunk into the open nodes
    - Finally the RUE is treated
    - A MLD session may last from 30 to 60 minutes, depending on the amount of tissue fibrosis

PHYSICAL AGENTS AND MECHANICAL MODALITIES

♦ Contraindications for use of compression include acute infections, arterial wounds, ABI<0.8, cardiac edema, DVT, and allergy to any component of the bandage or garment
♦ Precautions include heart failure, diabetes, decreased sensation, and paresis
♦ Compression bandaging
  - Bandage supplies need to be organized prior to application
  - The arm is clean and dry, and lotion is applied
  - The first bandage layer is stockinette, which serves to absorb moisture from the skin and to protect the skin from chaffing
  - Padding layers follow, with attention to making the arm as cylindrical as possible to maintain even tension in the bandages
  - Specialized bandages are used to wrap the fingers and hand
  - Short stretch bandages are next, with increasing width from distal to proximal
  - The number of bandages used is based on the volume and fibrosis in the arm
  - The compression gradient is checked after application of each bandage, making sure that pressure

increases distal to proximal
  - Bandages are anchored with tape rather than clips to avoid potential skin pricks
  - Bandages are worn 23 hours a day during the active treatment phase
  - The patient or family member is instructed in bandaging techniques
♦ Compression garments
  - Garments are available ready-made or custom from a variety of vendors
  - They are ordered by Compression Class, with 20 to 30 mmHg generally used for grade 1 UE lymphedema, and 30 to 40 mmHg generally used for grade 2 UE lymphedema
  - Compression garments need to be replaced every 6 months
♦ Vasopneumatic compression devices
  - Pumps should provide sequential compression from distal to proximal
  - The arm is covered with stockinette to absorb moisture
  - Since lymphatic capillaries collapse at pressures greater than 60 mmHg,[48] the recommended compression cycle should not exceed 45 mmHg[10]

ANTICIPATED GOALS AND EXPECTED OUTCOMES

♦ Impact on pathology/pathophysiology
  - Edema and lymphedema are reduced as evidenced by reduction in RUE arm volume.
♦ Impact on impairments
  - Aerobic capacity, endurance, and muscle performance are increased, and patient tolerates a full work day without fatigue.
  - Integumentary integrity is improved, and erythemia in forearm area is reduced to WNL.
  - Relaxation is increased.
  - ROM is improved.
♦ Impact on functional limitations
  - Ability to independently perform physical actions, tasks, and activities related to ADL/IADL in self-care, home management, work, community, and leisure activities with compression bandages or garment is increased.
  - Tolerance of positions and work activities is increased.
♦ Risk reduction/prevention
  - Communication enhances risk reduction and prevention of infection.
  - Disability associated with chronic illness is reduced.
  - Risk factors for infection are reduced.

- Risk of recurrence of condition is reduced.
- Risk of secondary impairment is reduced.
- Self-management of symptoms through home MLD and compression bandaging is improved.

◆ Impact on health, wellness, and fitness
- Behaviors that foster prevention are acquired.
- Fitness is improved.
- Health status is improved.
- Physical function is improved.

◆ Impact on societal resources
- Documentation occurs throughout patient management and follows APTA's *Guidelines for Physical Therapy Documentation.*[21]

◆ Patient/client satisfaction
- Coordination occurs with equipment suppliers for purchase of bandages and garments.
- Patient's and family's knowledge and awareness of the diagnosis, prognosis, interventions, and understanding of anticipated goals and expected outcomes are increased.
- Sense of well-being is improved and return to previous social functions is enhanced.
- Stressors are decreased.

REEXAMINATION

Reexamination is performed throughout the episode of care.

DISCHARGE

Mrs. Johnson is discharged from physical therapy after a total of 16 outpatient physical therapy sessions and attainment of her goals and expectations. These sessions have covered her entire episode of care. She is discharged because she has achieved her goals and expected outcomes. Since lymphedema requires life-long management, she may return to therapy for additional episodes of care.

PSYCHOLOGICAL ASPECTS

Lymphedema affects the quality of life of breast cancer survivors,[49-51] and quality of life improves with complex decongestive therapy.[52]

Case Study #2: Chronic Venous Insufficiency

Mr. Ted Conner is a 67-year-old male with chronic venous insufficiency and secondary lymphedema in the lower extremities, left greater than right.

PHYSICAL THERAPIST EXAMINATION

HISTORY

◆ General demographics: Mr. Conner is a 67-year-old white male. He is left-hand dominant. He has a high school education.

◆ Social history: Mr. Conner is married and is the father of five children and grandfather of 10 children. He lives with his wife.

◆ Employment/work: He is retired from labor/construction work. He was primarily a plasterer, requiring long hours standing on his feet.

◆ Living environment: He lives in a one-story house with his wife, with four steps to get into the house with a handrail.

◆ General health status
- General health perception: Mr. Conner reports the status of his health to be fair.
- Physical function: He reports that walking is limited by excessive weight, LE swelling, and pain in both knees from arthritis. He has difficulty wearing shoes because of swelling of his feet and difficulty reaching his feet because of his protuberant abdomen.
- Psychological function: Mr. Conner states concern about the increased swelling in his legs that seems to be getting worse.
- Role function: Husband, father, grandfather.
- Social function: He meets with a group of retired men regularly for lunch.

◆ Social/health habits: Mr. Conner used to smoke a pack of cigarettes a day for the past 20 years, but finally quit 5 years ago. His weight increased when he quit smoking. He drinks two beers daily with friends or at home. He has never exercised on a regular basis. His diet is "meat and potatoes."

◆ Family history: His father died from a heart attack at age 70. His mother died from a stroke at age 72.

◆ Medical/surgical history: Mr. Conner has a 12-year history of bilateral LE edema, L>R, that was precipitated from long hours standing on his feet as a plasterer. He used to wear "elastic socks" when he worked, but has not done so since he retired 2 years ago. With the decrease in activity since retirement, his weight has increased, and he is short of breath when walking short distances. He does not see a doctor on a regular basis.

◆ Prior hospitalizations: He has never been hospitalized.

◆ Preexisting medical and other health-related conditions: He has a moderate increase in BP and cholesterol that are partially controlled with medication. He is overweight.

- Current condition(s)/chief complaint(s): Mr. Conner was seen in the hospital clinic 1 week ago, and the doctor was concerned about the edema in his legs and sent him to physical therapy. He would like to have the swelling decreased but was not aware that anything could be done to change it.

- Functional status and activity level: Mr. Conner has poor foot and lower leg hygiene because he cannot reach his toes. He is able to independently do LE dressing with difficulty but only wears slip-on shoes or house shoes. He is unable to ambulate community distances due to shortness of breath. He states that he gets short of breath after one block of walking. He can independently climb four or five stairs at a slow pace while using a handrail.

- Medications: Mr. Conner is taking Procardia (20 mg tid), a calcium channel blocker for high BP, and lipitor (30 mg daily) for cholesterol.

- Other clinical tests: His bilateral ABI is 0.9. This test provides a ratio of the systolic BP of the LE compared with the UE. Normal ABI is 1.00, with 0.8 to 1.00 indicating mild peripheral arterial occlusive disease.[12]

SYSTEMS REVIEW

- Cardiovascular/pulmonary
  - BP: 135/90 mmHg (with medication)
  - Edema: Present in both lower legs, feet, and toes, L>R
  - HR: 75 bpm
  - RR: 17 bpm
- Integumentary
  - Presence of scar formation: No scars
  - Skin color: Hemosiderin (dark areas on skin indicative of increased deposition of iron in the tissue) mid shin to ankles L>R
  - Skin integrity: Very thick yellow soles with cracks in both heels, papillomas on posterior left calf
- Musculoskeletal
  - Gross range of motion
    - WFL hip and knees
    - Limited at ankles
  - Gross strength: Decreased in ankles
  - Gross symmetry: Both lower legs, ankles, and feet are swollen, L>R
  - Height: 6'2" (1.88 m)
  - Weight: 280 lbs (127.3 kg)
- Neuromuscular
  - Balance: WNL
  - Locomotion, transfers, and transitions: Slow, but independent and safe
  - Communication, affect, cognition, language, and learning style

- Communication, affect, and cognition: Has difficulty understanding complex concepts
- Open to learning
- Learning preferences: Visual and verbal learner

TESTS AND MEASURES

- Aerobic capacity and endurance
  - 6-Minute Walk test[15]
    - He was able to walk 560 feet (170.7 meters) in 6 minutes with dyspnea on Borg Scale that increased from 8/19 at rest to 13/19 after walk[16]
    - Range for 6-Minute Walk test distance is reported to be from 1312 to 2297 feet (400 to 700 meters) in healthy adults, and approximately 1903 feet (580 meters) for healthy men
  - Mr. Conner is generally deconditioned
- Anthropometric characteristics
  - BMI[17]=weight (kg) divided by height^2 (meters) (127.3 kg/3.53)
    - BMI=36 kg/m^2 which indicates that he is obese
  - Circumferential girth measurements in cm
    - First metatarsal phalangeal: R=27.9, L=28.0
    - Base of fifth metatarsal: R=29.0, L=29.5
    - 10 cm from heel (foot at 90 degrees): R=33.5, L=35
    - 20 cm: R=40.3, L=44.2
    - 30 cm: R=47.8, L=52.6
    - 40 cm: R=45.3, L=48.8
    - 50 cm: R=60.3, L=63.1
    - 60 cm: R=70.0, L=73.5
  - Pitting edema 2+ in dorsum of both feet
  - Nonpitting edema with fibrosis present in mid right calf to ankle and entire left lower leg[10]
  - Stemmer skin fold sign positive bilaterally (thickened cutaneous folds on the dorsum of the toes when compared to the opposite side)[1]
- Arousal, attention, and cognition: WNL but difficulty with complex tasks
- Assistive and adaptive devices: None
- Circulation
  - Decreased venous and lymphatic circulation in both LE secondary to work history, obesity, and inactivity
  - Bilateral dorsalis pedis and posterior tibial arteries WNL
- Cranial and peripheral nerve integrity
  - Peripheral nerve integrity
    - Decreased sensation to light touch over the left ankle and shin secondary to thickened skin tissue
    - Normal on RLE
- Environment, home, and work barriers

- Has four steps to enter home, but has handrail so no home barriers
- Gait, locomotion, and balance
  - Able to walk on level surfaces independently without assistive devices
  - Gait is wide based and slow due to edema and overall endurance
  - Gait pattern is shuffling due to lack of dorsiflexion range and poor push off
- Integumentary integrity
  - Edema does not change with elevation of right or left legs
  - Skin characteristics
    - No heat noted on palpation right and left
    - Color
      - Hemosiderin bilateral shin to ankle right and left
      - Hemosiderin is the rust brown color that results from the lysis of red blood cells that have been deposited in the interstitial space due to venous insufficienty[12]
    - Very thick yellow soles on both feet
    - Hyperkeratosis with heel fissures present both heels, L>R
- Muscle performance
  - MMTs revealed the following deviations from normal:
    - Hip extension: R and L=4/5
    - Knee extension: R and L=4/5
    - Ankle dorsiflexion: R and L=3+/5
- Orthotic, protective, and supportive devices
  - He is in need of appropriate supportive and protective shoes
- Pain
  - Pain intensity bilateral knees secondary to arthritis rated 3/10 using the NPS where 0=no pain and 10=worst possible pain[16]
  - Pain only present with weight bearing activities like walking and stair climbing
- Posture
  - Observational assessment done from all perspectives
    - Revealed forward head, thoracic kyphosis increased in the upper thoracic spine, mildly flexed hips and knees
- Range of motion
  - Bilateral hip flexion: AROM and PROM=0 to 90 degrees, early capsular end feel, no pain
  - Bilateral knee extension to flexion: AROM and PROM=0 to 110 degrees, soft tissue end feel, no pain

- Bilateral ankle dorsiflexion AROM and PROM=0 degrees, soft tissue end feel, no pain
- Self-care and home management
  - He states difficulty wearing shoes because of swelling in both feet
  - He has difficulty reaching his feet because of his protuberant abdomen and therefore has poor foot and lower leg hygiene
  - He is able to independently do LE dressing with difficulty, but only wears slip-on shoes or house shoes
  - He needs to rest following a shower and dressing
  - He gets short of breath after climbing four or five stairs
- Work, community, and leisure integration or reintegration
  - He gets short of breath after walking the distance of a community block or from the car to the store

EVALUATION

Mr. Conner is a 67-year-old male with a 12-year history of LE edema secondary to venous insufficiency. This long history of edema without treatment has compromised the lymphatic system, indicated by the facts that edema does not reverse with elevation of the legs and has a fibrotic component. Decreased overall endurance is both a cause and a result of inactivity. Health behaviors including smoking, drinking, diet, and lack of exercise have contributed to obesity that further impedes his endurance.

There is 2+ pitting edema in the feet and nonpitting edema with hard fibrosis in the lower legs and calf L>R. This combination of venous and lymphatic pathology has been termed phlebo-lymphostatic edema.[3] His lymphedema is classified as Stage II and III, or Grade 2 and elephantiasis, due to fibrosis and skin changes.[10] There is a decrease in ROM and strength in the right and left ankles due to edema, which impact his gait pattern. His inability to reach his toes, more due to obesity than to ROM deficits, impacts self-care, cleanliness of his feet, and independence in applying compression to his legs. He lives with his wife, and she has agreed to assist him with compression bandaging. Skin care will be an important component of his intervention to prevent wound development. He has had no focused treatment for his leg edema. There are no contraindications for MLD or compression therapy.

DIAGNOSIS

Mr. Conner has a 12-year history of lower leg edema with both a venous and a lymphatic component, and he has pain. He has impaired: aerobic capacity/endurance; anthropometric characteristics; circulation; peripheral nerve integrity;

gait, locomotion, and balance; integumentary integrity; muscle performance; posture; and range of motion. He is functionally limited in self-care and home management and in work, community, and leisure actions, tasks, and activities. He is in need of appropriate supportive and protective footwear. Because of the chronic nature of his edema, he is at risk for both venous ulcers and infection in both LEs. His poor endurance during functional activities is related to his inactivity. These findings are consistent with placement in Pattern H: Impaired Circulation and Anthropometric Dimensions Associated With Lymphatic System Disorders, and also in Pattern B: Impaired Aerobic Capacity/Endurance Associated With Deconditioning and in Integumentary Pattern A: Primary Prevention/Risk Reduction for Integumentary Disorders.[21] The pain, impairments, functional limitations, and equipment and device needs will be addressed in determining the prognosis and the plan of interventions.

PROGNOSIS AND PLAN OF CARE

Over the course of the visits, the following mutually established outcomes have been determined:

- Ability to perform physical activities related to dressing and walking is improved
- Behaviors that foster healthy habits, wellness, and prevention are acquired
- Edema is reduced
- Integumentary integrity is improved
- Health status is improved
- Patient knowledge of diagnosis, prognosis, interventions, goals, and outcomes related to edema management is increased
- Patient knowledge of personal factors associated with decreased endurance is increased
- Physical function is improved
- Risk of recurrence of condition is reduced
- Risk of secondary impairment is reduced
- Self-management of symptoms is improved
- Sense of well-being is improved

To achieve these outcomes, the appropriate interventions for this patient are determined. These will include: coordination, communication, and documentation; patient/client-related instruction; therapeutic exercise; self-care and home management; manual therapy techniques; and physical agents and mechanical modalities.

Treatment of the edema is the primary focus with the improvement in overall endurance and instructions in skin care as components of the edema management. Based on the diagnosis and prognosis, Mr. Conner will be seen for 24 visits over 6 weeks. He has good support from his family and is motivated to improve his condition.

INTERVENTIONS

RATIONALE FOR SELECTED INTERVENTIONS

Therapeutic Exercise

The rationale for therapeutic exercise for people with lymphedema is presented in Case Study #1. Following are additional considerations for this case.

Active exercise of the knee, ankle, and foot will increase flexibility in the respective joints and activate a muscle pump to facilitate venous return. Exercise done without compression bandages may allow for better increase in ROM. Exercises done with short stretch compression bandages will facilitate both venous and lymphatic return.[27]

Aerobic exercise will be an important component of increasing endurance, overall fitness, and weight control.

Manual Therapy Techniques

The rationale for manual therapy for people with lymphedema is presented in Case Study #1. Following are additional considerations for this case.

In phlebolymphostatic edema, the lymph nodes are intact and may be utilized to absorb fluid from the ipsilateral involved leg. The trunk is treated prior to the extremity to move fluid from the leg into the general lymphatic circulation.[3]

Physical Agents and Mechanical Modalities

The rationale for compression for people with lymphedema is presented in Case Study #1. Following are additional considerations for this case.

Compression is the hallmark treatment for venous insufficiency.[12] Bandages may only be needed to the knee, which may improve adherence to the treatment. Compression varies in the amount of support needed from low compression (18 to 24 mmHg) to high compression (40 to 50 mmHg).[12] Bandages are used during the active treatment phase until edema is reduced, and compression stockings are used to maintain the decreased edema. Vasopneumatic sequential compression pumps may be useful in decreasing the venous components of phlebolymphostatic edema.

COORDINATION, COMMUNICATION, AND DOCUMENTATION

Communication will occur with family members, equipment suppliers for compression supplies, and the physician. Referral will be made for nutritional counseling and weight control. All elements of the client's management will be documented.

PATIENT/CLIENT-RELATED INSTRUCTION

The patient will be instructed in the pathophysiology of venous insufficiency as it relates to home management. With the assistance of family members, he will be independent in performing self-MLD, compression bandaging, exercise, and in donning and doffing compression stockings. Risk factors for infection, for worsening of edema, and for development of wounds will be discussed. Skin care rationale and procedures will be discussed and practiced.

This patient had minimal knowledge of his problem at the time of initial evaluation and demonstrated difficulty in understanding concepts that were discussed. He appeared ready to learn about his problem. Verbal demonstration, handouts, and audiovisual material will be used in patient education. The role of his wife in understanding and assisting in home management skills is essential for positive outcomes from the interventions.

Therapeutic Exercise

♦ Aerobic capacity/endurance conditioning
  • Patient will be screened for CAD prior to beginning a moderate exercise program due to risk factors including age, weight, smoking history, family history, high cholesterol, high BP, and sedentary lifestyle. A cardiac stress test would be useful in determining exercise parameters.
  • Mode
    ▪ Walking, treadmill, elliptical, climbing machine, bicycle
    ▪ Aerobics classes
  • Duration
    ▪ 15 minutes or more, but may begin with less and increase as tolerated
  • Intensity
    ▪ 60% to 80% of THR or less if necessary; 12 to 16 range on Borg scale of perceived exertion
  • Frequency
    ▪ Three to five times a week
  • Precautions
    ▪ Initial cardiac status must be determined and monitored as program progresses
♦ Flexibility exercises
  • Stretching exercises should be done after warming up, using a slow and steady stretch accompanied by deep breathing, and building hold up to 30 seconds
  • Active and passive exercises for foot and ankle ROM and for knee ROM
    ▪ Ankle pumps, toe curls, circumduction
    ▪ Supine heel slides
    ▪ Sitting knee flexion and extension
    ▪ Seated gastrocsoleus stretches, (knees extended and knees slightly flexed) using a towel to pull ankles into dorsiflexion
    ▪ Standing gastrocsoleus stretches (knees extended and knees slightly flexed)
    ▪ Hip flexion stretches in Thomas position

FUNCTIONAL TRAINING IN SELF-CARE AND HOME MANAGEMENT

♦ Self-care and home management
  • Demonstrate LE dressing skills and provide assistive devices as needed
  • Demonstrate proficiency in home MLD and bandaging
  • Demonstrate ability to don and doff compression stockings
  • Demonstrate ability to maintain appropriate lower leg and foot hygiene

FUNCTIONAL TRAINING IN WORK, COMMUNITY, AND LEISURE INTEGRATION OR REINTEGRATION

♦ Community
  • Improved comfort with walking
  • Ability to walk five community blocks without tiring

MANUAL THERAPY TECHNIQUES

♦ MLD
  • Precautions for use of MLD include untreated acute infections, untreated malignancies, uncontrolled bronchial asthma, cardiac edema, renal edema, acute DVT, and aortic aneurysm
  • MLD is directed to the superficial fascia tissue layer with a light stretching pressure on the skin
    ▪ The strokes have a working "pressure on" stage and a resting "pressure off" stage
    ▪ Treatment initiates centrally with diaphragmatic breathing and specific MLD strokes to the venous angles to open the central lymph channels
    ▪ The ipsilateral inguinal nodes are treated next, followed by the thigh, knee, calf, ankle and foot
    ▪ A MLD session may last from 30 to 60 minutes, depending on the amount of tissue fibrosis[3]

PHYSICAL AGENTS AND MECHANICAL MODALITIES

♦ Compression
  • Contraindications for use of compression include acute infections, arterial wounds, ABI <0.8, cardiac

edema, DVT, allergy to any component of the bandage or garment
  - Precautions include heart failure, diabetes, decreased sensation, and paresis
- Compression bandaging
  - Short stretch bandages are applied in layers as discussed in Case Study #1
  - Bandaging will include the toes, foot, and lower leg to the knee
- Compression garments
  - Garments are available ready-made or custom from a variety of vendors
  - They are ordered by Compression Class, progressing 25 to 35 mmHg to 40 to 50 mmHg
  - The least amount of compression that controls the edema is selected
  - Edema with a lymphedema component generally requires higher compression
  - Compression garments need to be replaced every 6 months
- Vasopneumatic compression devices
  - Pumps should provide sequential compression from distal to proximal
  - The leg is covered with stockinette to absorb moisture and elevated in a comfortable position
  - Maximum pressure is set to tolerance without exceeding diastolic BP
  - It is generally in the range of 45 to 60 mmHg
  - Treatment time is 2 to 4 hours, one to two times daily[53]

ANTICIPATED GOALS AND EXPECTED OUTCOMES

- Impact on pathology/pathophysiology
  - Edema and lymphedema are reduced as determined by decrease in girth measurements.
- Impact on impairments
  - Aerobic capacity and endurance are increased as evidenced by increased distance with less exertion as measured by the Borg scale.
  - Integumentary integrity and texture are improved.
  - Muscle performance is increased.
  - Pain is decreased
  - ROM is improved.
- Impact on functional limitations
  - Ability to independently perform physical actions, tasks, and activities related to ADL/IADL in self-care, home management, community, and leisure activities with or without assistive devices and equipment is increased.

- Ability to perform physical activities related to walking exhibits improved speed and cadence.
- Risk reduction/prevention
  - Communication enhances risk reduction and prevention of infection.
  - Disability associated with chronic illness is reduced.
  - Risk factors are reduced.
  - Risk of recurrence of condition is reduced.
  - Risk of secondary impairment is reduced.
  - Self-management of symptoms is improved.
- Impact on health, wellness, and fitness
  - Behaviors that foster prevention are acquired.
  - Fitness is improved.
  - Health status is improved.
  - Physical function is improved.
- Impact on societal resources
  - Documentation occurs throughout patient management and follows APTA's *Guidelines for Physical Therapy Documentation.*[21]
- Patient/client satisfaction
  - Coordination occurs with equipment suppliers.
  - Patient's and family's knowledge and awareness of the diagnosis, prognosis, interventions, and understanding of anticipated goals and expected outcomes are increased.
  - Sense of well-being is improved.
  - Stressors are decreased

REEXAMINATION

Reexamination is performed throughout the episode of care.

DISCHARGE

Mr. Conner is discharged from physical therapy after a total of 24 outpatient physical therapy sessions and attainment of his goals and expectations. These sessions have covered his entire episode of care. He is discharged because he has achieved goals and expected outcomes.

REFERENCES

1. Weissleder H, Schuchhardt C, eds. Lymphedema diagnosis and therapy. *Viavital Verlag GmbH.* Koln; 2001:26-29, 50, 52-89.
2. Wittlinger G, Wittlinger H. *Textbook of Dr. Vodder's Manual Lymph Drainage. Vol 1. Basic Course.* Brussels: Haug International; 1995.
3. Foldi E, Foldi E, Kubik S, eds. *Textbook of Lymphology for Physicians and Lymphedema Therapists.* English ed. Munchen: Elsevier GmbH; 2003.

4. Bannister L, Berry M, Collins P, et al, eds. *Gray's Anatomy.* 38th ed. New York, NY: Churchhill Livingstone; 1995:1605-1626.

5. Vander A, Sherman J, Luciano D. *Human Physiology: The Mechanisms of Body Function.* 8th ed. Boston, Mass: McGraw Hill; 2001:416-426.

6. Foldi E, Foldi M, Clodius L. The lymphedema chaos. *Plast Surg.* 1989;22:505-515.

7. Pain S, Purushotham A. Lymphoedema following surgery for breast cancer. *Br J Surg.* 2000;87(9):1128-1141.

8. Meek A. Breast radiotherapy and lymphedema. *Cancer.* 1998; 83(12 Suppl American):2788-2797.

9. Sener S, Winchester D, Martz C, et al. Lymphedema after sentinel lymphadenectomy for breast carcinoma. *American Cancer Society.* 2001;92:748-752.

10. Kelly D. *A Primer on Lymphedema.* Upper Saddle River, NJ: Prentice Hall; 2002:36-37, 112.

11. Rockson S. Lymphedema. *Am J Med.* 2001;110(4):288-295.

12. Sussman C, Bates-Jensen B. *Wound Care.* 2nd ed. Gaithersburg, Md: Aspen Publications; 2001.

13. Tiwari A, Cheng KS, Button M, et al. Differential diagnosis, investigation, and current treatment of lower limb lymphedema. *Arch Surg.* 2003;138(2):152-161.

14. Nguyen TV, Pocock N, Eisman JA. Interpretation of bone mineral density measurement and its change. *J Clin Densitom.* Summer 2000;3(2):107-119.

15. Enright PL, Sherrill DL. Reference equations for the six-minute walk in healthy adults. *Am J Respir Crit Care Med.* 1998; 158(5):1384-1387.

16. Borg G. *Borg's Perceived Exertion and Pain Scales.* Champaign, Ill: Human Kinetics; 1998.

17. USDA Center for Nutrition Policy and Promotion. Body mass index and health. *Nutrition Insight.* 2000;March.

18. Sander A, Hajer N, Hemenway K, Miller A. Upper-extremity volume measurements in women with lymphedema: a comparison of measurements obtained via water displacement with geometrically determined volume. *Phys Ther.* 2002;82(12):1201-1212.

19. Johansson K, Ohlsson K, Ingvar C, et al. Factors associated with the development of arm lymphedema following breast cancer treatment: a match pair case-control study. *Lymphology.* 2002;35(2):59-71.

20. Werner R, McCormick B, Petrek J, et al. Arm edema in conservatively managed breast cancer: obesity is a major predictive factor. *Radiology.* 1991;180:177-184.

21. American Physical Therapy Association. Guide to physical therapist practice. 2nd ed. *Phys Ther.* 2001;81:9-744.

22. Foldi E. The treatment of lymphedema. *Cancer.* 1998;83(12 Suppl American):2833-2834.

23. Leduc O, Leduc A, Bourgeois P, Belgrado JP. The physical treatment of upper limb edema. *Cancer.* 1998;83(12 Suppl American):2835-2839.

24. Lerner R. Complete decongestive physiotherapy and the Lerner Lymphedema Services Academy of Lymphatic Studies (the Lerner School). *Cancer.* 1998;83(12 Suppl American):2861-2863.

25. Kasseroller RG. The Vodder School: the Vodder method. *Cancer.* 1998;83(12 Suppl American):2840-2842.

26. Casley-Smith JR, Boris M, Weindorf S, Lasinski B. Treatment for lymphedema of the arm—the Casley-Smith method: a noninvasive method produces continued reduction. *Cancer.* 1998;83(12 Suppl American):2843-2860.

27. Brennan M, Miller L. Overview of treatment options and review of the current role and use of compression garments, intermittent pumps, and exercise in the management of lymphedema. *Cancer.* 1998;83(12 Suppl American):2821-2827.

28. Cohen S, Payne D, Tunkel R. Lymphedema: strategies for management. *Cancer.* 2001;92(4 Suppl):980-987.

29. Havas E, Parviainen T, Vuorela J, Toivanen J, et al. Lymph flow dynamics in exercising human skeletal muscle as detected by scintography. *J Physiol.* 1997;504(Pt 1):233-239.

30. Segar ML, Katch VL, Roth RS, et al. The effect of aerobic exercise on self-esteem and depressive and anxiety symptoms among breast cancer survivors. *Oncol Nurs Forum.* 1998; 25(1):107-113.

31. Pinto BM, Clark MM, Maruyama NC, Feder SI. Psychological and fitness changes associated with exercise participation among women with breast cancer. *Psychooncology.* 2003; 12(2):118-126.

32. Kolden GG, Strauman TJ, Ward A, et al. A pilot study of group exercise training (GET) for women with primary breast cancer: feasibility and health benefits. *Psychooncology.* 2002;11(5):447-456.

33. Kennedy RJ, Bradley J, Parks RW, Kirk SJ. Prospective evaluation of the morbidity of axillary clearance for breast cancer. *Br J Surg.* 2001;88(6):114-117.

34. Network NL. 18 Steps to Prevention: Upper Extremities. Available at: www.lymphnet.org. Accessed January 19, 2005.

35. Petrek JA, Pressman PI, Smith RA. Lymphedema: current issues in research and management. *CA Cancer J Clin.* 2000; 50(5):292-307.

36. Harris S, Niesen-Vertommen S. Challenging the myth of exercise-induced lymphedema following breast cancer: a series of case reports. *J Surg Oncol.* 2000;74(2):95-98.

37. McKenzie D, Kalda A. Effect of upper extremity exercise on secondary lymphedema in breast cancer patients: a pilot study. *J Clin Oncol.* 2003;21(3):463-466.

38. Turner J, Hayes S, Reul-Hirche H. Improving the physical status and quality of life of women treated for breast cancer: a pilot study of a structured exercise intervention. *J Surg Oncol.* 2004;86(3):141-146.

39. Ahmed RL, Thomas W, Yee D, Schmitz KH. Randomized controlled trial of weight training and lymphedema in breast cancer survivors. *J Clin Oncol.* 2006;24(18):1-8.

40. Williams AF, Vadgama A, Franks PJ, Mortimer PS. A randomized controlled crossover study of manual lymphatic drainage therapy in women with breast cancer-related lymphoedema. *Eur J Cancer Care.* 2002;11(4):254-261.

41. Erickson VS, Pearson ML, Ganz PA, et al. Arm edema in breast cancer patients. *J Natl Cancer Inst.* 2001;93(2):96-111.

42. Harris S, Hugi M, Olivotto I, Levine M. Clinical practice guidelines for the care and treatment of breast cancer: 11. Lymphedema. *CMAJ.* 2001;164(2):191-199.

43. Dini D, Del Mastro L, Gozza A, et al. The role of pneumatic compression in the treatment of postmastectomy lymphedema. A randomized phase III study. *Ann Oncol.* 1998;9(2):187-190.

44. Cheville AL, McGarvey CL, Petrek JA, et al. Lymphedema management. *Semin Radiat Oncol.* 2003;13(3):290-301.

45. Kocak Z, Overgaard J. Risk factors of arm lymphedema in breast cancer patients. *Acta Oncol.* 2000;39(3):389-392.

46. Ridner S. Breast cancer lymphedema: pathophysiology and risk reduction guidelines. *Oncol Nurs Forum.* 2002;29:1285-1292.

47. Norman S, Miller L, Erikson H, et al. Development and validation of a telephone questionnaire to characterize lymphedema in women treated for breast cancer. *Phys Ther.* 2001;81(6):1192-1205.

48. Miller GE, Seale J. Lymphatic clearance during compressive loading. *Lymphology.* 1981;14(4):161-166.

49. Kwan W, Jackson J, Weir LM, et al. Chronic arm morbidity after curative breast cancer treatment: prevalence and impact on quality of life. *J Clin Oncol.* 2002;20(20):4242-4248.

50. Velanovich V, Szymanski W. Quality of life of breast cancer patients with lymphedema. *Am J Surg.* 1999;177(3):184-188.

51. Beaulac SM, McNair LA, Scott TE, et al. Lymphedema and quality of life in survivors of early-stage breast cancer. *Arch Surg.* 2002;137(11):1253-1257.

52. Mirolo BR, Bunce IH, Chapman M, et al. Psychosocial benefits of postmastectomy lymphedema therapy. *Cancer Nurs.* 1995;18(3):197-205.

53. Hayes KW. *Manual for Physical Agent*s. 5th ed. Upper Saddle River, NJ: Prentice Hall Health; 2000:83-89.

Abbreviations

2-D ECHO=two-dimensional echo

AACVPR=American Association of Cardiovascular and Pulmonary Rehabilitation
Aa-DO$_2$=alveolar-arterial oxygen difference
AAROM=active assistive range of motion
ABG=arterial blood gas
ABI=ankle brachial index
ACCP=American College of Chest Physicians
ACE=angiotensin converting enzyme
ACL=anterior cruciate ligament
ACSM=American College of Sports Medicine
ADL=activities of daily living
A-fib=atrial fibrillation
A-flutter=atrial flutter
AIDP=acute inflammatory demyelinating polyradiculopathy
AIMS=Alberta Infant Motor Scale
ALI=acute lung injury
ANF=atrial natriuretic factor
ANP=atrial natriuretic peptide
AP=arterial pressure
APTA=American Physical Therapy Association
ARDS=acute respiratory distress syndrome
ARF=acute respiratory failure
AROM=active range of motion
ASD=atrial septal defect
AST=aspartate aminotransferase
ATS=American Thoracic Society
ATT=alpha1-antitrypsin
AV=atrial ventricular
a-VO$_2$ diff=arteriovenous oxygen difference

BE/BD=base excess/base deficit
BIPAP=bilevel positive airway pressure
BLE=bilateral lower extremities
BMI=body mass index
BNP=B-type peptide
BP=blood pressure
BPD=bronchopulmonary dysplasia
bpm=beats per minute
bpm=breaths per minute
BUE=bilateral upper extremities
BUN=blood urea nitrogen

CAD=coronary artery disease
CBC=complete blood count
CDC=Centers for Disease Control and Prevention
CHD=coronary heart disease
CHF=congestive heart failure
CI=cardiac index
CK=creatine kinase
CK-MB=creatine kinase-myocardial band
CMV=cytomegalovirus
CO=cardiac output
CO$_2$=carbon dioxide
COPD=chronic obstructive pulmonary disease
CP GXT=cardiopulmonary graded exercise testing
CPAP=continuous positive airway pressure
CPR=cardiopulmonary resuscitation
CPT=chest physical therapy
CRP=C-reactive protein
CT=computed tomography
CVP=central venous pressure
CWE=chest wall expansion
CXR= chest radiograph (x-ray)

DEXA=dual-energy X-ray absorptiometry
DJD=degenerative joint disease
DMD=Duchenne's muscular dystrophy
DO$_2$=oxygen delivery
DVT=deep vein thrombosis

ECG=electrocardiogram
ECHO=echocardiography
ECMO=extracorporeal membrane oxygenation
ED=emergency department
EDV=end-diastolic volume
EEG=electroencephalogram
EF=ejection fraction
EIA=exercise-induced asthma
ELBW=extremely low birth weight
EPS=electrophysiologic test
ERS=European Respiratory Society
ESR=erythrocyte sedimentation rate

FDA=Food and Drug Administration
FEV=forced expiratory volume

FHP=Farmer's Hypersensitivity Pneumonitis
FiO_2=fraction of inspired oxygen
FRC=functional residual capacity
FVC=forced vital capacity
FWC=functional work capacity

GBS=Guillain-Barré syndrome
GCS=Glasgow Coma Scale
GERD=gastroesophageal reflux disease
GM-IVH=germinal matrix-intraventricular hemorrhage
GXT=graded exercise test or stress test

HbA1C=hemoglobin A1C
Hct=hematocrit
HD=hemodynamic
HDL=high-density lipoprotein
Hgb=hemoglobin
HR=heart rate
HRCT=high resolution computed tomography
HTN=hypertension

IAD=implantable atrial defibrillator
IADL=instrumental activities of daily living
ICU=intensive care unit
IHD=ischemic heart disease
IL=interleukins
IMST=inspiratory muscle strength training
INR=international normalized ratio
IPL=infant problem list
IPPV=intermittent positive pressure ventilation
IV=intravenous
IVH=intraventricular hemorrhage

JVD=jugular vein distension

LAD=left anterior descending
LCA=left circumflex artery
LDH=(serum) lactic dehydrogenase
LDL=low-density lipoprotein
LE=lower extremity
LLE=left lower extremity
LUE=left upper extremity
LVAD=left ventricular assist device
LVEDP=left ventricular end-diastolic pressure
LVEF=left ventricular ejection fraction
LVF=left ventricular failure
LVH=left ventricular hypertrophy
LVRS=lung volume reduction surgery

MAP=mean arterial pressure
MAS=meconium aspiration syndrome
MEP=maximal expiratory pressure
MET=metabolic equivalent

MHR=maximal heart rate
MI=myocardial infarction
MIP=maximal inspiratory pressure
MLD=manual lymphatic drainage
MMT=manual muscle test
MMV=maximal voluntary ventilation
MRI=magnetic resonance imaging
MSAF=meconium-stained amniotic fluid
MUGA=multigated acquisition
MV=minute ventilation
MVO_2=myocardial oxygen consumption

NCH=normocapnic hyperpnea
NDT=neurodevelopmental treatment
NG=nasogastric
NHLBI=National Heart, Lung, and Blood Institute
NICHD=National Institute of Child Health and Human Development
NICU=neonatal intensive care unit
NIDCAP=Newborn Individualized Developmental Care and Assessment Program
NIH=National Institutes of Health
NIPS=Neonatal Index of Parent Satisfaction
NIV=noninvasive ventilation
NMES=Neuromuscular electrical stimulation
NPPV=noninvasive positive pressure ventilation
NPS=numeric pain rating scale
NSAIDs=nonsteroidal anti-inflammatory drugs
NSR=normal sinus rhythm
NYHA=New York Heart Association

O_2=oxygen
OA=osteoarthritis
ODTS=Organic Dust Toxic Syndrome
OEET=oral endotracheal tube
OOB= out of bed
ORD=Office of Rare Diseases

PAC=premature atrial contraction
$PaCO_2$=partial pressure of carbon dioxide in arterial blood
PAD=peripheral arterial disease
PaO_2=partial pressure of oxygen in the arterial blood
PAP=pulmonary artery pressure
PAT=paroxysmal atrial tachycardia
PAWP=pulmonary artery wedge pressure
PCA=postconceptional age
PCO_2=arterial pressure of carbon dioxide
PCWP=pulmonary capillary wedge pressure
PDA=patent ductus arteriosus
PDA=posterior descending artery
PDMS-2=Peabody Developmental Motor Scales
PEEP=positive end-expiratory pressure
PEFR=peak expiratory flow rate

PET=positron emission tomography
PFPL=primary care team and family identified problem list
PFT=pulmonary function test
PH=pulmonary hypertension
PIP=peak inspiratory pressure
Plts=platelets
PPHN=persistent pulmonary hypertension of the newborn
PRE=progressive resistive exercises
PROM=passive range of motion
PT=prothrombin time
PTCA=percutaneous transluminal coronary angioplasty
PTT=partial thromboplastin time
PVC=premature ventricular contraction
PVD=peripheral vascular disease
PWC=physical work capacity

RAH=right atrial hypertrophy
RAP=right atrial pressure
RCA=right coronary artery
RDS=respiratory distress syndrome
RHR=resting heart rate
RLE=right lower extremity
RNA=radionuclide angiogram
RNV=radionucleotide ventriculogram
ROM=range of motion
ROP=retinopathy of prematurity
RPE=rate of perceived exertion
RPP=rate pressure product
RR=respiratory rate
RUE=right upper extremity
RVEF=right ventricular ejection fraction
RVHR=right ventricular heart failure

SA=sinoatrial
SaO$_2$=arterial oxygen saturation

SD=standard deviation
SDS=simple descriptive scale
SHBD=alpha-hydrokybutyrate dehydrogenase
SIMV=synchronized intermittent mechanical ventilation
SO$_2$=oxygen saturation
SOB=shortness of breath
SOFA=sequential organ failure assessment
SpO$_2$=pulse oxygen saturation
SV=stroke volume
SvO$_2$=oygen saturation of venous blood
SVR=systemic vascular resistance
SVT=supraventricular tachycardia

TEE=transesophageal echo
THR=target heart rate
TIMP=Test of Infant Motor Performance
TNF-a=tumor necrosis factor a
Total Chol=total cholesterol
TPL=therapist problem list
TV=tidal volume

UBE=upper body ergometer
UE=upper extremity
US=ultrasonography

VAS=visual analog scale
VC=vital capacity
VO$_2$=oxygen consumption
VRI=Ventilatory Response Index

WBC=white blood cell count
WFL=within functional limits
WHO=World Health Organization
WNL=within normal limits

Brand Name Drugs and Products

Abbokinase (Abbott Labs, Abbott Park, Ill)

Accolate (AztraZeneca, Wilmington, Del)

Actonel (Procter & Gamble Pharmaceuticals, Cincinnati, Ohio)

Activase (Hoffmann-La Roche, Nutley, NJ)

Adalat (Bayer Healthcare, Morristown, NJ)

Advil (Wyeth Consumer Healthcare, Richmond, Va)

Aerobid (Forest Pharmaceuticals, St. Paul, Minn)

Aerolate (Fleming & Company, Fenton, Mo)

Aldactone (Pfizer, New York, NY)

Aleve (Bayer Healthcare, Morristown, NJ)

Alupent (Boehringer Ingelheim Pharmaceuticals, Ridgefield, Conn)

Ancef (GlaxoSmithKline, Philadelphia, Pa)

Apresoline (CIBAVision, Duluth, Ga)

Astramorph (AztraZeneca, Wilmington, Del)

Ativan (Wyeth Pharmaceuticals, Philadelphia, Pa)

Atretol (Novartis, Cambridge, Mass)

Atrovent (Boehringer Ingelheim Pharmaceuticals, Ridgefield, Conn)

Azmacort (Kos Pharmaceuticals, Cranbury, NJ)

Benadryl (Pfizer, New York, NY)

Bentyl (Marion Merrell Dow, Kansas City, Mo)

Betapace (Berlex, Wayne, NJ)

Bronkaid Mist (Bayer Healthcare, Morristown, NJ)

Carbatrol (Shire Pharmaceuticals, Wayne, Pa)

Calan (Searle Labs, Searle Labs Skokie, Ill)

Calciparine (Sanofi-Aventis, Bridgewater, NJ)

Capoten (Bristol-Myers Squibb, New York, NY)

Cardizem (Kos Pharmaceuticals, Cranbury, NJ)

Cartrol (Abbott Labs, Abbott Park, Ill)

Cipro (Bayer Healthcare, Morristown, NJ)

Clorpres (Bertek Pharmaceuticals, Morgantown, WV)

Colace (Purdue Pharma, Stamford, Conn)

Combivent (Boehringer Ingelheim Pharmaceuticals, Ridgefield, Conn)

Coumadin (Bristol-Myers Squibb, New York, NY)

Cytoxan (Bristol-Myers Squibb, New York, NY)

Darvocet (Eli Lilly & Co, Indianapolis, Ind)

Darvon (Eli Lilly & Co, Indianapolis, Ind)

Deponit (Schwarz Pharma, Milwaukee, Wisc)

Digitaline (Proctor & Gamble Pharmaceuticals, France)

Dilacor (Watson Pharmaceuticals, Corona, Calif)

Dilaudid (Knoll Pharamaceuticals, North Chicago, Ill)

Diovan (Novartis, Cambridge, Mass)

Dobutrex (Eli Lilly & Co, Indianapolis, Ind)

Dopastat (Pfizer, New York, NY)

Duragesic (Ortho-McNeil, Titusville, NJ)

Duramorph (Baxter Healthcare, Deerfield, Ill)

Dyrenium (WellSpring Pharmaceuticals, Neptune, NJ)

Flovent (GlaxoSmithKline, Philadelphia, Pa)

Foradil (Schering-Plough, Branchburg, NJ)

Garamycin (Schering-Plough, Branchburg, NJ)

Hep-Lock (Baxter Healthcare Corporation, Deerfield, Ill)

HydroDIURIL (Pfizer, New York, NY)

Hydrostat IR (Shire Pharmaceuticals, Wayne, Pa)

Imdur (Schering-Plough, Branchburg, NJ)

Inderal (Wyeth Pharmaceuticals, Philadelphia, Pa)

Infumorph (Elkins-Sinn, Cherry Hill, NJ)

Intal (Fisons, Bedford, Mass)

Ismo (Wyeth Pharmaceuticals, Philadelphia, Pa)

Isoptin (Abbott Labs, Abbott Park, Ill)

Isordil (Wyeth Pharmaceuticals, Philadelphia, Pa)

Isuprel (Withrop Pharmaceuticals, New York, NY)

Jenamicin (W.E. Hauck, Alpharetta, Ga)

Keflex (Dista, Indianapolis, Ind)

Lanoxin (Vatring Pharmaceuticals, Wytheville, Va)

Lasix (Sanofi-Aventis, Bridgewater, NJ)

Levatol (Schwarz Pharma, Milwaukee, Wisc)

Levbid (Schwarz Pharma, Milwaukee, Wisc)

Lincocin (Pfizer, New York, NY)

Lincorex (Hyrex Pharmaceutical, Memphis, Tenn)

Lipitor (Pfizer, New York, NY)

Liquaemin (Organon, Roseland, NJ)

Lopressor (Novartis, Cambridge, Mass)

Lovenox (Sanofi-Aventis, Bridgewater, NJ)

Maxair (Merck, Whitehouse Station, NJ)

Medrol (Pfizer, New York, NY)

Midamor (Merck, Whitehouse Station, NJ)

Miradon (Schering-Plough, Branchburg, NJ)

Monoket (Schwarz Pharma, Milwaukee, Wisc)

Motrin (Pfizer, New York, NY)

Mucomyst (Bristol-Meyers Squibb, New York, NY)

Mucosil (Novartis, Cambridge, Mass)

Neurontin (Pfizer, New York, NY)

Nitrek (Bertek Pharmaceuticals, Morgantown, WV)

Nitro-Bid (Marion Laboratories, Kansas City, Mo)
Nitrocot (C.O. Truxton, Bellmawr, NJ)
Nitro-Dur (Schering-Plough, Branchburg, NJ)
Nitro-Par (ParMed Pharmaceuticals, Niagara Falls, NY)
Nitrogard (Forest Pharmaceuticals, St. Louis, Mo)
Nitrostat (Pfizer, New York, NY)
Norvasc (Pfizer, New York, NY)
OxyContin (Purdue Pharma, Stamford, Conn)
Primaxin IV (Merck, Whitehouse Station, NJ)
Procardia (Pfizer, New York, NY)
Proventil (Schering-Plough, Branchburg, NJ)
Pulmicort (AztraZeneca, Wilmington, Del)
Qvar (Teva Pharmaceuticals, North Wales, Pa)
Reglan (Schwarz Pharma, Milwaukee, Wisc)
Respbid (Boehringer Ingelheim Pharmaceuticals, Ridgefield, Conn)
Retavase (PDL BioPharma, Fremont, Calif)
Riopan (Altana Pharma, Germany)
Roxanol (aaiPharma, Wilmington, NC)
Seldane (Sanofi-Aventis, Bridgewater, NJ)
Serevent (GlaxoSmithKline, Philadelphia, Pa)
Singulair (Merck, Whitehouse Station, NJ)
Slo-bid (Rhone-Poulenc Rorer Pharmaceuticals, Collegeville, Pa)
Slow-Mag (Purdue Products, Stamford, Conn)
Sorbitrate (AztraZeneca, Wilmington, Del)
Spiriva (Pfizer, Cambridge, Mass)
Streptase (ZLB Behring, King of Prussia, Pa)

Tegretol (Novartis, Cambridge, Mass)
Tenoretic (AztraZeneca, Wilmington, Del)
Tenormin (AztraZeneca, Wilmington, Del)
Thalitone (Monarch Pharmaceuticals, Bristol, Tenn)
Theo-dur (Schering-Plough, Branchburg, NJ)
Tilade (Fisons, Cheshire, UK)
Toprol (AztraZeneca, Wilmington, Del)
Tylenol (McNeil Consumer, Fort Washington, Pa)
Uni-dur (Schering-Plough, Branchburg, NJ)
Uniphyl (Purdue-Frederick, Norwalk, Conn)
Vancocin (Eli Lilly & Co, Indianapolis, Ind)
Vasodilan (Apothecon, Princeton, NJ)
Vasotec (Merck, Whitehouse Station, NJ)
Ventolin (GlaxoSmithKline, Philadelphia, Pa)
Wellbutrin (GlaxoSmithKline, Philadelphia, Pa)
Zocor (Merck, Whitehouse Station, NJ)

PRODUCTS

Acapella (DHD Healthcare, Wampsville, NY)
Cough Assist In-Exsufflator (JH Emerson, Cambridge, Mass)
Curves (Curves International, Waco, Tex)
Flutter (Axcan Pharma, Birmingham, Ala)
Passey Muir (Irvine, Calif)
SmokEnders (Kensington, Md)
StairMaster (Nautilus, Vancouver, Wash)
ThAIRapy Vest (Hill-Rom, St. Paul, Minn)

Index

Acapella™ device
  for asthma, 209, 210
  for bronchitis and emphysema, 106, 107
  for cystic fibrosis, 102
  for Guillain-Barré syndrome, 185
accessory muscles of respiration, 6, 166
ACE inhibitors, 125, 127
activity tolerance reports, 139–140
activity/workload monitoring, 133
acute respiratory distress syndrome (ARDS), 193
  pathophysiology of, 197–198
  SOFA classification of, 197, 198
acute respiratory dysfunction, 194, 195
acute respiratory failure (ARF)
  evaluation and diagnosis of, 213–214
  examination for, 211–213
  interventions for, 214–220
  pathophysiology of, 193–195
  positioning effects in, 225
  prognosis and plan of care for, 214
  psychological aspects of, 221
  reexamination and discharge for, 220–221
  SOFA classification of, 197, 198
aerobic capacity/endurance
  with cardiovascular pump dysfunction/failure, 115–159
  in cystic fibrosis, 90
  impaired, associated with deconditioning, 37–77
aerobic deconditioning, 37–38
aerobic/endurance conditioning
  for acute respiratory failure, 214–215, 218
  for chronic venous insufficiency, 278, 279
  for lymphedema, 272, 273
  for metabolic syndrome, 71
aging, prevention related to, 3–4
airway clearance
  dysfunction of, 83–108
  techniques of
    for acute respiratory failure, 217
    for asthma, 209–210
    for bronchitis and emphysema, 106, 107–108
    for congestive heart failure with complicated myocardial infarction, 139, 144
    for cystic fibrosis, 92–95, 96, 100, 102
    for Guillain-Barré syndrome, 183, 185–186

    for meconium aspiration syndrome, 261
    for neonatal respiratory distress, 252, 253
    for obesity-related shortness of breath, 16
    for respiratory failure, 228
    for right ventricular heart failure, 154, 156–157
    for ventilatory pump dysfunction/failure in Duchenne's muscular dystrophy, 174–175
airways, 6–7, 84
  mucociliary blanket in, 85–86
American Association of Cardiovascular and Pulmonary Rehabilitation (ACCVPR) risk factors, 116
analgesics, 43, 169
angina, 115
anthropometric measurements
  in chronic venous insufficiency, 276
  in lymphedema, 270
  in obesity-related shortness of breath, 12
  in shortness of breath and post-debridement of right knee, 19
antianxiety agents, 198
antiarrhythmics, 125–129, 128
antibiotics
  for airway clearance dysfunction, 89
  for cardiopulmonary disease, 11
  for Duchenne's muscular dystrophy, 168
  for respiratory failure, 198–199
anticholinergic agents, 43, 88–89
anticoagulants, 128, 129, 169
antihyperlipidemic agents, 128
anti-inflammatory agents
  for cardiovascular pump dysfunction/failure, 128, 129
  for emphysema, 197
  for respiratory failure, 199
antimicrobials, 168, 169
antithrombolytics, 128
antivirals, 199
apnea, neonatal, 238, 241–242
arrhythmia, 118, 151
aspirin, 128
assistive/adaptive devices
  for cystic fibrosis, 90, 98, 101
  for Guillain-Barré syndrome, 180, 183, 185
  for respiratory failure, 226
  for ventilatory pump dysfunction/failure, 173–174, 176

asthma
    interventions for, 203–210
    pathophysiology of, 195–196
    pharmacological management of, 195–196
atherosclerosis, 117
atrial fibrillation, uncontrolled episodes of, 153
atrial natriuretic peptide (ANP), release of, 121
atrial septal defects
    case study of, 147–159
    events leading to hospitalization for, 149–150
    interventions for, 152–159
    prognosis and plan of care for, 152
    tests and measures for, 148–151
autogenic drainage, 94

bed mobility, 226
bed rest deconditioning, 38–41
benzopyrones, 268
beta-adrenergic agonists
    for airway clearance dysfunction, 88
    for asthma, 196
    for deconditioning, 43
beta-adrenergic blockers, 126, 129
bilevel positive airway pressure (BIPAP), 216, 219–220, 221
blood gases
    arterial, 9, 125
    deconditioning and, 40
    in metabolic syndrome, 42–43
blood pressure monitoring, 155
body mass index (BMI), 10
bradycardia of prematurity, neonatal, 241–242
breast cancer survivors, lymphedema in, 269–270, 275
breathing, anatomy and physiology of, 83–84, 166
breathing techniques
    active cycles of, 94, 102, 106, 209, 228
    for acute respiratory failure, 217
    for asthma, 205, 208, 209–210
    for bronchitis and emphysema, 107
    for congestive heart failure with complicated myocardial infarction, 144
    for cystic fibrosis, 92, 102
    for Guillain-Barré syndrome, 185–186
    for respiratory failure, 228
    for right ventricular heart failure, 154, 156–157
    slow deep breathing, 215
    for ventilatory pump dysfunction/failure, 176–177
bronchial artery embolization/cauterization, 97
bronchitis, 103–108
bronchodilators
    for airway clearance dysfunction, 88–89
    for asthma, 196
    for deconditioning, 43
    for Duchenne's muscular dystrophy, 168
    for exercise-induced asthma, 206

    for Guillain-Barré syndrome, 169
    for respiratory failure, 199
bronchopulmonary dysplasia
    diagnostic criteria of, 240
    imaging for, 241
    in preterm neonate, 238–239
bronchoscopy, 88
bronchospasm, 206
Buteyko breathing techniques, 205

calcium channel blockers, 126, 129
calcium supplements, 11
capillaries, Starling's law of, 267
cardiac glycosides, 127
cardiac muscle pump, 115, 116
    imaging and laboratory tests for, 122–125
    pathophysiology of, 115–122, 130–159
        pharmacologic treatment of, 125–130
cardiac system, 9–10
cardiomyopathy, 10–11
cardiopulmonary disease, progression of, 83
cardiovascular deconditioning, 38–39
cardiovascular pump dysfunction/failure
classification criteria for, 119–120
    impaired aerobic capacity/endurance associated with, 115–159
    pathologic conditions contributing to, 118
cardiovascular system
    aerobic deconditioning effects on, 38–39
    anatomy of, 4–5, 7–8, 165–166
    disorders of, 10–11
        primary prevention of, 1–4
    imaging of, 11
    physiology of in ventilation and respiration, 166–167
catheterization, 122–123
central nervous system depressants, 199
central venous pressure, 122–123
chest expansion exercises, 144
chest pain, 118
chest percussion/vibration techniques
    for cystic fibrosis, 92–94, 96, 102
    for neonatal respiratory distress, 252
    for ventilatory pump dysfunction/failure in Duchenne's muscular dystrophy, 177
chest physical therapy, 92–94, 252
chest wall stretching, 173
    for asthma, 208
    for Guillain-Barré syndrome, 183, 185
    using vital capacity maneuver, 134
    for ventilatory pump dysfunction/failure, 176, 177
chest x-rays
    for airway clearance dysfunction, 88
    for cardiovascular pump dysfunction/failure, 123
    for cystic fibrosis, 97

for deconditioning and metabolic syndrome, 42
for Duchenne's muscular dystrophy, 168
for Guillain-Barré syndrome, 168
for respiratory dysfunction/failure, 194, 198
childhood, diseases of civilization during, 3
cholecystitis, lifestyle-related, 44–63
chronic obstructive pulmonary disease (COPD), 87
in acute respiratory failure, 213
asthmatic, 195–196
diagnosis of, 213–214
interventions for, 29, 214–220
chronic venous insufficiency, 268
diagnosis of, 277–278
evaluation for, 277
examination for, 275–277
interventions for, 278–280
prognosis and plan of care for, 278
reexamination and discharge for, 280
circulation
impairment of, 267–280
peripheral, 8
civilization, diseases of, 2–3, 77
coagulation test, 125
Combivent, 43
compression garments, 274, 280
compression therapy, 272–273, 274, 278, 279–280
computed tomography (CT)
for airway clearance dysfunction, 88
for cardiopulmonary disease, 11
for cardiovascular pump dysfunction/failure, 123
for deconditioning and metabolic syndrome, 42
for lymphedema, 268
for neonatal respiratory failure, 241
for respiratory failure, 198
conduction system, 7
congestive heart failure (CHF), 10–11
cardiovascular pump dysfunction and, 121
with complicated myocardial infarction, 130–146
diagnosis and prognosis for, 27
examination for, 25–27
interventions for, 27–31
psychological aspects of, 31, 146
rehabilitation intervention for, 145–146
risk stratification for exercise events in, 135
therapeutic exercise for, 28
controlled breathing, 157, 217
coordinated breathing, 144
coronary arteries, 8
coronary artery disease (CAD), 10, 115–116
coronary blood flow, 10, 115, 116
corticosteroids
for airway clearance dysfunction, 89
for asthma, 196
for cardiovascular pump dysfunction/failure, 128, 129

for deconditioning, 43
for neonatal respiratory failure, 242
for respiratory failure, 199
cough, physiology of, 166–167
cough assist devices, 185
cough/huff technique, assisted, 107, 228
cough reflex, 85–86
cough techniques
assisted, 166–167
for cystic fibrosis, 102
for Guillain-Barré syndrome, 184
for ventilatory pump dysfunction/failure, 176–177
for asthma, 209
modified, for CHF with complicated myocardial infarction, 144
for ventilatory pump dysfunction/failure, 174
cromolyn (Intal), 199, 206
cycle ergometer test-retest, 61–62
cycle ergometer tests, 47–49
cystic fibrosis
evaluation and diagnosis of, 91, 99
examination for, 89–91, 97–99
interventions for, 91–97, 99–103
pathophysiology of, 86–87
prognosis and plan of care for, 91, 99
reexamination and discharge for, 97, 103
cytokines, 194

deconditioning
cardiovascular and hemodynamic effects of, 38–39
case studies of, 44–77
endocrine and metabolic effects of, 41
gastrointestinal effects of, 40–41
hematologic effects of, 39
imaging and laboratory tests for, 42–43
immunological effects of, 41
impaired aerobic capacity/endurance associated with, 37–77
integumentary effects of, 41
lifestyle-related cholecystitis and, 44–63
musculoskeletal effects of, 40
neuromuscular effects of, 40
pathophysiology of, 38, 41–42
pharmacology for, 43–44
psychological effects of, 41
pulmonary effects of, 39–40
decongestants, 89
depression
in Duchenne's muscular dystrophy, 178
in Guillain-Barré syndrome, 187
developmentally supportive care
for meconium aspiration syndrome, 260
for neonatal respiratory distress, 248–250, 253
diaphragm, 5–6

diaphragmatic breathing, 83
    for acute respiratory failure, 215
    for right ventricular heart failure, 154
digitalis glycoside, 129
digitoxin, 127
digoxin, 11, 125–129, 127
dilated right atrium and ventricle, 147–159
diuretics
    for cardiovascular pump dysfunction/failure, 126, 129
    for lymphedema, 268
doxapram, 242
Duchenne's muscular dystrophy, 167
    acute shortness of breath in, 169–178
    imaging for, 168
    pharmacologic treatment of, 168

early mobilization
    for congestive heart failure with complicated myocardial infarction, 137–138
    postoperative for lifestyle-related cholecystitis, 56
    for respiratory failure, 225
echocardiography, 11, 123
electrocardiography, 123, 155
electrophysiologic testing, 123
electrotherapeutic modalities, 217
emphysema
    evaluation and diagnosis of, 105
    examination for, 103–105
    inspiratory muscle training for, 215–216
    interventions for, 105–108, 215
    pathophysiology of, 196–197
    prognosis and plan of care for, 105
    reexamination and discharge for, 108
end diastolic volume (EDV), 7, 9
endotracheal intubation, 226
exercise
    for acute respiratory failure, 214–216, 218–219
    adverse responses to, 138
    for asthma, 204–209
    ATS/ERS guidelines for, 215
    barriers to, 205
    blood biochemistry and, 43
    for bronchitis and emphysema, 105–107
    checklist before starting, 54
    for chronic venous insufficiency, 278, 279
    for congestive heart failure
        with complicated myocardial infarction, 136–143
        and pneumonia-related shortness of breath, 28–30
    for cystic fibrosis, 92, 95–96, 99–101
    for Guillain-Barré syndrome, 182–184
    for lifestyle-related cholecystitis, 55–59
    for lymphedema, 272, 273
    for meconium aspiration syndrome, 260
    for metabolic syndrome, 71–73

    for neonatal respiratory distress, 250–251, 253
    for obesity-related shortness of breath, 14–16
    for respiratory failure, 225–227
    for right ventricular heart failure, 152–156
    risk stratification for, 135
    for shortness of breath and post-debridement or right knee, 21–23
    for ventilatory pump dysfunction/failure, 173, 175–176
exercise-induced asthma, 195
    interventions for, 205–206
    suppressors for, 199
exercise testing
    for deconditioning and metabolic syndrome, 43
    graded, for cardiovascular pump dysfunction/failure, 123
    for lifestyle-related cholecystitis, 50
    for metabolic syndrome, 65
expectorants, 88
expiration muscles, 83, 166

family-centered care, neonatal, 254–255, 262
family support, in congestive heart failure, 146
Farmer's hypersensitivity pneumonitis (FHP), 103
fentanyl (Duragesic), 199
fetal circulation, 237
15-Count Breathless Score, 104
fitness promotion, 1–4
flexibility exercises
    for chronic venous insufficiency, 279
    for lymphedema, 273
forced expiratory technique
    for respiratory failure, 228
    for right ventricular heart failure, 156
Function, International Classification of, 39
functional training
    for acute respiratory failure, 219
    for asthma, 209
    for bronchitis and emphysema, 107
    for chronic venous insufficiency, 279
    for congestive heart failure and pneumonia-related shortness of breath, 30–31
    for congestive heart failure with complicated myocardial infarction, 143
    for cystic fibrosis, 96–97, 101
    for Guillain-Barré syndrome, 184
    in lifestyle-related cholecystitis, 59
    for lymphedema, 273–274
    for meconium aspiration syndrome, 260–261
    for metabolic syndrome, 73–74
    for neonatal respiratory distress, 251, 253
    for obesity-related shortness of breath, 16
    for respiratory failure, 225–228
    for right ventricular heart failure, 156
    for shortness of breath and post-debridement or right knee, 23–24

for ventilatory pump dysfunction/failure, 176–177

gas exchange
impaired, 165–187, 193–229
physiology and anatomy of, 84
gastroesophageal reflux disease (GERD), 195
germinal matrix-intraventricular hemorrhage (GM-IVH), 239, 241
glucose intolerance, 4
glycosides, 129
graded sensory motor stimulation, 253, 260
graded vestibular/kinesthetic stimulation, 250
Guillain-Barré syndrome
diagnosis of, 181
evaluation of, 181
examination for, 178–181
imaging for, 168
interventions for, 182–187
pathophysiology of, 167–168
pharmacologic treatment of, 169
prognosis and plan of care for, 181–182
psychological aspects of, 187
reexamination and discharge for, 187

heart
anatomy of, 7
deconditioning and functioning of, 40
development of, 237
loss of contractility in, 118
physiology of, 9
heliox, 196–197
hemodynamic monitoring, 122
high frequency chest wall compression or oscillation (HFCC), 95, 96, 101
high resolution computed tomography, 241
Holter monitoring, 123
hospitalization
events leading to with atrial septal defects, 149–150
psychological effects of, 41
hospital bed, 185
huff cough/sneeze techniques, 144
hypertension
in cardiovascular pump dysfunction, 117–118
prevention of, 2–4
hypoxemia
classification of severity of, 226
progression of, 193–194

imaging. *See* specific techniques
implantable atrial defibrillator, 153
inotropic agents, 127–128, 129
inspiration, physiology of, 166
inspiration muscles, accessory, 83
inspiratory muscle training, 215–216

inspiratory resistive training, 219
insufflation/exsufflation, mechanical, 174
insulin insensitivity, 41
intercostal muscles, 6, 83, 165–166
intermittent abdominal pressure ventilator, 174
ischemic heart disease (IHD), 1
in cardiovascular pump dysfunction, 117
prevention of, 4
isosorbide dinitrate, 130

knee debridement, shortness of breath after, 18–32
Krebs cycle, 37

larynx, 6, 84
lasix, 11
left ventricular failure, 120–121
leukotriene modifiers, 199
lifestyle factors, 2
lifestyle modifications, 146
lifestyle-related cholecystitis
evaluation and diagnosis of, 54
interventions for, 55–63
preoperative course for, 57
prognosis and plan of care for, 55
tests and measures for, 46, 47–49, 50–54
lipid-lowering agents, 129
loop diuretics, 129
lorazepam (Ativan), 198
lungs
in airway clearance, 83–84
anatomy and physiology of, 37, 165
deconditioning effects on, 40
development of, 237
distensibility of, 83
gas diffusion in, 84–85
hyperinflated, 168
injury to
acute, 197, 198
phases in development of, 195
SOFA classification of severity of, 198
neonatal disease of, 241, 242
positioning and perfusion in, 85
protein-rich edema of, 194
surface markings of, 84
lymph, 267
lymphangion contractions, 267
lymphatic fluid, 267–268
lymphatic system
anatomy of, 267
disorders of, impaired circulation and anthropometric dimensions associated with, 267–280
imaging of, 268
pathophysiology of, 268
in peripheral circulation, 8

lymphedema, 268
  with chronic venous insufficiency, 275–280
  diagnosis and evaluation of, 271
  examination for, 269–271
  interventions for, 272–275
  pharmacological management of, 268
  prognosis and plan of care for, 271
  psychological aspects of, 275
  reexamination and discharge for, 275
lymphoscintigraphy, 268

magnetic resonance imaging (MRI)
  for airway clearance dysfunction, 88
  for cardiopulmonary disease, 11
  for cardiovascular pump dysfunction/failure, 123
  for deconditioning and metabolic syndrome, 42
  of lymphatic system, 268
  for neonatal respiratory failure, 241
manual lymphatic drainage (MLD), 272, 274, 279
mast cell stabilizers, 199
meconium aspiration syndrome (MAS), 240–241
  diagnosis of, 259
  evaluation for, 258–259
  examination for, 255–258
  interventions for, 260–262
  prognosis and plan of care for, 259
  psychological aspects and patient/family satisfaction in, 262
  reexamination and discharge for, 262
meconium-stained amniotic fluid (MSAF), 240
metabolic syndrome, 41–42
  evaluation and diagnosis of, 70
  examination for, 63–70
  imaging and laboratory tests for, 42–43
  interventions for, 70–74
  prognosis and plan of care for, 70
  psychological aspects of, 77
  reexamination and discharge for, 74–77
methylxanthines, 241–242
minute ventilation (MV), formulas for, 8, 84
mobilization techniques
  for Guillain-Barré syndrome, 185
  progression of, 56
mucociliary clearance impairment, 39–40
mucokinetic agents
  for Duchenne's muscular dystrophy, 168
  for Guillain-Barré syndrome, 169
mucolytic agents, 88
MUGA, 123
muscle atrophy, 40
muscle testing, manual, 101
myocardial infarction, 10–11, 130–146
myocardial oxygen demand/supply, 115
  in cardiovascular pump dysfunction, 115

determinants of, 10, 115, 116
imbalanced, 115–116, 118

naturopathy, 205
nedocromil (Tilade)
  for exercise-induced asthma, 206
  for respiratory failure, 199
neonatal physical therapy, decision-making algorithms for, 244, 245, 249
neonatal respiratory distress
  diagnosis of, 248
  evaluation for, 247–248
  examination for, 242–247
  interventions for, 248–255
  prognosis and plan of care for, 248
  psychological aspects of, 254–255
  reexamination and discharge for, 254
neonate
  anatomy of, 237–238
  classification based on birth weight of, 238
  development of, 237
  full-term, respiratory failure in, 240–241
  imaging, 241
  preterm, respiratory failure in, 238–240
  respiratory failure in, 237–262
    pharmacologic treatment of, 241–242
nervous system, 7–8
neurodevelopmental treatment protocol, 250–251
neuromotor development training, 253, 260
neuromuscular electrical stimulation, 217, 220
New York Heart Association Functional Classification, 116, 117
Newborn Individualized Developmental Care and Assessment Program (NIDCAP) guidelines, 248–250
  nitrates, 44, 126, 129–130
nitroglycerin, 129–130
noninvasive interventions, 1, 197, 216
normocapnic hyperpnea, 216
nutritional rainbow, 72

obesity, 10, 19–24
obesity-related shortness of breath
  evaluation and diagnosis for, 13
  examination for, 11–13
  impact of impairment in, 17
  interventions for, 14–17
  prognosis and plan of care for, 13–14
  psychological aspects of, 17
  tests and measures for, 12–13
oral feeding transition, 251
oral-motor stimulation, neonatal, 251, 253, 261
Organic Dust Toxic Syndrome (ODTS), 104, 105
oropharyngeal suction, 177

orthotic/protective devices
    for Guillain-Barré syndrome, 180
    for meconium aspiration syndrome, 261
oscillatory airway clearance devices, 176
oxygen delivery determinants, 37
oxygen supplementation
    for acute lung injury, 197–198
    for acute respiratory failure, 216–217, 220
    for emphysema, 196
    low flow, for acute respiratory failure, 216
    for preterm neonatal respiratory failure, 238–239
    for ventilatory pump dysfunction/failure in Duchenne's
        muscular dystrophy, 176
oxygen transport, 37–38

paced breathing
    for bronchitis and emphysema, 107
    for congestive heart failure with complicated myocar-
        dial infarction, 144
    for cystic fibrosis, 102
    for ventilatory pump dysfunction/failure in Duchenne's
        muscular dystrophy, 177
pacing, temporary overdrive, 153
pain, in Guillain-Barré syndrome, 169, 180
paralytic ileus of bowel, 40–41
peak flow meter, 176
phlebolymphostatic edema, 278
phosphodiesterase inhibitors, 127
pleura, 7
pneumocytes, types I and II, 194–195
pneumonia-related shortness of breath, 25–31
positioning techniques
    for meconium aspiration syndrome, 261
    for neonatal respiratory distress, 253
    for respiratory failure, 228
positive airway pressure (PEP) device, 101
positive end-expiratory pressure (PEEP), 226
positive expiratory pressure, 94–95
positive pressure ventilation
    for emphysema, 197
    for Guillain-Barré syndrome, 183
    intermittent, 173–175
    nocturnal nasal intermittent, 174
    noninvasive, for emphysema, 197
positron emission tomography (PET)
    for cardiopulmonary disease, 11
    for cardiovascular pump dysfunction/failure, 123–124
    for neonatal respiratory failure, 241
    postural control training, 218
    postural drainage, 92, 93, 96, 100, 102, 108
    potassium-sparing diuretics, 129
preterm neonate
    extremely low birthweight, 247–248, 250
    respiratory failure in, 238–240

prevention, 1–4
PROM exercise, 261
protease inhibitors, 197
pulmonary capillary wedge pressure, 123
pulmonary edema, 120
pulmonary function test (PFT), 124
pulmonary hypertension, 120
pulmonary system
    aerobic deconditioning effects on, 39–40
    anatomy of, 5–7, 165–166
    disorders of, prevention of, 1–4
    in neonate *versus* adult, 237–238
    normal functioning of, 84–85
    physiology of, 8–9
    in ventilation and respiration, 166–167
pulse oximeter, 176, 185
pursed lip breathing, 144, 217

radiography
    for cardiopulmonary disease, 11
    for neonatal respiratory failure, 241
    for respiratory failure, 198
radionucleotide angiography, 122
relaxation training, 216, 219
renal dysfunction, 41
respiration
    anatomy and physiology of, 83–84
    impairment/dysfunction of, 89–108, 165–187, 193–229
    normal, 84–85
    pathophysiology of, 167–168
respiratory distress syndrome, neonatal, 242
respiratory dysfunction, continuum of, 193–194
respiratory failure
    anatomy and physiology of, 193
    evaluation and diagnosis of, 203, 224
    examination for, 200–203, 221–224
    in full-term neonate, 240–241
    imaging for, 198
    impaired ventilation and respiration/gas exchange asso-
        ciated with, 193–229
    interventions for, 203–210, 225–229
    in neonate, 237–262
    pathophysiology of, 193–198
    pharmacologic treatment of, 198–199
    in preterm neonate, 238–240
    prognosis and plan of care for, 203, 224–225
    psychological aspects of, 210–211
    reexamination and discharge for, 210, 229
respiratory muscles, 5–6, 83
    categories of, 165–166
    performance tests for, 124
    physiology of, 166
    training, 173, 183, 184
respiratory support, 196

retinopathy of prematurity (ROP), 239
right heart failure, 120–121
right ventricular heart failure, 152–159
ROM training, 225

salbutomol, 196
salmeterol, 206
scalene muscles, 165
segmental breathing, 144
sequential organ failure assessment (SOFA) score criteria, 197, 198
shortness of breath
    acute, 169–178
    case study of, 18–24
    interventions for, 21–24
    obesity-related, 11–17
    pneumonia-related, 25–31
6-Minute Walk test
    for acute respiratory failure, 212
    for chronic venous insufficiency, 276
    for congestive heart failure and pneumonia-related shortness of breath, 26
    for cystic fibrosis, 98
    for lifestyle-related cholecystitis, 50, 51–53
    for lymphedema, 270
    for obesity-related shortness of breath, 12
    for shortness of breath and post-debridement of right knee, 19
skin breakdown, 41
soft tissue mobilization, 251–252, 253, 261
spirometry, 97
sputum culture, 97
stacked breathing, 102
status asthmaticus, 196, 203–210
strength/endurance training
    for acute respiratory failure, 214–215
    for lymphedema, 272, 273
stress test, 123
stroke, 4
support devices, for respiratory failure, 219–220
support services
    for Duchenne's muscular dystrophy, 178
    for Guillain-Barré syndrome, 187
surfactants, 242

Test of Infant Motor Performance (TIMP test), 257, 258–259
thallium imaging, 11
theophylline, 43, 241–242
thermodilution catheterization, 123
thiazides, 129
thorax, 5
    in airway clearance, 83–84
    bony, 165

thromboembolus, 38–39
thrombolytics, 128, 130
tidal volume (TV) formulas, 8–9
tilt-table challenge test, 43
tracheobronchial tree, 84
treadmill tests, 43, 66–69, 75–76
tricuspid valve regurgitation, 147–159

ultrasonography
    for deconditioning and metabolic syndrome, 42
    Doppler, for cardiovascular pump dysfunction/failure, 124
    of lymphatic system, 268
    for neonatal respiratory failure, 241

vasodilators
    for cardiovascular pump dysfunction/failure, 127, 130
    for deconditioning, 44
vasopneumatic compression devices, 272, 274, 278, 280
venous thromboembolic disease, 39
ventilation, 9
    anatomy and physiology of, 83–86
    for congestive heart failure with complicated myocardial infarction, 144
    for Guillain-Barré syndrome, 180
    impaired, 89–108
        imaging for, 87–88
        pathophysiology of, 86–87
        pharmacologic treatment of, 88–89
        with respiratory failure, 193–229
        with ventilatory pump dysfunction/failure, 165–187
    noninvasive, for acute respiratory failure, 216
    for preterm neonatal respiratory failure, 238–239
    respiratory failure with, 221–222
    for ventilatory pump dysfunction/failure in Duchenne's muscular dystrophy, 173–174
ventilation maximization techniques, 185
ventilation-perfusion matching, 9
ventilation-perfusion (V/Q) scan, 88
ventilator weaning
    for CHF with complicated myocardial infarction, 131
    for Guillain-Barré syndrome, 182–183, 184
    inspiratory muscle strength training for, 216
ventilatory muscle strength training, 226
ventilatory pump, 165–166
ventilatory pump dysfunction/failure
    case studies of, 169–187
    diagnosis of, 172–173, 181
    in Guillain-Barré syndrome, 167–168, 181–187
    imaging for, 168
    impaired ventilation and respiration/gas exchange associated with, 165–187
    interventions for, 173–178
    pharmacologic management of, 168–169

prognosis and plan of care for, 173
psychological aspects of, 173
Vest, 95–96, 101, 176
vital capacity maneuver, 134

weight control, for metabolic syndrome, 72
weight training, 59
wellness, promotion of, 1–4

yoga breathing techniques, 205, 208, 209–210

WAIT

...There's More!

SLACK Incorporated's Health Care Books and Journals offers a wide selection of products in the field of Physical Therapy. We are dedicated to providing important works that educate, inform and improve the knowledge of our customers. Don't miss out on our other informative titles that will enhance your collection.

Essentials in Physical Therapy Series

The *Essentials in Physical Therapy* series answers the call to what today's physical therapy students and clinicians are looking for when integrating the *Guide to Physical Therapist Practice* into clinical care.

Essentials in Physical Therapy is led by Series Editor Dr. Marilyn Moffat, who brings together physical therapy's leading professionals to produce the most anticipated series of books in the physical therapy market to cover the four main systems:

◆ Musculoskeletal
◆ Cardiovascular/Pulmonary
◆ Neuromuscular
◆ Integumentary

Written in a similar, user-friendly format, each book inside the *Essentials in Physical Therapy* series not only brings together the conceptual frameworks of the *Guide* language, but also parallels the patterns of the *Guide*.

In each case, where appropriate, a brief review of the pertinent anatomy, physiology, pathophysiology, imaging, and pharmacology is provided. Each pattern then details diversified case studies coinciding with the *Guide* format. The physical therapist examination, including history, systems review, and specific tests and measures for each case, as well as evaluation, diagnosis, prognosis, plan of care, and evidence-based interventions are also addressed.

Series Editor: Marilyn Moffat, PT, DPT, PhD, FAPTA, CSCS, *New York University, New York, NY*

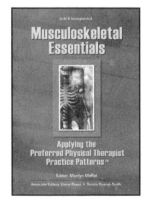

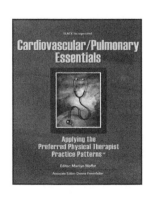

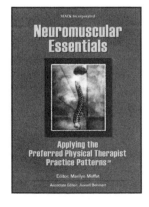

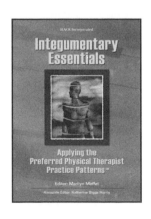

Essentials in Physical Therapy Series

Cardiovascular/Pulmonary Essentials: Applying the Preferred Physical Therapist Practice PatternsSM
Marilyn Moffat, PT, DPT, PhD, FAPTA, CSCS, *New York University, New York, NY* and Donna Frownfelter, DPT, MA, CCS, FCCP, RRT, *Rosalind Franklin University of Medicine and Science, North Chicago, IL*
400 pp., Soft Cover, February 2007, ISBN 1-55642-668-2, Order #46682, **$58.95**

Neuromuscular Essentials: Applying the Preferred Physical Therapist Practice PatternsSM
Marilyn Moffat, PT, DPT, PhD, FAPTA, CSCS, *New York University, New York, NY* and Joanell Bohmert, PT, MS, *University of Minnesota, Twin Cities, MN*
400 pp., Soft Cover, June 2007, ISBN 1-55642-669-0, Order #46690, **$58.95**

Integumentary Essentials: Applying the Preferred Physical Therapist Practice PatternsSM
Marilyn Moffat, PT, DPT, PhD, FAPTA, CSCS, *New York University, New York, NY* and Katherine Biggs Harris, PT, MS, *Quinnipiac University, Hamden, CT*
160 pp., Soft Cover, June 2006, ISBN 1-55642-670-4, Order #46704, **$50.95**

Musculoskeletal Essentials: Applying the Preferred Physical Therapist Practice PatternsSM
Marilyn Moffat, PT, DPT, PhD, FAPTA, CSCS, *New York University, New York, NY*; Elaine Rosen, PT, DHSc, OCS, FAAOMPT, *Hunter College, New York, NY*, and Sandra Rusnak-Smith, PT, DHSc, OCS, *Queens Physical Therapy Associates, Forest Hills, NY*
448 pp., Soft Cover, June 2006, ISBN 1-55642-667-4, Order #46674, **$58.95**

Please visit

www.slackbooks.com

to order any of these titles!
24 Hours a Day...7 Days a Week!

Attention Industry Partners!
Whether you are interested in buying multiple copies of a book, chapter reprints, or looking for something new and different — we are able to accommodate your needs.

Multiple Copies
At attractive discounts starting for purchases as low as 25 copies for a single title, SLACK Incorporated will be able to meet all your of your needs.

Chapter Reprints
SLACK Incorporated is able to offer the chapters you want in a format that will lead to success. Bound with an attractive cover, use the chapters that are a fit specifically for your company. Available for quantities of 100 or more.

Customize
SLACK Incorporated is able to create a specialized custom version of any of our products specifically for your company.

Please contact the Marketing Manager of the Health Care Books and Journals for further details on multiple copy purchases, chapter reprints or custom printing at 1-800-257-8290 or 1-856-848-1000.

*Please note all conditions are subject to change.

CODE: 328

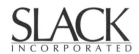

SLACK Incorporated • Health Care Books and Journals
6900 Grove Road • Thorofare, NJ 08086

1-800-257-8290 or 1-856-848-1000
Fax: 1-856-853-5991 • E-mail: orders@slackinc.com • Visit www.slackbooks.com